Chiropractic Pediatrics

This text is lovingly dedicated to the memory of my great friend and colleague Dr Adam Hyland, to whom we said goodnight at the age of 32 as we began preparing to undertake this project together.

See you in the morning my friend.

For Elsevier

Commissioning Editor: *Claire Wilson*
Development Editor: *Helen Leng*
Project Manager: *Gopika Sasidharan*
Designer/Design Direction: *Stewart Larking*
Illustration Manager: *Gillian Richards*

Chiropractic Pediatrics

A Clinical Handbook

SECOND EDITION

Edited by

Neil J. Davies DC Cert Clin Chiro Paeds FICC FACC

Chief Executive Officer, Kiro Kids Pty Ltd, Ballarat, Australia;
Course Leader, MSc (Paediatrics) Program, McTimoney College of Chiropractic, Abingdon, United Kingdom

Consultant

Joan Fallon DC FICCP

Chief Executive Officer, Curemark LLC, Rye, New York, USA

Dr Joan Fallon is a member of the ICA Pediatrics Council Board of Directors and is the current immediate past Council Chairperson. Dr Fallon has been committed to chiropractic pediatrics for many years and more recently has been awarded a patent for her enzyme therapy treatment for ADD, ADHD and autism by the US Patent and Trademark Office. Dr Fallon was recently officially recognized by the New York State Senate for her research and development of pancreatic enzyme therapy. She is a compassionate caring chiropractor who has made a substantial contribution to the development of the field of chiropractic pediatrics through research, publication and clinical care.

Foreword by

Dana J. Lawrence DC MMedEd

Senior Director, Center for Teaching and Learning, Palmer College of Chiropractic, Davenport, Iowa, USA

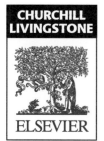

CHURCHILL LIVINGSTONE

ELSEVIER

Edinburgh London New York Oxford Philadelphia St Louis Sydney Toronto 2010

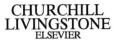

First edition © Harcourt Publishers Limited 2000
Second edition © 2010, Elsevier Limited. All rights reserved.

ISBN 9780702031298

British Library Cataloguing in Publication Data
A catalogue record for this book is available from the British Library

Library of Congress Cataloging in Publication Data
A catalog record for this book is available from the Library of Congress

Notice
Knowledge and best practice in this field are constantly changing. As new research and experience broaden our knowledge, changes in practice, treatment and drug therapy may become necessary or appropriate. Readers are advised to check the most current information provided (i) on procedures featured or (ii) by the manufacturer of each product to be administered, to verify the recommended dose or formula, the method and duration of administration, and contraindications. It is the responsibility of the practitioner, relying on their own experience and knowledge of the patient, to make diagnoses, to determine dosages and the best treatment for each individual patient, and to take all appropriate safety precautions. To the fullest extent of the law, neither the publisher nor the editor assumes any liability for any injury and/or damage to persons or property arising out of or related to any use of the material contained in this book.

The Publisher

Printed in the United States of America
Transferred to Digital Printing, 2013

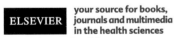

Contents

Avril V. Brereton BEd DipECD
Centre for Developmental Psychiatry, Monash Medical Centre, Melbourne, Australia

Thelma Buchanan BA(Hons)(Psych) DipTeaching GradDipSpecEd GradDipCouns
School Counsellor, Department of Education and Training, NSW, Australia

Neil Cox BSc(Hons) MSc(Chiro) DC
Private Practice, Exeter, United Kingdom

Maurice K. Easton MBBS FRACP
Head, Paediatrics Department, Ballarat Health Services, Ballarat, Victoria, Australia; Associate Tutor, Clinical Paediatrics Melbourne University, School of Medicine Melbourne, Victoria, Australia

Kylie M. Gray BA GradDipEdPsych PhD
Centre for Developmental Psychiatry & Psychology, School of Psychology and Psychiatry, Monash University Melbourne, Australia

Philip J. Parry BSc(Hons)Chiro MScChiro(Paeds) DipChildPsy MMCA FCC
Paediatric Chiropractor, Piyavate Hospital, Bangkok; Board Member of Kids Ark Foundation, Chiang Mai, Thailand

Kyla Sheridan BN DipMid
Registered Midwife (Clinical Nurse Specialist), Ballarat Health Services, Victoria, Australia

Allan G. J. Terrett MAppSc(Chiro) FIACN FACCS
Associate Professor, RMIT University, Melbourne, Victoria, Australia

Bruce J. Tonge MBBS MD DPM MRCPsych FRANZCP
Centre for Developmental Psychiatry, Monash Medical Centre, Melbourne, Australia

Kimberley Tuohey B(App) Sci(Clin) BChiroSc
Private Practice (Paediatrics), Ballarat, Victoria, Australia

Robert Turner-Jensen BSc(Chiro) MCSc(Chiro Paeds)
Chiro Care for Kids North Strathfield, Sydney, New South Wales, Australia

Ailsa van Poecke MSc(Chiro) DC MScChiro(Paeds) FEAC(Paeds)
Private Practice, Deventer, The Netherlands

Sarah E. Whyatt BHSc MChiro MScChiro(Paeds)
Private Practice, Adelaide, South Australia, Australia

Foreword

It was 33 years ago, just over a single generation, that a young student went to a local public library to locate resources about a field into which he had just been accepted to begin his studies. His search was not only fruitless but distressing; only a single book about chiropractic was to be found in that library, and it was entitled "In the Public Interest: The Case against Chiropractic"(Smith 1969). Astute readers will recognize this as a volatile piece of anti-chiropractic propaganda, but the state of our art, such as it was in 1976, was that we had few resources available and fewer to be found from outside our profession.

I was that person then. Flash forward to 2009. In the intervening 33 years, much has happened. Chiropractic blossomed into the vital health care field it is today. It has a growing and important body of evidence to support its clinical interventions. It has a world-wide presence, and a cadre of critical researchers, academics and clinicians. It has specialty disciplines: orthopedics, radiology, family practice, rehabilitation, sports medicine, and the quickly growing discipline of pediatrics. In that discipline it has some truly high-quality practitioners. Neil Davies stands out among them all. Dr. Davies has published a critical text within chiropractic, and I am pleased to see that this update is now complete.

Pediatric chiropractic is growing at a fast rate. On an informal basis, each term I ask my students at Palmer College of Chiropractic how many will specialize in this discipline, and each term I find that at least 20 people (mostly, but not exclusively, women) plan to take further study in pediatrics. Because of that interest, both American professional organizations offer advanced training- what is termed diplomate training- in pediatrics, and at least one private organization does as well. There are other top-quality texts on pediatrics, each with its own strengths to offer. There are journals devoted to the discipline.

For it is important to note that children are not just smaller versions of adults. They are unique, have unique problems and need to be understood for what they are. We live in an evidence-based and an evidence-informed world, and that requires the members of our profession to be conversant with what that evidence suggests. But we need also to stay mindful that evidence is not just what we see from clinical trials, though of course this is critically important information. Evidence also exists in the procedures we use daily in practice; in fact, it was Sackett who noted that evidence-based practice is "the conscientious, explicit and judicious use of current best evidence in making decisions about the care of individual patients" (Sackett & Rosenberg 1995). It requires the integration of the clinical evidence, practitioner expertise and patient values.

Chiropractic pediatrics has not been without its share of controversy, but this comes from outside our profession from anti-chiropractic crusaders who claim that we lack that evidence. But here it is, in this textbook, writ large for all to see. There is a wealth of information to be read here, a profession's worth of experience on the diagnosis, treatment and management of the conditions affecting children. Here, in this text, we demonstrate to all the full strength of what we do, our professional skill and our collective wisdom. This text is a service to our profession and the smallest of whom we treat.

Dana J. Lawrence, DC, MMedEd

References

Smith, R.L., 1969. In the public interest: the case against chiropractic, Pocket Books, New York, NY.

Sackett, D.L., Rosenberg, W.M., 1995. The need for evidence-based medicine. J. R. Soc. Med. 88, 620–624.

Over 10 years has passed since the writing of the first edition of this text. Much has changed in that time and many of those changes are reflected in this second edition. As was the case with the first edition, the purpose of this book has been to seek to define both the boundaries of safe clinical practice and the most appropriate way to practice inside those boundaries. The constant theme of this book is the irrevocable intertwining of orthodox diagnostic practice and 'subluxation-based' chiropractic management to produce a 'best available evidence' approach to every subject considered.

I make no pretence that this text is an exhaustive treatise on the subject of pediatric health care, as it has been constrained by both time and space to those subjects that are most likely to be encountered by the family practice chiropractor or are of such clinical importance they simply could not be left out. The aim of each chapter is to offer the family practice chiropractor and specialist alike practical guidance in diagnosis and clinical decision-making, identifying as far as possible safe solutions to common clinical problems. In the years since the publication of the first edition, a wide range of educational DVD products have been produced by the Kiro Kids company in Australia. These include presentations by several medical specialists and chiropractors practicing in the pediatric field which are both companion to this text and additional to the subject matter covered. These educational products are available for purchase online at www.neuroimpulse.com.

Finally, it is my sincere hope that this text will continue to support the endeavors of chiropractic educators as they seek to give to their students the best possible understanding of chiropractic in the pediatric field. If it becomes instrumental in assisting future generations of chiropractors to care for children in a safe and competent manner, it will have achieved its purpose and the effort will be well worthwhile.

Neil J. Davies
Ballarat

Acknowledgments

I would like to express my sincere gratitude to some very special people who selflessly gave of themselves and their time to make this text a reality:

To my good friend and constant mentor Dr Maurice Easton, whose friendship and unfaltering commitment to professionalism has long been my inspiration.

To Associate Professor Allan Terrett, Ms Thelma Buchanan, Dr Ailsa van Poecke, Dr Kylie Gray, Dr Bruce Tonge, Ms Avril Brereton, Dr Philip Parry, Dr Neil Cox, Dr Sarah E. Whyatt, Dr Robert Turner-Jensen and Ms Kyla Sheridan.

To Dr Kimberley Tuohey, my beautiful daughter, who was a chiropractic student during the writing of the first edition and has now blossomed into a compassionate and deeply caring pediatric chiropractor, a colleague, a contributor, but most of all a wonderful friend.

To my grandchildren and little patients who so patiently endured my endless photographic sessions.

To Dr Sheila Bonnett, who came to Australia at the height of the work on the text to undertake a pediatric training program and left having contributed so much technically to the chapters and their references.

To my patients and their parents, the best teachers of them all.

To Ms Kristin Holland, my long-suffering personal assistant, whose cheerful and happy disposition lightened the load on many occasions.

To my lovely wife Robyn, who willingly and without complaint sacrificed so much to allow me to bring this volume into existence – you are the wind beneath my wings.

Finally, to the Lord Jesus Christ, in whose grace and mercy I live, move and have my very being.

Chiropractic in the pediatric field

Neil J. Davies

*And let the beauty of the Lord our God be upon us,
and establish the work of our hands for us; yes,
establish the work of our hands.*

Psalm 90.17 (New King James Version)

History of pediatrics

The practice of pediatrics is based on the dictum that children are not little adults and cannot be treated as such. Pediatrics began to emerge as a medical specialty late in the 19th and early 20th centuries in response to the growing appreciation that the health problems affecting children are different from those affecting the adult population. Not only are the health problems of children different from those of adults, but they also differ between different cultures and nations around the world. Factors which contribute to these differences are 'the prevalence and ecology of infectious agents and their hosts; climate and geography; agricultural resources and practices; educational, economic and sociocultural considerations; and, in many instances, the gene frequencies for some disorders. These factors are often interrelated' (Vaughan 1987).

Initially the field of pediatrics was dominated by research in the fields of immunology and infection control. In the late 19th century in the United States, of every 1000 children born alive 200 might be expected to die before the age of 1 year from such conditions as dysentery, pneumonia, measles, diphtheria, whooping cough, and the like. The efforts of pediatricians, combined with those of immunologists and pioneers in public health, have led to such better understanding of the origins and management of many problems of infants that in the past half-century infant mortality in the United States has fallen from around 75/1000 live births in 1925 to about 10.9 in 1983.

The advent of medical discoveries such as penicillin and other antibiotics has had a profound influence on the clinical outcome of diseases affecting large numbers of children. This is reflected in the extremely low mortality rates in the developed world in comparison to those in countries where such medical care is less available.

As early as the first decade of the 20th century, medical scientists such as Arnold Gesell began to evaluate childhood development over time using scientific methods (Levine et al 1999). This led to the development of well child clinics, a practice that has persisted to the present time and one which fits comfortably into the chiropractic wellness paradigm. In the latter half of the 20th century, the discipline of pediatrics has increasingly focused attention on conditions that affect relatively small numbers of children (i.e. leukemia, cystic fibrosis, congenital disease, etc.) as well as the developmental, behavioral and social aspects of child health.

Chiropractors have treated children in the course of their general practice since the inception of the chiropractic profession. It is only after a century of chiropractic care of infants and children that pediatrics is beginning to emerge as a systematic and structured specialty discipline in chiropractic practice. Pediatric education at undergraduate level appeared in the curriculum of some chiropractic colleges as early as 1915. That chiropractors have always seen well child care as a fundamental role of chiropractic in the pediatric field is shown in a 1918 patient education brochure produced by the Eastern College of Chiropractic (Newark, NJ) which advocates 6-monthly check-ups for all children. The authors of this pamphlet clearly demonstrate, even at an early stage of its development, their understanding of the preventive value of chiropractic care, by stating 'One adjustment in the child is worth fifty in the adult' (Callender et al 1998).

While undergraduate education in chiropractic pediatrics was part of college curricula for most of the 20th century, postgraduate specialist training was singularly lacking until the School of Chiropractic at Phillip Institute of Technology in Australia introduced its Certificate in Chiropractic Paediatrics course in 1987. This course comprised 200 hours of self-directed learning plus required residential training schools. The course was designed and constructed by the author of this

DOI: 10.1016/B978-0-7020-3129-8.00001-3

text in conjunction with a number of medical specialists and other educators within the Australian university system. This course became the forerunner of an Australian university accredited Master of Chiropractic Science degree (MCSc), a short version of what is now a full-length Master of Science (MSc) degree accredited by a major university in the United Kingdom. This course has been available since 2003 and is currently offered worldwide as the first university-accredited MSc degree in chiropractic pediatrics to be made available to the chiropractic profession in its 100 plus years of existence, thus filling a void in specialist training. Parallel to the development of this degree has been the implementation in the 1990s of two certification courses in chiropractic pediatrics in the United States, one by the International Chiropractic Pediatrics Association founded by Dr Larry Webster (1937–1997) and the other by the International Chiropractic Association.

The principle which underpins all efforts in pediatric health care, and which fits comfortably into the chiropractic paradigm, is perhaps best summed up by Behrman et al (2007): 'The goal in the medical management of the child is to permit him to come into adulthood at his optimal state of development, physically, mentally and socially, so that he can compete at his most effective level.'

The chiropractic subluxation in children

According to Palmer (1910), the chiropractic subluxation is the result of insult(s) to the nervous system caused by any one or a combination of physical trauma, chemical irritants or 'mental' (emotional) stresses. Since the time of Dr Palmer, numerous attempts have been made to define the chiropractic subluxation. For the purposes of this text, a slightly modified version of the definition proposed by the Association of Chiropractic Colleges (ACC) will be employed to identify the lesion treated by chiropractors. The ACC definition of the chiropractic subluxation includes the following core statements:

> Chiropractic is concerned with the preservation and restoration of health and focuses particular attention on the subluxation.
>
> A subluxation is a complex of functional and/or structural and/or pathological articular changes arising from compromised neural integrity and may influence organ system function and general health.
>
> A subluxation is evaluated, diagnosed, and managed through the use of chiropractic procedures based on the best available rational and empirical evidence.

While the sincere and scholarly work of many others who have published on this subject (Gatterman 1995) is recognized and acknowledged, no credible reason is seen to warrant a departure from the use of historical chiropractic terminology, provided such terminology is adequately defined.

The development of the subluxation is distinctively chiropractic and reflects in a unique way the clinical practice of chiropractic. Common to all concepts of subluxation are some form of both neurological and kinesiological dysfunction. The proposed model of subluxation used in this text (Fig. 1.1) addresses the issues of chiropractic in a uniquely chiropractic way while remaining understandable to other health care professionals. Neuropathology is shown at the apex of the model since cortical dysafferentation forms the bedrock of a modern understanding of the subluxation complex. The other factors shown (kinesiopathology, myopathology, connective tissue pathology, etc.) all derive from, and are a reflection of, the

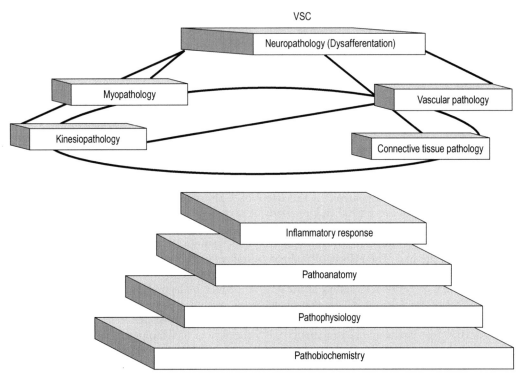

Figure 1.1 • Conceptual model of the chiropractic vertebral subluxation complex (VSC). (Adapted and modified from Lantz C 1995 The vertebral subluxation complex. In: Gatterman MI (ed) Foundations of chiropractic: subluxation. Mosby, St Louis, p. 152.)

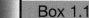

patterns of aberrant neurological function commonly referred to as dysafferentation. Chapter 21 provides a more complete and detailed discussion of this phenomenon.

The chiropractic paradigm

The subluxation forms the absolute basis of the chiropractic paradigm. The precursor of identifiable disease is *dis*-ease, a state in which the body is 'not at ease' or as Selye (1956) put it: 'the syndrome of just being sick.' It is the assertion of fundamental chiropractic principle that this state is the direct result of physiological imbalance caused by diminished functional neurological integrity and, indirectly, immunological function which is so vital to the preservation of homeostasis. The profound relationship between the nervous and immune systems in maintaining homeostasis is becoming better understood as a result of recent research and publication (Brooks et al 1982; Gatterman 1990, 1995; Haas & Schauenstein 1997; Ito et al 2008; Nakanishi & Furuno 2008; Smith & Blalock 1988).

The role played by the chiropractor in pediatric health care delivery has little to do with the direct, interventional treatment of disease as is the case in allopathic medicine. The 'therapeutic' role of the chiropractor is, simply stated, to identify patterns of neurological dysfunction, make as precise and complete a correction of all the factors involved as possible, monitor the clinical outcome over time (including the parameters of disease) and teach parents how to implement preventive health care strategies with their children. Heilig (1949), who noted that the longer the period of osseous development during which asymmetrical forces are acting on the spine and pelvis, the greater will be the frequency, duration and extent of spinal damage, illustrates the importance of the early implementation of chiropractic care.

Commenting on the absence of spinal pain syndromes in children who demonstrate neurological imbalance, Anderson-Peacock (1996) notes that in one study of asymptomatic children 15.8% had cervical subluxations and 40% had pelvic subluxations. She further points out that it has been estimated that by age 2 some 80% of all children are out of neurological balance. This estimate concurs with a survey carried out by staff and senior chiropractic student interns at two Melbourne secondary colleges on 13- and 14-year-old children in 1982, in which it was shown that 83% of all the children examined had postural deviation and other physical findings consistent with neurological dysfunction. Health promotion through well child maintenance care is an invaluable contribution which

Box 1.1

Key developmental ages at which children should be evaluated for both developmental progress and neurological dysafferentation

- 6 weeks
- 3 months
- 4–5 months
- 6 months
- 9 months
- 12 months
- 18 months
- 24 months
- Every 6 months thereafter until school entry

chiropractic can make to the health and well-being of the developing child. Box 1.1 sets out the frequency of well-being chiropractic visits recommended to candidates for the University of Wales validated Master of Science (Paediatrics) degree offered by McTimoney College of Chiropractic, based on the key developmental ages identified in the various screening instruments available to health care providers (Eu 1986, Frankenburg et al 1971, Illingworth 1987) and the recommendations made in the publication *The Child Patient: A Matrix for Chiropractic Care* by Fallon (2005). This frequency is considered the basic minimum for well children. Additional chiropractic neurological assessments should be made in the event a child suffers any traumatic event, receives a vaccination, becomes infected or manifests any change in demeanor, feeding or sleeping habits.

Even after the advent of identifiable disease and the movement of the individual patient into the interventionist medical paradigm, the chiropractic focus on the subluxation remains unchanged. This unwavering therapeutic focus, however, does not excuse or exempt the chiropractic clinician from the responsibilities of practicing the science and art of orthodox physical diagnosis. It remains the emphatic responsibility of the chiropractic clinician to identify where on the health–disease continuum (Fig. 1.2) the patient is in order to make the most appropriate clinical decision as to which paradigm the patient should be placed in, and to what extent each patient should be managed alone or in concert with other health care providers. To this extent, the chiropractor is, generically speaking, a practitioner of complementary medicine as opposed to an 'alternative' practitioner, a term which implies an isolationist 'them and us' attitude (Kleynhans 1994).

In the health care continuum it can be readily seen that chiropractic and western modern medicine have quite different, if often overlapping, roles to play in providing patient care. The fundamental principle upon which chiropractic is based

Well-being	Physiological dis-ease	Pathophysiology	Pathology	Death
	No identifiable pathology	Measurable physiological change	Identifiable disease	
Functional balance	**Functional imbalance**		**Tissue/system dysfunction**	
(Homeostasis)	(The chiropractic wellness paradigm)		(The interventionist medical paradigm)	
	Chiropractic		**Chiropractic + Medicine**	

Figure 1.2 • The relationship of the chiropractic and medical paradigms to the health care continuum from wellness to death. The two paradigms must be seen not to interface but to overlap, the latter implying the need for clinical co-management.

is that of restoration and maintenance of homeostasis by correcting neurological dysfunction. This definition is in keeping with that proposed by the founding father of chiropractic, Dr Daniel David Palmer, who described health as 'that condition of the body in which all the functions are performed in a normal degree' (Palmer 1910). In contrast to chiropractic, the basic principle of medicine is the identification of and direct intervention in the disease process, primarily using drugs and surgery.

Except when clinical contraindications can be demonstrated, chiropractic has, to a large degree, a critical role to play in the management of the patient who clearly belongs in the medical paradigm (pathophysiology and pathology), since disease is a 'battle to maintain the homeostatic balance of tissues despite damage' (Gatterman 1990). By contrast, medicine has little role to play in the management of the patient who fits within the chiropractic wellness paradigm because of the lack of an identifiable pathology. Even preventive measures such as prophylaxis for asthma are dependent for their implementation upon the demonstration of the presence of the disease in the first place.

Etiology of the subluxation complex in children

The three categories of stress factors, physical, chemical and emotional, which produce the subluxation (Palmer 1910) apply equally to both children and adults. In children, however, they are perhaps more identifiable as each pediatric age group has its special peculiarities of life experiences. For example, in the neonate and infant, physical trauma is all but isolated to the birth process and handling errors, while in the school-age child such injury may arise from a wide range of sources, including general play and organized sports.

Physical trauma

Birth trauma is obviously the most common form of physical trauma in the infant. While much attention has been focused by the chiropractic profession on the use of forceps and suction extraction, it would appear that the potential for subluxation development may occur much earlier in the delivery process than previously thought. This is evidenced by the fact that many infants who had a 'normal' occiput anterior, non-instrumental delivery demonstrate clinically significant neurological dysfunction as early as the first day of life and commonly within the neonatal period (birth to 6 weeks). After consultation with two gynecologists associated with the development of the MSc (Paediatrics) degree program mentioned earlier, it has been hypothesized that the upper cervical subluxation, particularly the anterior occiput, extended atlas and posterior axis may be a result of deflexion of the cervical spine which often occurs during the first stage of labor. This is not to deny the importance of the necessarily forceful, or sometimes injudicious, use of forceps or suction devices.

Injury incurred through handling, both accidental and intentional, is a well-recognized cause of subluxation in children. Such handling errors can occur during bathing or parent–child play (such as throwing the baby up and catching them under the arms), from the use of poorly designed papoose carriers, dressing with tight clothing (especially around the neck), neck position during feeding, prolonged periods in car seats, bypassing the crawling phase of gross motor development and falls from tables, beds and high chairs which do not have restraint capability.

In the preschool-age period, subluxation may result from the use of walker frames, jolly-jumpers, trampolines, traction on the arm and shoulder from parents pulling the child by the arm, falls resulting from play and other activities, and inappropriately forceful spanking practices. The chiropractic subluxation is also a common outcome of infectious illness, presumably from a combination of decreased muscle tone and coughing.

Chemical trauma and irritants

Palmer (1910) identifies the importance of chemical irritants or 'poisons' as a general category of neurological stress. A typical statement from *The Chiropractor's Adjuster: The Science, Art and Philosophy of Chiropractic* reads: 'Displacements of the osseous framework of the body are directly caused by injuries and accidents. Indirectly through poisons which contract the fibers of the nervous system, which in turn act on muscles, thereby drawing bones out of alignment.' With the limited knowledge of neurophysiology at the time he was writing, it is remarkable that Palmer was able to identify the importance of chemical stresses in the etiology of the chiropractic subluxation.

Exposure to chemical irritants may begin in utero with the fetus exposed to substances capable of producing a neurotoxic effect. Recreational substances and some prescribed medications exert such an effect (Table 1.1). In particular, it is worth noting that alcohol consumption is most dangerous during the organogenic period of the first trimester of pregnancy and as little as two glasses of standard wine per day is capable of creating developmental abnormality and deformity (Hankin 2002, Rosett et al 1983). Indeed, current opinion is that zero is the only safe limit for alcohol consumption during pregnancy (Ethen et al 2009, Golbus 1983). On the matter of smoking, one study demonstrated that women who used marijuana during pregnancy delivered smaller infants who were nearly five times more likely to have features compatible with those seen in fetal alcohol syndrome (Hingson et al 1982).

After birth, environmental and food allergens are common irritants which result in development of the chiropractic subluxation via the viscerosomatic pathways (Budgell 1998, Homewood 1981). Principally, the environmental irritants to which children are commonly exposed are seasonal pollens, air and water pollution, and environmental noise pollution, while the offending food substances are principally dairy products, various sugars, food additives and colors, and wheat-derived products (gluten and yeast). The subject of allergy and substance intolerance is more fully discussed in Chapter 18.

Emotional factors

Maternal bonding

An understanding of the emotional stresses experienced by children is extremely important to an understanding of many

Table 1.1 Recreational substances and prescribed medications which may have a neurotoxic effect on the fetus and contribute to both developmental anomalies and the development of neurological dysafferentation in the unborn child

Substance	Known clinical effects
Antibiotics	Generally very safe, but tetracycline discolors deciduous teeth and competes with and displaces calcium in the teeth and bones
Cancer drugs	Highly neurotoxic drugs associated with gross developmental anomalies
Thyroid function drugs	Some of these produce scalp deformities, fetal goiter, deflexed heads at birth and cretinism
Progesterone	Cardiac defects may arise, especially if contraceptive medication is continued after conception has occurred
Anticonvulsant drugs	In particular, phenytoin may produce growth and mental retardation, microcephaly, ptosis and hypoplasia of the distal phalanges
Coumarin-derived drugs	This category of drug has been shown to cause a flat nasal bridge with resultant mechanical breathing difficulty, mental retardation, abnormal brain development and optic atrophy
Alcohol	Some of the more common effects of fetal alcohol syndrome are tetralogy of Fallot, ventricular septal defect, pulmonary stenosis, cleft palate, retarded psychomotor development, persistent ductus arteriosus, failure-to-thrive syndrome, microphthalmia, transposition of the great arteries, cerebral palsy, cerebral atrophy, gastroesophageal reflux, cataracts, temporal lobe epilepsy, myopia, developmental retardation and abnormal facial configuration
Smoking	Light-for-date baby, prematurity, increased rate of perinatal mortality, addiction and features typically seen in fetal alcohol syndrome (marijuana)

Box 1.2

The four essential factors involved in successful bonding

- Holding the infant close to the mother's body
- Maintaining sustained eye contact
- Smiling and making soothing sounds
- Constant light sensory stimulation of the infant by the mother

of the clinical presentations with which the chiropractor will be confronted. At the earliest point of life, the newborn baby becomes psychologically bonded to its mother and henceforth dependent upon her not only for nutrition, but for comfort, safety, warmth, nurture and a sense of well-being. Until very recently the notion of a wordless, psychological bond between mother and baby which ultimately had a significant bearing on the baby's physical well-being was generally regarded to be the product of the overactive imagination of 'cranks and extremists' and lacking any scientific foundation. That impression has largely changed now and bonding is a well understood phenomenon that has been defined as 'a non-verbal form of psychological communication, an intuitive rapport that operates outside of or beyond ordinary rational, linear ways of thinking or perceiving' (Pearce 1977). It may be that specific hormones are involved in bonding, and breastfeeding is absolutely essential if bonding is to be full and complete.

In one study on infantile autism (Zaslow & Breger 1969), the investigators concluded that there are four essential factors involved in successful bonding (Box 1.2). 'The issue of bonding is not sweet sentiment. The issue is intelligence, the ability of the brain to process sensory information, organize muscular responses and interact with the environment' (Pearce 1977). It can surely be readily appreciated what effect unsuccessful bonding would have in creating aberrant neurological function.

In his book *Magical Child*, Pearce (1977) recounts the following:

> Jean MacKellar told me of her years in Uganda where her husband practiced medicine. Local mothers brought their infants to see the doctor, often standing patiently in line for hours. The women carried the tiny infants in a sling next to their bare breasts. Older infants were carried on their back papoose style. The infants were never swaddled, nor were diapers used, yet none of them were ever soiled when they finally saw the doctor. Puzzled by this Jean finally asked some of the women how they managed to keep their babies so clean without diapers and such. Oh, the women answered, we just go to the bushes. Well, Jean countered, how do you know when to go to the bushes? The women were astonished at her question. How do you know when you need to go they exclaimed.

Needless to say, these mothers and babies were bonded.

Domestic disharmony and maternal distress are very quickly picked up by the infant and translated into irritability, crying and unsettledness. The negative effect on muscle tone, sleeping and feeding patterns is a major contributor to cortical dysafferentation in young children, particularly those who are breastfed. Maternal counseling may play a very important role in the management of such situations.

Fear and other negative emotions

Beyond the first year of life when a greater separation of mother and child begins to occur, fear and other negative emotions may begin to impinge upon normal neurological function. Feelings of fear, anxiety and insecurity become stored in the brain as memories and may be activated at any time as thought processes to re-establish previously subjugated patterns of neurological dysfunction. 'Once memories have been stored in the nervous system, they become part of the processing mechanism. The thought processes of the brain compare new sensory experiences with the stored memories which help to select the important new sensory information and to channel this into important storage areas for future use or into motor areas to cause bodily responses' (Guyton & Hall 2005). The physical end result is like pulling out a previously recorded tape and replaying it. This process in part explains why patterns of neurological dysfunction are often recurrent.

So profound is the mind–soma relationship that 'with a proper technique it is possible to analyze a personality solely by a study of muscular behavior, in the same way and with the same results as by a study of mental processes alone' (Homewood 1981). Muscular tone is modified by the emotion, whatever it is, producing a typical aberrant posture which may lead to neurological dysfunction. Repeated exposure to the emotion, such as a child who regularly witnesses violence at home or is subjected to bullying at school, not only creates recurrent patterns of neurological dysfunction but imprints the nervous system which, in turn, as a now stored memory, bears on the processing of new sensory information.

As a consequence of civilization and an increasingly fast-paced lifestyle which is more and more sedentary and less and less physical, stimulation of the sympathetic 'fight or flight' mechanism which demands an expression of fear in muscular activity (Homewood 1981) is inadequately managed by the body. How, for instance, does one fight the threat of war or atomic attack? Yet the 'fight or flight' mechanism remains built into the body and continues to demand an appropriate response to the stimulus that has aroused the emotion of fear. The end result is alteration in autonomic function (tachycardia, hypertension, decreased peristalsis, sleep disturbance, etc.) and recurrent patterns of neurological dysfunction. In more recent times, since the September 2001 attacks on the World Trade Center in New York, with its repeated showing on worldwide television and the constantly talked about threats of further terrorist attacks, psychologists have identified an increase in anxiety in children resulting from a non-specific fear of being the victim of such an attack. Some have even labeled it the 9/11 syndrome.

Conversely, the subluxation, which may have originally derived from either physical trauma or chemical irritation, may have the effect of disturbing the emotional or mental stability and well-being of individuals until they are no longer capable of coping with the emotional stress of their environment (Homewood 1981). The art, therefore, of restoring functional integrity to the nervous system is in a very real sense psychosomatic per se, as it removes that which is responsible for the nerve irritation which in turn may affect a particular organ or gland.

> Every nerve infringement within the vertebral column is an incipient pathological state involving some concurrent psychic infringement. The initial malformation may readily lead to a true psychosomatic condition if the patient centrally superimposes upon this localized neural irritation invoking specific regional pain and the additional generalized or widely distributed weight of fear in any one of its protein forms. Thus, increased by a remoter reinforcement from another power area or energy source, the pain is necessarily paralleled by a corresponding growth in fear, worry or anxiety and the slow nibbling away of a sufferer's psyche goes on apace.
>
> (Homewood 1981)

In summary, while it may be possible to identify a single subluxation initiating factor, in reality the chiropractor will be dealing with a constellation of factors which, for the most part, can only ever be partially addressed. The real value of a detailed search for etiological factors in children lies in the ability such knowledge bestows upon the practitioner to effectively teach and counsel the parents and their child in terms of prevention.

Clinical decision-making in chiropractic pediatrics

Pediatric patients are unique in many ways. For the most part they cannot verbally interact in the clinical consultation and therefore often become uncooperative; it takes a great deal of innovation and imagination on the part of the clinician when treating them; they experience a high incidence of sudden-onset illness which often looks much worse than it actually is; they are not 'little adults' and cannot be treated as such. Twenty-four hours in the life of a child can be a very long time (Hewson & Oberklaid 1994). Pediatrics, and especially the care of the very young, is an unusual and sometimes threatening clinical milieu in which to work for the chiropractor unaccustomed to seeing large numbers of children as patients.

The typical adult chiropractic practice seldom involves confrontation with rapidly fulminating, life-threatening disease or situations in which patients are in imminent physical danger within their home environment. Such is not the case, however, with children, who are by and large brought to chiropractors for very different reasons than adults. Spigelblatt et al (1994), in a study of parents' motives for bringing their children to alternative practitioners (chiropractors and others), identified the main reasons as being respiratory tract disorders (27%), ear, nose and throat disorders (24%), allergies (15%), skin conditions (6%), gastrointestinal disorders (6%) and preventive care (5%). In any similar survey of adult patients consulting chiropractors, an overwhelming percentage would cite musculoskeletal disorders, particularly low back pain, neck pain and headache, as the reason for seeking care. This high percentage of children brought to chiropractors with organic disease and dysfunction demands of the clinician an equally high diagnostic skill level and a thorough knowledge of the natural history of the conditions likely to be encountered. A 'simple' viral infection of the upper respiratory tract, for example, may progress to acute otitis media, pneumonia or meningitis, or a baby with colicky symptoms may have serious substance intolerance, gastroenteritis or even intussusception – conditions which may be encountered by chiropractors according to Spigelblatt et al (1994).

When consulting children, the chiropractic clinician is well advised to diligently follow a clinical framework of history-taking, physical examination and clinical investigation which will identify as many of the symptoms and signs of serious illness as possible. A suggested framework to follow is shown in Table 1.2.

A word about visit frequency is probably in order. For children receiving the benefits of well child evaluations, the suggested frequency of care is designed to coincide with key developmental stages. In the sick child, however, frequency of visits should be far greater until there is unequivocal evidence of recovery, at which time care frequency can be returned to well child levels. There are two reasons for implementing a greater frequency in overtly sick children: firstly, disease progression in children can be extremely rapid, in some instances making even daily visits too widely spaced to allow for identification of the clinical signs of serious illness at an early enough stage; and secondly, active illness, especially

Table 1.2 Framework for the clinical evaluation of a pediatric patient in a chiropractic primary care setting

Presenting patient	Chiropractic paradigm	Possible outcomes
Clinical history-taking	Presenting complaint Review of systems Social history Family history Psychological screening Developmental history Immunization status	Specialist referral or Proceed to physical examination
Physical examination	Assessment of growth Developmental screening Head and neck Cardiovascular Respiratory Abdomen Neurological Orthopedic Immunological	Specialist referral or Proceed to investigations or Proceed to chiropractic subluxation assessment
Investigations	Radiological Laboratory Other	Specialist referral or Proceed to chiropractic subluxation assessment

Subluxation assessment	Kinesiopathology
	  Motion palpation
	  Posture
	  X-ray mensuration
	Myopathology
	  Static palpation
	  Muscle testing
	  Orthopedic tests
	  Range of motion
	Connective tissue pathology
	  Static palpation
	  Orthopedic tests
	  Range of motion
	Vascular pathology
	  Skin temperature
	    instrumentation
	  Static palpation (i.e.
	    blanching tests)
	Neuropathology
	  Skin temperature
	    instrumentation
	  Myotomes
	  Dermatomes
	  Muscle stretch
	  Reflexes
	  Pathological reflexes
	    (e.g. Shimizu,
	    Babinski)
		Commence chiropractic management
		or
		Arrange for cooperative management

infection, causes recurrence of the dysafferentation in as little as a few hours. Maintenance of neural balance is essential to the best possible clinical outcome in the shortest possible time frame in childhood illness. In the great majority of cases this

increased level of visit frequency will be necessary for only 2–3 days. For a scholarly and detailed discussion of care frequency for children in chiropractic practice, readers are referred to *The Child Patient: A Matrix for Chiropractic Care*, by Fallon (2005).

In the more chronically ill child, visit frequency will be best determined by the level of stability that can be obtained in subluxation correction. In some cases, such as plagiocephaly from birth trauma, for example, visit frequency will be quite low, while in other cases where there is active disease, such as asthma, visit frequency will be governed not only by the stability of the subluxation correction, but also by the frequency of the periods of symptomatic exacerbation. In all except the acutely ill child, the dictum 'less is better' is a sound clinical rule to follow in the chiropractic management of children.

Legal considerations in chiropractic pediatrics

With the rise of chiropractic pediatrics as a specialty practice and the increased frequency with which the population at large are turning to chiropractic for their children's health care, certain legal issues have taken on increasing importance to the chiropractor. The most significant of these issues appear to be informed consent, failure to diagnose, failure to inform, failure to warn, and patient confidentiality.

Informed consent

The notion of informed consent has been an ever-escalating issue from the mid 20th century onward. Earlier that century, in 1914 in the USA, Justice Benjamin Cardozo had summed up the principle of an individual's right to self-determination in his judgment in the case of *Schloendorff v. Society of New York Hospital* with the following words: 'Every human being of adult years and sound mind has the right to determine what should be done with his own body' (Schloendorff v. Society of New York Hospital 1914). While self-determination is a key issue, the other element underpinning the principle of informed consent is that of professional negligence. It is the duty of care of every clinician to their patient to inform them about their condition, their treatment options, what the clinician recommends as being the most appropriate approach and why, material risks, and the known possible or potential reactions to such treatment. A clinician who fails to take such care may be found guilty of negligence and therefore liable to compensate the patient for any injury caused by the failure to give appropriate information (Plueckhahn et al 1994).

Following the conclusion of World War II, the issue of the individual's right to self-determination took on great and urgent significance in response to a number of highly publicized studies in which the rights of human research subjects were clearly violated by Nazi doctors. The initial response to this gross and inhumane abrogation of the rights of the individual was the formulation in 1947 of the Nuremberg Code. This outlined 10 principles governing medical research designed specifically to protect research subjects. After the formation of the United Nations in 1948, the Universal Declaration of Human Rights was adopted by the UN General Assembly and its first article declares that 'All human beings are born free and equal in dignity and rights.' Since that time a number of other laws protecting research subjects have arisen, including the Declaration of Helsinki in 1964, the National Research Act (USA) of 1974 and the Belmont Report of 1979 (Swisher & Krueger-Brophy 1998).

Gradually, informed consent has become a critical issue for all those involved in medical research, clinical education and private practice. A succinct definition of informed consent is needed to better understand the issue at the clinician–patient interface.

Informed consent is a process, not a signed piece of paper. It is based on discussion between the doctor and patient about the condition, treatment options, and the information the patient needs to know about these in order to make an informed choice. There is no ideal process and it needs to be tailored to each individual patient's situation. The process is necessarily dependent upon each individual's ability to understand and comprehend what is being discussed including the possible risks associated with the suggested treatment that they, as an individual, would deem to be significant.

Informed consent has been defined as an exchange of information between a therapist and a patient that enables a patient to make an informed choice about treatment options. The basis of informed consent is the patient's right to self-determination – that is, the right to make decisions about what happens to one's body. Informed consent should not be viewed by the therapist merely as a form to be completed, but rather as a substantive, ongoing dialogue with the patient that reflects changes in the therapeutic regimen and anticipated outcomes.

(Swisher & Krueger-Brophy 1998)

In chiropractic pediatric practice, as in all other forms of health care, informed consent must be obtained before proceeding with treatment. The basic elements of informed consent have a dual focus. Firstly, the chiropractor must inform the patient or legal guardian of all aspects of the proposed care that other professionals would consider necessary. This is referred to as the *reasonable doctor standard* (Nisselle 1997). Secondly, the chiropractor must share all the information about the proposed care that the patient would deem necessary in order to make an informed decision. In general, the basic elements should include the diagnosis, nature of treatment to be given, any material decisional risks involved, the expected benefits or outcomes of treatment, and any available alternatives. Informed consent also requires that such verbal intercourse between clinician and patient be in plain language which is readily understood by the patient and any questions should be answered simply and honestly. This is referred to as the *reasonable patient standard* (Nisselle 1997). Thirdly, and finally, there is all the information that this particular patient has requested (the individual patient level) (Nisselle 1996).

Verbal consent is a legally acceptable standard, provided what was discussed is entered into the clinical record in detail. However, written signed consent is usually more appropriate as it affords evidence that the patient agrees that they have been informed about their condition and provided with the opportunity to ask questions, and that those questions have been answered to their satisfaction. Written consent helps to ensure an understanding between the clinician, the patient and any other party who may at some later stage become involved in providing care to that particular patient.

Since the law regarding informed consent is very 'jurisdictional', it is recommended that each individual chiropractor consult with a legal practitioner as well as local chiropractic regulatory bodies when designing a form for use in the particular location where he or she practices.

An important issue growing out of informed consent is the matter of clinical record-keeping. Clinical records should contain clear, concise information detailing diagnosis, management plan, precautions, any special problems, contraindications, clinical goals, anticipated progress and plan for re-evaluation. In addition, any patient reaction to treatment must be carefully noted. Common problems related to clinical record-keeping include failure to date or sign notes, failure to identify the patient, use of vague terms, and erasure or obliteration of clinical notes. Changes to a clinical note should be done by drawing a single line through the note, writing the word 'error' next to it and then dating and signing the entry (Swisher & Krueger-Brophy 1998).

In addition to, and possibly growing out of, the issue of informed consent are the problems of failure to diagnose, failure to inform, and failure to warn.

Failure to diagnose

Failure to make a diagnosis renders the clinician, chiropractic or otherwise, legally culpable. To use the argument that chiropractors do not treat disease, so why diagnose it, is naïve and unscientific since accurate diagnosis allows the chiropractor to make the critical decision of which paradigm the patient belongs in (Modde 1985). In chiropractic pediatrics, such a decision may save, or cost, a life.

Failure to inform

As noted earlier, under the law, patients are guaranteed the inalienable right to self-determination and therefore must be fully and completely informed by their health care provider. The burden on doctors is not just to give full warnings about the possible consequences of the proposed treatment but also to fully inform the patient generally – for example, but not limited to, how the diagnosis was made, the range of therapeutic options, the merits or otherwise of each option, the doctor's recommendation and the reasons for that recommendation (Nisselle 1996).

Failure to warn

'Failure to warn' is essentially an act of omission by the chiropractor to identify potential harm that may arise from the proposed treatment. The essential legal argument is that 'even if the treatment negligence asserted in all the previous items is not supported by the court, then failure to warn of the complication was negligent and led to damage because the plaintiff would not have proceeded with the treatment even if warned' (Nisselle 1996).

Patient confidentiality

By way of succinct definition, patient confidentiality describes the expectation that clinicians will not, without the express written consent of their patient, disclose to any third party information acquired by reason of their professional relationship. The existence of a family relationship between the patient and the person to whom the disclosure is made does not exonerate clinicians from the consequences of their obligation to maintain secrecy (Plueckhahn et al 1994).

The notion that a child should have the same rights to confidentiality is well established in law. With the clear exception of that which is illegal, the chiropractor is duty bound to maintain in confidence that which has been conveyed by a child regardless of age. If it is deemed absolutely necessary to inform a parent or guardian of something that has transpired during the course of a consultation, the child's permission must first be obtained and an appropriate file note made. Obviously, confidentiality does not extend to cover statements by patients, child or adult, that give the chiropractor knowledge of a criminal or other illegal activity, either before or after the fact.

As a final remark on the issue of confidentiality, it is seldom ever appropriate to dismiss the child from a consultation in order to discuss the case with a parent or guardian. Such an action creates an atmosphere of mistrust on the part of the patient, especially teenagers (Green 1998).

References

Anderson-Peacock, E.S., 1996. Chiropractic adjustment of children. Can. Chiropractor 1 (2), 21–26.

Behrman, R.E., Jenson, H.B., Nelson, W.E., et al., 2007. Nelson Textbook of Pediatrics, eighteenth ed. WB Saunders, Philadelphia.

Brooks, W.H., Cross, R.J., Roszman, T.L., et al., 1982. Neuroimmunomodulation: neural anatomical basis for impairment and facilitation. Ann. Neurol. 12, 56–61.

Budgell, B., 1998. A Neurophysiological Rationale for the Chiropractic Management of Visceral Disorders. Seminar Proceedings of the International College of Chiropractic Friday Forum Series, February 6, Sydney, Australia.

Callender, A.K., Plaugher, G., Anrig, C.A., 1998. Introduction to chiropractic pediatrics. In: Anrig, C.A., Plaugher, G. (Eds), Pediatric Chiropractic. Williams & Wilkins, Baltimore.

Ethen, M.K., Ramadhani, T.A., Scheuerle, A.E., et al., 2009. Alcohol consumption by women before and during pregnancy. Matern. Child Health J. 13 (2), 274–285.

Eu, B.S.L., 1986. Evaluation of a developmental screening system for use by child health nurses. Arch. Dis. Child. 61 (1), 34–41.

Fallon, J., 2005. The child patient: a matrix for chiropractic care. J. Clin. Chiropractic Pediatr. Suppl. 6 (3), 1–14.

Frankenburg, W.K., Camp, B.W., van Natta, P.A., 1971. Reliability and stability of the Denver Developmental Screening Test. Child Dev. 42 (5), 1315–1325.

Gatterman, M.I., 1990. Chiropractic Management of Spine Related Disorders. Williams & Wilkins, Baltimore.

Gatterman, M.I. (Ed.), 1995. Foundations of Chiropractic: Subluxation. Mosby, St Louis.

Golbus, M., 1983. Drugs in pregnancy. Audio-Digest Foundation. Obstet. Gynecol. 30 (4).

Green, M., 1998. Pediatric Diagnosis: Interpretation of Symptoms and Signs in Children and Adolescents, sixth ed. WB Saunders, Philadelphia.

Guyton, A.C., Hall, J.E., 2005. Textbook of Medical Physiology, eleventh ed. WB Saunders, Philadelphia.

Haas, H.S., Schauenstein, K., 1997. Neuroimmunomodulation via limbic structures – the neuroanatomy of psychoimmunology. Prog. Neurobiol. 51 (2), 195–222.

Hankin, J.R., 2002. Fetal alcohol syndrome prevention research. Alcohol Res. Health 26 (1), 58–65.

Heilig, D., 1949. Osteopathic pediatric care in the prevention of structural abnormalities. J. Am. Osteopath. Assoc. 48, 478–481.

Hewson, P., Oberklaid, F., 1994. Recognition of serious illness in infants. Mod. Med. Aust. (July) 32–37.

Hingson, R., Alpert, J., Day, N., et al., 1982. Effects of maternal drinking and marijuana use on fetal growth and development. Pediatrics 70 (4), 539–546.

Homewood, A.E., 1981. Neurodynamics of the Vertebral Subluxation. Valkyrie Press, St Petersberg, Florida.

Illingworth, R.S., 1987. The Development of the Infant and Young Child: Normal and Abnormal, ninth ed. Churchill Livingstone, Edinburgh.

Ito, A., Hagivama, M., Oonuma, J., 2008. Nerve–mast cell and smooth–muscle mast cell interaction mediated by cell adhesion molecule-1, CADM1. J. Smooth Muscle Res. 44 (2), 83–93.

Kleynhans, A.M., 1994. The naming of a multidisciplinary university department. Chiropractic Journal of Australia 24, 63–69.

Lantz, C., 1995. The vertebral subluxation complex. In: Gatterman, M.I. (Ed.), Foundations of chiropractic: subluxation. Mosby, St Louis.

Levine, M.D., Crocker, A.V., Carey, W.B., 1999. Developmental–Behavioral Pediatrics. WB Saunders, Philadelphia.

Modde, P.J., 1985. Chiropractic Malpractice. Hanrow Press, Columbia, Maryland.

Nakanishi, M., Furuno, T., 2008. Molecular basis of neuroimmine interaction in an in vitro coculture approach. Cell. Mol. Immunol. 5 (4), 249–259.

Nisselle, P., 1996. Medical Negligence. Crisis or Beat-up? Business Law Education Centre, South Melbourne.

Niselle, P., 1997. Informed Consent. Medical Protection Society, Leeds.

Palmer, D.D., 1910. The Chiropractor's Adjuster: the Science, Art, and Philosophy of Chiropractic. Portland Printing House, Portland, Oregon.

Pearce, J.C., 1977. Magical Child – Rediscovering Nature's Plan for Our Children. EP Dutton, New York.

Plueckhahn, V.D., Breen, K.J., Cordner, S.M., 1994. Law and ethics in medicine for doctors in Victoria. VD Plueckhahn, Geelong, Victoria.

Rosett, H.L., Weiner, L., Edelin, K.C., 1983. Treatment experience with pregnant problem drinkers. J. Am. Med. Assoc. 249 (15), 2029–2033.

Schloendorff v Society of New York Hospital, 1914. 105 NE 92, 93.

Selye, H., 1956. The Stress of Life. McGraw-Hill, New York.

Smith, E.M., Blalock, J.E., 1988. A molecular basis for the interactions between the immune and neuroendocrine systems. Int. J. Neurosci. 38 (3–4), 455–464.

Spigelblatt, L., Laine-Ammara, G., Pless, B., et al., 1994. The use of alternative medicine by children. Pediatrics 94, 811–814.

Swisher, L.L., Krueger-Brophy, C., 1998. Legal and Ethical Issues in Physical Therapy. Butterworth-Heinemann, Boston.

Vaughan, V.C., 1987. The field of pediatrics. In: Behrman, R.E., Vaughan, V.C. (Eds) Nelson Textbook of Pediatrics. thirteenth ed. WB Saunders, Philadelphia.

Zaslow, R.W., Breger, L.A., 1969. A Theory and Treatment of Autism: Clinical Cognitive Psychology, Models and Integration. Prentice-Hall, Englewood Cliffs, NJ.

The pediatric history

2

Neil J. Davies

The clinical value of an effective patient history must never be underestimated. Not only can a good interview technique provide an effective method of obtaining information critical to forming a diagnostic impression, it can also be a therapeutic tool in itself.

> A unique feature of pediatrics is that the history represents an amalgam of parents' objective reporting of facts (e.g. fever for 4 days), parents' subjective interpretation of their child's symptoms (e.g. an infant crying that is interpreted by parents as abdominal pain), and for older children their own history of events. Parents and patients may provide a specific and detailed history, or a vague history that necessitates more focused probing. Parents may or may not be able to distinguish whether symptoms are caused by organic illness or a psychological concern. It is often helpful to ask specifically what problems the parents wish to address in order to determine what really prompted the clinical visit. Some visits are occasioned by problems at school, such as low grades or troublesome peer relationships. Understanding the family and its hopes for and concerns about the child can help in the process of distinguishing organic illness from emotional or behavioral conditions, thus minimizing unnecessary testing and intervention.
>
> (Hay et al 2007)

Hughes & Griffith (1984), in commenting on the importance of the clinical history, identified the following five fundamentals of diagnosis:

1. skilful history-taking
2. careful physical examination
3. keen powers of observation
4. wise selection of laboratory and other technical procedures
5. good analytic judgment.

The ability to obtain a thorough clinical history and to conduct an adequate physical examination is not only basic to the diagnosis of disease but is also essential in the evaluation of the normal child, especially the child who has slight deviations from the usual but still falls within the normal range (Barness 1994). Despite this obvious need, more errors are made because of inadequate history-taking and superficial physical examinations than any other cause. In terms of the clinical history, clinicians of all kinds fall into two distinct categories, those who are logical and strategic in pursuing the history as potential diagnoses dictate and those who take a scatter-gun, all inclusive history – the mindless fact collector (Pang & Newson 2005). The latter approach results in a collection of data that are a mixture of relevant and irrelevant facts and increases the likelihood of a wrong diagnostic conclusion, unnecessary investigations and inappropriate treatment.

More than in any other area of chiropractic practice, it is with pediatrics that the doctor of chiropractic must demonstrate scientific curiosity about people, and utilize every communication skill possible. These skills include:

- observation of the patient and caregiver(s)
- listening
- touching
- empathizing.

The ultimate goal is to develop the ability to 'read' the patient. Barness (1994) advises that, during the interview, it is important to convey to the parent interest in the child as well as the illness. The parent is allowed to talk freely at first and to express concerns in their own words. The interviewer should look directly at the parent or the child intermittently, and not only at the writing instruments. A sympathetic listener who addresses the parent and child by name frequently obtains more accurate information than does a harried, distracted interviewer. Careful observation during the interview frequently uncovers stresses and concerns that otherwise are not apparent.

While the information that follows in this chapter can provide you with the necessary tools to conduct an effective clinical interview, it must be remembered that it is essentially an intuitive process.

As a chiropractic clinician you should be aware that all patients, particularly young children, will scrutinize you for evidence of your attitude. Your facial expression and body

© 2010, Elsevier Ltd, Inc, BV
DOI: 10.1016/B978-0-7020-3129-8.00002-5

language can help to facilitate the effectiveness of a clinical interview. It is important not only to listen to what the patient or caregiver/historian is telling you, but also to be sure that your facial expression and body language never reflect your personal judgment of what may be being told to you.

Because of your role as a primary contact health care provider, your patient has the right to present to you with any problem or combination of problems. The most effective interview techniques are those that focus on one problem at a time and utilize open-ended questions to generate meaningful information (Green 1998).

It is sometimes difficult to generate a complete historical database at the first interview owing to the sensitive nature of some information occasionally pertaining to the pediatric patient. Parents and children are often not forthcoming in matters such as family finances, sexuality, domestic harmony, etc. (Bouchier & Morris 1982). The astute chiropractic clinician will recognize this and accept that as care is given over time and the patient/parents gain confidence in the chiropractor, further information may be progressively elicited.

The manner in which you begin the interview process will to some extent depend upon the structure of your clinic. In some cases a chiropractic assistant may place the patient in a room where relevant personal information is gathered, and then the doctor may enter to commence the interview. In other cases the chiropractic assistant may take the patient into the doctor's office, and in still other cases the doctor may personally take the patient from the waiting room.

All cases allow for an exchange of pleasantries and essential introductions. This is a valuable opportunity to create rapport and begin building relationship. It is important to establish how your patient wishes to be addressed, and for you to set the ground rules as to how you prefer to be addressed, be it your first name or title.

Observation of the patient and caregiver

Much can be learnt about the patient, family dynamics and attitude towards you as a chiropractor by observing the patient and caregiver(s) during history-taking. The following are good clues to watch for (Green 1998):

- perspiration, blushing or paling
- controlled, uneven or blocked speech
- talking in a whisper
- the patient's gait on entering the room
- frequent swallowing, tenseness, fidgeting, a preoccupied air or avoidance of eye contact
- sudden glance at the interviewer or someone else in the family following a statement or question
- clenching, rubbing, wringing hands
- scratching or nail-biting
- the kind of clothing worn – dark clothes may be a sign of depression in an adolescent
- sudden request by parent or adolescent for permission to smoke

- reddening of the eyes or crying
- frowns, a smile
- apparent concern or unconcern about symptom(s)
- double messages (i.e. mother laughing while telling the child to behave or smiling when talking about the child's bad behavior)
- the light that seems to go on in a patient's mind when a significant association or new insight is achieved
- interactions between parents and child, parent and parent, and between child and physician during the visit
- developmentally inappropriate behavior (e.g. older child on parent's lap, difficulty in separating child from parent, or the mother laying a young infant on the examination table then walking away)
- the way in which the infant or young child is held or helped during the interview and physical examination
- the mother's parenting presence
- the child's response to parental requests
- the child's play and activity.

Listening to the patient and caregiver

Children can be apprehensive and fearful about a visit to the chiropractor and sometimes a remark like 'I'll bet you were a little nervous about coming here' may be most helpful in breaking the ice. It may also be useful to offer the child a tongue depressor or other harmless object to play with while the history is being taken.

Introduce yourself and explain what it is a chiropractor does, but, especially, be yourself – a special doctor who is interested in helping children. Give the child a few moments to get acquainted with you and the surrounding chiropractic equipment. Your comfortable friendliness will place most children at ease. It is usually very profitable to spend a few minutes playing with the child to gain their confidence.

Do not leave the child out of the interview process. The child is, after all, the patient and the success of your management may depend upon the rapport you establish on the initial visit.

Attempt to dispel any anxiety the parents may feel about chiropractic. Emphasize its safety and gentleness in particular. A doctor standing over a small child in the manner required by some common chiropractic procedures can look quite threatening. A parent will also sometimes need to be reassured about 'doing the right thing' by consulting a chiropractor. Family and community attitudes toward chiropractic management of young children can be quite intimidating to parents.

Dealing with fear

Try to minimize any fears the child may be exhibiting about being adjusted. The following mechanisms may prove helpful in this regard:

- Ask about school, kindergarten, etc.
- Use a teddy bear as a substitute patient and turn him into a 'talking teddy'.

- Talk to the child about his perception of what the problem is.
- Above all, be natural and do that which is 'you' in establishing rapport with the patient.

As the interviewer, you need to hear and receive what the patient is trying to convey. Note the order in which problems are mentioned and any recurrent references. In particular, listen carefully to the patient's first and last statements as they frequently convey exactly what the patient wants you to know (Green 1998).

When a patient says, 'I don't see what that has to do with my problem', it is probably clinically relevant (Green 1998). Note whether the patient/caregiver avoids a question by subtly changing the subject or appears to misunderstand while feigning an eagerness to answer. If you believe an answer to a question to be not entirely honest, rephrase the question or return to it later. Sometimes a question to which a patient initially chooses not to respond may be answered later or in a subsequent consultation.

Non-stop talking should be interpreted as a cover for anxiety, perhaps serving as a defensive screen so as to preclude the opportunity for you to ask embarrassing questions (Green 1998).

Although most patients come with the desire and expectation of receiving help, they may have reservations about both. They may have their own agenda of concerns and ideas as to what would be helpful. A lifetime of 'medical conditioning' will sometimes create an attitude of reserve in some caregivers about the value of chiropractic care for young children. These considerations may condition or bias the success of the visit.

It is not uncommon for patients and caregivers to withhold information or fail even to disclose the primary or real reason for coming until convinced that the chiropractor will be empathetic and genuinely interested in their well-being. The patient who feels that you understand will usually, if given a chance, share real concerns and problems in addition to those presented as the chief complaint.

You should always remember that patients and caregivers may be wholly unaware of what is self-evident to you as a clinician (Hull & Johnston 1987). The way patients perceive symptomatic events may be very different from how you, or even another of the patient's family members, see them. Patients and caregivers should never be given reason by their chiropractor to feel embarrassed about their lack of understanding of a health problem. The time necessary to offer a full and complete explanation should never be denied a patient.

Some definite taboos

- Never be critical of another practitioner's diagnosis or treatment suggestions.
- Never allow a child who has been brought for treatment to leave without it. Be sure you do what you must, despite any protestation the child may make.
- Never allow a child to be rewarded for being sick. If the parents want to buy the child something as a comfort, encourage them to give it when the child recovers. This reinforces the positive value of being well.

Interviewing the uncooperative patient

Some patients and caregivers present with an attitude towards the chiropractor which makes it difficult to build a constructive doctor–patient relationship or gain an accurate clinical history. There are many reasons, most of which are not immediately evident, why patients present to doctors with such an attitude. A young patient, for example, may demonstrate an angry or even insulting attitude as a manifestation of anxiety or cockiness, a compensation for insecurity, or a cover for hostility. This inappropriate behavior may derive from stress in previous relationships with authority figures such as teachers, police, counselors, etc. If you sense at the beginning of the interview that patients are angry, try to disarm them by conveying your understanding of how they feel, and be careful not to be perceived as being critical, irritated or condescending.

With patients who display inappropriate behavior you should attempt to maintain calmness in your attitude and resist the desire to retaliate in any way. It may be useful to make a sympathetic statement such as, 'There must be something pretty awful going on to make you so upset – would you like to tell me about it?' At the same time, no chiropractor should be expected to accept abuse from a patient or caregiver.

Compulsive or highly self-centered patients are difficult to help. They see no merit in changing their behavior or in accepting the suggestions of others, and are rarely proactive in their health management. Some patients may be unable to form a trusting relationship with you, while others' expectations of chiropractic may be so great or unrealistic that they cannot be satisfied. Some patients will display no overt emotion at all and respond with parsimonious, almost telegraphic answers that tend to conceal more than they reveal, while other patients talk incessantly but assiduously avoid revealing their real feelings.

Green (1998) suggests that the following expressions may be useful when dealing with an angry or otherwise uncooperative patient:

- How did you manage?
- They must have made you angry (sad, happy).
- That must have been a trying time for you.
- You must have been hurt (upset).
- It's hard to talk about this.
- People don't seem to understand how you feel.
- You seem to be receiving a lot of unwanted advice.
- You seem to be kind of hard on yourself.
- I'd guess you find it difficult to trust anyone.
- The death of someone so close is hard to deal with.
- I suppose you were scared that you might lose (son, daughter).
- This has been kind of a secret fear, I take it.

In addition, an understanding nod may convey that you are 'with them'.

Discussing difficult subjects

There are many topics of discussion that may arise during a clinical interview which the patient or caregiver may find difficult to discuss openly, such as sexuality, child abuse, serious disease, psychological etiology, suicide, divorce, drug addiction, peer issues, etc. It is always appropriate to ask permission to seek information on any topic during a clinical interview. Such a request shows respect for the patient's privacy and dignity. A question such as, 'I need to ask you some personal questions, is that OK?' or 'I know some things are a bit difficult to talk about and I really wish I didn't have to ask, but I need to know about . . ., is that alright?' would be an appropriate opener.

It is imperative that patients being asked difficult questions are not made to feel pressured for an answer or hurried in any way. A statement such as, 'Take all the time you need, I know this is difficult for you' is reassuring to the patient and shows understanding on your part.

On occasion, it may be your experience that the roles will be reversed and you, as the clinician, will be the one in the difficult position. Some patients will preface their remarks with 'I want to talk to you about something, but I want to be sure you will not tell anyone'. Such a request for unconditional confidentiality is unreasonable and potentially dangerous. A clinician faced with such situations should respond by informing patients that they can be assured of confidentiality provided what they are about to tell you is not concerning a criminal or otherwise illegal activity. Finally, professional clinicians should never entertain questions from patients about their private lives, families, etc. Patients who make such inquiries should be politely told that the private or domestic life of the chiropractor has no bearing on their case and therefore will not be discussed.

Drawing the history-taking time to a conclusion

In the practice of chiropractic pediatrics, the interview is concluded when the clinical database either identifies a presumptive diagnosis or demands a particular aspect of physical examination (e.g. neurological examination).

While it is axiomatic that when you conclude the interview and indicate to the patient and caregivers that it is the time to proceed to examination, then the interview is ended, be aware of last minute 'throw away' lines at this time, as this may represent the real reason you have been consulted in the first place. It is wise at this time to pursue these remarks as they may bear significantly on the investigations ordered (e.g. X-ray series), final diagnosis and potentially the whole chiropractic management program.

Recording the pediatric history

Personal details

All pediatric records in a chiropractic clinic should contain the following personal details:

- name
- current address and telephone number
- age and date of birth (DOB)
- name(s) of parent(s)
- name(s) and age(s) of sibling(s).

Reliability of the historian

Any person providing historical data is termed an historian and should be described by name and/or relationship to the patient. It is not uncommon for different family members to accompany the patient on different visits and for adolescents to be accompanied by friends rather than parents. Clinicians often forget who came with the patient on the previous visit and frequently a different member of the health care team takes responsibility for the patient at a subsequent visit.

Therefore, it is quite helpful to identify each historian explicitly. With clinical records it is important to record whether or not one believes that the historians are reliable, that is, that their reports are complete and accurate. Any inadequacies should be clearly identified and the nature of the inadequacies should be mentioned on the file. For example, the information may be incomplete, vague or disorganized. Alternatively, it may be presented in chronological order that does not seem logical or be distorted in another consistent or significantly patterned way.

Also, the suspected reason for the problem as offered by the historian should be noted. Some parents say, 'I don't know' as a way to avoid discussing personal or unsettling issues. For others, the inadequate information they offer may be a result of intellectual limitations, psychological problems (psychosis, depression, anxiety), drugs, alcohol or other organic brain problems which interfere with perception and recall. Additionally, the stress of the health care visit itself may interfere with the motivation or attention of the child or parent/caregiver, if, for instance, they are frightened or angry (Bouchier & Morris 1982, Lott Ferholt 1980).

The presenting complaint

While acknowledging the danger of a reductionist attitude in clinical practice (that which turns a patient into a pathology), a priori reasoning in the history-taking process cannot be overemphasized. The history should be as complete a factual record as possible of the health issue at stake which will allow you, from knowledge of the presentation and natural history of disease, to draw logical diagnostic conclusions from which a course of action can be planned and executed.

A fundamental aspect of good history-taking is to know or define what patients mean when they employ terminology (Table 2.1). It is also important, in reading pediatric literature and understanding developmental differences, to know what is meant by the terminology used in defining age periods (Table 2.2).

Finally, the process of a priori reasoning is greatly enhanced by pursuing the following mnemonic (M.K. Easton, personal communication, 1987) to narrow the diagnostic categories

Table 2.1 Comparison of the frequency terms used by patients to the percentage time the reported symptom is actually present

Term used	Percentage of time the symptom is actually present
Always	100
Almost always	75–100
Usually	35–100
Frequently	42–93
Often	28–92
Occasionally	0–42
Infrequently	0–28
Rarely	0–17
Never	0

Table 2.2 Chronological age range to which the terms used for descriptive age in pediatrics refer

Period	Age range
Neonatal	0–4 weeks
Infancy	0–1 year
Toddler	1–2 years
Preschool	2–5 years
School	5–15 years
Adolescent	13–19 years
Childhood	1–15 years

the patient may fit into, and in making your questions more specific, goal oriented and systematic:

Clinical	Congenital – genetic/in utero
Instruction	Infection
In	Injury – mechanical/thermal/chemical
Chiropractic	Mechanical
Must	Metabolic
Cover	Circulatory
Every	Endocrine
Disease	Degenerative
kNown	Neoplastic
About	Autoimmune

A direct quotation from the historian is the preferred manner of recording the symptom(s) of concern. Details of the history should then ideally follow the outline below.

Location

A precise location should be identified, preferably with the patient or caregiver pointing to the area of concern. Inquiry should be made as to whether or not the child always points to the same location, or if it varies from day to day. Of particular interest with the younger child is the ability to be specific about location rather than indicating a more general area.

Timing

The time of the day the symptom appears and when it is at its most severe are important. Relationship to other events in the daily cycle should be noted (e.g. tummy pains when it is time to go to school, etc.).

Factors which produce exacerbation or remission of symptoms

Those factors that relieve or worsen the symptoms should be identified. Inquiry in relation to these factors should identify response to treatment, timing, daily routine, and possible psychological causes.

Associations

An attempt should be made to identify all factors that are deemed, by either the patient or the parent, to be associated with the symptoms. These might include such items as school toilet phobias, environmental allergic factors, family issues, reaction to particular foods, etc.

Onset

Any details about the onset of the symptom(s) are most helpful (e.g. pain in the knee started after a bicycle fall, etc.). A defining incident, or knowledge of the circumstances surrounding the onset, provides valuable information which can be integrated into the clinical picture.

Response to previous or current treatment

This information will assist in determining the accuracy of a previous diagnosis and the appropriateness of current treatment. Persisting symptoms in children should be regarded as being due to incorrect diagnosis until it can be conclusively proven otherwise.

Severity, nature and effects

It is helpful, if practicable, to attempt to identify the severity of a symptom and its nature or character. Usually by age 6–7, children can begin to give reliable information of this sort. In younger children, the description of the effects of the symptom on the child by the parent or caregiver is usually the only reliable information available.

Direct quotations of descriptive terms used by caregivers who have had opportunity to observe the child are usually most helpful.

The past clinical history

The past clinical history should include such detail as the age of the mother at delivery, previous miscarriages or stillbirths, the number of current siblings, clinical history of maternal hypertension or proteinuria, alcohol consumption during pregnancy, smoking habits including both tobacco and marijuana,

15

use of prescribed and over-the-counter medications, and X-ray or ultrasound investigations, mother's diet during pregnancy and a general survey of maternal health.

Perinatal

This section will include details of the actual birth as follows:

- length of gestation
- drugs employed during labor, if any
- type of delivery/presentation (i.e. vaginal or caesarean)
- duration of first and second stage of labor
- details of membrane rupture (i.e. spontaneous or physician induced).

Neonatal

Details of the patient's health at birth are recorded here as follows:

- whether the child need to be respirated
- feeding mode and pattern in first week and subsequently (i.e. breastfed, artificially fed, development of colic, etc.)
- sleep patterns
- weight at birth and hospital discharge (available from documents given to the mother by the hospital)
- head circumference and supine length at birth (also available from documents given to the mother by the hospital).

It is usual to measure the Apgar score at 1 and 5 minutes following birth and these values should be recovered from the perinatal record and entered into the case history.

Childhood illnesses

Details should include such items as:

- feeding history beyond the neonatal period
- timing and success or otherwise of the introduction of solids
- dental eruption patterns
- immunization record
- record of any 'childhood diseases'
- physical development (i.e. weight gain, head circumference, length, fontanel closure, developmental survey)
- general health status of the patient.

Previous illness and immunization status

The clinical record should include a summary of the so-called 'childhood diseases' the patient has experienced as well as which immunizations have been administered. Unless information is volunteered by the historian in relation to the less common childhood illnesses, one should ask about:

- measles
- rubella
- roseola
- exanthem subitum
- erythema infectiosum
- meningitis/encephalitis
- chickenpox.

Allergies

Inquiry should be made about seasonal, environmental and substance allergy/hypersensitivity reactions. Evidence of allergy would include discharge from the eyes and nose, sneezing, allergic 'shiners' (dark rings under the eyes), macular skin rashes, changes in gastrointestinal motility, abdominal bloating, frequent passage of flatus, scratching, and a transverse line across the nose.

Inquiry into the allergy status of siblings and parents is most useful. Hypersensitivity to protein and wheat products, for example, has a very strong familial orientation.

Trauma and injuries

The cause and extent of any injuries should be explored. Of particular concern would be multiple fractures or bruising, particularly if the bruising has a particular shape, is located in a body area unlikely to be traumatized by daily living, or is multiple and at differing stages of healing. All these factors suggest intentional injury.

Hospitalizations and surgery

The dates, diagnoses and clinical outcomes of any hospitalizations or surgery should be recorded.

Nutrition and dietary factors

Inquiries should be made as to the method of feeding for infants and whether or not any problems are or have been encountered.

In bottlefed babies, both the name of the formula and the concentration being used should be recorded. Some babies will be exhibiting symptoms from allergy to a particular formula, while in others inappropriately low concentration quickly produces symptoms which mimic protein hypersensitivity.

In older children, a survey of the food categories consumed should be made. Particular attention should be paid to the amount of refined and 'junk foods' being consumed as well as the level and type of fluid intake. Excessive consumption of any food is significant, as it is typical for children to crave foods that they are actually allergic to (Rapp 1991).

Growth and development

Where possible, the results of previous screenings should be obtained, including measurements of head circumference, length, weight and fontanel diameter. A comment on the achievement of age-appropriate milestones should be entered on the clinical record (Table 2.3).

While successful milestone achievement is comforting to the clinician, an appropriate developmental screening procedure such as the Woodside (Eu 1986) or Denver (Hughes & Griffith 1984, Kliegman et al 2007) systems should be routinely administered when consulting all preschool-age children. Special training programs are needed to qualify you to administer a Denver Developmental Screening Test (DDST). The Woodside screening system is less complicated and requires no special training to administer.

Table 2.3 Essential milestones of development (reproduced with kind permission from Illingworth 1983)

Birth	Prone – pelvis high, knees under abdomen Ventral suspension – elbows flex, hips partly extended
4–6 weeks	Smiles at mother. Vocalizes 1–2 weeks later
6 weeks	Prone – pelvis flat
12–16 weeks	Turns head to sound Holds object placed in hand
12–20 weeks	Hand regard
20 weeks	Goes for objects and gets them without the object being placed in the hand
26 weeks	Transfers objects from one hand to another Chews Sits, hands forward for support Supine – lifts head up spontaneously Feeds self with biscuit

Family and social history

This should include details of the physical characteristics of the home, progress at school, family economic situation, domestic harmony, etc. A detailed family history should be performed and recorded using standard genetic symbols (Fig. 2.1).

As part of the social history, an attempt should be made to estimate the intellectual development of the patient. This may be done by employing the Goodenough Draw-A-Man test, Gessell/Binet/Bender/Gestalt drawings and age-appropriate tasks with 1-inch cubes. These tests are all detailed in Chapter 8.

Review of systems

General considerations

The pediatric review of systems consists of a series of global questions about observations the historian may have made relating to the body systems. The information gleaned in the case of an infant, toddler or preschool-age child is necessarily not as descriptive or as qualitative as that expected from the older child, adolescent or adult. This fact, however, should not be seen as trivializing the information that can be derived.

Before investigating particular systems, general information should be sought on topics such as appetite, activity and energy level, sleep patterns, fever, days of missed school, growth and development concerns, etc.

Head and neck

Some of the typical symptoms experienced in the head and neck region about which inquiry should be made are as follows:

Head

Headache, dizziness, dysmorphic features, trauma.

Eyes

Alignment, problems with vision, corneal/conjunctival irritation.

Ears

Dizziness, recurrent infection, hearing deficit, tinnitus, discharge.

Nose

Irritation, bleeding, discharge, snoring.

Mouth/throat

Enlarged or painful lymph nodes, previous thyroid problems, masses, head held to one side, thrush infection, discomfort or difficulty nursing on one side, tongue protrusion, and difficulty swallowing.

Skin

Productive inquiry would include rashes, birthmarks, the recent appearance of a new lesion, changes in color, masses/swellings, bruises, petechiae, purpura, fine brittle hair that falls out and brittle nails that split or break easily.

Breasts

Questions related to developmental staging, asymmetry (the rule rather than the exception during the developmental period), pain, masses or nipple discharge may be asked.

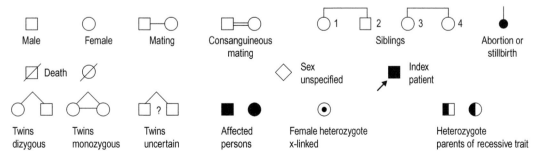

Figure 2.1 • Genetic or pedigree symbols used for recording a family health history (reproduced with kind permission from Hull & Johnston 1987).

Respiratory

Important facets to inquire about include dyspnea, cough, hemoptysis, recurrent infection, a history of asthma and loud adventitious breath sounds.

Cardiovascular

In chiropractic pediatric practice, it is important to appreciate the possibility of a primary presenting symptom being of cardiovascular origin. Signs including cyanosis of the skin, mucous membranes and tongue, edema over the sacrum or at the ankles, or an obvious precordial thrill. Together with a history of murmur, cardiac abnormality or hypertension, any of these signs would raise the suspicion index of underlying pathology.

Gastrointestinal

The gastrointestinal system in small children is capable of producing a constellation of signs and symptoms. At history, it would be important to explore the conditions associated with the presence of abdominal pain, nausea, vomiting, changes in motility, soiling, food intolerances, abdominal bloating with excessive passage of flatus, hernia, jaundice, hematemesis, melena, rectal bleeding and hepatitis.

Genitourinary

Pain on urination, changes in frequency, a sense of urgency, daytime incontinence in older children, dysuria, recurrent infection, resumption of enuresis after a prolonged dry period, and uremia all need to be inquired about.

In addition, carefully phrased questions about the genital anatomy should be asked. In the male, one would seek information about hernia, undescended testes, hypospadias, circumcision, testicular pain or swelling, age of pubertal onset, penile discharge and, on occasion, sexual issues.

In the female, vaginal discharge or irritation, unexpected bleeding, age of pubertal onset, details of the menstrual cycle and occasionally sexual issues need to be inquired about.

Given the current statistical data on early adolescent sexuality, it will be pertinent to inquire about exposure to AIDS and other sexually transmitted diseases in some cases. Considerable discretion about which cases warrant such questioning is strongly recommended.

Orthopedic

Information related to previous chiropractic care, joint or limb pain, swelling and/or edema, congenital abnormalities, sports injuries, previous podiatric treatment, scoliosis, limping and other abnormalities of gait should be sought.

Neurological

Neurological presentations can be very confusing in children, with wide-ranging manifestations. The neurological history should seek information about: the characteristics of the baby's cry, hypopigmented (achromatic) areas and hyper-pigmented (café-au-lait) skin lesions, cutaneous hemangiomas, irritability, seizures, personality changes, numbness, paresthesia, symmetry of limb movement, jerky movements, tremors, dysgraphia, changes in muscle tone and/or strength, CNS infection, developmental delays, poor school achievement, balance/coordination problems, maintenance of fixed posture (e.g. frog leg, scissoring), fisting with thumb adduction in infants, facial and eyelid ptosis, proptosis, dilated or constricted pupils, and sustained opisthotonos.

Psychological

Affective development

Questions to the child or caregiver in this area would seek information related to the child's mood, general behavior, socialization, temperament, attitude, response to authority and utilization of free time.

Cognitive development

Exploration of intellectual development, language acquisition and school progress is an appropriate line of inquiry.

Lifestyle

It may be appropriate to explore such areas as habits (biting nails, head banging, etc.), sexual awareness and experience, substance abuse, sleep patterns, degree of attainment of bowel and bladder control, sports in which the patient is engaged, etc.

Family health history

The chiropractic clinician should endeavor to obtain as accurate a three-generation family history as possible, in an attempt to ascertain whether or not a genetic or familial factor exists. This aspect of the history should explore all cousins, siblings of parents and grandparents. It is appropriate to record this aspect of the history using standard genetic symbols (see Fig. 2.1). A good example of how a detailed, well recorded family pedigree can assist in making a diagnosis is shown in Fig. 2.2.

The clinical history as part of the therapy

As chiropractors, we often think of the management of a particular case as a chronological sequence commencing with history-taking and examination, followed by formulation of a differential diagnosis, appropriate diagnostic investigations, final diagnosis, implementation of chiropractic management and measurement of clinical outcome. Many families who have a child in need of chiropractic care will not necessarily arrive at the consultation with the same perspective. They will come

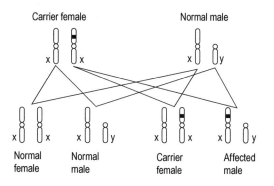
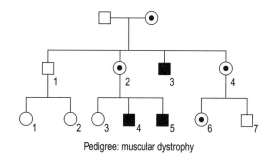

Figure 2.2 ● Family health history of two male siblings suffering from muscular dystrophy which has sex-linked recessive inheritance (reproduced with kind permission from Hull & Johnston 1987).

because they will have perceived that their child has a health problem and they are often anxious because it may turn out to be serious. In the chiropractic clinic they will be in a foreign environment that may well have frightening associations for them. They may not know what exactly you are, or in fact whether you are the best person to help them with their child's problem.

You can ease much of this anxiety by explaining who you are and what you do in language they will understand. You should express to them that you are genuinely interested in their concerns for their child and that you value their insights into what may be the cause. Always give clear, easily understood explanations of what you think the child's problem is and be gentle and caring during the examination. Always carefully explain the reason why you want to order investigations, including what they may reveal and how they may bear on management planning. In this way you will help to obtain the family's confidence and trust, which in turn will improve their willingness to cooperate with the plan of investigation and treatments.

You will not acquire all these skills overnight, but learning them is rewarding and fun, and you will be a much more effective doctor for children and their families at the end of the process (Lissauer & Clayden 2007).

References

Barness, L., 1994. Principles and Practice of Pediatrics, second ed. JB Lippincott, Philadelphia.

Bouchier, I.A.D., Morris, J.S., 1982. Clinical Skills: A System of Clinical Examination, second ed. WB Saunders, London.

Eu, B.S.L., 1986. Evaluation of a developmental screening system for use by child health nurses. Arch. Dis. Child 61 (1), 34–41.

Green, M., 1998. Pediatric Diagnosis: Interpretation of Symptoms and Signs in Children and Adolescents, sixth ed. WB Saunders, Philadelphia.

Hay, W.W., Levin, M.J., Sondheimer, J.M., et al., 2007. Current Pediatric Diagnosis and Treatment, eighteenth ed. Lange Medical Books/McGraw Hill, New York.

Hughes, J.S., Griffith, J.F., 1984. Synopsis of Pediatrics, sixth ed. Mosby, St Louis.

Hull, D., Johnston, D., 1987. Essential Paediatrics, second ed. Churchill Livingstone, Edinburgh.

Illingworth, R.S., 1983. The Development of the Infant and Young Child: Normal and Abnormal, eighth ed. Churchill Livingstone, Edinburgh.

Kliegman, R.M., Behrman, R.E., Jenson, H.B., et al., 2007. Nelson Textbook of Pediatrics, eighteenth ed. Saunders Elsevier, Philadelphia.

Lissauer, T., Clayden, G., 2007. Illustrated Textbook of Paediatrics, third ed. Mosby Elsevier, Edinburgh.

Lott Ferholt, J.D., 1980. Clinical Assessment of Children: A Comprehensive Approach to Primary Pediatric Care. JB Lippincott, Philadelphia.

Pang, D., Newson, T., 2005. Paediatrics. Mosby, Edinburgh.

Rapp, D., 1991. Is This Your Child? Discovering and Treating Unrecognised Allergies in Children and Adults. William Morrow, New York.

The pediatric physical examination

Neil J. Davies

The physical examination of children in the context of the chiropractic paradigm serves two purposes. Firstly, it is a tool for supplying specific clinical information about the health status of the child and, secondly, it facilitates the development of the chiropractor–patient relationship. Certainly, confidence in the chiropractor is inspired in parents when a thorough physical examination is conducted before an opinion about the child's condition is expressed or management options are discussed.

In the practice of chiropractic pediatrics, the assessment commences the moment the parents and child enter the consultation room. Observation of children's behavior during the clinical interview is an important tool in assessing the relationship they have with their parents, level of confidence in the presence of a stranger, and the presence of important symptoms such as a cough or wheeze, gait dysfunction, postural deformity, etc.

It is an imperative that the chiropractor addresses children by their first name from the outset in order to convey an attitude of caring and concern. Even young children are capable of quickly recognizing insincerity in a clinician, particularly if the clinician appears rushed and impatient. The chiropractor can often gain a patient's cooperation by learning to anticipate the reactions normal to age and personality type. For example, most teenagers are seldom openly forthcoming about what may be wrong with them when they first meet you, while the majority of preschool-age children are frank and open about their visit.

The child's temperament should be taken into account when first attempting to establish a chiropractor–patient relationship. The child with a 'slow to warm up' temperament may best be initially approached vicariously by using a stuffed toy such as a teddy to do the talking. On the other hand, children with the 'quick to warm up' temperament may well sit on your knee as you talk to them. It is important to quickly assess your patient's likely temperament with a question such as, 'How are you today?' The child's initial reaction will most likely be an accurate guide to his or her subsequent behavior during the consultation.

If the child appears friendly and unconcerned, the chiropractor may begin the examination on the table. It is usually best, however, to perform as much of the examination as possible with the child on the mother's lap. This tends to create a secure, familiar environment while offering the best opportunity for cooperation. In a child who is persistently resistant to examination, it is often fruitful to examine their teddy first and even allow the child to use your stethoscope or tongue depressor to examine teddy.

Being able to handle the chiropractor's diagnostic equipment often relieves the child's fear about it. As a last resort, it may sometimes be necessary to apply manual constraint in the event that the child's moving about may cause injury, such as when performing otoscopy or using a tongue depressor to examine the pharynx.

It is always wise to remember that children are not little adults and frequently find a visit to the chiropractor very frightening, particularly if they have not previously accompanied one of their parents to a consultation. In the adult patient, physical examination generally follows a well-structured format, usually on a system-by-system basis. In the child, depending on the level of cooperation and apprehension, it is often necessary to alter the order of the examination routine in order to accommodate the emotional state of the child.

General appearance

The physical examination really begins the moment the chiropractor meets the child. It should be noted if the child appears generally well or is exhibiting obvious signs of illness such as pallor, dyspnea, lassitude, cyanosis or jaundice. Any obvious evidence of physical abnormality and the demeanor of the child should also be noted. A concise file note, such as those below, should be entered into the patient record (Lott Ferholt 1980).

Example 1: Healthy looking female toddler with obvious right out-toeing.

DOI: 10.1016/B978-0-7020-3129-8.00003-7

Example 2: Male infant appears unwell with fever and nasal flaring.

Example 3: Female toddler appears frightened and clinging to mother's dress.

Assessment of growth and vital signs

Longitudinal assessment of growth is fundamental to chiropractic pediatrics. On the initial visit, and subsequently at key developmental ages, the chiropractor should measure, record and plot on anthropometric charts the dimensions of head circumference, length/height, weight and anterior fontanel diameter.

Head circumference

This is measured at the maximum occipitofrontal circumference (Fig. 3.1) and plotted on the appropriate anthropometric chart according to age and gender (Appendix 1). The head circumference should be considered 'normal' when the plotted value is located on the percentile graph in a position consistent with those for height and weight. In the case of a head circumference that is high on the graph compared with height and weight, the head circumference of both parents should be obtained and plotted on the adult graph (Appendix 2), and compared to the position of the child's before a conclusion of macrocephaly is reached.

Weight

The child's weight should be measured and plotted on the appropriate anthropometric chart according to age and gender. For children weighing less than 30 kg, accurately calibrated baby scales should be used (Fig. 3.2), while for children weighing over 30 kg, commercially available bathroom scales are

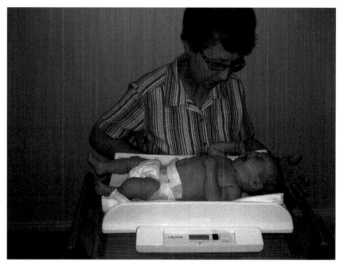

Figure 3.2 • Technique for weighing babies under 30 kg using digital scales.

appropriate for use provided they are placed on a hard floor surface. Inaccurate measurement will result if the scales are placed on a carpeted floor.

Length/height

The length of children up to 3 years of age should be measured with the child in the supine position, preferably using a stadiometer. Commercially produced flat stadiometers are readily available through standard medical supply companies. The child's head is held firmly against the headboard, the knees are held by the examiner in full extension and the feet are brought into an anatomically neutral position. The child's length is then read off the stadiometer with the slide positioned against the heels (Fig. 3.3). The child's length/height

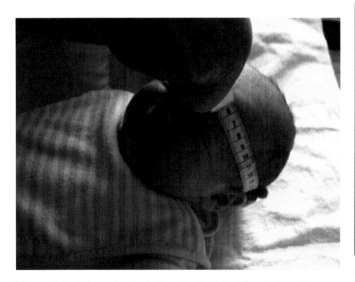

Figure 3.1 • Measuring technique for the infant head circumference. The maximum occipitofrontal diameter should be obtained for comparison with normal percentile charts.

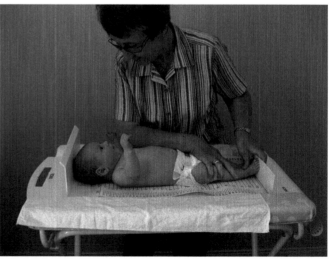

Figure 3.3 • Measuring technique for infantile length in the supine position using a horizontal pad-type stadiometer. The head is touching the headboard, the knees are fully extended and the feet are at 90° to the lower leg before the measured value is determined.

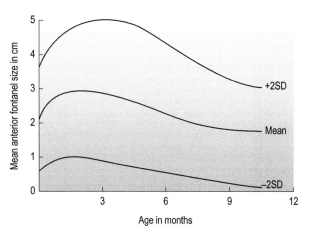

Figure 3.4 • Percentile chart against which measured values for the diameter of the anterior fontanel are compared (reproduced with kind permission from Popich & Smith 1972).

Table 3.1 Normal respiratory and heart rates at different ages

Age	Heart rate (beats/min)	Respiratory rate (breaths/min)
Premature	120–170	40–70
0–3 mo	100–150	35–55
3–6 mo	90–120	30–45
6–12 mo	80–120	25–40
1–3 yr	70–110	20–30
3–6 yr	65–110	20–25
6–12 yr	60–95	14–22
12 yr	55–85	12–18

should be plotted on the appropriate anthropometric chart according to age and gender.

Once a child reaches 3 years of age, their length should be measured as standing height using a standard wall-mounted measuring device.

Anterior fontanel

The diameter of the anterior fontanel should be determined by averaging the measurements taken along the coronal and sagittal sutures. The stage of closure can be estimated by plotting the value on the percentile graph (Fig. 3.4). Early closure of the fontanel that is associated with a small head circumference and ridged sutures may be due to craniosynostosis, while a large fontanel diameter associated with an increasing head circumference may be due to hydrocephalus.

Pulse rate

The pulse rate may be determined by palpating either the radial or carotid pulses. The number of beats per minute and any irregularity of rhythm should be noted. Once the child's pulse rate has been determined, it should be compared to established normal ranges (Table 3.1).

Respiratory rate

The respiratory rate may be measured by either observing the abdominal excursions associated with the respiratory cycle or by auscultation. Once the child's respiratory rate has been determined, it should be compared to established normal ranges (see Table 3.1).

Temperature

This is most reliably measured in the ear canal using a digital thermometer. While 36.8°C is a common average in older children, temperature control is not as well regulated in babies

and toddlers who may demonstrate temperatures >39°C with only very minor infection. Young children who are very active may also exhibit temperatures >38.5°C at the end of the day (Barness 1981).

Blood pressure

Blood pressure in children is infrequently measured by most chiropractors because of a false presupposition that it is either too difficult to obtain the level of patient cooperation necessary to derive an accurate value or that children do not have blood pressure problems at all. When the child is familiarized with the sphygmomanometer and stethoscope, and an appropriate technique is used, it is usually possible to produce an accurate result.

There are a number of cuff sizes to suit varying ages commercially available through medical supply companies. To obtain an accurate measurement, the cuff must cover 80% of the brachium. This will produce a measurement which can be reliably compared to standardized tables of values for age and gender (Appendix 3). As a useful guide in the clinical setting, the normal ranges for systolic blood pressures in children by age have been published by Roberton & South (2006) and are shown in Table 3.2. The use of a cuff which covers less than half the width of the brachium tends to

Table 3.2 Normal range for systolic blood pressure in children by age

Age	Normal range for systolic pressure (mmHg)
Newborn	50–75
1 week–3 months	50–85
3 months–2 years	60–100
2–10 years	70–110
>10 years	85–120

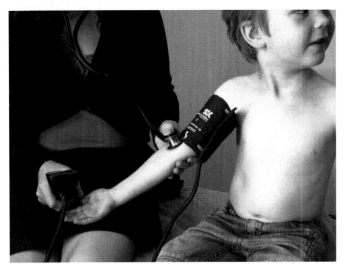

Figure 3.5 • Technique for measuring blood pressure in a toddler. Note how the examiner's left hand is holding the child's arm into full extension in order to prevent contraction of the biceps muscle.

artificially elevate the values obtained. The chiropractor should hold the patient's arm in full extension as the stethoscope is placed over the brachial artery in the antecubital fossa, leaving the other hand free to work the pressure bulb (Fig. 3.5).

It is sometimes necessary to obtain a measurement of lower limb blood pressure when there is a question of impaired blood flow arising from a congenital anomaly such as coarctation of the aorta. In such a case, the cuff should be placed on the patient's thigh, the knee maintained in full extension and the stethoscope placed over the popliteal pulse. If blood pressure is difficult to obtain at this location, it is appropriate to place the cuff over the lower leg and auscultate over the dorsalis pedis pulse.

The definition of 'normal' when making a clinical interpretation of a pediatric blood pressure should be arrived at only after three consecutive measurements have been compared with established standardized percentiles and are shown to be consistent between themselves, all values being below the 90th percentile and above the 10th (Barness 1981, Kliegman et al 2007). Several studies have shown that a bigger body size in pediatrics is associated with higher blood pressure values. The clinician should always use height as opposed to weight when considering the effect of body size as obesity is usually associated with elevated blood pressure (Rosner et al 1993). Hypertension in children and adolescents continues to be defined as systolic and/or diastolic blood pressure that is above the 95th percentile on three or more consecutive measurements. Blood pressures that lie between the 90th and 95th percentile are generally considered to be 'high normal', but to remain consistent with the Seventh Report of the Joint National Committee on the Prevention, Detection, Evaluation and Treatment of High Blood Pressure, this level of blood pressure is now termed 'prehypertensive' and represents grounds for advice on lifestyle modification (National High Blood Pressure Education Program Working Group on High Blood Pressure in Children and Adolescents 2004).

On the basis of developing evidence, it is now apparent that hypertension is detectable in young children and indeed occurs commonly. Given that the long-term health risks of uncontrolled hypertension in children and adolescents is substantial, it is incumbent upon chiropractors seeing children to show due diligence in evaluating their blood pressure so that appropriate preventive strategies can be implemented at the earliest possible time.

Integument

Inspection of the integument should include an assessment of the condition of the skin, mucous membranes, nails and hair.

Skin and mucous membranes

The oral mucosa is readily visualized and should be assessed for moisture and general color (Bickley & Szilagyi 2008). Central cyanosis is best appreciated at the tongue and the anemic child will usually exhibit paleness in the mucosa. The skin should be assessed for color, local temperature changes, pigmented markings (café-au-lait spots, etc.), general turgor, rashes, inflammation, bruises, scratches, scars, contusions, and other marks which may indicate intentional injury. The possible clinical significance of commonly encountered skin changes is shown in Table 3.3.

When assessing skin turgor, it is useful to roll a section of skin from the abdominal wall between the thumb and forefinger to determine its consistency, the degree of subcutaneous tissue present and the hydration. The skin in well-hydrated infants and small children will return to its original position immediately it is released, while in a dehydrated child there will be a delay in return. This phenomenon is termed 'tenting'.

The color of the skin in a newborn is red, often resembling that of a 'boiled lobster', which gives way to the usual pink color after about 34 hours (Maxwell 1977). Mottling will also occur in response to cooling and is particularly noticeable on the trunk, arms and legs. Acrocyanosis is present at birth and generally persists for the first week or so of life. It commonly recurs in infancy in response to cooling and is of no significance unless it persists for several hours, especially in the feet. The child in whom it persists in such a manner should be sent for investigation of the cardiovascular system for congenital anomaly (Barness 1981, Maxwell 1977).

Nails

Fingernails and toenails should be inspected for evidence of thrush infection, brittleness and clubbing. Clubbing is an evidence of serious cardiac, pulmonary and in some cases gastrointestinal disease (Barness 1981), and is caused by edema under the nailbed which subsequently changes the angle between the terminal digit of the finger and the nail (Fig. 3.6).

Table 3.3 The clinical significance to the chiropractor of commonly seen skin and mucous membrane changes

Skin and mucous membrane	Possible clinical significance
Macular rash over upper trunk, neck, face, fossae, hair line, skin folds and anogenital region	This rash is commonly associated with cow's milk allergy and forms one part of the triad of signs that form the diagnostic paradigm for this particular syndrome. This rash may also be a result of heat stress
Café-au-lait spots	Small café-au-lait spots are a common finding and when they exist singly have no clinical significance. Six or more spots having a diameter of 1.5 cm or greater are considered a hallmark of neurofibromatosis
Nappy rash	Erythematous rash over the buttocks and anogenital region. This rash is occasionally due to congenitally low pH and responds well to having an alkali such as powdered antacid placed on each new nappy liner
Koplik's spots	These are an enanthem on the buccal and pharyngeal mucosa which is pathognomonic of measles (rubeola). They are small crystalline white spots that resemble grains of sugar. They occasionally have erythematous margins
Eczematous rash	This typical rash is most often seen in skin folds and body fossae
Bruises	Multiple bruising is common and to be expected on the lower limbs of ambulatory children. Bruising, especially multiple bruises at varying stages of healing in body areas not likely to suffer trauma, is highly suggestive of non-accidental trauma
Milia	Milia are pinhead-sized, smooth, raised areas that are white in color and are free of surrounding erythema. They appear mostly on the nose, cheeks and forehead. They are caused by the retention of sebum in the openings of the sebaceous glands, spontaneously resolve over several weeks, and are of no clinical significance
Miliaria rubra	These are vesicles situated on an erythematous base and located variously about the trunk and face. They are due to blockage of sweat gland ducts
Erythema toxicum	These lesions are seen in the neonatal period, usually appearing on the second or third day of life. The lesions look quite like insect bites as erythematous macules with a central vesicle. The lesions will appear all over the body and generally last about 1 week then spontaneously disappear
Capillary hemangiomas	These are irregularly shaped red patches that appear on the forehead, upper eyelids, the upper lip and over the occipital area. They are common and disappear by the end of the first year of life

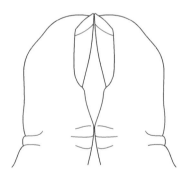

Figure 3.6 ● In clubbing, the normal diamond-shaped space between the nail beds, as shown above, is closed up.

Hair and scalp

The child's hair should be inspected for bald patches (alopecia areata), dryness and splitting of the ends. The scalp should be inspected to determine the presence of 'cradle cap' rashes, lesions, heaping or ridging of the sutures (craniosynostosis), and any other marks.

Examination of the eyes

The most commonly reported symptoms of eye disease encountered in general practice are redness, tearing, discharge, pain and photophobia (Eisenbaum 1997).

The eye examination is difficult to perform on children, especially neonates and infants. The order of the examination is not particularly important and will usually be dictated by the demeanor of the patient at the time. The examination of the eyes by a chiropractor must include, however, the following components.

- inspection
- visual screening tests
- palpation
- ophthalmoscopy.

Inspection

A survey of the orbits, lids, sclera, irides and pupils should be carried out. This may be done with the child on the mother's lap or in the supine position and note should be made of any masses, scars, abrasions, obvious hemorrhage or other marks.

Table 3.4 The clinical significance of important conditions that may be encountered during routine examination of the eye

Eye sign/ condition	Clinical significance
Pupillary asymmetry	Pupillary asymmetry is not uncommon in infants, but should be considered clinically significant if it persists as a constant over time. Inequality of pupillary diameter is seen as one component in either complete (miosis/ anhidrosis/ptosis) or partial (miosis/anhidrosis) Horner's syndrome
Ptosis	Ptosis of one or both lids is a serious sign and may be associated with a congenital defect of the levator palpebrae, oculomotor nerve paralysis with frontalis overaction, Möbius syndrome, neuroblastoma and other tumors, Homer syndrome, myasthenia gravis, the muscular dystrophies, drug use (e.g. vincristine) and occasionally hysteria
Proptosis	Proptosis, which is a forward bulging of the eye, is also a serious sign which may be associated with craniosynostosis, Crouzon's disease (craniofacial dysostosis), orbital tumors such as neuroblastoma, osteoma, retinoblastoma, rhabdomyosarcoma, neurofibroma, histiocytosis X, etc., orbital hemorrhage, orbital cellulitis, cavernous sinus thrombosis, thyrotoxicosis and aneurysm
Setting-sun sign	The setting-sun sign is associated with raised intracranial pressure as in hydrocephalus. This sign may sometimes be seen in otherwise normal neonates, albeit briefly

Pupillary asymmetry, ptosis of one or both lids, any degree of proptosis in addition to any evidence of the so-called 'setting-sun sign' all represent clinical evidence implicating pediatric referral (Table 3.4).

The infant may then be held in vertical suspension in order to assess extraocular movements. The child is rotated about the y-axis with the head held in the midline by the examiner. It is normal for the child's eyes to look in the same direction as rotation and, when the rotation is stopped, for the eyes to look to the opposite direction following momentary, unsustained nystagmus. Definitive following movements are not usually seen until the child is several weeks old (Barness 1981).

Visual screening tests

A common presentation to chiropractic clinics is the child with strabismus, otherwise referred to as a squint, lazy eye or turned eye. Strabismus is a condition where there is lack of parallelism of the visual axes resulting in disconjugate fixation. The two most likely mechanisms are:

* two images are received by the visual cortex of which one is suppressed to avoid diplopia
* images of unequal clarity are received at the visual cortex.

The result is that one eye becomes 'lazy' and stops functioning, which, in time, adversely affects its visual acuity. The 'lazy' eye will tend to adopt a consistent position of ocular deviation either away from the central axis (*exotropia*) or toward the midline from the central axis (*esotropia*). The screening tests which may be used in the chiropractic clinic to identify ocular deviation caused by extraocular muscle weakness are Hirschberg's corneal reflex test, the cover–uncover test, and the alternate cover test (Barness 1981, Eisenbaum 1997, Green 1986, Olitsky et al 2007).

Hirschberg's test requires the use of a light source. The child is asked to maintain visual fixation on a light source held 30–35 cm away while the examiner looks over the top of the light source at the reflection from each pupil (Fig. 3.7). In a patient free from strabismus, the reflection pattern should be symmetrical and right out of the center of the pupil. In the case of esotropia, the lazy eye will demonstrate reflection from the lateral margin of the pupil while in exotropia the reflection in the lazy eye will be from the medial margin of the pupil.

The cover test (Barness 1981), or cross-cover test as it is sometimes referred to, is performed by asking the patient to maintain visual fixation on the light source as in Hirschberg's test. The examiner then covers one of the patient's eyes as the opposite eye is observed for movement (see Fig. 3.7). No movement will occur in a normal child, movement from lateral to medial will be noted in exotropia and medial to lateral in esotropia.

On occasion, latent deviation will be present. Latent deviation is not obvious on either casual observation or Hirschberg's test, but may be demonstrated using the cover–uncover test. This test is carried out in an identical manner to the cross-cover test except that the examiner covers one eye and then observes as it is uncovered (see Fig. 3.7). The normal eye will not move as it is uncovered, but remain fixed with its pair on the light source. In exophoria, the eye will move from medial to lateral as it is uncovered and in esophoria it will move from lateral to medial (Eisenbaum 1997, Green 1986).

There is important clinical significance for the chiropractor in carefully assessing the strabismus patient in this manner. Strabismus, identifiable by Hirchberg's test and the cross-cover test, is sometimes able to be resolved quite satisfactorily by the use of chiropractic methods, while the case involving latent deviation seldom responds favorably to chiropractic and should thus be referred to an ophthalmologist without delay. Uncorrected strabismus is one of the two most common causes of amblyopia and anopsia, the other being aniso-metropia, a condition in which one eye has a refractive error 1.5 diopters greater than its pair (Bickley & Szilagyi 2008).

Visual acuity is difficult to assess with any kind of precision in children under the age of 3 years. The best the chiropractic clinician can hope to achieve is to evaluate gross visual capacity by using the miniature or Kendall toy test. The child is given a set of miniature toys and the chiropractor has an identical set. The chiropractor sits some 3 meters from the child and holds up one of the toys. The child should then be asked to hold up the same toy from the set they have. The test is repeated with each eye covered alternately by the mother or a chiropractic assistant. In children over 3 years of age, a Snellen chart can be used and will yield an accurate evaluation of visual acuity.

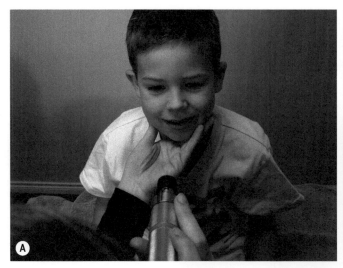

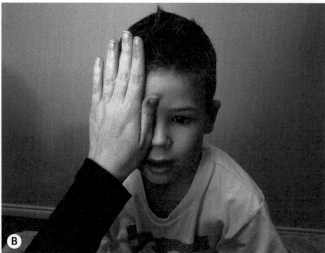

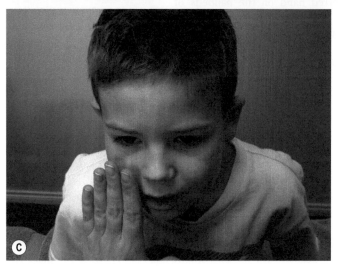

Figure 3.7 ● Technique for evaluating strabismus. (A) Hirschberg's test. The child is asked to look directly at the light source while the examiner looks over the top of it to the reflection coming from the pupils. (B) Cross-cover test. The examiner carefully watches one eye as the opposite eye is covered. (C) Cover–uncover test. The examiner watches one eye, covers it and then observes for horizontal movement as it is uncovered.

The examiner should also attempt to identify refractive error when using the Snellen eye chart. This is done by simply asking the child to look at an image at the level of predetermined visual acuity, then placing a card with a pinprick size hole in it in front of the eye and asking them to look through it to the image. If it is much clearer the child has long-distance refractive error. Normal values for visual acuity in children by age are found in Table 3.5.

Table 3.5 Normal values for visual acuity in children (reproduced from Hay et al 1997 *Current diagnosis and treatment*, 13th edn, with permission of the McGraw-Hill Companies)

Age	Visual acuity
3 years	20/40
4 years	20/30
5 years	20/20

Similarly, for short-distance refractive error, have the child read a few words from a page of writing, then have them do it again looking through the pinhole. If the image is clearer, the child has short-distance refractive error. The significance of determining refractive error is simple. If it remains uncorrected despite the child doing otherwise well with chiropractic management, they need to be referred to an optical professional as persistent refractive error, otherwise known as anisometropia, may lead to amblyopia or anopsia.

Nystagmus is a common and normal finding in a neonate, but has considerable clinical significance when it persists beyond this period. Nystagmus can only be reliably tested in a child who has adequately developed following movements. Nystagmus may be defined as an involuntary rapid movement of the eye, which may be in a horizontal, vertical, rotary or mixed direction. Even in the child with developed following movements, nystagmus should be considered 'physiological' if it can only be demonstrated outside a conical arc >30° from the z-axis of the body with a focal point at the pupil of the eye being examined. Rotary nystagmus is a common single neurological finding in children who are exhibiting a functional cranial fault, and consistently disappears immediately following cranial correction.

The chiropractor can test for nystagmus by simply asking the child to visually fix upon the forefinger which is then slowly moved in a horizontal plane, then a vertical plane, and finally in a circle. The rapid flicking type of movement characteristic of nystagmus is quite difficult to misinterpret (Barness 1981).

Palpation

It is appropriate to palpate the closed eyes of a child to determine the possibility of raised intraocular pressure. The technique is performed by overlaying the tips of the middle and index fingers of the non-preferred hand on the nailbeds of the corresponding middle and ring fingers of the preferred hand. The pad of the middle finger is placed over the orbital arch to create stability while the pad of the index finger is placed over the midpoint or pole of the eyeball. Gentle pressure is generated by the index finger of the non-preferred hand while the examiner appreciates the resistance in the eyeball with the pad of the index finger that is in contact with the eye (Fig. 3.8).

Ophthalmoscopy

The use of the ophthalmoscope is at its most difficult in very young patients. If a successful examination is to be performed, then patience on the part of the examiner is of the essence. The general technique of ophthalmoscopy is the same as for the adult in that the examiner begins with an assessment of the red light reflex, direct and consensual pupillary reflex, and then, using the highest diopter settings first to view the outer surface of the eye, gradually working toward the back of the eye by reducing the diopter settings. While the general

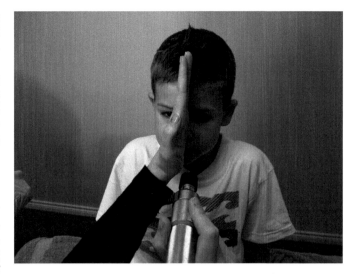

Figure 3.9 ● Technique for examining the pupillary reflexes in the eye. Direct pupillary reflex is obtained by watching the eye being light stimulated, while the consensual reflex is obtained by watching the non-stimulated eye.

technique does not vary, the actual approach to the patient differs significantly (Bickley & Szilagyi 2008).

The attending caregiver should hold the child's head firmly in the midline and as still as possible during the ophthalmoscopic examination. There are four distinct and separate steps in performing a thorough ophthalmoscopic examination. Firstly, the direct pupillary reflex is obtained by watching for pupillary constriction as a bright light is flashed tangentially across the outer surface of the eye. The consensual reflex is obtained by simply observing one eye while the light is flashed across its pair (Fig. 3.9). The usual color of the pupillary reflex is red. A white pupillary reflex is generally a serious sign and necessitates immediate pediatric referral for investigation. Some of the more important causes of a white light reflex are shown in Box 3.1.

Secondly, the ophthalmoscope is placed at 45° to the central axis of the eye and the cornea is studied carefully for any marks such as scratches or scars (Fig. 3.10). This is a naked eye examination.

Box 3.1

Important causes of the white pupillary reflex in childhood

- Cataracts
- Retinoblastoma
- Colobomas
- Retrolental fibroplasia
- Chorioretinitis
- Organized vitreous hemorrhage
- Congenital retinal fold
- Intraocular foreign body
- Retinal detachment
- Metastatic retinitis and enophthalmitis

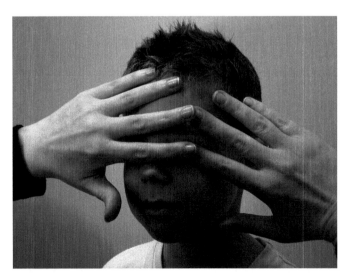

Figure 3.8 ● Technique for palpating intraocular pressure in the eye.

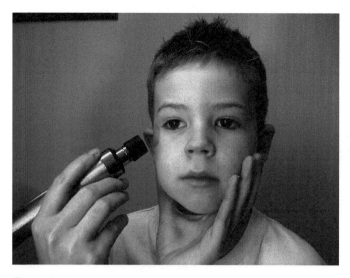

Figure 3.10 • Examination of the cornea for scratches, scars and other lesions.

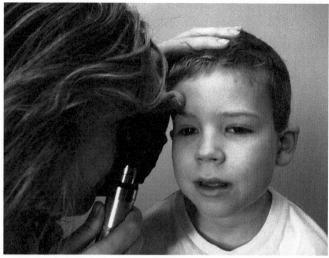

Figure 3.12 • Technique for examining the internal structures of the eye with the ophthalmoscope. The higher diopter settings focus on the more anterior structures such as the lens while the lower diopters bring to focus the retina and its features.

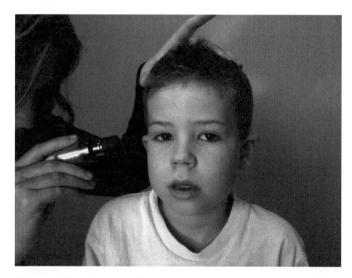

Figure 3.11 • Tangential light examination for increased intraocular pressure.

Thirdly, the ophthalmoscope is placed to shine light tangentially across the surface of the eye (Fig. 3.11). This is done to see if the entire iris lights up, which is the expected response. Increased intraocular pressure may cause only the temporal side to light up due to increased sphericity of the eye surface from the increased pressure.

Fourthly, and lastly, the ophthalmoscope is positioned to shine light into the pupil angled at 15° toward the nasal side of the eye (Fig. 3.12). This position will offer the best possibility of sighting the optic cup and keep the light from falling directly on the macula. Young children will look around all over the place during the ophthalmoscopic examination and the key to obtaining useful information is to remain still in order to catch a glimpse of the structures as they become momentarily visible. The older child is a little easier to manage in that the examiner can involve the child by asking them to look up, look down, look sideways, etc., thus obtaining the widest possible view of the fundus.

From the ophthalmoscopic examination, it may be possible to see a dislocation of the lens. This has the appearance of a crescent-shaped line at the top of the eye in downward dislocation and at the bottom of the eye in upward dislocation. Upward dislocation is seen in Marfan syndrome while downward dislocation is seen in homocysteinuria.

Cataracts may also be visualized at the depth of the lens (Bickley & Szilagyi 2008). While it is possible to identify the reason why a child has cataracts in some cases, in about 50% of cases it will not be possible to identify a cause.

The features of papilledema are the same in children as they are in the adult patient. Papilledema is commonly associated with raised intracranial pressure, which may result from a number of causes. Whatever its cause, it represents an unequivocal implication for pediatric referral (Hughes 1974, Kliegman et al 2007).

Some of the known causes of cataracts in children are shown in Box 3.2 and the diagnostic characteristics of papilledema in Box 3.3.

Box 3.2

Some of the known causes of cataracts in children
- Intrauterine rubella
- Trauma
- Drugs – especially corticosteroids
- Rheumatoid arthritis
- Diabetes mellitus
- Down syndrome
- Hypoparathyroidism
- Galactosemia
- Galactokinase deficiency
- Glaucoma

Diagnostic characteristics of papilledema

- Elevation of the optic disc
- Veins distended with loss of the normal visible pulsation
- Red discoloration of the optic disc
- Blurred disc margins (nasal margins are sometimes blurred in normal subjects)
- Deflection of the vessels as they pass over the margins of the disc
- Hemorrhages near the disc
- Enlargement of the blind spot
- Diminution of visual fields
- Gradual loss of visual acuity

Table 3.6 Differential clinical characteristics of mastoiditis and otitis externa

Mastoiditis	Otitis externa
Tenderness over mastoidal antrum	Diffuse tenderness
Loss of the posterior auricular sulcus	Posterior auricular sulcus preserved
No lymphadenopathy	Pre- and postauricular lymphadenopathy
No tragal tenderness	Tragal tenderness commonly noted
Bony change on X-ray common	No radiological change demonstrated
Mucopurulent discharge	Discharge containing a large amount of epithelial debris

Examination of the ears

The examination of the ears is of great importance in chiropractic practice owing to the frequency with which children who have ear problems present for chiropractic care. Ear infection, normally well managed by chiropractors, is the single most frequent reason for the prescription of antibiotics in preschool-age children (Fireman 1997). Careful ear examination, together with the nose, throat and neck, permits the chiropractor to determine if referral for antibiotic therapy is necessary and also provides vital information for monitoring the success or otherwise of chiropractic care.

Inspection

Inspection of the pinna and surrounding areas should be carried out. Occasionally, malformation of the pinna, infection of local skin, or a foreign body in the outer canal may be seen.

Palpation

The tragus should be routinely palpated prior to the performance of otoscopy. Depress the tragus gently inwards and observe or ask children, according to age, if they experience pain. Pain on tragal palpation is suggestive of either an outer canal infection or the presence of a foreign body (Barness 1981). Introduction of the otoscope speculum into the outer canal, therefore, should be done with great caution.

Palpation of the auricular lymph nodes, the tonsillar node and posterior chain should always be carried out, as these nodes are frequently enlarged in cases of middle ear infection. Resolution of nodular enlargement is often 7–10 days behind that of the patient's symptoms.

Percussion

Following palpation, gentle percussion of the mastoid processes should be performed to check for tenderness, which may indicate infection of the air cells. If there is obvious discharge from the ear, a sample should be inspected as its

characteristics provide valuable information about the possible source of infection. The clinical characteristics which facilitate differentiation of mastoiditis and outer ear infection are shown in Table 3.6.

Hearing assessment

The manner in which the hearing assessment is carried out is dependent upon the age of the child and the degree of cooperation that can be gained. In an infant and toddler, the aural–palpebral or startle reflex offers the examiner a gross estimate of hearing intactness. This reflex is seen as blinking of the eyes in response to a single clap made in the vicinity of one ear. Each ear is tested separately and the examiner should stand outside the child's direct line of vision in order to reduce the possibility of visual stimulus producing the blink response (Fig. 3.13). In a sublimated child, this response may be subdued or even absent despite the fact the hearing is intact. It is therefore not wise to draw conclusions from a test

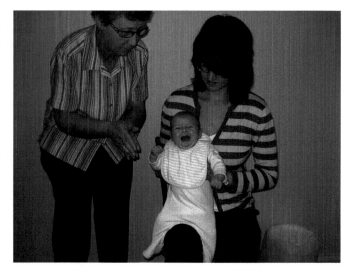

Figure 3.13 • Technique for performance of the startle reflex.

conducted on a baby that has just been fed or woken from sleep. The startle reflex is appropriate up to 13 months of age (Barness 1981).

From 13 months to about 3 years of age, a sound stimulus such as a rattle or cellophane paper being slowly crushed in the examiner's hand will cause the child to turn the head to the source of the sound.

By age 3 years, most children demonstrate the cognitive ability to recognize play items such as a set of plastic animals and respond to commands given in a low voice from a distance of 3 m to identify certain of the animals. Each command should be at a slightly lower tone. It is helpful to have an assistant block the hearing in one ear at a time in order to focus the assessment.

By the time a child begins school, it should be possible to accurately perform Schwabach's, Rinne's and Weber's tests using a tuning fork (Barness 1981). Schwabach's test is performed by comparing the length of time a child and examiner can hear the tuning fork when it is placed over the mastoid process. If the child hears the sound for less time than the examiner, then bone conduction is impaired, indicative of sensorineural hearing loss. If the child hears the sound for longer than the examiner, then air conduction is impaired.

The Rinne and Weber tests are used to compare air and bone conduction in the patient (Maran 1988). Firstly, the tuning fork is placed over the mastoid process as before. When the sound can no longer be heard the tuning fork is placed about 3 cm immediately lateral to the pinna. Air conduction is heard for approximately twice the length of time as that of bone conduction (Rinne test). Secondly, the vibrating fork is placed over the midline of the forehead and the child is asked to identify in which ear the sound is loudest. In unilateral conductive deafness, the sound lateralizes to the affected ear, whereas in sensorineural deafness the sound will lateralize to the unaffected ear.

Otoscopy

Finally, otoscopy should be performed. The purpose of this examination is to directly inspect the outer canal and tympanic membrane. In addition, pneumatic otoscopy allows for assessment of the function of the tympanic membrane. There are a number of steps associated with pediatric otoscopy that should be routinely followed in order to minimize the possibility of causing injury and to yield the maximum possible information.

Firstly, the largest possible speculum should be used, 3 mm being the absolute minimum (Barness 1981). Secondly, the pinna in young children should be tractioned downward to straighten the canal before the speculum is inserted. In older children, the canal is more adult-like and needs to be tractioned up and posteriorly in order to straighten it. Thirdly, the otoscope should be held much like a pencil with the fingers of the hand holding it pressed against the child's head. This prevents damage being done to the canal in the event the child unexpectedly moves during the examination. Fourthly, the outer canal should be carefully inspected first, to ensure that there are no foreign bodies or pathology such as furuncle, vesicle, etc. present. It is very distressing for a

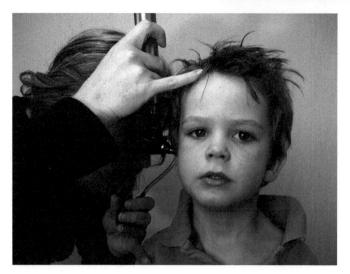

Figure 3.14 • Technique for pneumatic otoscopy in a toddler. Note how the barrel of the otoscope is held in a vertical up position much as one would hold a pencil.

child if a speculum is pressed against such a lesion. Lastly, pneumatic examination should be carried out only after all the structures have been inspected (Fig. 3.14).

On inspection of a normal ear, the tympanic membrane is usually gray to white in color and translucent or opalescent (Maran 1988). The handle of the malleus may be visualized as a small white streak running posteriorly and inferiorly to end at the umbo. The short process of the malleus appears as a small white projection at its upper end. Inferiorly to the umbo is the cone or circle of light. The appearance of the normal tympanic membrane is illustrated in Fig. 3.15.

When effusion is present in the middle ear, these structures are obliterated from view as the tympanic membrane bulges outwardly. In this case the membrane is usually quite reddened with very prominent blood vessels. When there is negative pressure in the middle ear, the tympanic membrane is drawn inwardly making these structures more prominent. The color of the tympanic membrane in this case usually remains grayish, but may, depending on the reason for the

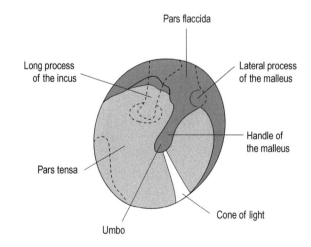

Figure 3.15 • Appearance of the normal tympanic membrane as visualized on otoscopic examination.

negative pressure, appear very dull red, indicating the presence of blood in the middle ear (Maran 1988).

Pneumatic otoscopy is based on the physiological principle that, in a normally aerated ear, the pressure is at standard atmospheric pressure (atm) on either side of the drum. When the air pressure is momentarily elevated in the outer canal by sharply squeezing the pneumatic bulb, the tympanic membrane moves first inwardly, and then as the air rushes out, temporarily reducing the pressure in the outer canal below 1 atmosphere, the membrane moves outwardly before returning to its neutral position. Observation of this phenomenon permits the examiner to deduce that normal aeration of the middle ear is present and therefore there is no effusion or adhesive disease such as chronic serous otitis media (Maran 1988).

Care must be taken when performing pneumatic otoscopy as false-positive results may be obtained if the speculum fails to form an adequate seal with the wall of the outer canal (Berman & Chan 1997).

The absence of normal movement indicates the presence of fluid (middle ear effusion), negative pressure in the middle ear from eustachian tube dysfunction, tympanic perforation, a mass in the middle ear such as a cholesteatoma or a normally functioning tympanostomy tube in situ.

Examination of the nose and sinuses

The nose and sinuses are routinely examined in any child who presents with upper respiratory tract or ear infection. The nose is examined with the assistance of a wide-diameter otoscopic speculum. The child's head is held steady by the examiner and the tip of the nose is distended with the examiner's thumb in a cephalad direction. Inspection of the nasal cavity is then accomplished using the otoscope (Fig. 3.16).

Polyps and evidence of local or diffuse infection are the most common conditions seen on nasal examination (Barness 1981). Hyperostotic inferior turbinate, while not common,

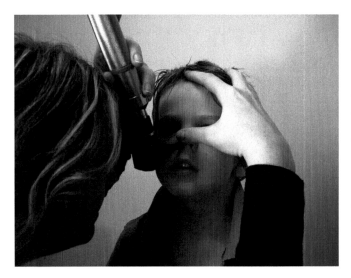

Figure 3.16 • Technique for examination of the nose by direct instrumental inspection using the otoscope and a large-diameter speculum.

presents a clinical scenario in which the resultant narrowing of the nasal passage acts as a mechanical obstruction and therefore a site of recurrent infection. These children usually snore loudly. Such a condition warrants referral for specialist opinion as surgery is often required.

The sinuses are first examined by palpation, then by percussion. Any sense of tenderness is suggestive of infection or effusion and indicates the need for further diagnostic investigation, usually in the form of an X-ray and specific management.

Examination of the oral cavity

The oral cavity examination is accomplished by inspection using a tongue depressor and light source. Firstly, the lips and teeth should be inspected without the introduction of a tongue depressor. Secondly, the patient is asked to open the mouth and protrude the tongue as far as possible. The examiner lifts first one side of the tongue and then the other in order to visualize the floor of the mouth as far posteriorly as the lingual tonsils, as this is the most common location in the oral cavity in which to find a tumor such as lymphoma. Next the buccal mucosa is inspected, followed by the tonsillar arch, the uvula and finally the oropharynx. Table 3.7 lists some of the more important clinical conditions which may be visualized on inspection of the oral cavity.

Examination of the neck

While it only takes a short time to perform, the neck examination is nonetheless very important since a wide range of diseases affect the neck area. Initially the neck should be visually inspected for size and symmetry. The neck of a newborn appears very short and it does not begin to lengthen until around 3 years of age.

Some of the more common causes of persistent short neck in infants are shown in Box 3.4. Asymmetry may be the result of edema, swelling such as that seen in mumps infection, or congenital anomaly.

Pulsations in the anterior neck may sometimes be seen. These are mostly arterial and due to increased activity or anxiety in the patient. Arterial pulsations, however, may be due to aortic insufficiency. Venous pulsations, as they are obliterated by light jugular pressure, are always abnormal if seen in the upright child. In a child where heart failure may be present, pressure applied over the liver will cause the neck veins to bulge. This sign represents a dire clinical emergency and the child should be sent to hospital immediately (Barness 1981).

Next, the structures of the neck are palpated. Firstly, the lymph nodes should be examined following a systematic method. The location of the lymph nodes and the structures they drain are shown in Table 3.8. A lymph node with a diameter exceeding 1 cm in a child can reasonably be considered enlarged (Barness 1981).

The salivary glands are not routinely palpated during the neck examination. When enlarged, the parotid gland usually extends down into the anterior and lateral aspects of the neck (Barness 1981).

Table 3.7 Clinical significance of common and important conditions which can be visualized in the oral cavity

Condition	Clinical significance to the chiropractor
Oral thrush	Usually seen on the tongue and buccal membranes, but may on occasion also be seen further back in the mouth on the soft palate and uvula. Oral thrush must always be directly treated or it tends to persist. The nursing mother should also be advised to treat her nipple and areolar areas
Ulcers	Mouth ulcers tend to indicate a lowered immune status and this should be adequately addressed as part of the chiropractic management plan
Herpes simplex	Herpes stomatitis and 'cold sores' tend to suggest the need for nutritional immune support
Follicular tonsillitis	Punctuate white lesions on a reddened tonsillar surface suggest the need for antibiotic therapy
Membranous tonsillitis	A yellow or whitish membrane over the tonsils strongly suggests infectious mononucleosis. It is imperative to carry out a liver, spleen and lymphatic examination in children with this presentation
Unilaterally enlarged tonsil	Lymphoma must be considered when a palatine tonsil is unilaterally enlarged to the midline
Bifid uvula	Normal anatomical variant
Salivary pooling	Children who exhibit salivary pooling, an apparent inability to swallow, and have a fever must be referred to the nearest hospital with a tentative diagnosis of acute epiglottitis. Under no circumstances should a spatula be used to examine this child's oral cavity

Box 3.4

Some causes of a short neck in infants

- Platybasia
- Morquio syndrome
- Cretinism
- Gargoylism
- Klippel–Feil syndrome

Table 3.8 Lymph node locations and the anatomical structures they drain

Location of lymph node	Structure drained
Submental	Anterior oral cavity
Submandibular	Sublingual area
Tonsillar (at the angle of mandible)	Palatine tonsillar area
Anterior cervical chain	Pharynx
Supraclavicular	Mediastinum
Posterior chain	Pharynx and ears
Suboccipital	Scalp
Postauricular	Ears and scalp
Preauricular	Ears and parotid gland

Occasionally, a hard mass will be encountered high in the anterior midline of the neck. This presentation often causes much anxiety in patients and parents but is usually due to a thyroglossal cyst (Maran 1988). If this mass can be demonstrated to move superiorly when the patient swallows and when the examiner gently pulls the tongue out of the mouth, it can be concluded that it is indeed a thyroglossal cyst. It remains only to reassure the patient that this lump is of no significance and is not in need of any intervention.

Hard, non-tender lumps which cannot be demonstrated to move against underlying tissue should be viewed suspiciously as being metastatic or due to malignant disease of the salivary glands (Bickley & Szilagyi 2008).

The sternocleidomastoid muscle (SCM) is the next structure to be palpated. A mass in the lower one-third of the SCM in a child who is holding the head to the same side is associated with congenital torticollis. Barness (1981) reports an association between gastroesophageal reflux and torticollis where the histology of the SCM is normal. These children commonly have upper cervical subluxation, impairing neurological integrity of the muscle and the balance of the sympathetic–parasympathetic systems in the upper gastrointestinal tract.

Smooth oval-shaped masses usually found anterior to the upper one-third of the SCM will be due to branchial cyst formation. Those arising from the first branchial cleft are seen mostly above the level of the mandible while those arising from the second branchial cleft are seen mostly directly under the mandible, close to the SCM. These cyst formations sometimes show a fistula. These children are in need of referral to a pediatric surgeon.

The trachea should now be palpated. Firstly, palpate along the anterior surface with the index finger, and secondly, palpate the anterolateral borders by gently compressing the trachea between the thumb and forefinger. The trachea is normally positioned slightly right of the midline. Positional shift should raise the suspicion of a mediastinal tumor, a neck mass or a pneumothorax (Bickley & Szilagyi 2008). The palpatory sense of a thud that may also be heard on auscultation suggests the presence of a foreign body.

The thyroid is the next structure to be examined by palpation. While it may be appropriate to examine the infant in a supine position on the mother's lap, it is best to examine the older child in the seated position. Stand behind the child and first feel the thyroid isthmus. Secondly, feel both sides of the thyroid cartilage. The thyroid will move superiorly as the child swallows. Next, estimate the space between the thyroid cartilage and the SCM on each side. Unilateral enlargement of the thyroid will obliterate this space on the involved side. Assess any mass size, shape and position in relation to surrounding structures, mobility and tenderness (Barness 1981).

Venous pressure can be estimated by measuring the distance from the upper border of the clavicle to the most superior level of visual venous distension in the neck with the child sitting (Bickley & Szilagyi 2008, McMillan et al 1977).

After the palpatory examination of the anterior and lateral structures of the neck has been completed, auscultation should be performed in order to ascertain if any murmurs or bruits are present.

Examination of the chest

The order of examination in children, unlike in the adult patient, is relatively unstructured and pursued on the basis of patient cooperation. It should not be considered at all inappropriate to listen with the stethoscope as the first step in the examination if the child is initially cooperative or not crying.

The lungs

Review of functional anatomy

The gross anatomy of the pulmonary system that is clinically relevant to the examiner called upon to make an assessment of respiratory function is shown in Fig. 3.17.

Observation

The shape of the chest is noted, particularly any asymmetries. At birth, the chest is round with the anteroposterior diameter being the same as the transverse diameter. As the child grows, the chest shape becomes more like that of an adult, with the transverse diameter becoming greater than the anteroposterior diameter (Barness 1981). Certain diseases will cause the chest to change shape (Table 3.9).

The circumference of the chest should be measured and compared to the previously measured head circumference. In the first 2 years of life, these two measurements should be approximately the same. Any major variance will normally be due to macrocephaly and requires careful investigation. Beyond the age of 3 years the chest circumference becomes larger than the head circumference.

The breathing pattern should be noted as being predominantly either abdominal or thoracic. Up to school age, most of the respiratory effort is abdominal and the examiner will see considerable rising and falling of the abdomen. Beyond school age, the respiratory effort becomes increasingly thoracic

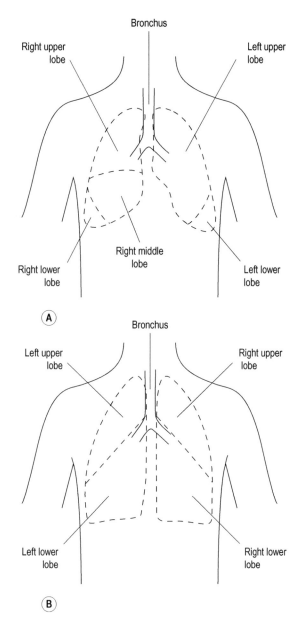

Figure 3.17 ● Functional gross anatomy of the pulmonary system: (A) anterior to posterior view and (B) posterior to anterior view.

in origin. Noticeable intercostal and supraclavicular retraction during inspiration should always raise the suspicion of underlying pulmonary disease, or peritonitis if the child is young (Barness 1981). When significant retraction is present, it should be noted if it is unilateral or bilateral. Breath rate may be measured by observing the rise and fall of the abdomen. The normal ranges of breath rates according to age are shown in Table 3.1.

The mechanics of the normal respiratory cycle involve simultaneous chest expansion, increase of the sternal angle and descent of the diaphragm on inspiration. These movements are reversed in expiration. The chest is seen to collapse on inspiration over any area of pneumothorax, a condition referred to as paradoxical breathing (Barness 1981).

Table 3.9 Diseases which can cause a change in normal chest shape

Description of chest shape	Disease with which this shape is associated
The funnel-shaped chest is characterized by sternal depression	This is normally a congenital anomaly
Pigeon breast is characterized by protrusion of the sternum	This shape can be due to a congenital anomaly, but is often associated with osteoporosis or rickets
An increased transverse diameter	This is often normal in the child who fits the profile of a typical endomorph. It may also be due to Morquio syndrome
The barrel chest is characterized by persisting equality of the anteroposterior and transverse diameters	This is often associated with chronic pulmonary disease. This child may also demonstrate Harrison's sulcus, seen as a transverse groove at the point where the diaphragm leaves the chest wall
Flaring is seen at the lower margins of the rib cage, immediately below what would be described as a depression	Flaring is so frequently seen in normal children that its diagnostic value is dubious. If the flaring is extreme, it may imply underlying pulmonary disease or possibly rickets
Rachitic rosary is seen as small lumps over the costochondral junctions	Rickets
The angle formed by the lower rib margin with the sternum should be 45°	A greater angle suggests pulmonary disease such as asthma, while a smaller angle is seen in children suffering malnutrition

Finally, the scapulae are inspected for symmetry of elevation and flaring. In Sprengle's deformity, one scapula rides visibly higher than its pair. Winging of the scapula is a condition where the inferior angle adopts a much more lateral position than its pair and demonstrates excessive motion. This is frequently due to paralysis of the long thoracic nerve and consequently weakness of the serratus anterior muscle.

The stage of breast development should be assessed using standardized percentile charts (Tanner 1962). Examples of these charts can be found in Appendix 1.

It should be noted that asymmetrical development is quite normal and usually begins with a lump or bud forming under the areola, frequently giving rise to some anxiety in the patient and caregiver (Green 1986). Certain endocrine disease states may produce alterations to the rate of development of breast tissue, making the assessment of secondary sexual characteristic staging an important part of the physical examination. Some of the more common causes of precocious and delayed breast development are listed in Box 3.5.

Box 3.5

Some of the more common causes of precocious and delayed breast development

Precocious development
- Ovarian and adrenal tumors
- Hyperthyroidism
- Hypothyroidism

Delayed development
- Pituitary disease
- Anorexia
- Gonadal dysgenesis
- Adrenal disease

Palpation

The palpatory examination is performed first to confirm your impression made on observation of such things as rachitic rosary, asymmetries, etc. Next, the body of each clavicle should be lightly palpated to determine if there is any fracture present. This is particularly important in infants where birth trauma may have caused a fracture, in a situation where the baby has been accidentally traumatized, such as a fall from a change table, and when intentional injury is suspected. The clavicle is the most frequently fractured bone in the first year of life and when fractured will be associated with reduced and often painful glenohumeral abduction.

The lymph nodes in the axilla should be examined. This is best performed with the child seated with the arm hanging loosely by the side. The examiner palpates with a flat hand first against the medial wall of the axilla, reaching as high as possible and then pulling the tissue down against the wall of the chest. It is usual to feel two or three small lymph nodes of about 3–4 mm in diameter in a normal child when performing this maneuver. The lateral, anterior and posterior wall of each axilla should be examined in a similar fashion (Barness 1981, Easton 2004).

Vocal fremitus is the next aspect of the palpatory examination. The examiner, with the fingers hyperextended at the metacarpophalangeal joints, palpates the chest wall in a systematic pattern with the heads of the metacarpal bones as these provide a sensitive reception to vibratory sense. The older child is asked to repeat the number 99 to provide the vocal fremitus while in the younger child the examination is best carried out while the child is crying (Green 1986).

Airway obstruction from mucus and other causes in the lower respiratory tree and plural effusion will decrease vocal fremitus, while the presence of mucus high in the respiratory tract will increase it. Fremitus assessment is notably unhelpful in identifying pneumonia or space-occupying lesions.

Finally, the intercostal spaces should be examined during respiration. Excessive movement indicates increased respiratory activity while a lack of absence of movement suggests intercostal muscle paralysis or decreased respiratory activity (Barness 1981).

Percussion

The purpose of percussion of the lung fields is to determine the position of underlying organs (i.e. heart and liver) and to evaluate the aeration of the lung lobes. Alterations to the normal tympani expected over the lung fields are sometimes helpful in determining the presence of consolidation such as that seen with pneumonia (hyporesonance) or the presence of excessive air in the chest such as would occur with emphysema (generalized hyperresonance) or pneumothorax (localized hyperresonance) (Easton 2004).

The technique of percussion, which has the most applicability to general chiropractic practice with children, is referred to as the indirect method. This technique is performed by placing the middle or index finger of one hand firmly against the chest wall while the middle finger of the opposite hand acts as a percussive hammer. The action of percussion is produced by dorsiflexion of the hand followed by a smooth, free flowing falling of the hand so that the tip of the percussive finger strikes the distal phalanx of the palpating finger in a distinct, crisp manner similar to the staccato note in music. The resultant sound is referred to as the percussive note (Bickley & Szilagyi 2008).

Auscultation

The use of the stethoscope is often frightening for a small child. The best cooperation is usually gained by allowing the child a brief time to play with the instrument and perhaps listen to teddy's chest. It may even be appropriate in a very anxious and frightened child for you to listen to teddy's chest in order to let the child see how the examination is conducted.

In the infant, the breath sounds are much louder and harsher than those heard in the adult. This is because the source of the sounds in the respiratory tree is in much closer proximity to the head of the stethoscope in a child and also because there is usually much less muscular and other soft tissue to listen through. It is also best to try to examine the child with the head in a midline position. When an infant's head is turned to one side, the breath sounds on the opposite side are often diminished.

Breath sounds in infants usually exhibit an irregular pattern, being slow and shallow, then rapid and deep. The astute examiner will be patient and opportunistic when attempting to evaluate the breath sounds of the very young. It should also be noted that fine crackles are often heard on late inspiration in infancy as a normal finding. The breathing patterns of older children, while continuing to be harsh and loud, are more regular than in the infant. When a child consistently moves their head on respiratory examination, especially into extension, significant airway disease should be suspected.

The pattern of auscultation that should be routinely followed is based on the physiological principle that each lung

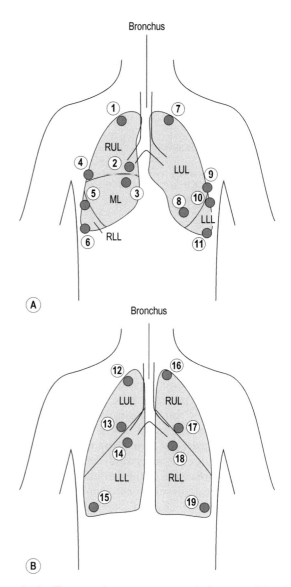

Figure 3.18 • The auscultatory pattern used when examining the lung fields of a pediatric patient: (A) anterior to posterior view and (B) posterior to anterior view. LLL=left lower lobe; LUL=left upper lobe; ML=middle lobe; RLL=right lower lobe; RUL=right upper lobe.

lobe should be auscultated at its base anteriorly, posteriorly and laterally as well as at its apex (Fig. 3.18). When auscultating a child's lung fields, the apex and base of each lobe should be routinely examined anteriorly, laterally and posteriorly. The anatomical locations that provide best access to these structures are described in Table 3.10. Be sure to listen long enough at each location to determine the intensity of the breath sound throughout inspiration and early expiration (Green 1986). It is common for the latter two-thirds of expiration to be silent. Note any added (adventitious) sounds such as wheezes, crackles, rubs and thuds, timing them according to when they are heard in the respiratory cycle.

Table 3.10 Anatomical locations used for auscultating the pediatric chest

Description of anatomical location	Area of lung being auscultated
1. Suprasternal areas – right and left	Apices of the upper lobes
2. 3/4 intercostal space – right and left anteriorly	Base of the upper lobes
3. Over the fifth rib – right only	Middle lobe
4. Immediately above the costal margins in the midaxillary line – right and left	Base of the lower lobes laterally. This is the most common site in which consolidation will be heard
5. 5/6 intercostal space at the midaxillary line – right and left	Apex of the lower lobes laterally
6. In the axilla above the fifth rib – right and left	Base of the upper lobes laterally
7. 3/4 intercostal space between the spine and scapula – right and left	Base of the upper lobes posteriorly
8. 4/5 intercostal space between the spine and scapula – right and left	Apex of the lower lobes posteriorly

The heart

Review of functional anatomy

The anatomy of the heart beyond the neonatal period reflects that seen in the adult (Fig. 3.19). Neonatal circulation differs significantly from that of the older child as it reflects the fetal circulation that has been dependent upon the role of the

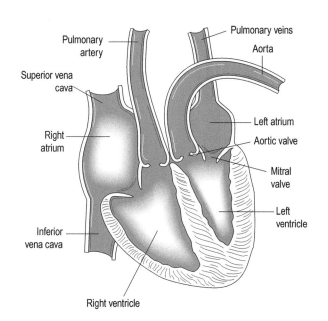

Pulmonary artery

Pulmonary veins

Aorta

Superior vena cava

Left atrium

Aortic valve

Right atrium

Mitral valve

Left ventricle

Inferior vena cava

Right ventricle

Figure 3.19 • Functional anatomy of the heart and great vessels in the child beyond the neonatal period.

placenta. In the fetus, systemic resistance to blood flow is low owing to the fact that the placenta offers little resistance to the flow of blood, while pulmonary resistance is relatively high because pulmonic arterioles are relatively constricted and therefore offer considerable resistance to blood flow through the lungs. This situation changes rapidly after birth as the placenta is severed from the neonate causing a sudden increase in resistance in the systemic circuit while the advent of breathing increases the oxygen tension in the vicinity of the small pulmonic arterioles, thus releasing much of the constriction. Indeed, shortly after birth, systemic resistance to blood flow is seen to be greater than pulmonic resistance. As a result of this rapid change of resistance, most of the blood flow in the left outflow tract now bypasses the ductus arteriosus and enters the descending aorta, resulting in functional closure of the ductus arteriosus shortly after birth. The ductus arteriosus, which is a patent communication between the ascending aorta and the pulmonic artery in the fetus, closes anatomically at approximately 3 months of age and the anatomy of the heart and great vessels becomes adult-like.

In the fetus, the foramen ovale is a one-way valve made up of a tissue flap that permits the flow of blood between the right and left atria. At birth, as the systemic resistance to flow rises dramatically, the pressure in the left atrium literally holds the valve closed, thus preventing any communication of blood between the right atrium and the left. The foramen ovale, while it remains functionally closed throughout life, may remain patent in about 25% of patients.

Although the greatest change from fetal to adult circulation occurs immediately after birth, changes do continue throughout the first 6–12 months of life. This progressive change appears to be due to the developmental changes in the structure of the pulmonary arterioles (Wolfe et al 1997).

Observation

The observational items described in the section on respiratory examination are equally applicable to the cardiovascular assessment. In addition, any evidence of precordial bulging or visible cardiac impulse, also termed ventricular impulse (Lissauer & Clayden 2007), should be noted. With the exception of very thin children, or a child who appears very excited and hyperactive, a visible cardiac impulse should be considered abnormal (Barness 1981).

Palpation

The palpation examination is used to assess the peripheral pulses, identify thrills, and locate the point of maximal impulse (PMI) and apex beat.

Pulse assessment should determine *rate*, *rhythm* and *synchronicity* with other pulses. Excitement, fever, poor exercise tolerance due to heart disease, infection and toxicity such as seen with some forms of thyroid disease may significantly increase the pulse rate in children (Barness 1981). It should be noted that the pulse rate will increase by approximately 10 beats per minute for each degree the temperature is elevated and, in cases involving lower airway disease such as bronchitis, the pulse rate may reach 300 beats per minute (Barness 1981). On some occasions, children with cranial and upper cervical subluxation may present with idiopathic tachycardia and following correction of the subluxation complex the heart rate will return to normal.

Several variations to the usual even pulse rhythm may be seen. *Paroxysmal auricular tachycardia* may be seen in children with congenital heart disease or infection where toxicosis is an issue. Tachycardia may reach rates exceeding 300 beats per minute in such cases (Barness 1981). *Pulsus alternans* is a situation where one pulse is strong and the following pulse is weak. This is a sign of severe heart strain. Slow heart rate or bradycardia is indicative of a congenital condition such as atrial septal defect, infection or hypothyroidism. On occasion, children with cranial and upper cervical subluxation involving evidence of cord pressure such as a Shimizu reflex and a hyperactive pectoral reflex will present with bradycardia, which is thought to be due to raised intracranial pressure. In such cases, normalization of the heart rate quickly follows correction of the subluxation complex.

Corrigan's pulse, otherwise known as *waterhammer pulse*, is a very forceful beat, usually felt at the femoral or radial arteries (Barness 1981). It is commonly associated with congenital heart disease causing a very wide pulse pressure. Pulse pressure in children is best appreciated by plotting the blood pressure values on standard percentile charts. In widened pulse pressure, systole will have a high percentile value, while diastole will have a low percentile value. A pulse that is fast, weak and intermittent to palpation is generally referred to as *thready*. A child with a thready pulse is experiencing shock or heart failure (Barness 1981) and needs emergency hospitalization. *Pulsus paradoxus* is a pulse that undergoes a change in amplitude synchronous with the respiratory cycle. It is only rarely abnormal, but in all children who exhibit this pulse who also have asthma, multiple, rapidly repeated blood pressure measurements should be obtained to determine the variation in pulse pressure. Variation in pulse pressure exceeding 30 mmHg is a serious clinical sign.

Finally, it is both extremely common and entirely normal for children and adolescents to exhibit a *sinus arrhythmia* where the pulse rhythm has a predictable, repeated pattern of irregularity (Barness 1981).

As part of the routine cardiovascular examination, the synchronicity of upper and lower pulses should be assessed by simultaneously palpating the radial and femoral pulses, checking for timing and pulse volume. In cases of uncertainty, assessment of blood flow may be made by simultaneously applying digital pressure to the hand and foot to produce a blanching response. Normally, blanching will disappear at the same rate in both the foot and hand. In the event that blood flow is impaired, usually to the lower limb, there will be a noticeable delay in the return of normal color in the affected limb. Weakness of the femoral pulses in young children suggests coarctation of the aorta, which requires surgical intervention without unnecessary delay (McMillan et al 1983).

The palpation examination is completed by identifying the position of the PMI, which is almost always found at the position of the apical beat. Palpation is carried out using the pads of the fingers applied very lightly to the chest wall. The PMI is often difficult to palpate in infants and toddlers unless the heart is enlarged or the subcutaneous fat is minimal (Green 1986). The PMI is usually found at the left 4/5 rib interspace medial to the nipple (midclavicular line) in children up to 7 years of age. From 7–8 years of age the PMI is located in the left 5/6 rib interspace, again medial to the nipple; and from age 8 onwards it is found in the adult position at the left 6/7 interspace. Any child who has a PMI lateral to the nipple and lower than it should be for age has, by definition, cardiomegaly and should be referred without delay for specialist investigation.

Percussion

Percussion is used essentially to assess the left border of the heart. It may be performed using the same method as that described for the lung fields earlier in this chapter, or alternatively, using the scratch method. To use the scratch method, place the stethoscope over the sternum and listen for the change in note as you make parallel scratches down the left side of the chest (Barness 1981). It is also appropriate to listen with the stethoscope as you tap the chest, listening for the change in sound as the left border of the heart is reached.

Auscultation

The stethoscope is utilized in cardiac auscultation in much the same manner as that employed for the respiratory examination. The child should be auscultated in both the sitting and the supine position with both the bell and the diaphragm of the stethoscope. Again, as with the lungs, there is a definite pattern of listening points and these are identified in Table 3.11 and shown diagrammatically in Fig. 3.20.

When listening at each point identified above, the following should be noted (Easton 2004, Green 1986):

- first, second and, if audible, the third heart sound
- splitting of the second heart sound (normal on full inspiration)
- added sounds such as valvular opening snaps or friction rubs.

The heart sounds

The first heart sound (S1), which signals the beginning of systole, is heard as a single event and is caused by closure of the mitral and tricuspid valves. The second heart sound (S2), which signals the end of systole and the beginning of diastole, is produced by closure of the aortic and pulmonic valves which may occur at slightly different times, heard with the stethoscope as a 'split' sound. This is a very common and normal finding in children and is best heard at the 2/3 intercostal space against the left border of the sternum. Since deep inspiration delays pulmonic valve closure, this splitting phenomenon is widened when the child breathes in fully and narrows as the child breathes out fully (Barness 1981, Bickley & Szilagyi 2008). The relationship of the first and second heart sounds to systole and diastole is shown in Fig. 3.21.

Table 3.11 Anatomical locations used for auscultation of the heart

Anatomical location of listening point	Structure/pathology from which sound is generated
2/3 intercostal space to the right of the sternum	Where the aortic valve is best heard
2/3 intercostal space to the left of the sternum	Where the pulmonic valve is best heard
3/4 intercostal space to the left of the sternum	Where aortic diastolic murmurs are best heard
At the 4/5 intercostal space at the right margin of the sternum	Where the tricuspid valve is best heard
At the apical beat in the 5/6 interspace lateral to the sternum	Where the mitral valve is best heard
Halfway between the apical beat and the left sternal margin	Functional murmurs often heard here
Just left of the sternal border at the 3/4 intercostal space	Functional murmurs often heard here
At the 3/4 and 4/5 intercostal spaces several centimeters to the left of the sternum	Murmurs here are largely produced by patent ductus arteriosus and aortic coarctation
Above the clavicle in the anterior cervical triangle	Venous hum (functional murmur) and radiation of sound from various pathological murmurs
In the axillae, along the midaxillary line, below the scapulae and in the space between the clavicles and spine	Radiation of sound from various pathological murmurs. Coarctation of the aorta is the only pathology to radiate sound to the interscapular space

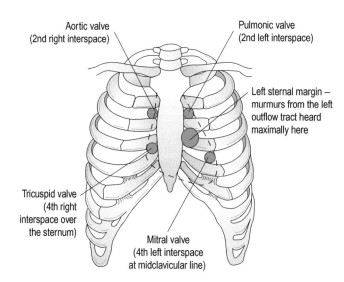

Figure 3.20 ● Diagrammatic representation of the cardiac auscultatory locations. The exact anatomical descriptions and the source of the sounds heard at each point are found in Table 3.10.

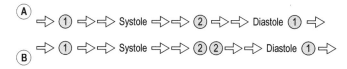

Figure 3.21 ● The relationship of the first and second heart sound to systole and diastole where the second sound is (A) a single phenomenon, and (B) a split phenomenon.

Narrow splitting of the second heart sound which conforms to a predictable physiological pattern is normal at all pediatric age levels. Reasons to consider referral for specialist investigation include wide splitting within the normal physiological pattern, fixed splitting throughout both inspiration and expiration, and paradoxical splitting (wider splitting in expiration). Any splitting of the first heart sound also represents good reason for referral.

On occasion, a third heart sound (S3) may be heard early in diastole. This sound is produced by vibration of the muscular wall of the left ventricle (Barness 1981). It is not often heard and is a normal finding. The rhythm produced when the third heart sound is audible can be better understood if the examiner says the word 'Kentucky' as 'Ken-tuck-y', with each verbal sound corresponding to one of the heart sounds. This diagnostic trick will assist in clarifying the rhythm as due to an audible third heart sound and not a gallop rhythm that is pathological and implies that the heart is failing. Further confirmation of the innocence of the rhythm can be taken from the fact that a gallop rhythm will be associated with other signs of cardiac failure such as pallor, a palpable thrill, a normal-sized liver in which the inferior margin is located more than two fingerwidths below the costal margin, etc.

Murmurs

The heart murmur is of considerable diagnostic importance in pediatric cardiovascular assessment. Innocent murmurs are frequently heard in normal children, principally at the base of the heart, along the left sternal margin, or over the pulmonic auscultatory area (Green 1986). The intensity of innocent murmurs is increased significantly by exercise and febrile illness (Barness 1981). Serious cardiovascular disease in children seldom presents without an organic murmur, making its recognition by the chiropractor of utmost importance. The innocent or functional murmur is generally a result

Table 3.12 Congenital heart conditions responsible for organic murmurs in children in order of frequency of presentation – the list below accounts for just over 85% of all congenital heart disease (adapted from Kliegman et al 2007 with permission)

Defect	Frequency
Ventricular septal defect	28.3%
Atrial septal/AV canal defects	10.3%
Pulmonary stenosis	9.9%
Patent ductus arteriosus	9.8%
Tetralogy of Fallot	9.7%
Aortic stenosis	7.1%
Coarctation of the aorta	5.1%
Transposition of the great arteries	4.9%

Table 3.13 Criteria used for estimating the intensity of a cardiac murmur

Grade	Description of diagnostic criteria
1	The most faint murmur it is possible to hear and may, in fact, not necessarily be heard in all positions
2	Quiet, but heard immediately after placing the stethoscope on the patient's chest
3	Moderately loud
4	Loud
5	Very loud – may be heard with the stethoscope partly off the chest
6	May be heard with the stethoscope completely off the chest

of turbulence in the left or high-pressure outflow tract while the origin of pathological murmurs depends on the nature of the pathology (e.g. valvular stenosis) or malformation (e.g. tetralogy of Fallot). The innocent murmur invariably occurs during systole, while the organic or pathological murmur can occur anywhere within the cardiac cycle. In addition, any murmur that is found in association with other signs of cardiac disease, such as valvular clicks, precordial thrills, edema, clubbing, blood and pulse pressure changes, cyanosis, etc., must always be considered pathological and the child referred accordingly. Congenital heart conditions and the frequency with which they are responsible for the presence of organic murmurs are shown in Table 3.12.

There are seven steps to fully and completely assess a heart murmur, these being the description of timing, shape, location of maximal intensity, radiation to other locations (Fig. 3.22), intensity, pitch and quality (Newell & Darling 2008, Hay et al 2007). Table 3.13 offers a guide to the evaluation of intensity of cardiac murmurs. The responsibility of the chiropractor, however, is much like that of the general medical physician and other primary contact health providers in that the murmur must be first recognized and then identified as to whether or not it meets the criteria for being categorized as functional. There are six essential clinical characteristics required to be identified to categorize a murmur as innocent (Pang & Newson 2005). These minimum clinical criteria are summarized in Table 3.14. As a sound clinical guideline, if it cannot be determined with complete confidence that a murmur is functional, the child should be referred for investigation.

Table 3.14 Diagnostic characteristics of functional cardiac murmurs (adapted from Lissauer & Clayden 2007 with permission)

Murmur characteristic to be assessed	Diagnostic finding
Timing	Functional murmurs are only ever heard during systole. A murmur can be confidently placed in systole once it can be determined that it is heard immediately prior to the heart sound which splits with inspiration (S2)
Location of maximal intensity	The great majority of functional murmurs are heard in the following two locations: 1. Halfway between the apical beat and the left sternal margin, and 2. Just left of the sternal border at the 3/4 intercostal space Pathological murmurs generally have a point of maximal intensity that corresponds with the anatomical site from which the murmur originates
Radiation	Functional murmurs do not radiate to other anatomical locations
Intensity	A murmur intensity exceeding 3 is usually pathological and therefore a pediatric specialist should assess all murmurs at this level and above. The diagnostic criteria for grading murmurs are described in Table 3.13
Response to change of position	Functional murmurs are generally only audible in the supine position. Disappearance of a murmur once the patient is placed in a sitting position is a characteristic of critical diagnostic importance
Response to exercise	The intensity of functional murmurs significantly increases after exercise while that of pathological murmurs tends not to change

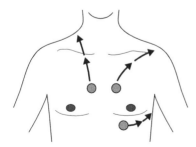

Figure 3.22 • Pathological murmurs frequently radiate to predictable locations as shown above. Innocent or functional murmurs never radiate from the point of sound source.

Added sounds

A *pericardial friction rub* produces a grating sound that increases when the stethoscope is pushed more firmly against the chest. The presence of such a sound requires immediate referral for further assessment and is usually caused by pericarditis.

Listen for systolic ejection clicks which are heard immediately after S1, systolic clicks which may be heard anywhere during systole, or diastolic opening snaps which occur immediately after S2 (Barness 1981, Bickley & Szilagyi 2008). All such noises should be considered pathological and the patient referred for further assessment.

Examination of the abdomen

The order of examination in the abdomen should be inspection, auscultation, percussion, superficial palpation and finally deeper palpation (Easton 2004, Lissauer & Clayden 2007).

Observation

The shape of the abdomen should be noted. In prepubertal children a 'pot belly' appearance is normal (Green 1986), particularly when viewed laterally in the standing child. This is thought to be due to the fact that the abdominal musculature in children is thinner than in the adult and that children tend to stand in such a way that the lumbar lordosis is exaggerated.

Distension is a common and clinically significant finding. It is generally caused by air or fluid in the bowel or peritoneal cavity, but may be due to obesity and a number of less common causes such as tumors (Barness 1981). The differentiation of distension is effected by the technique of percussion and will be discussed under that heading later in this chapter.

Respiration has a significant abdominal component in the very young. The patient should be observed in the supine position for symmetry and degree of abdominal movement on respiration. In a child in whom respiration appears to be entirely abdominal, lung pathology should be considered, while lack of abdominal movement suggests an intra-abdominal cause such as peritonitis, excessive gaseous accumulation in the bowel, paralytic ileus, diaphragmatic paralysis or appendicitis (Barness 1981). Lack of movement or excessive movement both require very careful investigation and, when accompanied by other signs such as abdominal and rebound tenderness, distension, fever, pallor, etc., should be referred for specialist care.

The umbilicus, linea alba and inguinal areas should be inspected for evidence of hernia. Increasing intra-abdominal pressure generally makes a hernia more prominent and in the case of a lump in the groin area may assist in differentiating a hernia from an undescended testicle (Easton 2004). A central umbilication in the umbilical hernia is predictive of resolution without surgical intervention and the parents should be so advised. All other hernias, however, will require surgical correction.

A diastasis recti is noted as a longitudinal midline protrusion usually extending from the xiphoid to the umbilicus in a great many children and is without any clinical significance. Parents who express concern about a diastasis recti should be reassured of its normality.

Peristalsis can be seen in small children by inspecting with the eye at the level of the abdomen as light is shone tangentially across the area to be inspected. Visible peristalsis is seen as shadows moving across the abdomen and is considered indicative of a diagnosis of obstruction until it can be positively ruled out. *Reverse peristalsis (movement from left to right across the upper abdomen)* followed by projectile vomiting at the time of feeding is consistent with a diagnosis of pyloric stenosis.

Finally, a simple test for peritonitis can be carried out by holding the hand several centimeters from the child's abdomen and asking the patient to 'push their tummy up' to touch your finger. To do so, the intra-abdominal pressure must be increased and in the presence of peritonitis this maneuver will cause pain (Easton 2004). Sometimes the muscular guarding is so severe as to disallow even an effort at this maneuver.

Auscultation

Auscultation of the abdomen must precede either palpation or percussion in order to avoid disturbing the peristaltic pattern, thus producing a false clinical impression. Auscultation should be performed with the diaphragm of the stethoscope placed gently over the abdominal midline just below the umbilicus or over each of the four quadrants. Peristalsis is variously described as producing a metallic, tinkling, clicking or gurgling sound. Bowel sounds are deemed to be normal if heard within a 40-second period of auscultation. Before a decision that there is absence of bowel sounds is made, however, the examiner should listen continuously for at least 3 minutes (Barness 1981).

Hyperperistalsis is sometimes heard as a loud gurgling sound described by the patient as 'tummy rumbles' and is referred to as borborygmi. While this is frequently a clinically meaningless phenomenon, hyperperistalsis may accompany peritonitis, gastroenteritis, diarrhea or early bowel obstruction. Absence of bowel sounds, especially if associated with generalized muscular guarding, may suggest the onset of peritonitis as a result of recent rupture of an abdominal organ such as would occur with a perforated appendix or intentional blunt injury to the abdomen.

It is also appropriate to listen with the stethoscope over the aorta and the renal and iliac arteries. The appropriate auscultatory locations are illustrated in Fig. 3.23. The renal arteries should be auscultated from both the anterior and posterior. A bruit may be heard over the aorta in children with coarctation and similarly over the renal arteries in systolic hypertension.

Percussion

Percussion of the abdomen is most helpful in determining the cause of distension. Should the cause of the distension be fluid accumulation, then two maneuvers are appropriate. Firstly, have an assistant place a hand firmly against the abdomen in the midline as the examiner palpates one side of the abdomen with the free hand, then strike the abdomen sharply on the opposite side (Fig. 3.24) to create a fluid wave which will be appreciated as a thrill on the opposite side of the abdomen.

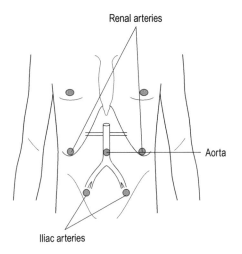

Figure 3.23 • Anatomical locations for auscultation of the aorta, renal and iliac arteries.

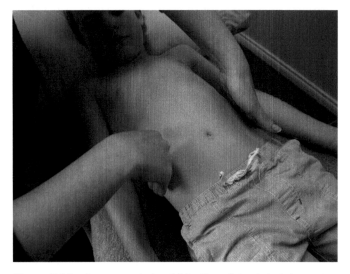

Figure 3.24 • Assessment of a child with a distended abdomen to determine if the cause of the distension is fluid, fat or gas.

Secondly, fluid level may shift by changing the patient's position. To demonstrate this shift, follow the three steps of examination described below (Easton 2004):

Step 1
Percuss from the midline of the abdomen to the lateral aspect of the abdomen until the normal tympanic note becomes dull. Mark this point with a skin pencil.

Step 2
Roll the patient toward the side of the abdomen until the normal tympanic note becomes dull. Mark this point with a skin pencil.

Step 3
Repeat step 1 and mark the point of dullness. If fluid accumulation is causing distension, the second mark will be closer to the abdominal midline than the first.

The presence of accumulated fluid in the abdomen of a child is a serious sign and such children should always be referred for specialist investigation. Gaseous accumulation, on the other hand, generally does not have the same degree of clinical significance and is frequently due to aerophagia (air swallowing) and substance hypersensitivity reactions, especially to gluten, lactose and cow's milk protein. In older children, excessive gaseous accumulation with frequent passage of flatus, low weight-to-height ratio, foul and flocculent stools, increased lumbar lordosis and gluteal atrophy is the usual combination of signs and symptoms associated with celiac disease, an enteropathic malabsorption syndrome which results from the inability of the gut to cope with gluten. Such children always require a blood test followed by a biopsy for diagnostic confirmation. Celiac disease was quite rare towards the end of the last century but the incidence in the past 10–15 years has been escalating, possibly due to the increase in gluten density in wheat grown using genetically modified growing techniques.

Percussion is also used to assist in delineating the position of intra-abdominal organs as well as defining the position and size of solid masses. This aspect of percussion will be discussed later in this chapter.

Palpation

Abdominal palpation can yield a great deal of important clinical information and should be performed with considerable care and attention to detail. While the technique of examination of the infant and young child has many similar characteristics to that of the adolescent and adult, the manner in which patient response is understood and interpreted is considerably different.

The first step in the abdominal examination is a general, superficial scan of all abdominal quadrants. The patient should be supine with the examiner to the right side. The examiner's elbow must be kept below the level of the hand and palpation is carried out with the pads of the fingers. Palpation pressure on the abdomen is generated by slowly and deliberately flexing the metacarpophalangeal joints (Easton 2004). A deep probing, circular movement with the tips of the fingers is never appropriate. The examiner first feels for softness or rigidity of the abdominal wall, then notes any areas of tenderness.

In the young child, tenderness is noted by observing the face for wincing, crying or a change in the pitch of the cry. The eyes should also be carefully observed when attempting to locate the point of maximal tenderness. When a truly tender area is touched, the child's pupils will constrict. It is useless to ask a child, 'Does this hurt?' unless the child is old enough to give a reliable answer.

Muscular rigidity and resistance to palpation should always alert the examining chiropractor to underlying pathology. Diffuse or poorly localized tenderness may be due to serious respiratory infection, mesenteric adenitis, peritonitis, rheumatic fever, measles, leukemia or emotional distress. The differential of muscle soreness from intra-abdominal tenderness is effected by asking the child to raise the head from the examination table. If the cause of the tenderness is muscle soreness, tenderness to palpation will increase with this maneuver, while it will decrease if the cause is intra-abdominal. The clinical significance of localized tenderness in the pediatric abdomen is illustrated in Fig. 3.25.

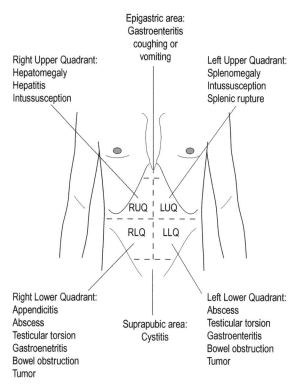

Epigastric area:
Gastroenteritis
coughing or
vomiting

Right Upper Quadrant:
Hepatomegaly
Hepatitis
Intussusception

Left Upper Quadrant:
Splenomegaly
Intussusception
Splenic rupture

RUQ | LUQ

RLQ | LLQ

Right Lower Quadrant:
Appendicitis
Abscess
Testicular torsion
Gastroenetritis
Bowel obstruction
Tumor

Suprapubic area:
Cystitis

Left Lower Quadrant:
Abscess
Testicular torsion
Gastroenteritis
Bowel obstruction
Tumor

Figure 3.25 • Clinical significance of localized tenderness in the pediatric abdomen.

After completing the superficial palpatory examination, the abdominal organs should be evaluated. The structures that should be carefully palpated are the liver, spleen, kidneys, small and large bowel, bladder, ovaries, testes, anogenital region and, when appropriate, the rectum.

Liver

The liver may enlarge as far as the right iliac fossa as a result of left heart failure causing engorgement via the hepatic vein. Infectious and malignant disease may also cause enlargement, albeit of a lesser magnitude, and is usually accompanied by tenderness. Hyperinflation of the lungs such as occurs in obstructive airway disease may cause a liver of normal vertical span to be pushed into the abdomen. It is therefore important to locate the inferior margin of the liver by both palpation and percussion as well as the upper margin by percussion so that the vertical span and position of the liver can be evaluated. A liver with a normal vertical span in which the inferior margin is well below the costal arch suggests intrathoracic pathology, while a liver with an upper margin in the expected position and an increased vertical span placing the lower margin below the costal arch should be considered enlarged and the reason sought by investigation.

When examining the liver, the upper margin should be located by percussing along the midclavicular line at successive intercostal spaces. The percussive note changes from tympanic to dull when the liver is encountered. This location should be marked with a skin pencil as it will be used as a reference point to measure the vertical span of the liver once the lower margin has been located.

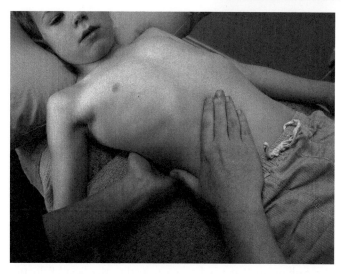

Figure 3.26 • Technique for palpation of the pediatric liver. Note how the examiner lifts the right side of the child's abdomen to make the liver margin more prominent and therefore more accessible to palpation.

The lower margin is located by palpation. The examiner places the superior hand under the lower rib cage posteriorly and slightly lifts the patient. Palpation with the inferior hand, which is placed on the abdomen with the index finger parallel with the line of the costal margin, begins in the right lower quadrant and proceeds up the midclavicular line in small increments, feeling for the inferior margin of the liver (Fig. 3.26). The inferior margin should be palpated for position, consistency, tenderness, and the presence of any pulsations.

An alternative technique for palpation of the lower margin of the liver is for the examiner to stand further up the table towards the patient's head and reach across the costal margin with the fingers, palpating gently upwards until the liver is felt (Fig. 3.27).

Once located, the position should be confirmed by percussion. This is carried out by percussing in the midclavicular line, beginning well below the point identified by palpation as the

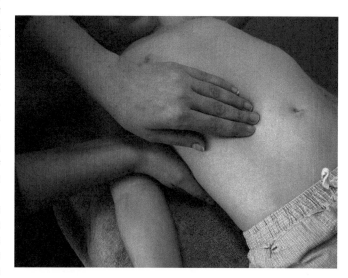

Figure 3.27 • An alternative technique for palpation of the inferior liver margin.

lower margin of the liver, progressing upward in small increments until the usual tympani heard over the abdomen changes to dullness normally heard over a solid mass. The point should coincide with that found on palpation.

The distance between the two points identified on examination is measured and this represents the vertical span of the liver, which should be compared to the percentile chart to check for normality (Fig. 3.28). It is usual for the lower margin of the liver in a child to be located up to 3 cm below the costal arch, this measurement being made in the midclavicular line (Easton 2004).

Spleen

In order to palpate the spleen, the examiner reaches across the supine patient, placing the superior hand under the lower rib cage posteriorly in order to lift the left upper abdomen in similar fashion to that used when palpating the liver. Palpation with the inferior hand should commence in the right lower abdominal quadrant since it is not uncommon for the spleen to enlarge across the midline of the abdomen (Fig. 3.29). The fingers of the palpating hand should point towards the left upper quadrant and be moved in small increments obliquely across the abdomen in that direction (Fig. 3.30). The size of the spleen should be noted and also whether or not it is tender. It should be noted that the spleen will sometimes enlarge down the lateral aspect of the abdominal wall and, as such, the palpation examination should be extended right across to the lateral wall (Easton 2004).

Splenomegaly is seen in such conditions as infection (e.g. Epstein–Barr virus), septicemia, leukemia and hemolytic jaundice. The enlarged spleen is felt as a superficial mass in the left upper quadrant that has a sharp straight border with a notch on the medical aspect. The presence of this notch formation assists the examiner in differentiating the enlarged spleen from other masses such as that which may be caused by lymphoma (Barness 1981). The normal spleen can be palpated in some 30% of children up to 13 months of age, beyond

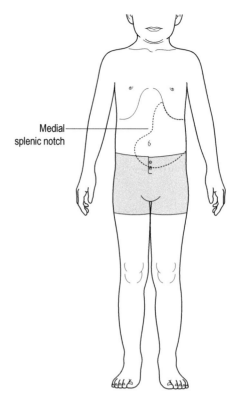

Figure 3.29 • It is not uncommon for the spleen in children to enlarge across the abdominal midline into the right lower quadrant. Note in the illustration above the presence of the medial splenic notch, a key landmark when attempting to differentiate splenomegaly from other abdominal masses.

which the spleen is palpable only when enlarged (Easton 2004). It should be noted that the floating ribs may be mistaken on palpation for the spleen. Differentiation can usually be positively made by percussion, employed in similar fashion to that used to confirm the position of the inferior margin of the liver.

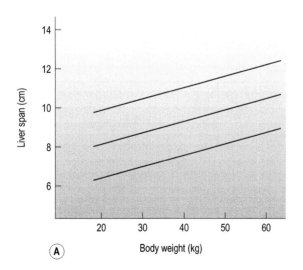
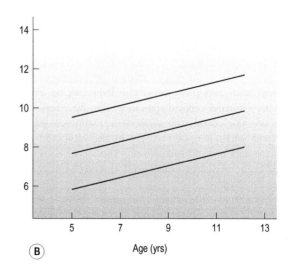

Figure 3.28 • Percentile values for normal liver span in children by (A) body weight, and (B) age (adapted from Younoszai & Mueller 1975 with permission).

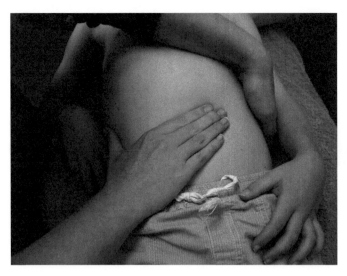

Figure 3.30 • Technique for palpating the spleen. Note how the examiner lifts the left side of the child's abdomen to make the splenic margin more prominent and therefore more accessible to palpation.

Figure 3.32 • Technique for palpation of the kidney in a school-age child and adolescent.

Kidneys

Both kidneys in the infant may be palpated by compressing the lateral aspect of the abdomen immediately below the costal arch between the thumb and forefinger (Fig. 3.31). The forefinger of the palpating hand is placed in the costovertebral angle at the back and, as the infant's leg is brought up into flexion at the hip, is forced as deeply as possible into the soft tissues overlying the kidneys in order to feel as much of the organ as possible. It is more common to be able to feel the right kidney as it sits slightly lower than the left.

An enlarged kidney, or a mass overlying the kidney with an irregular outline, is usually due to infection, tumor or congenital anomaly. In any event, children with such a finding must be referred for specialist investigation in order to determine the nature of the mass.

In older children, the kidneys are palpated using the technique of ballottement (Fig. 3.32). This is performed by applying bimanual palpation over the kidney. The examiner makes a quick 'flick' with the hand on the abdomen. If a ballottable mass such as a kidney underlies the area being examined, the palpation hand will feel a rebound sensation similar to a ball striking the hand (Barness 1981, Bickley & Szilagyi 2008).

Bladder

The bladder is best palpated by using a cupped hand (Fig. 3.33), the examiner pressing gently downward into the abdomen, beginning at the umbilical level and moving towards the pubis in small increments until the upper margin of the bladder is encountered (Easton 2004). Percussion may confirm

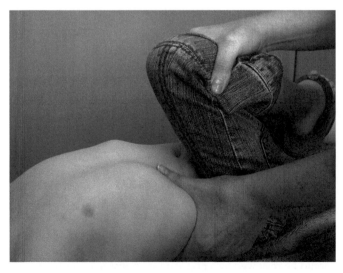

Figure 3.31 • Technique for kidney palpation in a child from birth up to preschool age depending upon size and fatness.

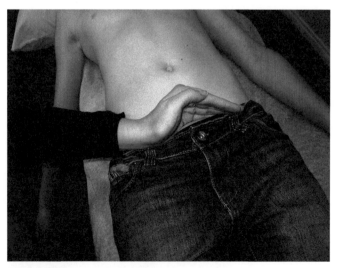

Figure 3.33 • Technique for palpation of the upper margin of the bladder. Note how the examiner utilizes a cupped hand, feeling with the medial margin of the fifth digit.

the position of the bladder. It is sometimes useful, having determined the position of the bladder before micturition, to reassess immediately afterwards. The fully emptied bladder cannot normally be palpated or percussed, and therefore the ability to do so after micturition strongly suggests incomplete emptying.

The large bowel

Palpation of the large bowel is an important part of the abdominal examination as it permits the examiner to determine the presence of fecal and other masses. The examiner holds the lateral wall of the abdomen with the superior hand while the inferior hand applies pressure downward and laterally (Fig. 3.34). The contents of the colon are gently compressed and examined between the two hands. It is unusual to feel fecal material in the cecum or ascending colon.

The technique for palpation of the descending colon is shown in Fig. 3.35. This technique is the same as that used for palpation of the cecum and ascending colon in that the superior hand is placed against the lateral wall of the abdomen while the inferior hand applies a compressive pressure downward and laterally, gently compressing and examining the contents of the descending colon and sigmoid between the two hands. It is normal to feel fecal material when a considerable period of time has elapsed since the last bowel evacuation. When a considerable period of time has elapsed since the last bowel evacuation, such as in constipation, fecal material may be felt throughout almost the entire left side of the abdomen (Fig. 3.36).

The small bowel

Once superficial examination has been completed, the four quadrants of the abdomen should now be more deeply palpated, taking note of any tenderness and, in particular, any masses. The small bowel will be palpated in each of the four quadrants.

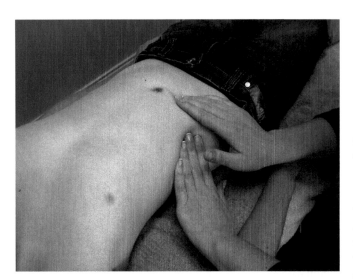

Figure 3.34 • Technique for palpation of the cecum and ascending colon.

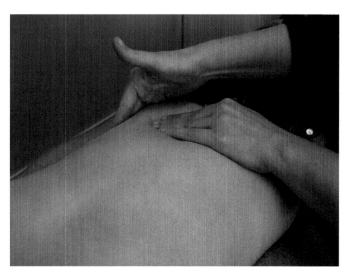

Figure 3.35 • Technique for palpation of the descending colon and sigmoid.

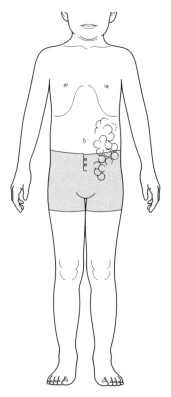

Figure 3.36 • The area of the abdomen throughout which fecal material may be palpated in a child who has not had a bowel evacuation for several days.

Evaluation of an abdominal mass

When a mass is encountered on palpation of the abdomen, its characteristics should be as thoroughly described as possible. Once it has been determined beyond reasonable doubt that the mass is not an enlarged organ or fecal material, the child should be reviewed by a pediatric specialist in order to identify the nature of the mass. The characteristics of a mass in the abdomen that one should endeavor to identify are listed in Box 3.6.

Diagnostic characteristics of an abdominal mass which requires palpatory evaluation

- Anatomical position
- Size
- Shape
- Color of overlying abdominal wall
- Temperature
- Tenderness/pain
- Movement against surrounding tissues
- Consistency
- Surface contour (smooth or nodular)
- Margins (smooth or irregular)

The ovaries

The ovaries in preadolescent patients rarely need clinical assessment. Beyond puberty, ovarian cysts are sometimes encountered, and these are palpated in the same manner as would normally be used for an adult.

The genitalia

Examination of the female genitalia by a chiropractor is limited to inspection of the labia majora and minora. In order to carry out this examination, the labia are gently separated and the structures inspected. It is not uncommon to see a thin membrane joining the labial edges and, while this is easily lysed with a cotton swab, it should be considered outside the scope of chiropractic practice to do so.

The principal reason that a chiropractor would perform this examination at all is to determine the presence of infection such as candida that will not require referral, or to confirm the impression of sexual abuse, should such a diagnosis be suspected from the clinical history.

Examination of the male genitalia involves inspection of the penis and scrotal contents, performance of the cremasteric reflex, and examination of the inguinal lymph nodes. The cremasteric reflex is performed by stroking the proximal one-third of the medial aspect of the thigh and watching for the testis on that side to elevate, sometimes completely into the inguinal canal. Absence of this reflex may accompany a low spinal cord lesion, but it is often absent in otherwise normal boys. The inguinal lymph nodes are readily palpated in young children as small, highly mobile lumps <1 cm in diameter in the groin area (Barness 1981).

To examine the penis, the foreskin should be retracted in order to allow visualization of the glans and external urethral meatus. The position of the meatus should be noted in addition to any signs of tethering of the foreskin or inflammation/infection.

Since the testes in young boys are highly retracted, the examiner should have the child sit in a cross-legged position in order to 'trap' the testes in the scrotal sac for examination.

A diagnosis of undescended testes can only be reliably made after such a maneuver. The truly undescended testis is normally palpable and sometimes visually obvious in the inguinal canal. While it is certainly appropriate to show the child's parents how to manually manipulate the undescended testes towards the scrotum, it should be remembered that many such cases will require surgical correction.

Acute painful swelling of the testes has a number of causes, the most common being torsion of the spermatic cord, orchitis or epididymitis (Barness 1981). Torsion is a surgical emergency as such cases may develop infarction within a few hours. A patient with a painfully swollen scrotum should be referred for emergency surgical opinion.

The anus and rectum

This examination involves inspection and palpation of the sacrococcygeal region, the buttocks, the perianal skin and the anus. The rectum is examined only in children in whom lower gastrointestinal disease is suspected.

If a mass is encountered over the sacrococcygeal area, it may be a tumor. Tufts of hair suggest underlying malformation such as spina bifida and children exhibiting this finding should be neurologically assessed with great care. Pilonidal sinus is a visual finding which maybe more obvious when viewed under magnification and direct lighting using an ophthalmoscope.

The examination of the anus and perianal skin is accomplished by spreading the child's legs comfortably apart and then separating the buttocks with both hands in order to permit visualization. An anal fissure is readily identified as a cut or tear that causes the mucosal folds to appear asymmetrical. Examination in this manner may cause actual bleeding. Children with an anal fissure are often very irritable and the cause of their distress may sometimes be put down to 'colic'. Anal fissure is one of the most common causes of constipation and rectal bleeding in infants up to 3 years of age. Small mucosal tabs have no clinical significance, while the presence of large flat skin tabs should raise the suspicion of sexual abuse. These tabs are referred to as condylomas (Barness 1981).

In case presentations to a chiropractor involving either suspected sexual abuse or acute abdominal pain, it will be necessary to conduct a digital examination of the rectum. The three major findings which will require emergency referral are decreased anal tenesmus, a palpable mass, and blood on the palpating finger that is not due to an anal fissure. The best position in which to perform this examination is probably with the child lying on one side with the legs drawn up into flexion. The fifth finger is used as it is the smallest and the gloved hand should be adequately lubricated. To gain access to the rectum, the tip of the finger is pressed very gently against the anal orifice until the sphincter can be felt slowly relaxing. Insertion of the finger should be slow and deliberate, noting the degree of tenesmus and any discomfort as demonstrated by facial expression. An insertion depth of 2–3 cm should be adequate. Any palpable mass must be noted and the palpation finger inspected for the presence of blood once the examination is completed.

Hernias

Hernias in children may be noted at the umbilicus, just above the umbilicus (supraumbilical), in the groin and rarely in the linea alba between the xiphoid process and the umbilicus. The examination of a hernia does not vary from that performed on an adult in that the examiner palpates the herniation and feels for enlargement as the patient increases the intra-abdominal pressure.

As a general rule, all hernias in infants will require surgical repair except those arising from within the umbilicus which demonstrate a central umbilication. These will spontaneously resolve with time and require no intervention.

The neurological and orthopedic examinations per se are not covered in this chapter as they are considered specific to those body systems and are therefore detailed in the chapters dealing with neurological and orthopedic conditions respectively.

References

Barness, L.A., 1981. Manual of Pediatric Physical Diagnosis, fifth ed. Yearbook Publishers, Chicago.

Berman, S., Chan, K., 1997. Ear, nose and throat. In: Hay, W.W., Groothius, J.R., Hayward, A.R. et al. (Eds), Current Pediatric Diagnosis and Treatment, thirteenth ed. Appleton & Lange, Stamford.

Bickley, L.S., Szilagyi, P.G., 2008. Bates Guide to Physical Examination and History Taking, tenth ed. Lippincott Williams & Wilkins, Baltimore.

Easton, M.K., 2004. Examining the Paediatric Patient (DVD). Kiro Kids, Adelaide.

Eisenbaum, A.M., 1997. In: Hay, W.W., Groothius, J.R., Hayward, A.R., et al. (Eds), Current Pediatric Diagnosis and Treatment. thirteenth ed. Appleton & Lange, Stamford.

Fireman, P., 1997. Otitis media and its relation to allergic rhinitis. Allergy Asthma Proc. 18 (3), 135–143.

Green, M., 1986. Pediatric Diagnosis, Interpretation of Symptoms and Signs in Different Age Periods, fourth ed. WB Saunders, Philadelphia.

Hay, W.W., Groothius, J.R., Hayward, A.R. et al. (Eds), 1997. Current Pediatric Diagnosis and Treatment, thirteenth ed. Appleton & Lange, Stamford.

Hay, W.W., Levin, M.J., Sondheimer, J.M., et al., 2007. Current Diagnosis and Treatment in Pediatrics, eighteenth ed. McGraw Hill, New York.

Hughes, J.G., 1974. Synopsis of Pediatrics, fourth ed. Mosby, St Louis.

Kliegman, R.M., Behrman, R.E., Jenson, H.B., et al., 2007. Nelson Textbook of Pediatrics, eighteenth ed. Saunders Elsevier, Philadelphia.

Lissauer, T., Clayden, G., 2007. Illustrated Textbook of Paediatrics. Mosby Elsevier, Edinburgh.

Lott Ferholt, J.D., 1980. Clinical Assessment of Children: A Comprehensive Approach to Primary Pediatric Care. JB Lippincott, Philadelphia.

McMillan, J.A., Nieburg, P.I., Oski, F.A., 1977. The Whole Pediatrician Catalogue: A Compendium of Clues to Diagnosis and Management. WB Saunders, Philadelphia.

McMillan, J.A., Stockman, J.A., Oski, F.A., 1983. The Whole Pediatrician Catalogue. A Compendium of Clues to Diagnosis and Management. WB Saunders, Philadelphia.

Maran, A.G.D. (Ed.), 1988. Logan Turner's Diseases of the Nose, Throat and Ear, tenth ed. John Wright, London.

Maxwell, G.M., 1977. Principles of Pediatrics. University of Queensland Press, Brisbane.

National High Blood Pressure Education Program Working Group on High Blood Pressure in Children and Adolescents, 2004. The fourth report on the diagnosis, evaluation and treatment of high blood pressure in children and adolescents. Pediatrics 114 (2), 555–576.

Newell, S.J., Darling, J.C., 2008. Lecture Notes Paediatrics, eighth ed. Blackwell, Oxford.

Olitsky, S., Hug, D., Smith, L.P., 2007. In: Kliegman, R.M., Behrman, R.E., Jenson, H.B., et al. (Eds), Nelson Textbook of Pediatrics. eighteenth ed. Saunders Elsevier, Philadelphia.

Pang, D., Newson, T., 2005. Paediatrics. Mosby, Edinburgh.

Popich, G.A., Smith, D.W., 1972. Fontanels: range of normal size. J. Pediatr. 80 (5), 749–752.

Roberton, D.M., South, M., 2006. Practical Paediatrics, sixth ed. Churchill Livingstone Elsevier, Edinburgh.

Rosner, B., Prineas, R.J., Loggie, J.M.H., et al., 1993. Blood pressure nomograms for children and adolescents, by height, sex and age, in the United States. J. Pediatr. 123 (6), 871–886.

Tanner, J.M., 1962. Growth at Adolescence. Blackwell, London.

Wolfe, R.R., Boucek, M., Schaffer, M.S., et al., 1997. In: Hay, W.W., Groothius, J.R., Hayward, A.R., et al. (Eds), Current Pediatric Diagnosis and Treatment. thirteenth ed. Appleton & Lange, Stamford.

Younoszai, M.K., Mueller, S., 1975. Clinical assessment of liver size in normal children. Clin. Pediatr. (Phila) 14 (4), 378–380.

Recognizing the seriously ill child

4

Neil J. Davies

Acute life-threatening illness is only rarely encountered in general chiropractic practice with either adult or pediatric patients. In the first instance, such patients do not belong within the chiropractic paradigm. Ethical and scientific necessity demand that patients with these types of presentation be urgently transferred to a hospital facility where clinicians are both adequately trained and technologically equipped to handle such emergency cases.

While recognition of an acute illness which imminently threatens life is frequently obvious in the adult patient, it is often far less so among children, and particularly infants. As a general rule, it is reasonable to say that the younger the child the more difficult is the task of identifying serious, life-threatening illness.

Hewson & Oberklaid (1994) have proposed a concise system of disease markers designed to assist general clinicians to recognize the presence of serious illness in infants. The system is based on a combination of the work of McCarthy et al (1982) at Yale, who investigated the markers of serious illness in children aged between 3 and 36 months, and the Baby Illness Research Project Team in Cambridge and Melbourne, who are investigating bacterial illness in children from birth to 6 months of age. These investigators have identified two classes of signs and symptoms that apply to serious illness. Firstly, there are those which are commonly associated with serious illness such as drowsiness, dyspnea, decreased fluid intake, etc., and secondly, there are those which are less common, but which when present are associated with a higher incidence of serious illness.

Even the experienced chiropractor, competent in the basic clinical skills of history-taking, physical examination and disease recognition, may find serious illness in infancy extremely difficult to identify. The purpose of this chapter is to present a step-by-step approach, built around the model proposed by Hewson & Oberklaid (1994), which can be readily applied in general practice by the chiropractor to identify the 'red flags' which would demand pediatric referral for further assessment. Given the fulminating capacity of many of the acute diseases which may possibly present initially to the chiropractor, the

referral criteria proposed in this chapter are necessarily conservative in nature, leaving as wide a margin as possible for error.

Within the framework of the routine clinical history and physical examination, the basic elements of assessment in an infant where the possibility of serious illness must be addressed include the following:

- core body temperature
- state of arousal
- ease with which the patient can breathe
- state of peripheral circulation
- amount of fluids taken in and excreted on a 24-hour basis and, where possible, measurement of acute body weight loss as an estimate of the extent to which dehydration has occurred.

Assessment of fever

An assessment of core body temperature is best made in the ear canal using electronic instrumentation. This method is quick, easy to perform, non-invasive and accurate. A reliable estimate of core body temperature can be achieved within seconds in the chiropractic clinic and, when interpreted in conjunction with a serious illness observation scale, provides invaluable information in the total assessment of the infant and toddler who may have serious illness.

McCarthy et al (1982) have proposed a series of observation scales to identify when serious illness is the cause of raised core body temperature in a febrile child. In a multicentered six-item trial involving 312 children, their proposed model was found to be suitably specific, sensitive and predictive of serious illness in febrile children. The six observational items (Table 4.1) in this model may be readily assessed in a chiropractic clinic and represent a valuable tool in guiding the chiropractic clinical decision-making process in cases where infantile fever is a presenting feature. The clinical importance of fever is often misunderstood or grossly exaggerated by

© 2010, Elsevier Ltd, Inc, BV
DOI: 10.1016/B978-0-7020-3129-8.00004-9

Table 4.1 Predictive model for serious illness in febrile children: six observation items and their scales. For the chiropractic clinician, any child with a score exceeding 10 should be considered as a candidate for specialist referral. (Reproduced with permission from McCarthy et al 1982, p. 806)

Observational item	Normal score = 1	Moderate impairment score = 3	Severe impairment score = 5
Quality of cry	Strong with normal tone or content and not crying	Whimpering or sobbing	Weak or moaning or high pitched
Reaction to parent stimulation	Cries briefly then stops or content and not crying	Cries off and on	Continual cry or hardly responds
State variation	If awake → stays awake or if asleep and stimulated → wakes up quickly	Eyes close briefly → awake or awakes with prolonged stimulation	Falls to sleep or will not rouse
Color	Pink	Pale extremities or acrocyanosis	Pale, cyanotic or ashen
Hydration	Skin and eyes normal, mucous membranes moist	Skin and eyes normal AND mouth slightly dry	Skin doughy or tented AND dry mucous membranes AND/OR sunken eyes
Response (talk, smile) to social overtures	Smiles OR alerts (≤2 months)	Brief smile OR alerts briefly (≤2 months)	No smile, face anxious, dull, expressionless OR no alerting (≤2 months)

clinicians and therefore careful observation of the six-item scale in febrile cases may save needless referrals and much parental anxiety.

In febrile children who had an observational score of 10, only 2.7% had a serious illness, while in children whose score was 16, serious illness was present in 92.3%. While an observational scale such as this one is strongly recommended for use in chiropractic practice, it should be noted that its use is not a substitute for an adequate clinical history and physical examination, but a valuable adjunct.

In clinical practice, the observational scales are used by simply watching the febrile infant during the consultation and then assigning the number from the descriptors that best suits the individual case. Simply add up the six scores and make a clear entry into the patient record.

Assessment of arousal

The baby should be observed during history-taking and physical examination for signs of drowsiness, hypotonia and response to stimulation such as that provided during the neurological examination. Should the baby cry during the interview or examination, note of the characteristics of the cry should be made and entered into the clinical record. The cry of an acutely ill infant tends to be of a weak, whimpering nature and appears to require undue effort.

Assessment of breathing

A key element in identifying dyspnea in an infant is recession of the sternum and chest wall during the respiratory cycle. In addition, nasal flaring may also accompany the sternal and chest recession. Tachypnea as an isolated finding is not indicative of serious illness (Hewson & Oberklaid 1994).

Assessment of peripheral circulation

Poor peripheral circulation is seen as generalized pallor. Parents are usually able to indicate that the lack of pink color of their baby's body represents a change from before the child became symptomatic. While coldness of the feet and hands and mottling of the skin have little or no relationship to serious illness, cold lower legs from the knee down must be considered as a potential sign of serious illness.

Estimation of fluid intake and loss

The nursing mother should be asked to make an assessment in percentage terms of any decrease in the baby's fluid intake over the preceding 24 hours. Obviously, the bottlefeeding mother should be able to provide very accurate information in this regard. It should be considered a serious sign if a baby is ingesting 50% of the normal fluid intake.

If a mother is uncertain as to how much milk her baby usually consumes in a 24-hour period, an estimate based on average figures shown in Table 4.2 is a useful guide to assist in the estimation of necessary fluid levels in a healthy baby. For example, in a baby weighing 5.4 kg, fluid intake in the range 750–850 ml would be considered normal average intake. Obviously, if the intake has been considerably less over the previous 24-hour period, then that would have to be considered a serious sign.

The mother should also be asked if she has noticed a decrease in the number of wet diapers (nappies) since the child became symptomatic. As a general rule, four wet diapers or fewer per 24 hours should be considered an indicator of serious illness (Hewson & Oberklaid 1994).

Table 4.2 Range of average water requirements of children at different ages under ordinary conditions (reproduced with kind permission from Behrman & Vaughan 1987)

Age	Average body weight in kg	Total water in 24 hours (ml)	Water per kg body weight in 24 hours (ml)
3 days	3.0	250–300	80–100
10 days	3.2	400–500	125–150
3 months	5.4	750–850	140–160
6 months	7.3	950–1100	130–155
9 months	8.6	1100–1250	125–145
1 year	9.5	1150–1300	120–135
2 years	11.8	1350–1500	115–125
4 years	16.2	1600–1800	100–110
6 years	20.0	1800–2000	90–100
10 years	28.7	2000–2500	70–85
14 years	45.0	2200–2700	50–60
18 years	54.0	2200–2700	40–50

Estimation of acute body weight loss (Figs 4.1 and 4.2; Case studies 4.1 and 4.2)

One of the principal clinical crises likely to confront the chiropractor actively engaged in providing care for infants and toddlers is that of dehydration. Dehydration, one of the more serious complications of febrile and other disease, is produced by a combination of reduced fluid intake and insensible water loss such as that produced by coughing, sweating, tachypnea, etc. The extent to which dehydration has occurred is probably best appreciated by the patient during the course of the illness. When the acute body weight loss has reached 5%, the child should be referred for hospital care regardless of all other clinical findings.

When attempting to estimate acute body weight loss, the four steps below should be followed:

Step 1
Using the patient's anthropometric chart and the weight measurements taken during previous well baby check-ups, establish the percentile the baby's weight development is following.

Step 2
Locate the 'normal' or expected value on the percentile chart for weight that matches the baby's present age. This is done by simply extrapolating previously measured data to the appropriate age line.

Step 3
Measure and plot the baby's current weight.

Step 4
The difference between the two points on the percentile graph represents the magnitude of the acute body weight loss. This value is of little clinical use until it is converted to a percentage. In order to arrive at a percentage weight loss, simply divide the weight loss by the expected well baby weight (step 2) and multiply by 100.

Previous weight measurements will not always be available and, when such is the case, a clinical estimation of the extent of dehydration should be made. A child who is dehydrated may exhibit any number of the following signs (Mackenzie et al 1989) and when these are present should be referred for hospital care:

- poor peripheral perfusion. This is measured by holding the child's hand at the level of the heart with the child in the seated position; compress the hand to produce blanching and measure the time it takes for the normal color to reappear. Anything over 2 seconds should be considered as slow peripheral perfusion. The further from 2 seconds the measured value, the more serious the level of dehydration
- dry mucous membranes and skin
- rapid, weak pulse
- pallor or ashen/gray discoloration of the skin
- soft, sunken eyeballs
- depressed fontanel
- poor tissue turgor (able to 'tent' the skin)
- lethargy
- seizures (occurring only occasionally).

Boys 0–3 years Weight Percentile Chart

Weight should be taken in the nude, or as near thereto as possible.
If a surgical gown or minimal underclothing (vest and pants) is worn,
then the estimated weight (about 0.1 kg) must be subtracted before
weight is recorded. Weights are conveniently recorded to the completed
0.1 kg above the age of 6 months. The bladder should be empty.

Date	Age	Length	Weight	Head circum.
	Birth		3800 gm	
	6 wks		5200 gm	
	4 mnths		7400 gm	
	6 mnths		8700 gm	
	9 mnths		9000 gm	
	Extrapolated value for 9 mnths		10 kg	

DATE OF BIRTH _____ / _____ / _____

Simplified calculation of body surface area (BSA)

$$BSA\ (m^2) = \sqrt{\frac{Ht\ (cm) \times Wt\ (kg)}{3600}}$$

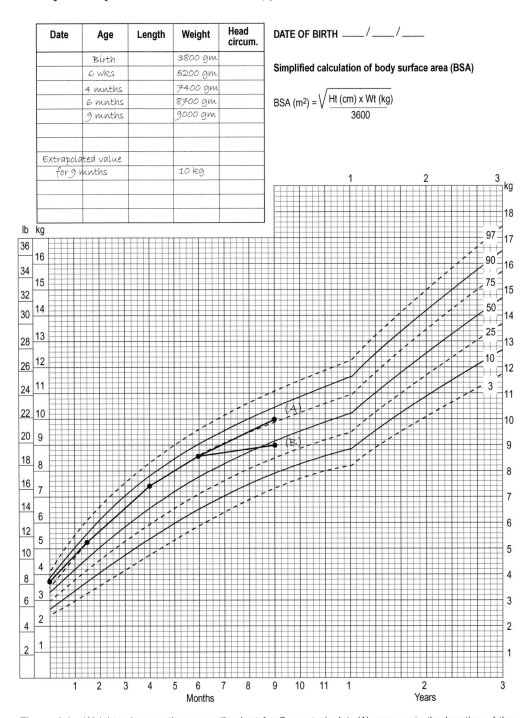

Figure 4.1 • Weight values on the percentile chart for Case study 4.1: (A) represents the location of the expected value based on an extrapolation of previously recorded data, and (B) is the actual weight measurement at presentation. The difference between (A) and (B) represents the acute body weight loss.

Boys 0–3 years Weight Percentile Chart

Weight should be taken in the nude, or as near thereto as possible.
If a surgical gown or minimal underclothing (vest and pants) is worn,
then the estimated weight (about 0.1 kg) must be subtracted before
weight is recorded. Weights are conveniently recorded to the completed
0.1 kg above the age of 6 months. The bladder should be empty.

Date	Age	Length	Weight	Head circum.
	Birth		3200 g	
	3 mnths		5800 g	
	5 mnths		7200 g	
	7 mnths		8200 g	
	9 mnths		8640 g	
	Extrapolated value			
	for 9 mnths		9,000 g	

DATE OF BIRTH ____ / ____ / ____

Simplified calculation of body surface area (BSA)

$$BSA\ (m^2) = \sqrt{\frac{Ht\ (cm) \times Wt\ (kg)}{3600}}$$

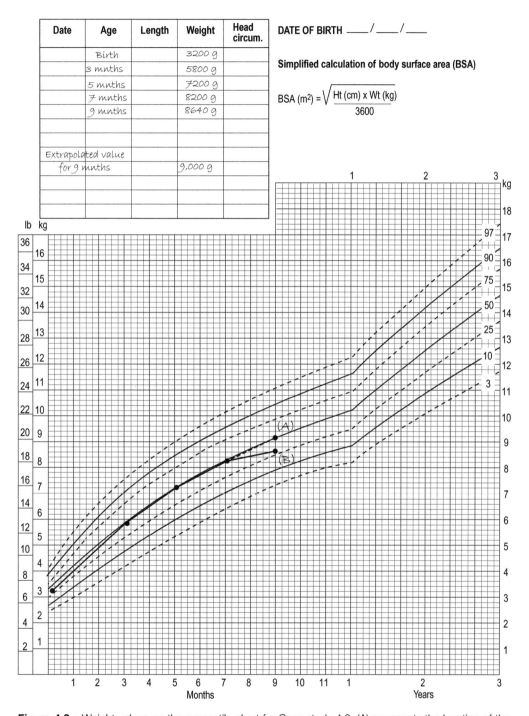

Figure 4.2 • Weight values on the percentile chart for Case study 4.2: (A) represents the location of the expected value based on an extrapolation of previously recorded data, and (B) is the actual weight measurement at presentation. The difference between (A) and (B) represents the acute body weight loss.

Case study 4.1

Ben

Ben has had bronchitis for 2 days. At each previous well baby check-up, his weight measurements have been at the 75th percentile. On the day of presentation, his weight at the 75th percentile would have been 10 kg. His actual weight, however, is 9 kg (see Fig. 4.1). The magnitude, therefore, of his acute body weight loss is 1 kg. The percentage body weight loss is calculated as follows:

$$1 \times 100 \div 10 = 10\%$$

An acute body weight loss of 10% represents a clinically serious case of dehydration and would require immediate referral. The presence of dehydration at this level overrides the need to check such items as observational scales and other aspects of illness assessment since it demands hospital-based rehydration procedures.

Box 4.1

Uncommon but high-risk signs of illness in infants (adapted from Hewson & Oberklaid 1994 with permission)

- Bile-stained vomiting
- Convulsions, particularly the first event (reduction or cessation of seizure disorders under chiropractic care has been reported in the literature)
- Apnea
- Respiratory grunting
- Central cyanosis
- A lump greater than 2 cm in diameter (apart from hydrocele or umbilical hernia)
- A petechial rash
- Fecal blood without visible cause

Less common high-risk signs of serious illness

Some clinical signs and symptoms (Box 4.1) are uncommon and therefore will not be seen very often in a chiropractic setting. They are important to document, however, as when they are present they are associated with a high risk of serious illness.

Applying the principles of serious disease recognition

During the clinical history it is important initially to attempt to identify any risk factors such as the reliability and vigilance

of the historian, significant past illness, prematurity, nutritional status, understanding of the parents, failure to thrive and, in particular, whether or not the child has been prescribed antibiotics (Lott Ferholt 1980). As a sound conservative clinical rule, if a child is currently taking antibiotics and presents with signs of serious illness, a pediatric referral should be made in order for the necessary investigations to be carried out without delay (Hewson & Oberklaid 1994).

The clinical history should always be thorough, following a structured format such as that outlined in Chapter 2. Similarly, the physical examination should follow a system-by-system method such as that suggested in Box 4.2. Where serious illness is a possibility, the following information about

Case study 4.2

Aaron

Aaron is 9 months old and has symptoms consistent with bronchiolitis. He has been sick for 3 days and his mother has brought him in for chiropractic care to assist with his recovery. Mother has recorded Aaron's temperature as 39.5°C on a number of occasions over the past 24 hours and reports that he is frequently coughing and seems to have a bit of trouble breathing. Mother is breastfeeding and reports no real difference in frequency or duration of nursing in the past 48 hours. She further states that Aaron has a wet diaper (nappy) each time he is changed.

On examination, Aaron appears listless but does not cry and is alert as he is handled by his mother. His body color is pale pink but shortly after undressing takes on a mottled appearance with the feet and hands losing their pinkish color. There are no sternal or chest recessions and nasal flaring is not in evidence. Fine crackles are heard across all lung fields associated with an obvious wheeze. Temperature is 38.7°C, pulse rate 114, respiratory rate 36 and blood pressure 100/60. There are no other clinically significant signs.

The anthropometric record for weight is shown in Fig. 4.2. In making a clinical assessment of Aaron, the key factors to bear in mind are the following:
- At present he has a fever consistent with that expected to accompany respiratory infection of viral origin such as that seen in bronchiolitis.

- Arousal is marginally affected.
- Breathing is unaffected.
- Peripheral circulation is within normal limits.
- Fluid intake and discharge have remained within normal limits. His observational items score is 6 and the acute body weight loss is 4%, being calculated from the percentile chart (see Fig. 4.2) as follows:

$$0.36 \times 100 \div 9.00 = 4\%$$

Clearly, Aaron has a viral infection that is already 48 hours old with which he is coping well physiologically. This child should be adjusted, and relevant home-based measures implemented and monitored each day. The natural history of bronchiolitis should see this particular case begin to improve rapidly within 24–48 hours. Failure to improve within this period, symptomatic progression or the appearance of diagnostic signs indicative of serious illness would all represent sound reasons to seek pediatric review. This mother should be given several copies of the Parents' check sheet for developing signs of serious illness' (see Fig. 4.3), shown how to use it at home and asked to report by telephone at regular intervals until such time as the infection is resolved.

Box 4.2

Outline of physical procedures to be performed in a child who presents with symptoms suggestive of serious illness

History

Vital signs

- Pulse rate
- Respiratory rate
- Temperature
- Blood pressure
- Head circumference
- Length
- Weight
- Fontanel diameter

Neurology

- Dermatomes
- Myotomes
- Muscle stretch reflexes
- Cranial nerves
- Primitive reflexes
- Pathological reflexes
- Upper motor neuron signs

Gastrointestinal/ genitourinary

- Inspection
- Auscultation
- Palpation
- Percussion
- Rebound testing
- Chemical urine analysis

Skin

- Inspection
- Palpation for tone
- Palpation for elasticity
- Palpation for dryness
- Mucous membranes

Respiratory

- Inspection
- Palpation
- Percussion
- Auscultation
- Peak flow estimation

Ear, nose and throat

- Inspection
- Palpation
- Percussion
- Instrument inspection of nose, oral cavity, ears
- Pneumatic otoscopy

Cardiology

- Inspection
- Palpation
- Percussion
- Auscultation

---

each of the body systems will prove fruitful and should always be sought as the basic minimum (see also Fig. 4.3).

General questions which will apply to most of the body systems include the following:

- Is your baby refusing fluids?
- Has your baby continued to have the usual number of wet nappies?
- Does your baby have a fever? Did it come suddenly? Has the temperature been measured?
- Does your baby appear restless, apprehensive or anxious?
- Is your baby difficult to arouse?
- Do your baby's arms or legs feel cold?
- Do you think your baby is having difficulty breathing?
- Has your baby been vomiting?
- Is your baby currently taking antibiotics?

Respiratory system

Croup, pneumonia and bronchiolitis are probably the most common serious respiratory illnesses to present initially to a chiropractor (Box 4.3). The following represent some of the more important questions to ask at history:

- Is there a history of respiratory infection within the past 3 days?
- Is there any coughing?
- Is there a history of chest disease?
- Is there any evidence of wheezing?
- Has your baby been excessively drooling and not able to swallow?
- Is your baby bottlefed or breastfed? (Breastfeeding reduces the incidence density ratio of respiratory infection (Beaudry et al 1995).)

Genitourinary system

Urinary tract infection can present with any of the symptoms described in the general section above. Any child meeting the criteria for having potentially serious illness will need a microscopic urine analysis and culture. There are no particular questions at history, other than those listed in the general section above, that will prove useful in the diagnosis of urinary tract infection.

Neurological system

Encephalitis and meningitis (Box 4.4) are probably the most common serious neurological illnesses to present initially to a chiropractor. The following represent some of the more important questions to ask at history if either encephalitis or meningitis is suspected:

- Is your baby drowsy or irritable?
- Does your baby look pale?
- Have you noticed any jaundice?
- Does your baby's abdomen appear to be bloated?
- If there has been a convulsion, particularly a first convulsion:
  - Is the baby under 6 months of age?
  - Did the convulsion last longer than 10 minutes? (Febrile seizures rarely last longer than 10 minutes.)
  - Was the baby pale or ill before the convulsion?
  - Is the baby on antibiotics for another condition?
  - Did the postictal phase last longer than 30 minutes?

Gastrointestinal system

Gastroenteritis, appendicitis, intussusception and pyloric stenosis (Box 4.5) are probably the most common serious abdominal illnesses to present initially to a chiropractor. The following represent some of the more important questions to ask at history if any of the above is suspected:

- Has your child been exposed to pig meats, canned fish, canned mushrooms, eggs, dried egg powder, milk or shellfish in the past 48 hours (Davies 1987)?
- Does your child fondle and kiss a household pet (especially turtles)?

Baby's name: _____   Date of birth: _____

Time observation made: _____

For you to do at home:

Listen carefully to the way your baby cries

What to look for (☑ the appropriate box):

My baby's cry is:
- ☐ Strong and normal
- ☐ Whimpering or sobbing
- ☐ Weak, moaning or high pitched

Observe how your baby responds to you
or to stimulation such as stroking,
speaking softly, massaging, etc.

My baby's response is to:
- ☐ Cry briefly then stop
- ☐ Continue to cry on and off
- ☐ Cry continually
- ☐ Not respond to me at all

Watch to see how your baby's state
of wakefulness changes both spontaneously
and as you provide stimulation

My baby tends to:
- ☐ Stay awake once awake
- ☐ Wake up from sleep when stimulated
- ☐ Wake up after closing eyes briefly
- ☐ Wake only after prolonged stimulation
- ☐ Not rouse from sleep

Study your baby's unclothed body

My baby's color is:
- ☐ Pink
- ☐ Pale in arms and legs
- ☐ Pale and cold below the knees
- ☐ Blue or ashen (whitish-gray color)

Gently pinch your baby's skin and lift it up a
little to make the shape of a tent, then press
gently on the eyes with the lids closed to feel
if the eyes are firm or soft and then look at the
inside of the cheeks in the mouth to see if they
are moist or dry

My baby has:
- ☐ Skin which feels normal to me
- ☐ Moist cheeks inside the mouth
- ☐ Slightly dry cheeks inside the mouth
- ☐ Skin that makes a little tent
- ☐ Dry cheeks inside the mouth

Talk softly to your baby and smile as you
make eye contact

My baby's response is:
- ☐ To smile back or become alert
- ☐ Only briefly smiles
- ☐ Only remains briefly alert
- ☐ Doesn't smile at all
- ☐ Seems anxious
- ☐ Has no facial expression

Fig. 4.3 • Parents' check sheet for developing signs of serious illness.

Box 4.3

Key diagnostic features of pneumonia and bronchiolitis in infants and toddlers

Pneumonia

- History of respiratory tract infection for a few days preceding sudden onset of fever
- Chills, cough and fever (older children and adolescents)
- Restlessness and apprehension
- Cyanosis and respiratory distress (nasal flaring/chest and sternal recession)
- Tachypnea and sometimes tachycardia

- A dull tympanic sound in one area of the lung fields
- Bronchial breathing, heard over the affected lobe

Bronchiolitis

- History of respiratory tract infection for a few days preceding
- Cough
- Wheeze
- Respiratory distress (nasal flaring/chest and sternal recession)
- Widespread crackles on auscultation

Box 4.4

Key diagnostic features of encephalitis and meningitis in infants and toddlers

Encephalitis

Early signs commonly include:
- Headache
- Abdominal distress
- Nausea and vomiting
- Screaming spells in infants

Later developing signs commonly include:
- Mental dullness eventuating to stupor
- Bizarre movements/convulsions
- Mild nuchal rigidity
- Focal neurological signs such as facial paralysis, tongue deviation, etc.
- Occasional bowel/bladder incontinence

Meningitis

Common signs in the neonate and infant:

- Jaundice
- Respiratory distress (nasal flaring/chest and sternal recession)
- Hepatomegaly
- Abdominal distension
- Anorexia and vomiting
- Lethargy
- Usually no evidence of bulging fontanel or nuchal rigidity

Common signs in the older child:
- Several days of respiratory or gastrointestinal symptoms
- Anorexia, nausea and vomiting
- Photophobia
- Nuchal rigidity
- Positive Brudzinski and Kernig signs
- Headache due to raised intracranial pressure

Box 4.5

Key diagnostic features of gastroenteritis, appendicitis, intussusception and pyloric stenosis in infants, toddlers and young children

Gastroenteritis

- Acute abdominal cramping
- Nausea and vomiting
- Diarrhea
- Chills
- Dizziness
- Headache

Appendicitis

- Abdominal pain beginning at the periumbilical area and moving to the right lower quadrant within hours
- Diarrhea
- Occasionally nausea and vomiting
- Dysuria
- Tachycardia and low-volume pulse
- Rapid, shallow breathing
- Ascites and hypoactive bowel sounds
- Rebound tenderness and muscular rigidity
- Pain increased by stretching the abdomen, coughing or moving about
- Tenderness at McBurney's point
- In infancy, there is a tendency to lie with the hips flexed in fetal position

Intussusception

- Sudden-onset pallor which becomes persistent
- Inactivity and unwillingness to be handled, bathed, massaged, etc.
- Episodic inconsolable crying
- Vomiting
- Occasionally rectal bleeding

Pyloric stenosis

- Increasingly severe vomiting which becomes projectile in nature
- Acute body weight loss
- Visible peristaltic waves across upper abdomen

- Does your child complain of abdominal pain? Point to where.
- Has your child developed diarrhea?
- Is it painful for your child to urinate?
- Has your child's breathing become rapid and shallow?
- Is your child's pain worsened by coughing, stretching, moving, etc.?
- Has your child starting lying with the hips flexed?
- Has your child suddenly become and remained pale?
- Is your child inactive?
- Is your baby having episodes of inconsolable crying?

- Has your child been vomiting? Is it projectile?
- Is your baby bottlefed or breastfed? (Breastfeeding reduces the incidence density ratio of gastrointestinal infection.)

Summary of referral criteria

In cases of potentially serious illness in infants and toddlers, the 'absolute bottom line' in clinical practice must surely be at what point a specialist pediatric referral should be made. Each case, of course, will be different and the only reliable guide is common sense and conservative estimation of the degree of illness the child is experiencing using the clinical information from this chapter.

As a matter of principle, the following guidelines may be helpful to the chiropractor trying to determine if a referral is necessary. In infants presenting with any of the following, a pediatric referral should be made in the first instance:

- acute body weight loss of 5% or greater
- observational items score >10 (See Table 4.1)
- any combination of poor arousal, circulation or dyspnea
- decreased fluid intake or excretion
- persistent bile-stained vomiting
- a first convulsion
- periods of apnea
- respiratory grunting or central cyanosis
- a lump >2 cm diameter (except hydrocele and umbilical hernia)
- a petechial rash
- blood evident in the feces
- fever of >3 days' duration in a child who is on antibiotics.

References

Beaudry, M., Dufour, R., Marcoux, S., 1995. Relation between infant feeding and infections during the first six months of life. J. Pediatr. 126, 191–197.

Behrman, R.E., Vaughan, V.C. (Eds), 1987. Textbook of Pediatrics. thirteenth ed. WB Saunders, Philadelphia.

Davies, N.J., 1987. Chiropractic management of the acute febrile paediatric patient. Journal of the Australian Chiropractors' Association 17 (4), 126–130.

Hewson, P., Oberklaid, F., 1994. Recognition of serious illness in infants. Mod. Med. Aust. (July) 32–37.

Lott Ferholt, J.D., 1980. Clinical Assessment of Children: A Comprehensive Approach to Primary Pediatric Care. JB Lippincott, Philadelphia.

McCarthy, P.L., Sharpe, M.R., Spiesel, S.Z., et al., 1982. Observation scales to identify serious illness in febrile children. Pediatrics 70, 802–809.

Mackenzie, A., Barnes, G., Shann, F., 1989. Clinical signs of dehydration in children. Lancet 2 (8663), 605–607.

The irritable baby

Neil J. Davies

5

The constantly irritable infant is often referred to by primary health care providers in a somewhat offhanded way as being colicky, as if that somehow represents the final word on the subject. 'Infantile colic' is a term which is used by various health care professions to describe the persistent, often violent crying which sometimes characterizes an otherwise healthy and thriving baby. As many as 1 in 5 parents report a problem with infant irritability or crying in the first 3 months of life but less than 1 in 20 with problem crying have an organic cause (Hiscock & Jordan 2004).

Although there have been a number of theories proposed as to the etiology of colic, the literature remains fraught with difficulties in definition, methodological problems and numerous claims as to both etiology and management that are anecdotal (Hewson et al 1987). Various medical authors believe colicky behavior to be a reaction pain, probably of intestinal origin (Behrman et al 2007, Hull & Johnston 1987, Illingworth 1985). That this characteristic irritable behavior attributed to colic which is uncomplicated by other disease is a result of pain is also supported by researchers within both chiropractic and medicine (Biedermann 1992, Gutmann 1987, Kloughart et al 1989, Nilsson 1985). While the exact mechanisms for this pain remain to some extent obscure, the work of Sato (1980) and Budgell (1998) has shed considerable light on the subject, suggesting a neurophysiological mechanism that supports the clinical observations of Kloughart et al (1989) in their multicentered research trial which demonstrated a striking success rate for resolution of colicky symptoms in young infants after chiropractic management.

Infantile colic probably remains best conceptualized as the end result of a complex transaction between the infant and their environment with multiple factors potentially responsible for the crying and distress (Hewson et al 1987). However, for a subgroup of infants, early excessive crying may evolve into a more generalized 'persistent mother–infant distress' syndrome (Leung & Lemay 2004). Taken together, these factors open the way for wide-ranging management options for the chiropractor.

Uncomplicated colic

The purpose of using the term 'uncomplicated colic' is to clearly signify in the clinical record that there are no factors such as protein intolerance, carbohydrate intolerance or obvious parenting errors that are complicating the colicky presentation. These complications are discussed later in this chapter.

Clinical presentation

The symptoms that are characteristic of the typical colicky infant begin abruptly: the cry is loud and more or less continuous, persisting for several hours at the same time each day, usually late in the afternoon or early in the evening; the face sometimes becomes flushed or circumoral pallor develops; the abdomen may be distended and tense with the legs drawn up; the feet are often found to be cold and the hands bunched into tightly held fists. The paroxysm may simply spontaneously terminate or relief is sometimes obvious after the passage of flatus or fecus (Barr 1998, Behrman et al 2007).

Diagnostic evaluation

Reaching a diagnostic conclusion of uncomplicated colic is a process of elimination. The child with colicky symptoms must be carefully evaluated for any clinical signs that may suggest underlying disease. The parents/caregivers must also be carefully questioned in order to establish that there are no parenting errors, environmental factors, feeding difficulties or family history that may be contributing to the child's irritable disposition. Only after all these factors have been taken into consideration and ruled out, can the chiropractor safely assume that the child indeed has a diagnosis of uncomplicated colic.

Table 5.1 lists some of the more common clinical conditions which may complicate the colicky presentation and their symptomatic characteristics.

© 2010, Elsevier Ltd, Inc, BV
DOI: 10.1016/B978-0-7020-3129-8.00005-0

Table 5.1 Clinical indicators that may imply underlying disease in irritable infant presentations

Body system	Symptom/sign	Associated condition
Integument	Maculopapular rash on trunk, neck, face and upper arms	Cow's milk or soy protein intolerance
	Excoriated erythematous skin on the buttocks and anogenital region	Congenitally low pH of urine and other body fluids
	Pustules over face and trunk with general lymphadenopathy	Congenital infection
	Erythematous rash which desquamates and forms pustules in an otherwise healthy term infant	Congenital candidiasis
Gastrointestinal	Bloating, frequent passage of flatus, constipation and/or diarrhea	Cow's milk or soy protein intolerance
	Sudden onset of paroxysms of severe colicky pain in a previously unaffected infant which get steadily worse over a few hours	Intussusception or other bowel obstruction
	Profuse, explosive diarrhea which has a sweet smell and tests positive for disaccharides	Lactose intolerance
	Projectile vomiting immediately following feeding preceded by 'golf ball' reverse peristaltic waves seen under tangential lighting of the upper abdomen	Pyloric stenosis
	Constant small-volume vomiting which has a sour smell	Gastroesophageal reflux
	Unchanged nappies (diapers)	Parenting error
	Swallowed air	Nursing technique
	Overfeeding, underfeeding, or inappropriately clothed for the prevailing temperature	Parenting error
Respiratory	Crackles/wet sounds without obvious dyspnea	Cow's milk or soy protein intolerance
	Crackles with fever and dyspnea	Infection
Genitourinary	Fever with decreased fluids out	Renal infection
Head and neck	Hair in the child's eye	Corneal irritation
	Fever	Otitis
	Nasal congestion, postnasal drip and reddened tonsils	Chronic catarrh
	Head held constantly to one side	Congenital sternomastoid tumor

Chiropractic management

Clinical studies with pediatric patients presenting with visceral conditions in general have shown somewhat variable responses to chiropractic management (Ali et al 2002, Bronfort et al 2002, Fallon & Edelman 1998, Froehle 1996, Gemmell & Jacobson 1989, Lebouef et al 1991, Nilsson & Christiansen 1988, Reed et al 1994). In terms of infantile colic, a number of studies have reported that chiropractic is effective in producing symptomatic relief in a relatively short timeframe (Davies & Jamison 2007, Klougart et al 1989, Mercer & Nook 1999, Wiberg et al 1999). However, one controlled clinical trial conducted in Norway concluded that 'chiropractic spinal manipulation' was no more effective than placebo in the treatment of infantile colic (Olafsdottir et al 2001). The growing weight of evidence in the scientific literature suggests that chiropractic management is safe and certainly warranted in cases where the irritability of babies can be classified as 'uncomplicated colic'.

Once the diagnosis has been established with clinical certainty, there are two major aspects involved in chiropractic management. The first is to assess and precisely correct the patterns of neurological dysafferentation. In years past the focus of the chiropractic profession has been largely upon the upper cervical complex and the T8–T12 region as representing the most likely anatomical location of the subluxation in colicky babies (Anrig & Plaugher 1998, Davies 2000). Since the advent of a more neurological approach to chiropractic, it now needs to

be said that the anatomical location is less predictable than was first thought and driven more by patterns of cortical dysafferentation and the associated dural tension and cerebrospinal fluid flow dynamics rather than nerve root factors.

The second aspect of care is to counsel the parents and caregivers carefully in relation to feeding practices, positive reinforcement and the use of contingent music therapy. The correction of neurological dysafferentation, while having been shown to be effective in resolving the distressing symptoms associated with uncomplicated colicky presentations (Meadow & Smithells 1975), is not the totality of patient management as the important factors referred to above cause frustration for both the infant and mother, creating a positive feedback cycle which in turn perpetuates irritability and recurrence of the subluxation complex, presumably via the viscerosomatic, somatosomatic and psychosomatic reflex pathways. Provision of adequate, practical counseling to the nursing mother is an essential element in the chiropractic management program (Taubman 1990).

Use of contingent music and differential reinforcement

It has been shown by clinical research that there is a significant behavioral aspect to children with uncomplicated colic presentations that can be considerably varied by the use of contingent music and differential reinforcement (Larson & Ayllon 1990).

Parents with colicky children should be carefully counseled to turn on music when the infant is quiet and alert for a period exceeding 30 seconds. In addition, at such times, reinforcement should be given in the form of parental attention, including making eye contact, talking softly, rocking, walking, playing with the baby, and generally being loving and affectionate. When crying resumes, parents should turn off music and attend to the infant's needs. This behavioral approach, which is designed to compete with crying by reinforcing quiet alertness with music and parental attention, has been demonstrated to reduce crying time by as much as 75% (Larson & Ayllon 1990). This technique of behavioral modification therapy is simple to employ within the home environment and is a valuable adjunct to chiropractic management.

Protein intolerance and allergy

This syndrome, despite extensive research reported in the scientific literature, continues to be underdiagnosed, frequently misdiagnosed, and even more frequently mismanaged. All too often cow's milk intolerance is misdiagnosed as uncomplicated colic and subsequent management programs fail accordingly. In chiropractic, such a mistake in diagnosis leads to overadjusting with all the attendant problems that accompany that form of mismanagement. Physicians and chiropractors alike continue to tell mothers that breastfeeding protects their child from cow's milk allergy and intolerance despite the wealth of studies which have been available in the scientific literature for over a decade demonstrating both the presence and clinical effect of cow's milk protein in human breastmilk (e.g. Barau & Dupont 1994, Chandra 1997, deJong et al 1998, Goldborough & Francis 1983, Gustafsson et al 1992, Host et al 1988, McCarty & Frick 1983, Wilson et al 1990).

Pathophysiology

The physiology of the human gut in the first year of life varies significantly from that of the older child in that the permeability is much greater. By the end of the first year of life the permeability becomes rapidly more adult-like. Because of this increased permeability, during the first year of life, proteinaceous substances can make their way across the gut wall into the bloodstream where they can produce an IgE-mediated antigen–antibody response (Plebani et al 1990, Wilson & Hamburger 1988). There is no single substance in cow's milk that produces the allergenic reaction. Casein, alpha-lactalbumin and beta-lactalbumin all show a high proportion of positive reactions (Savilahti & Kuitunen 1992) with specific IgE antibodies to these substances having been recovered from infants allergic to cow's milk (Bjorksten et al 1983). It has been further demonstrated that children with cow's milk intolerance have an even greater permeability of the small intestine than is the case with non-atopic children of the same age (Schrander et al 1992). Some cases of cow's milk intolerance, however, cannot be shown to be IgE mediated and therefore it seems apparent that the child's symptoms arise from a non-immune source (Foucard 1985).

While intolerance to cow's milk is typically seen in babies where there is a positive family history of atopic disease (Foucard 1985, Wilson & Hamburger 1988), this is not necessarily always the case. Certainly, a negative family history does not automatically eliminate a diagnosis of cow's milk intolerance.

Clinical presentation

The presentation of cow's milk intolerance shows a consistent pattern of symptoms of which those related to the gastrointestinal system predominate. Allergic reactions involving the skin, respiratory system and neurological system are also common (Burr et al 1993; Businco et al 1985; Chandra & Hamed 1991; Chandra et al 1989; Iacono et al 1998; Kahn et al 1988, 1989; Lucas et al 1990; Nadasdi 1992).

Diagnosis

In order to make a presumptive clinical diagnosis of cow's milk allergy, a 'triad' of symptoms, which must include the gastrointestinal, respiratory and integumentary systems, must be present. The majority of children who end up with a confirmed diagnosis of cow's milk allergy will present initially with this typical 'triad' of symptoms, namely gastrointestinal disturbance, skin rash and respiratory 'wet sounds'. While a small number present atypically, it is probably safe to say that all children with cow's milk allergy will at least have gastrointestinal symptoms and one or more of the other symptoms shown in Table 5.2.

Once the possibility of cow's milk allergy is considered, it is wise to arrange appropriate allergy tests and an evaluation of total serum IgE. When found in combination, a positive radioallergosorbent test (RAST) to cow's milk and an elevated total serum IgE is as reliable as laboratory investigations get in assisting the clinician to confirm a diagnosis of cow's milk allergy. Certainly, a combination of typical symptomatic pattern and positive laboratory results will confirm the diagnosis in a good proportion of cases.

Table 5.2 Common symptoms associated with cow's milk allergy and intolerance in infants

Body system	Symptom/sign
Gastrointestinal	Bloating, frequent passage of flatus and intractable crying/distress with pulling up of the legs Chronic diarrhea, constipation or an alternating pattern of both
Integument	Maculopapular rash which may occur anywhere on the body, but is found most commonly on the face, neck, trunk, buttocks and upper arms. Sometimes it is only seen in body fossae and within the enclosed areas of skin folds Eczema
Respiratory	Crackles/wet sounds without obvious dyspnea Wheezing and rhinitis
Neurological	Disturbed sleep pattern with frequent waking, crying at night, short sleep cycles and long non-rapid eye movement stage 1 (NREM1) sleep

It should be borne in mind when performing laboratory tests, however, that a second type of reaction to cow's milk that is really a non-immune intolerance will return negative laboratory results while the symptomatic picture remains strongly evidential of the diagnosis. Under these circumstances, a clinical diagnosis should be made and the patient managed accordingly. A successful clinical outcome is all the diagnostic confirmation that is needed.

Management

Chiropractic management of the infant who reacts to cow's milk protein is the same for IgE-mediated and non-immune intolerances. In both cases, diagnostic confirmation is dependent upon clinical outcome. The management of the breastfed infant is simple. The mother is counseled to avoid all food substances containing dairy products and to ensure a fluid intake of approximately 1.5–2 liters per day for the trial period of 15 days. The baby should be evaluated for evidence of neurological dysafferentation twice a week and correction made when necessary. Recurrent subluxation patterns are common among babies who react to cow's milk protein, presumably owing to activation of the viscerosomatic reflex by the offending protein. If the neurological dysafferentation is left uncorrected, the child's symptoms may persist, confusing the clinical outcome of the dairy-free trial period. If the child is clinically improved after the 15-day trial period and the correction of the neurological dysafferentation is stable, the mother should be counseled in relation to adopting a dairy-free diet with adequate supplementation for the duration of her breastfeeding, since human milk offers the best protection for the cow's milk reactive infant (Arato et al 1996, Gruskay 1982).

Artificially fed infants are somewhat more difficult to manage. Most artificially fed infants who have cow's milk intolerance or allergy will require feeding with a fully hydrolyzed formula, making a 14–21-day trial on such a formula the ideal approach to diagnostic confirmation. However, in some jurisdictions, government health authorities require an initial trial on a soy-based formula prior to the trial on a fully hydrolyzed formula in order to permit the writing of a formal prescription for the hydrolyzed formula. A significant percentage of children who are allergic or intolerant to cow's milk protein can tolerate soy protein without developing atopic symptoms in the short term (Nadasdi 1992). There are, however, a proportion of children who have a cross-reactivity to soy in whom symptomatic relief will be apparent within the 14–21-day trial, only to relapse again within a few days. Relief comes as the offending cow's milk proteins are eliminated from the diet and exacerbation occurs as a new antigen–antibody response specific to the soy protein begins. It needs to be pointed out that prolonged use of soy infant formula is not a perfect solution; the known problems with such an approach are more fully discussed in Chapter 19.

If soy cross-reactivity is identified, the child should then be trialed on a hydrolyzed formula such as Nutramigen or Pregestimil. Hydrolyzed formulae consist of dried glucose syrup, casein hydrolysate, a variety of vegetable oils, and a range of vitamins, minerals and amino acids. Cross-reactivity of hydrolyzed formulae with cow's milk protein has been demonstrated (Ragano et al 1993) but the incidence is very low (Host & Samuelsson 1988, Rugo et al 1992). The major problem encountered with hydrolyzed formulae is rejection by the infant. Cross-reactive infants generally have a high incidence of chronic subluxation recurrence and therefore need to be assessed on a very regular basis during the period of dietary manipulation.

As an aside, casein hydrolysate formulae are much to be preferred for their hypoallergenic properties than formulae with whey hydrolysate, which demonstrates a greater cross-reactivity with cow's milk (Host & Samuelsson 1988, Rugo et al 1992).

Children who have been shown to be cow's milk allergic or intolerant should ideally be kept permanently on a dairy-free diet. While this strategy has not been demonstrated to completely prevent later development of atopic disease (Bishop et al 1990), there is persuasive evidence suggesting that dietary avoidance of cow's milk protein lessens the incidence of such problems (Schrander et al 1992, Strobel 1992).

Carbohydrate intolerance

Gastrointestinal intolerance to sugars is thought to affect most of the adults in the world (Bayless et al 1975) to a greater or lesser extent, and is also commonly encountered in infants and older children.

Pathophysiology

The principal carbohydrate in human milk is the disaccharide lactose, which is hydrolyzed in the small intestine by lactase phlorizin hydrolase, otherwise known as lactase (Buller et al 1991). The absence of lactase permits the passage of undigested lactose into the large intestine and is associated with the well-known syndrome referred to as lactose intolerance.

Clinical presentation

The most common presentation of lactose intolerance in infancy almost invariably follows a bout of acute gastroenteritis in which the gastrointestinal mucosa has become damaged. This condition is self-limiting and will improve over time, but it is worth treating in order to gain symptomatic relief.

In older children the symptoms of lactose intolerance usually develop gradually, beginning several years after birth and presenting with abdominal cramps, bloating, chronic diarrhea, and excessive passage of flatus related to the ingestion of dairy products (Mitchell et al 1975).

While lactose is by far the most common carbohydrate to cause the above symptom pattern, some children will experience similar symptoms of abdominal distress and severe diarrhea due to sucrase isomaltase deficiency. This condition is very uncommon and need be considered only in the event that management implemented for lactose intolerance fails.

Diagnosis

The diagnosis of lactose intolerance is a clinical one dependent on the recognition of the symptom complex described above and does not normally require any laboratory investigations. However, simple tests which can be carried out on the liquid portion of the diarrheal stool may be performed if there is doubt about the diagnosis. Immediately after collection, the liquid stool specimen is mixed with two parts water, and 15 ml of the resultant fluid is tested with two Clinitest tablets for the presence of reducing sugars, while another drop is applied to the glucose tester on a Clinistix strip. Glucose at 0.5% or less should be considered normal (Behrman et al 2007). In addition, it is worthwhile to test the pH, which will be 5.5 or less in lactose-intolerant individuals.

Management

In breastfed infants, neurological dysafferentation should be corrected and the mother strongly encouraged to continue nursing. Weaning to a lactose-free formula should be considered only in the most severe, protracted cases where there is demonstrable weight loss. In artificially fed infants, the formula should be changed to one that is lactose free.

Older children in whom lactose intolerance has made a gradual appearance should be placed on a dairy-free diet, provided with adequate nutritional supplementation, and have their patterns of neurological dysafferentation corrected and monitored at regular intervals. Symptomatic resolution will come quickly and permanently provided there are no 'binges' on dairy products in which as little as 8 ounces of milk (half a glass) may produce a flat blood sugar curve, bloating, cramps, loose stools or diarrhea (Mitchell et al 1975).

Gastroesophageal reflux

Gastroesophageal reflux (GER) is a common occurrence during infancy with most children having a small degree of reflux that is of little clinical consequence, usually requiring only minimal intervention in the event it causes harm (Catto-Smith 1998, Glassman et al 1995). This phenomenon is due to the fact that the intra-abdominal segment of the esophagus is virtually nonexistent at birth (Hull & Johnston 1987) and therefore no effective reflux barrier exists. This barrier is created over the first few months of life as the intra-abdominal esophageal segment lengthens. It is important to recognize that the natural history of GER in infants differs significantly from reflux in adults (Catto-Smith 1998). In children, reflux-induced injury can result from acid exposure, nutrient loss or respiratory complications.

GER has become a rather 'fashionable' diagnosis in recent years in infants that are irritable, with the emergence of the totally unfounded notion of 'silent reflux' in which it is hypothesized that acid reflux into the distal esophagus occurs without the visible evidence of frequent and excessive small-volume vomitus. This notion lacks any scientific evidence at all.

Clinical presentation

In true GER the gastrointestinal signs and symptoms are related directly to the exposure of the distal esophageal epithelium to refluxed gastric contents (Behrman et al 2007). The majority of children with GER have delayed gastric emptying, and vomiting may be forceful because of pylorospasm (Behrman et al 2007). In the vast majority of children, excessive vomiting occurs within the first week of life (Behrman et al 2007, Smith 1980). Vomiting due to GER can occur at any time, unlike normal posseting in which infants will bring up a little milk as they expel swallowed air after feeding.

Respiratory systems are common in children with GER, usually owing to aspiration of refluxed material. Symptoms include chronic cough, wheezing and recurrent pneumonia. To be safe, GER should always be considered as a likely etiology of recurrent respiratory symptoms in the first 2 years of life and appropriate diagnostic evaluation carried out.

In children with GER, growth and weight gain are usually adversely affected. This has been demonstrated in about two-thirds of all cases with confirmed GER (Behrman et al 2007).

Diagnosis

In mild cases, diagnosis is made on history and clinical assessment alone. Episodic vomiting beginning in the first 1–2 weeks of life should underpin a diagnosis of mild GER in infancy. Careful monitoring of the child's response to management will quickly confirm the diagnosis. In more severe cases, it is wise to refer the child to a pediatric specialist for esophagoscopy or barium esophagography under fluoroscopic control. Strictures, recurrent reflux and ragged mucosal outline suggestive of esophagitis are readily seen with barium esophagography; however, esophagoscopy with biopsy is the preferred technique for demonstrating esophagitis.

Management

In mild cases the infant should be neurologically managed and monitored for symptomatic change over a period of 2 weeks. In the event that the cause of the reflux symptoms is functional the child will show rapid improvement related directly to the sustainability of the correction of patterns of neurological dysafferentation. In cases in which improvement is not sustained and the dysafferentation patterns are recurrent, concurrent treatment with an antacid that does not contain aluminum hydroxide is recommended along with formula thickening in bottlefed infants.

In more intractable cases, it is appropriate to refer the affected child to the family general practitioner for the prescription of one of the upper gastrointestinal motility-enhancing agents which are generally available around the world today.

In cases involving retarded growth factors, respiratory symptoms or excessive intractable vomiting which fails to respond to conservative care, referral to a pediatric specialist should be made in order to arrange for appropriate clinical investigation and possible surgical intervention (Smith 1980).

Infantile hypertrophic pyloric stenosis

Infantile hypertrophic pyloric stenosis (IHPS) is the most common condition affecting infants that requires surgical intervention (St Peter & Ostlie 2008). The etiology of IHPS is yet to be fully elicited. Since the 1990s, a sharp decline in IHPS has been reported in various countries. A possible correlation has been suggested between the 'Back to Sleep' campaign and the falling incidence of IHPS as its decline parallels that of sudden infant death syndrome (SIDS). Recent research from Scotland, however, has shown that the beginning of the decline in the incidence of IHPS predated by some 2 years that of SIDS (which did follow the 'Back to Sleep' campaign), making a direct correlation unlikely (Sommerfield et al 2008).

Infants with pyloric stenosis generally present with vomiting beginning as early as the end of the first week of life and as late as the fifth month (Behrman et al 2007), with the usual time of onset being around the third week. The vomiting may not, at first, be projectile but will progress to that in time. The development of pyloric stenosis is a progressive and dynamic process. The rate of hypertrophy to the point of meeting diagnostic criteria is unknown and there are no data published in the literature regarding the role of repeat ultrasound in patients with persistent symptoms (Keckler et al 2008). The usual pattern of vomiting is a large-volume, forceful vomit following the appearance of an obvious peristaltic wave moving across the upper abdomen. The peristaltic wave is often referred to as 'golf ball peristalsis' as it has the appearance of a moving golf ball located within the abdomen. This wave phenomenon is best visualized by looking tangentially across the abdomen. An olive-shaped mass is also usually palpable midway between the umbilicus and the costal margin, just inferior to the liver border. This mass will normally be more readily palpable immediately following an episode of vomiting.

IHPS has been linked to inappropriate neuromuscular action, poor breastfeeding performance and maternal stress (Behrman et al 2007). The striking success that some children receive from chiropractic bears testimony to an etiology of subluxation complex-induced neuromuscular incoordination. The gastrointestinal tract receives sympathetic supply from T8–L1 and, with the exception of the distal colon, parasympathetic supply via the Xth cranial nerve. Neurological dysafferentation involving the upper cervical complex may affect the function of the Xth cranial nerve, possibly owing to the anatomical proximity of the inferior vagal ganglion (Lawrence 1991), the effect of increased dural tension and altered cerebrospinal fluid pressure gradients. The combination of these factors may potentially affect the function of the gastrointestinal tract. In addition, it has been reported by Wiles (1990) that palpatory evidence of reduced motion in the vertebral segments between T7 and T12 has been found in association with generalized gastrointestinal disease. The diagnosis is made clinically and there is usually no need for the diagnostic imaging procedures to be performed.

Care must be taken when making management decisions in relation to children with pyloric stenosis. As the vomiting continues, a progressive loss of fluid, hydrogen and chloride ions occurs which will, if not corrected, lead to hypochloremic metabolic alkalosis. Serum potassium levels usually remain unaffected, but in severe cases a total body potassium deficit may occur. Where no evidence of dehydration or physiological stress from biochemical deficiency can be demonstrated, chiropractic management can be safely instigated. The care program should include careful neurological assessment with correction of any dysafferentation and maternal counseling in relation to feeding procedures and stress reduction. If the likelihood is that the mother is probably not going to be able to significantly change her circumstances to reduce stress levels, a referral after subluxation correction to a hospital for both mother and child is appropriate. In the hospital environment, the mother will receive the help she needs to cope with the demands of her baby and may be able to get some much-needed rest if sleep deprivation has been an issue. Stabilization of the neurological dysafferentation may ultimately depend on correcting breastfeeding errors and reducing immediate stress levels (Homewood 1981).

In the event that there is little or no improvement in the very short term after neurological correction as been achieved, the child should be referred to a pediatrician for investigation and possible surgical intervention. IHPS, which is related to neuromuscular incoordination, generally responds quickly and permanently to neurological correction. Failure to do so clearly implies that there is another cause for the neuromuscular incoordination unrelated to the subluxation.

When it is clear that a child is demonstrating evidence of dehydration or physiological stress arising from biochemical deficiency, a pediatric specialist referral is essential. This state does not, however, contraindicate the delivery of chiropractic care, which should be carried out prior to the referral being effected. The usual medical treatment is preoperative correction of the fluid, acid–base and electrolyte losses followed by an operative approach utilizing the application of laparoscopic or circumumbilical techniques to facilitate the pyloromyotomy (Aldridge et al 2007, Ostlie et al 2004, St Peter et al 2006, St Peter & Ostlie 2008).

Intussusception

Intussusception is defined as 'invagination of bowel into an adjacent lower segment' (Hull & Johnston 1987). While not a particularly common condition in terms of incidence, it does represent the most frequent cause of bowel obstruction in the first 2 years of life. The typical symptom pattern is characterized by episodic, uncontrollable crying, inactivity, irritability and an unwillingness to be handled, sudden onset of pallor which becomes persistent, vomiting, and occasionally rectal bleeding which may be identified in digital examination of the rectum.

When a child presents with this confluence of symptoms along with a tender palpable mass in the abdomen which is usually located in the right upper quadrant or close to the left side of the umbilicus, pediatric referral should be made without performing any investigations. Intussusception is a clinical diagnosis. Children presenting to chiropractors with symptoms and signs consistent with this condition should be referred for urgent surgical care as bowel viability can be quickly lost (Hull & Johnston 1987).

Intussusception in a baby that has not been seen previously may be more readily recognizable than is the case with an irritable baby that is being given ongoing chiropractic care, particularly if the symptomatic response is favorable. The latter may be present in such a way that both mother and chiropractor are led into believing that the baby is simply undergoing another paroxysm of irritability caused by a recurrence of the neurological dysafferentation. The critical decision-making problem in this case is linked to the fact that the viscerosomatic reflex responsible for neurological dysafferentation with 'colic' may well be activated in an identical manner by the intussusception. To avoid making an incorrect clinical decision, the abdomen of the irritable baby should be carefully examined at each review consultation.

References

Aldridge, R.D., MacKinlay, G.A., Aldridge, R.B., 2007. Choice of incision: the experience and evolution of surgical management of infantile hypertrophic pyloric stenosis. J. Laparoendosc. Adv. Surg. Tech. A 17 (1), 131–136.

Ali, S., Hayek, R., Holland, R., et al., 2002. Effect of Chiropractic Treatment on the Endocrine and Immune System in Asthmatic Patients. Proceedings of the 2002 International Conference on Spinal Manipulation. Foundation for Chiropractic Education and Research, Des Moines, Iowa.

Anrig, C.A., Plaugher, G. (Eds), 1998. Pediatric Chiropractic. Williams & Wilkins, Baltimore.

Arato, A., Szalai, K., Tausz, I., et al., 1996. Favourable effect of breast feeding and late introduction of cow's milk in the prevention of suspected allergic symptoms in infancy. Orv. Hetil. 137 (36), 1979–1982.

Barau, E., Dupont, C., 1994. Allergy to cow's milk proteins in mothers' milk or in hydrolysed cow's milk infant formulas as assessed by intestinal permeability measurements. Allergy 49 (4), 295–298.

Barr, R.G., 1998. Crying in the first year of life: good news in the midst of distress. Child Care Health Dev. 24 (5), 425–39.

Bayless, T.M., Rothfield, B., Massa, C., et al., 1975. Lactose and milk intolerance: clinical implications. N. Engl. J. Med. 292 (22), 1156–1159.

Behrman, R.E., Jenson, H.B., Nelson, W.E., et al., 2007. Nelson Textbook of Pediatrics, eighteenth ed. WB Saunders, Philadelphia.

Biedermann, H., 1992. Kinematic imbalance due to suboccipital strain in newborns. J. Man. Med. 6, 151–156.

Bishop, A.M., Hill, D.J., Hosking, C.S., 1990. Natural history of cow milk allergy: clinical outcome. J. Pediatr. 116 (6), 862–867.

Bjorksten, B., Ahlstedt, S., Bjorksten, F., et al., 1983. Immunoglobulin E and immunoglobulin G4 antibodies to cow's milk in children with cow's milk allergy. Allergy 38 (2), 119–124.

Bronfort, G., Evans, R.L., Kubic, P., et al., 2002. Chronic pediatric asthma and chiropractic spinal manipulation: a prospective clinical series and randomized clinical pilot study. J. Manipulative Physiol. Ther. 24 (6), 369–377.

Budgell, B., 1998. A Neurophysiological Rationale for the Chiropractic Management of Visceral Disorders. Seminar Proceedings of the International College of Chiropractic Friday Forum Series, February 6, Sydney, Australia.

Buller, H.A., Ringe, E.H., Montgomery, R.K., et al., 1991. Clinical aspects of lactose intolerance in children and adults. Scand. J. Gastroenterol. Suppl. 188, 73–80.

Burr, M.L., Limb, E.S., Maguire, M.J., et al., 1993. Infant feeding, wheezing, and allergy: a prospective study. Arch. Dis. Child. 68 (6), 724–728.

Businco, L., Benincori, N., Cantani, A., et al., 1985. Chronic diarrhea due to cow's milk allergy: a 4- to 10-year follow-up study. Ann. Allergy 55 (6), 844–847.

Catto-Smith, A.G., 1998. Gastroesophageal reflux in children. Aust. Fam. Physician 27 (6), 465–469, 472–473.

Chandra, R.K., 1997. Five year follow up of high-risk infants with family history of allergy who were exclusively breast-fed or fed partial whey hydrosylate, soy, and conventional cow's milk formulas. J. Pediatr. Gastroenterol. Nutr. 24 (4), 380–388.

Chandra, R.K., Hamed, A., 1991. Cumulative incidence of atopic disorders in high risk infants fed whey hydrosylate, soy, and conventional cow milk formulas. Ann. Allergy 67 (2/1), 129–132.

Chandra, R.K., Singh, G., Shridhara, B., 1989. Effect of feeding whey hydrosylate, soy and conventional cow milk formulas on incidence of atopic disease in high risk infants. Ann. Allergy 63 (2), 102–106.

Davies, N.J., 2000. Chiropractic Pediatrics – A Clinical Handbook. Churchill Livingstone, Edinburgh.

Davies, N.J., Jamison, J.R., 2007. Chiropractic management of the irritable baby syndrome. Chiropractic Journal of Australia 37, 25–29.

deJong, M.H., Scharp-van der Linden, V.T., Aalberse, R.C., et al., 1998. Randomised controlled trial of brief neonatal exposure to cow's milk on the development of atopy. Arch. Dis. Child. 79 (2), 126–130.

Fallon, J., Edelman, M.G., 1998. Chiropractic care of 401 children with otitis media: a pilot study. Altern. Ther. Health Med. 4 (2), 93.

Foucard, T., 1985. Development of food allergies with special reference to cow's milk allergy. Pediatrics 75 (1/2), 177–181.

Froehle, R.M., 1996. Ear infection: a retrospective study examining improvement from chiropractic care and analyzing for influencing factors. J. Manipulative Physiol. Ther. 19 (3), 169–177.

Gemmell, H.A., Jacobson, B.H., 1989. Chiropractic manipulation of enuresis: time series descriptive design. J. Manipulative Physiol. Ther. 12 (5), 386–389.

Glassman, M., George, D., Grill, B., 1995. Gastroesophageal reflux in children: clinical manifestations, diagnosis, and therapy. Gastroenterol. Clin. North Am. 21 (1), 71–98.

Goldborough, J., Francis, D., 1983. Dietary management. In: Proceedings of the Second Fisons Food Allergy Workshop. Medicine Publishing Foundation, Oxford, pp. 89–94.

Gruskay, F.L., 1982. Comparison of breast, cow and soy feedings in the prevention of onset of allergic disease: a 15 year prospective study. Clin. Pediatr. (Phila) 21 (8), 486–491.

Gustafsson, D., Lowhagen, T., Andersson, K., 1992. Risk of developing atopic disease after early feeding with cow's milk based formula. Arch. Dis. Child. 67 (8), 1008–1010.

Gutmann, G., 1987. Blocked atlantal nerve syndromes in infants and small children. J. Man. Med. 25, 5–10.

Hewson, P., Oberklaid, F., Menahem, S., 1987. Infantile colic, distress, and crying. Clin. Pediatr. (Phila) 26 (2), 69–76.

Hiscock, H., Jordan, B., 2004. Problem crying in infancy. Med. J. Aust. 181 (9), 507–512.

Homewood, A.E., 1981. The Neurodynamics of the Vertebral Subluxation. Valkyrie Press, St Petersburg, Florida.

Host, A., Samuelsson, E.G., 1988. Allergic reactions to raw, pasteurized, and homogenized/pasteurized cow milk: a comparison. A double-blind placebo-controlled study in milk allergic children. Allergy 43 (2), 113–118.

Host, A., Husby, S., Osterballe, O., 1988. A prospective study of cow's milk allergy in exclusively breastfed infants: incidence, pathogenetic role of early inadvertent exposure to cow's milk formula, and characterisation of bovine milk protein in human milk. Acta Paediatr. Scand. 77 (5), 663–670.

Hull, D., Johnston, D., 1987. Essential Paediatrics, second ed. Churchill Livingstone, Edinburgh.

Iacono, G., Cavataio, F., Montalto, G., et al., 1998. Intolerance of cow's milk and chronic constipation in children. N. Engl. J. Med. 339 (16), 1100–1104.

Illingworth, R.S., 1985. Infantile colic revisited. Arch. Dis. Child. 60, 981–985.

Kahn A Francois, G., Scottiaux, M., et al., 1988. Sleep characteristics in milk-intolerant infants. Sleep 11 (3), 291–297.

Kahn, A., Mozin, M.J., Rebuffat, E., et al., 1989. Milk intolerance in children with persistent sleeplessness: a prospective double-blind crossover evaluation. Pediatrics 84 (4), 595–603.

Keckler, S.J., Ostlie, D.J., Holcomb III, G.W., et al., 2008. The progressive development of pyloric stenosis: a role for repeat ultrasound. Eur. J. Pediatr. Surg. 18 (3), 168–170.

Kloughart, N., Nilsson, N., Jacobsen, J., 1989. Infantile colic treated by chiropractors: a prospective study of 316 cases. J. Manipulative Physiol. Ther. 12, 281–288.

Larson, K., Ayllon, T., 1990. The effects of contingent music and differential reinforcement on infantile colic. Behav. Res. Ther 28 (2), 119–125.

Lawrence, D., 1991. Fundamentals of Chiropractic Diagnosis and Management. Williams & Wilkins, Baltimore.

Lebouef, C., Brown, P., Herman, A., et al., 1991. Chiropractic care for children with nocturnal enuresis: a prospective outcome study. J. Manipulative Physiol. Ther. 14 (2), 110–115.

Leung, A.K., Lemay, J.F., 2004. Infantile colic: a review. J. R. Soc. Health 124 (4), 162–166.

Lucas, A., Brooke, O.G., Morley, R., et al., 1990. Early diet of preterm infants and development of allergic or atopic disease: randomised prospective study. Br. Med. J. 300 (6728), 837–840.

McCarty, E., Frick, O., 1983. Food sensitivity: keys to diagnosis. J. Pediatr. 102 (5), 645–646.

Meadow, S.R., Smithells, R.W., 1975. Lecture Notes on Pediatrics, second ed. Blackwell Scientific Publications, Oxford.

Mercer, C., Nook, B.C., 1999. The efficacy of chiropractic spinal adjustments as a treatment protocol in the management of infantile colic. Proceedings of the 5th Biennial Congress, Auckland, New Zealand, May 17–22, pp 170–171.

Mitchell, K.J., Bayless, T.M., Paige, D.M., et al., 1975. Intolerance of eight ounces of milk in healthy lactose-intolerant teenagers. Pediatrics 56 (5), 718–721.

Nadasdi, M., 1992. Tolerance of a soy formula by infants and children. Clin. Ther. 14 (2), 236–241.

Nilsson, N., 1985. Infantile colic and chiropractic. Eur. J. Chiropractic 33, 624–625.

Nilsson, N., Christiansen, B., 1988. Prognostic factors in bronchial asthma in chiropractic practice. J. Aust. Chiropractic Assoc. 18, 85–87.

Olafsdottir, E., Forshei, S., Fluge, G., et al., 2001. Randomised controlled trial of infantile colic treated with chiropractic spinal manipulation. Arch. Dis. Child. 84 (2), 138–141.

Ostlie, D.J., Woodall, C.E., Wade, K.R., et al., 2004. An effective pyloromyotomy length in infants undergoing laparoscopic pyloromyotomy. Surgery 136 (4), 827–832.

Plebani, A., Albertini, A., Scotta, S., et al., 1990. IgE antibodies to hydrolysates of cow's milk in children with cow milk allergy. Ann. Allergy 64 (3), 279–280.

Ragano, V., Giampietro, P.G., Bruno, G., et al., 1993. Allergenicity of milk protein hydrolysate formulae in children with cow's milk allergy. Eur. J. Pediatr. 152 (9), 760–762.

Reed, W.R., Beavers, S., Reddy, S.K., et al., 1994. Chiropractic manipulation of primary enuresis. J. Manipulative Physiol. Ther. 17 (9), 596–600.

Rugo, E., Wahl, R., Wahn, U., 1992. How allergenic are hypoallergenic infant formulae? Clin. Exp. Allergy 22 (6), 635–639.

St Peter, S.D., Ostlie, D.J., 2008. Pyloric stenosis: from a retrospective analysis to a prospective clinical trial – the impact on surgical outcomes. Curr. Opin. Pediatr. 20 (3), 311–314.

St Peter, S.D., Holcomb III., G.W., Calkins, C. M., et al., 2006. Open versus laparoscopic pylorotomy for pyloric stenosis: a prospective, randomized trial. Nat. Clin. Pract. Gastroenterol. Hepatol. 4 (4), 196–197.

Sato, A., 1980. Physiological studies of the somatoautonomic reflexes. In: Haldemann, S. (Ed.), Modern Developments in the Principles and Practice of Chiropractic. Appleton Century Croft, New York.

Savilahti, E., Kuitunen, M., 1992. Allergenicity of cow milk proteins. J. Pediatr. 121 (5/2), S12–S20.

Schrander, J.J., Ousden, S., Forget, P.P., et al., 1992. Follow up study of cow's milk protein intolerant infants. Eur. J. Pediatr. 151 (10), 783–785.

Smith, H.L., 1980. Gastro-oesophageal reflux and hiatal hernia in children. N. Z. Med. J. 92 (666), 148–151.

Sommerfield, T., Chalmers, J., Youngson, G., et al., 2008. The changing epidemiology of infantile hypertrophic pyloric stenosis in Scotland. Arch. Dis. Child. 93 (12), 1003–1004.

Strobel, S., 1992. Dietary manipulation and induction of tolerance. J. Pediatr. 121 (5/2), S74–S79.

Taubman, B., 1990. Parental counselling compared with elimination of cow's milk or soy milk protein for the treatment of infantile colic syndrome: a randomized trial. Pediatrics 81 (6), 756–761.

Wiberg, J.M., Nordsteen, J., Nilsson, N., 1999. The short-term effect of spinal manipulation in the treatment of irritable baby syndrome: a randomized controlled clinical trial with a blinded observer. J. Manipulative Physiol. Ther. 22 (8), 517–522.

Wiles, M., 1990. Visceral disorders related to the spine. In: Gatterman, M.I. (Ed.), Chiropractic Management of Spine Related Disorders. Williams & Wilkins, Baltimore.

Wilson, N.W., Hamburger, R.N., 1988. Allergy to cow's milk in the first year of life and its prevention. Ann. Allergy 61 (5), 323–327.

Wilson, N.W., Self, T.W., Hamburger, R.N., 1990. Severe cow's milk induced colitis in an exclusively breastfed neonate: case report and clinical review of cow's milk allergy. Clin. Pediatr. (Phila) 29 (2), 77–80.

Abdominal pain and altered states of bowel motility

6

Maurice K. Easton   Neil J. Davies

Abdominal pain in general and altered states of bowel motility are fairly common pediatric presentations and can often be ongoing, relapsing and resistant to treatment. The purpose of this chapter is to examine options for chiropractic assessment and intervention in such cases.

Acute abdominal pain

The majority of children with acute abdominal pain will usually be taken directly to either a medical practitioner or a hospital emergency room. Some, however, will present to the chiropractic clinician. Careful assessment should be undertaken to find signs and symptoms that would warrant emergency referral. Causes of acute abdominal pain that may possibly be seen by a chiropractor are shown in Box 6.1.

The chiropractic approach to the child with acute abdominal pain

When a child is brought to a chiropractor and the presenting complaint is acute abdominal pain, the following clinical approach is recommended.

Case history

A thorough clinical history should be taken with particular emphasis on recent food and fluid intake and output. The description of the pain should include the anatomical site, any radiations, quality, time of onset and any periodicity.

Physical examination

A careful physical examination should be carried out to include all of the following:

- **Vital signs.** Temperature, respiratory rate, heart rate, blood pressure.

- **Abdominal.** Inspection for distension and pattern of movement; auscultation for bowel sounds and vascular bruits; palpation for increased abdominal pressure, areas of tenderness, guarding, organomegaly or other masses; percussion for ascites. Always include examination of the genitalia.
- **Cardiopulmonary.** Particular attention should be paid to identifying evidence of shock and dehydration. Auscultation and percussion of the lung bases for evidence or consolidation associated with pneumonia should always be carried out.
- **Growth.** Abdominal problems should be considered in the context of the nutritional and growth status of the child. The usual anthropometric measurements (length/height, weight, head circumference and fontanel diameter when appropriate) should be made and plotted on the appropriate growth charts.
- **Investigations.** A dipstick urine analysis will be appropriate in most cases. If positive for protein, blood, nitrites or leukocytes, then microscopy and culture will be required. Other investigations that may be needed include full blood examination, serum biochemistry, stool examination, chest and abdominal radiography, and ultrasonography.

Acute gastroenteritis

The key symptoms of acute gastroenteritis in children are fever, diarrhea, nausea, vomiting and abdominal cramping. The etiology of acute gastroenteritis may be due to infection from viruses, bacteria or parasites, or from the effects of toxins. Rotavirus infection tends to have acute onset with a mean duration of 6 days while bacteria tend to produce more abdominal pain with blood in the stools and a longer duration of 10–14 days.

Children with acute gastroenteritis are at risk of developing dehydration. It is important to evaluate the history of fluid

© 2010, Elsevier Ltd, Inc, BV
DOI: 10.1016/B978-0-7020-3129-8.00006-2

Box 6.1

Causes of acute abdominal pain which may possibly be encountered in a chiropractic clinical setting

Common causes of acute abdominal pain

- Acute appendicitis
- Bowel obstruction
- Constipation
- Gastroenteritis
- Intussusception
- Mesenteric adenitis
- Strangulated inguinal hernia
- Urinary tract infection

Less common causes of acute abdominal pain

- Abdominal migraine
- Diabetes
- Gallstones
- Henoch–Schönlein purpura
- Hepatitis
- Inflammatory bowel disease
- Meckel's diverticulitis
- Pancreatitis
- Primary peritonitis
- Testicular torsion

intake (type and amounts) and fluid output (vomitus, diarrhea and urine). Comparison of the child's weight with a recent known weight will help to assess the degree of dehydration. Repeated weight checks are useful to assess the child's progress and possible need for referral for rehydration. While many physical signs of dehydration are listed in the scientific literature, only three are consistently reliable. These are decreased peripheral perfusion, deep acidotic breathing, and decreased skin turgor evidenced by slow retraction of pinched skin (tenting). Most children recover from gastroenteritis without becoming dehydrated. For these children, standard electrolyte replacement solutions can be given or even a substitute such as lemonade (e.g. 7-up) at a dilution of 4 parts water to 1 part lemonade. Hypertonic dehydration, in which water loss is greater in proportion than sodium loss, occurs only rarely. In the past, hypertonic dehydration resulted from inappropriately high sodium solutions being given orally for treatment. In such cases, the plasma volume and therefore the peripheral perfusion are better preserved resulting in the degree of dehydration being underestimated.

While fluid maintenance remains the key clinical issue in children with acute gastroenteritis, the administration of chiropractic care both during the infection and immediately after symptomatic resolution is appropriate. The relationship between autonomic function and the subluxation has been well described in the scientific literature (Budgell 1998, Budgell & Sato 1996, Coote 1980, Sato 1980, Sato et al 1975) and symptomatic responses to chiropractic care defined by many authors (Biedermann 1992, Gutmann 1987, Kloughart et al 1989, Nilsson 1985). The primary purpose of chiropractic for children suffering with acute gastroenteritis is not so much to shorten the natural history of the infection as to maintain

neurological integrity which may have been disrupted by the toxic nature of the gut irritation producing a sensory overload via the visceral afferents.

Intussusception

The key symptoms and signs associated with intussusception are colicky pain lasting 2 or 3 minutes, occurring at intervals of about 15 minutes. Initially there may be screaming, but later there is only whimpering. Vomiting often occurs at the onset of the intussusception but commonly does not persist. Progressive pallor, tachycardia, lethargy and drowsiness are usually seen along with rectal bleeding, which is seen in 70% of presentations (Kuppermann et al 2000). This bleeding is traditionally referred to as a redcurrant jelly stool. A sausage-shaped mass either in the right hypochondrium or close to the umbilicus on the left side of the abdomen can be felt on light abdominal palpation. These principles are well illustrated in Case study 6.1.

While not particularly common, intussusception represents the most frequent cause of bowel obstruction in the first 2 years of life after the newborn period. Intussusception is a surgical emergency. While bowel infarction is uncommon in the first 24 hours, the risk increases after that. Air or barium enema reduction is successful in about three cases out of four. Unsuccessful cases are corrected surgically.

The only role for the chiropractor is diagnostic recognition and timely referral.

Appendicitis

The key symptom of acute appendicitis is abdominal pain beginning in the periumbilical area which then usually moves to the right lower abdominal quadrant within a few hours. The pain is increased by movement or coughing, so affected children tend to lie very still. Anorexia, nausea, a coated tongue, tenderness and guarding at McBurney's point, and a low grade fever are also seen.

Case study 6.1

Intussusception

A 4 month old male presented due to a return of colicky symptoms previously treated successfully with chiropractic care. At that time the subluxation was found at the upper cervical complex. There had been no further episodes of crying and pulling the legs up until the day of presentation 3 weeks after the adjustment. His mother said that his last bowel action had been the previous evening and he had become 'floppy and irritable' in the past few hours. The child was obviously distressed and pale. A right upper quadrant abdominal mass was found measuring approximately 2 cm in diameter, palpation of which appeared to cause him pain. There was no blood found on digital examination of the rectum. An abdominal X-ray suggested an intussusception, which was confirmed and successfully treated by air enema.

This case highlights the need for careful re-evaluation of infants on each visit since many abdominal conditions, whether serious or non-serious, may present with similar symptom patterns.

According to Hull & Johnston (1999), appendicitis is the most common cause of acute surgical emergency in childhood with approximately 4 children per 1000 undergoing appendectomy each year. The presentation in older children tends to follow the same pattern as that seen in adults where abdominal pain, fever, tenderness with muscle guarding in the right iliac fossa, and rebound tenderness are the key clinical signs. Appendicitis in a child with a retrocecally located appendix may have no localized guarding until later in the course of the illness. A diagnosis other than acute appendicitis may be suggested by signs such as vomiting, diarrhea or dysuria. In a young child who cannot describe the pain, appendicitis tends to present with fever, irritability, anorexia and vomiting.

When an appendix has ruptured, if the abscess has not been well walled off by omentum, the child will develop peritonitis. Initially, there will be a decrease in the pain, followed by signs which include decreased bowel sounds, generalized abdominal tenderness, guarding and evidence of shock.

Acute appendicitis is a surgical emergency and must be considered in the differential diagnosis of virtually every acute abdominal emergency in childhood. Clearly, the role of the chiropractor in such cases is to recognize the symptoms and signs suggestive of appendicitis and refer the child without delay.

Testicular torsion

Torsion of the testis is the most common cause of an acute scrotum at all age levels in pediatrics, but the peak incidence occurs in both infancy and adolescence. It is a painful condition, which in older children is caused by an abnormal fixation of the testis.

The presenting symptom is severe pain in the lower abdomen and scrotum which may come on suddenly or gradually. Clinical signs include scrotal swelling, with the testes tender, hard and swollen, and pulled up high in the scrotum.

Even if an alternative cause of the acute scrotum is considered likely, such as epididymo-orchitis or torsion of an appendix testis, urgent referral for consideration of surgical exploration is essential. Behrman et al (2007) report that surgical intervention performed within 6 hours of onset results in survival of the gonad in 90% of cases, while the survival rate decreases rapidly after that time.

Mesenteric adenitis

Mesenteric adenitis is the condition most likely to mimic appendicitis. Children with upper respiratory viral infections may develop associated lymphadenitis in the abdomen. The associated pain and tenderness is likely to be milder and less localized than in acute appendicitis. The presence of upper respiratory infection does not automatically exclude acute appendicitis. Appendicitis can and does occur during the course of other illnesses.

It is reasonable to manage children with mesenteric adenitis conservatively, with adequate fluids, analgesics and chiropractic care. The child should be reviewed regularly and, if the pain

should begin to localize to the right lower quadrant, immediate referral for a surgical opinion should be made. It is safer to find a normal appendix at laparotomy in a child with mesenteric adenitis than it is to delay surgical exploration of a child who later proves to have appendicitis.

Urinary tract infection

Infection of the urinary tract is common and presents differently at different ages. In infants and younger children, common symptoms include feeding problems with failure to thrive, vomiting, diarrhea, crying, irritability, prolonged neonatal jaundice, fever and septicemia. In older children, symptoms include urinary urgency and frequency, dysuria, pain in the abdomen or flank, fever, secondary nocturnal enuresis and gastrointestinal symptoms.

A child with one or more of these features in whom a urinary tract infection may be a possibility should be investigated with urinalysis and culture. In the office-based evaluation, if the urine is positive on a test strip for leukocytes, nitrites, blood or protein, then infection should be considered likely. However, a negative dipstick test for any of these does not necessarily exclude a urinary tract infection as a possible cause of the child's symptoms. Upper urinary tract infections are more likely in the child who appears to be more seriously ill and the implementation of antibiotic therapy without delay is essential in order to minimize the risk of permanent renal damage.

The chiropractic role in management of urinary tract infection is an important one. In conjunction with antibiotic therapy, the child should be assessed daily and adjusted when necessary. The toxic nature of the condition increases the likelihood of the development of cerebral dysafferentation via sensory overload from the affected site. Fluid intake and pain control measures should also be addressed. Since most urinary tract infections outside the newborn period are thought to be from ascending infection up the urethra, parents and caregivers should be counseled about the child's toileting hygiene. It may be appropriate to arrange for urinary tract imaging studies after resolution of the infection to check for both renal damage and an underlying anatomical cause for the infection in the first place.

Constipation and diarrhea

Under what conditions can a child be deemed to be constipated and what represents true diarrhea? The answers to these questions appear, at least on the surface, so obvious that time and space need not be devoted to answering them. In clinical practice, however, as the clinician responds to a complaint that a child is constipated, or has diarrhea, a clear understanding of the wide range of what represents normal bowel function is absolutely essential. In a study of 350 children aged 1–4 years, Weaver & Steiner (1984) found that the frequency of bowel actions for 96% of the study subjects was between one every second day and up to three each day. Clinical features of the patient's history in conjunction with physical findings and the appearance of the stool will allow you to make the correct diagnosis in about 75% of all cases involving diarrhea (McMillan et al 1977).

The key to determining that a child is actually constipated is related to excessively dry, hard to pass stools or a definite decrease in frequency. Chronic constipation is usually due to a functional disturbance that is sometimes associated with training errors. The most common cause, however, is from painful defecation causing voluntary withholding. In one study of 227 children with 'difficult defecation' it was found that 63% of the children presenting with fecal soiling from chronic constipation had a history of painful defecation beginning before 36 months of age (Partin et al 1992). As the 'portal of entry' clinician, the chiropractor is uniquely placed to both assess and successfully manage the constipated child. These children generally present with a complaint of constipation, abdominal pain or encopresis. Other associated problems include anorexia, poor weight gain and urinary tract problems. Children with chronic constipation have been reported to have daytime urinary incontinence (20%), nocturnal enuresis (33%), and recurrent urinary tract infections in girls (10%) (Loening-Baucke 1989). In another case series study on primary enuresis (van Poecke & Cunliffe 2009), constipation was identified as a clinical issue in 40% of the study sample.

The clinical history and examination should specifically seek answers to the following clinical questions.

Breastfed infants

In breastfed infants, the chiropractor needs to determine if there is indeed true constipation, or rather normal bowel actions every few days. Breastfed infants may have a normal bowel pattern within the range from one bowel evacuation every 2 weeks to 24 per day (Illingworth 1983, Ulshen 1996). Even though there are infrequent bowel actions, if the consistency remains loose and there is no difficulty passing them, then the child is not constipated.

Bottlefed infants

Clein (1954) found that 6% of children with allergy to cow's milk protein suffered from constipation that responded to withdrawal of cow's milk from the diet. In a double-blind study of 65 consecutive cases of chronic 'idiopathic' constipation, Iacono et al (1998) found that 44 had resolution of symptoms after withdrawal of cow's milk protein and reappearance of symptoms when challenged with cow's milk protein. Protein and carbohydrate hypersensitivity and allergy syndromes are more fully discussed in Chapter 5.

Occasionally, otherwise apparently well babies that are being bottlefed pass hard stools. In this situation the chiropractor should seek to discover if the baby:

- is getting sufficient fluid
- is sweating excessively
- is overclothed – especially during hot weather
- has passed any bright red blood – especially in a 'striped toothpaste' pattern indicating an anal fissure.

Toilet training errors

Have the parents begun a toilet training program which compels the child to 'sit on potty' against his or her will? This aberrant parental conditioning frequently results in troublesome constipation.

Dietary and genetic factors

Is there a family history of chronic constipation or loose stools? There may be a genetic tendency toward a short or prolonged intestinal transit time. Weaver & Steiner (1984) in their study of preschool children found a mean transit time of 33 hours.

Is the family diet appropriate? A dietary analysis is always appropriate when a child is suffering from true constipation. An excess of highly processed foods to the detriment of cereals, fruit, vegetables and adequate fluids is a common problem.

Medication schedule

Has the child been given laxatives over a protracted period? The child's medication schedule should always be checked against the current edition of a drug compendium for pharmacokinetics and known adverse reactions.

Polyuria

Does the child have a pattern of polyuria and polydipsia? If so, there may be a metabolic reason for the constipation, such as diabetes insipidus.

Psychological factors

Chronic bowel motility changes in a child may be caused by an abusive situation at home. Intentional injury and child maltreatment is thoroughly discussed in Chapter 16. Such patients require urgent referral to the appropriate authority or a child psychologist if there is reasonable concern arising from the history and physical assessment. Psychological problems may be involved in the initiation of the cycle of withholding and functional constipation. Many children become withdrawn, deny the soiling, and start defecating in inappropriate places. Poor self-esteem and poor peer relationships follow. These children may well benefit from referral to a child psychologist. These principles are illustrated in Case study 6.2.

The chiropractic approach to management

Children with constipation and their parents and caregivers need counseling and an explanation of the problem. They should be advised in relation to adequate hydration and the role of a balanced diet. They should be encouraged to have adequate vegetables and fruit and to avoid an excessive intake of refined carbohydrates. They should be encouraged to take adequate levels of laxative medication to maintain a regular

Case study 6.2

Constipation

A 6-year-old female, well known to the author, was brought in by her mother complaining of constipation. In the past few weeks this little girl had gone from twice-daily bowel movements to not having passed any stool for 5 days. During the interview, the patient, who had always previously been friendly and somewhat high-spirited, was noticeably withdrawn and clinging to her mother. In addition to the constipation, her mother reported that she had begun waking up because of nightmares, had gone off her food, and did not seem to have any energy. On further questioning, her mother broke down in tears and reported that the child's symptoms had begun at the same time that her husband had begun physically assaulting her in front of the child.

This case highlights the principle that constipation that has a definite timing to the onset usually has a definable cause. In this case, the common signs of abuse were present.

bowel pattern so the cycle of withholding and stool retention can be successfully treated.

The presence of small amounts of bright red blood may indicate an anal fissure. These are caused by small tears in the anal skin from the passage of a large, hard stool. Most fissures occur in the anterior or posterior midline. They heal quickly but can contribute greatly to the child's effort to withhold stool in order to avoid further pain. Many children have bright red blood loss without any cause being identified. This bleeding is commonly associated with congestion of the normal submucous venous plexus while straining at stool (Hutson et al 1992). If, however, there is persistent, unexplained bleeding, the child should be referred for proctoscopy and possible further investigation.

Hirschsprung's disease occurs in about 1 in 5000 infants. It results from the absence of ganglion cells in the bowel wall extending proximally from the anus for a variable distance. In a study of 203 consecutive cases of neonatal bowel obstruction (excluding imperforate anus) at the Royal Children's Hospital, Melbourne, it was found that 25% were due to Hirschsprung's disease (Hutson et al 1992). This condition should be considered in any child who has delayed passage of the first meconium stool beyond 48 hours, as 99% of all neonates will have passed meconium by then (Behrman et al 2007). Occasionally, children who have only a very short aganglionic segment of bowel may present later with chronic constipation, abdominal distension and failure to thrive. They may have stool palpable throughout the abdomen but with an empty rectum on digital examination. These children frequently have a history of chronic laxative use and frequent suppositories or enemas to achieve bowel actions. They need specialist investigation that may include manometry, radiology and rectal biopsy. Children with confirmed Hirschsprung's disease require surgical intervention.

Constipation in children is, in the main, however, a functional condition that responds favorably to chiropractic management (Biedermann 1992, Budgell 1998, Gutmann 1987) coupled with sensible parental counseling, as outlined above.

The correction of patterns of cerebral dysafferentation by the chiropractor may have a helpful effect in restoring normal gastrointestinal function. The authors' experience, however, is that successful outcomes, while they do occur regularly, remain sporadic and somewhat unpredictable on a case-by-case basis. Outcomes may possibly be linked with patient adherence to dietary advice and psychological management of the child. The use of laxatives should be encouraged in order to empty the colon and prevent reaccumulation of stool while normal function is being restored (Loening-Baucke 1989, Nolan et al 1991).

The child with chronic diarrhea

Many children are said by their mothers to have chronic diarrhea when in fact they have normal bowel function. There is a very wide range of normal bowel frequency and consistency. The stools of breastfed infants may range in color from yellow to bright green and may be explosive in nature and contain milk curd. It is appropriate to ask if there has been a marked increase in stool frequency, offensive smell, blood, pus or mucus noted. The presence of any of these features would suggest that the pattern is pathological. As children progress to a mixed food diet, their bowel action increasingly takes on adult characteristics. While the cause of acute diarrhea is usually infectious and short-lived, chronic diarrhea requires further consideration.

A clinical hypothesis of a functional increase in gastrointestinal motility owing to the effects of functional neurological imbalance is reasonable and evidence-based (Biedermann 1992, Budgell 1998, Gutmann 1987). Before the implementation of chiropractic care, however, one should determine that the following key clinical signs that indicate the need for specialist referral are not present.

Medication schedule

Drugs such as antibiotics may cause diarrhea. Check each medication against a standard drug compendium such as MIMS and refer to the family general practitioner for review if necessary.

Psychological factors

Chronic diarrhea, as with chronic constipation, may be due to the existence of an abusive situation at home and needs to be similarly referred. There may also be other emotional stress factors that need to be considered.

Pathological factors

Chronic diarrhea with significant bleeding, melena, mucus or steatorrhea is likely to have a pathological basis and needs referral for medical or surgical investigation. Conditions that need to be considered include Crohn's disease, ulcerative colitis, Meckel's diverticulitis and chronic infection.

The incidence of Crohn's disease has been steadily increasing (Armitage et al 2001) and is now around 1 in 2500 children (Roberton & South 2007). It may present with recurrent abdominal pain, anemia, anorexia or growth failure. The incidence of ulcerative colitis, the other inflammatory bowel disease commonly seen in children, has been static over the same time period at about 1 in 10 000 (Kirschner 1988). If children are thought to have either of these conditions, they should be referred for investigations such as endoscopy.

Celiac disease is a small intestinal inflammatory disorder characterized by an immune-mediated enteropathy triggered by the ingestion of gluten from wheat and related cereals in genetically predisposed individuals carrying the human leukocyte antigens (HLA)-DQ2 or -DQ8 (Abdullah et al 2007). In the latter decades of the last century, celiac disease, unlike Crohn's disease, was decreasing in many countries of the world and by the 1990s was considered to be a rare condition in childhood (Martin 2008, Rodrigo 2006). The incidence in the UK, for example, was estimated to be as low as 1 child in 11 000 (Challacombe et al 1997). The reason for this decreasing trend appeared to be associated with changing infant feeding practices characterized by later introduction of dietary gluten, increased use of baby rice and gluten-free foods for weaning, and an increased incidence of initial breastfeeding (Challacombe et al 1997). From the middle to late 1990s, however, this situation changed and the incidence of celiac disease is now increasing to the point that it is referred to in the scientific literature as one of the commonest lifelong disorders worldwide (Fasano 2005). The incidence is now cited by researchers as falling somewhere between 1 in 100 (Scherer 2008, See & Murray 2006) and 1 in 300 (Cardenas & Kelly 2002). Classically, the condition presented with malabsorption and failure to thrive in infancy, but this picture has now been overtaken by the much more common presentation in adults, usually with non-specific symptoms such as tiredness and anemia, disturbance in bowel habit, or following low-impact bone fractures (McGough & Cummings 2005). Diagnosis has been made so much easier by the development of serological testing for IgA autoantibodies to the enzyme tissue transglutaminase (tTG), a component of endomysium (Schuppan et al 2005, Sherer 2008). Serological testing for serum IgA tTG has very high sensitivity and specificity (Cardenas & Kelly 2002), meaning the test outcome has a high predictive value (Schuppan et al 2005), and is therefore the mainstay of disease screening. The diagnostic gold standard, however, remains duodenal biopsy (Cardenas & Kelly 2002, Rodrigo 2006).

Celiac disease should be considered in any child with failure to thrive and bowel symptoms that appear after ingestion of wheat products. These children may have anorexia, abdominal bloating, fatty stools and mouth ulcers. Celiac disease is a lifelong disease in which the patient shows intolerance to gluten with associated atrophy of the mucosal villi of the small intestine. There is no place for a trial withdrawal of gluten prior to diagnostic evaluation as this may cause false-negative blood tests and create other diagnostic difficulties, especially on duodenal biopsy. While the diagnostic test series is not negotiable, there is no obvious reason why an affected child cannot receive chiropractic care while undergoing the tests.

Substance hypersensitivity – a special clinical scenario

Cow's milk and soy protein allergy are common causes of diarrhea in the first year of life (Sondheimer 1997). These gut reactions, mediated as they are via the viscerosomatic reflex pathways, are highly neuroirritant and cause recurrent patterns of cerebral dysafferentation. Only those infants with weight loss or evidence of failure to thrive should be referred for specialist investigation in the first instance. Most patients respond quickly to chiropractic care and dietary manipulation. Management of patients with substance hypersensitivity and allergy is discussed in Chapter 5.

The chiropractic approach to management

When the cause of chronic diarrhea can confidently be identified as functional, it is appropriate to implement chiropractic care. In addition, parents should be carefully counseled in regard to the child's personal hygiene, diet and toileting procedures. Chronic, non-specific diarrhea syndrome of childhood is the most common cause of chronic diarrhea in children. In some instances, this is due to the consumption of apple juice that has been produced by enzymatic processing of apple pulp. During this processing operation, non-absorbable monosaccharides and oligosaccharides are produced which cause diarrhea. Freshly pressed and unprocessed 'cloudy' apple juice is less likely to produce diarrhea (Hoekstra et al 1995).

Intestinal parasite infestation

It is not uncommon for children, especially those who are at school or in day care centers, to contract a parasitic infestation. Generally, the child incessantly scratches the anal area, as the worms cause perianal and vulval pruritus. Other symptoms include weight loss from malabsorption, abdominal pain and, rarely, intestinal obstruction.

Threadworm (*Enterobius*) infestation is very common and may be readily diagnosed by asking the parents to inspect the anal orifice of the sleeping child. The mobile thread-like worms may be seen then, or recognized later in a stool sample. A perianal scotch tape test may be done to detect eggs on the perianal skin. Generally, the child with threadworm infestation scratches the perineum because of perianal and vulval pruritus caused by worms.

Roundworms (*Ascaris lumbricoides*) are contracted by ingesting eggs found normally in soil. They migrate by the portal system to the lungs and bronchus where they may cause pneumonitis and eosinophilia. Less commonly, they cause gut symptoms such as malabsorption syndrome and obstruction.

Hookworms (*Ancylostoma*) are found in children who live in hot, humid climates such as those encountered in tropical areas of the world. Hookworm infestation can be a serious cause of iron deficiency anemia in these areas that may be recognized by excessive tiredness, the presence of petechial hemorrhages, especially on the palate, bruising and pale mucous membranes.

The flagellate protozoan *Giardia lamblia* is contracted from infected children or from contaminated food and water. Infected children may have anorexia with abdominal pain, malabsorption and weight loss. More than one stool sample may need to be examined for *Giardia lamblia* cysts as they will not be seen on inspection of one stool sample in about 50% of affected children. A careful clinical history should raise the possibility of this condition in the clinician's mind.

Parasitic infestation always warrants aggressive interventional therapy that is best administered under medical care.

References

Abdullah, F., Arnold, M.A., Nabaweesi, R., et al., 2007. Gastoschisis in the United States 1998–2003: analysis and risk categorization of 4344 patients. J. Perinatol. 27 (1), 50–55.

Armitage, E., Drummond, H.E., Wilson, D.C., et al., 2001. Increasing incidence of both juvenile-onset Crohn's disease and ulcerative colitis in Scotland. Eur. J. Gastroenterol. Hepatol. 13 (12), 1439–1447.

Behrman, R.E., Jenson, H.B., Nelson, W.E., et al., 2007. Nelson Textbook of Pediatrics, eighteenth ed. WB Saunders, Philadelphia.

Biedermann, H., 1992. Kinematic imbalances due to suboccipital strain in newborns. J. Man. Med. 6, 151–156.

Budgell, B., 1998. A Neurophysiological Rationale for the Chiropractic Management of Visceral Disorders. Seminar Proceedings of the International College of Chiropractic, Friday Forum Series, February 6, Sydney, Australia.

Budgell, B., Sato, A., 1996. Modulations of autonomic functions by somatic nociceptive inputs. Prog. Brain Res. 113, 525–539.

Cardenas, A., Kelly, C.P., 2002. Celiac sprue. Semin. Gastrointest. Dis. 13 (4), 232–244.

Challacombe, D.N., Mecrow, I.K., Elliott, K., et al., 1997. Changing infant feeding practices and declining incidence of coeliac disease in west Somerset. Arch. Dis. Child. 77, 206–209.

Clein, N.W., 1954. Cow's milk allergy in infants. Pediatr. Clin. North Am. 4, 949–962.

Coote, J.H., 1980. Central organization of somatosympathetic reflexes. In: Haldemann, S. (Ed.), Modern Developments in the Principles and Practice of Chiropractic. Appleton Century Crofts, New York.

Fasano, A., 2005. Clinical presentation of celiac disease in the pediatric population. Gastroenterology 128 (4 Suppl. 1), S68–S73.

Gutmann, G., 1987. Blocked atlantal nerve syndrome in infants and small children. J. Man. Med. 25, 5–10.

Hoekstra, J., van den Aker, J.H., Ghoos, Y.F., et al., 1995. Fluid intake and industrial processing in apple juice induced chronic non-specific diarrhea. Arch. Dis. Child. 73 (2), 126–130.

Hull, D., Johnston, D., 1999. Essential Paediatrics, fourth ed. Churchill Livingstone, Edinburgh.

Hutson, J., Beasley, S., Woodward, A., 1992. Jones Clinical Paediatric Surgery: Diagnosis and Management, fourth ed. Blackwell Science Publications, Melbourne.

Iacono, G., Cavataio, F., Montalto, G., et al., 1998. Intolerance of cow's milk and chronic constipation in children. N. Engl. J. Med. 336 (16), 1100–1104.

Illingworth, R.S., 1983. Common Symptoms of Disease in Childhood, nineth ed. Blackwell, London, p. 90.

Kirschner, B.S., 1988. Inflammatory bowel disease in childhood. Pediatr. Clin. North Am. 35 (1), 189–208.

Kloughart, N., Nilsson, N., Jacobsen, J., 1989. Infantile colic treated by chiropractors: a prospective study of 316 cases. J. Manipulative Physiol. Ther. 12, 281–288.

Kuppermann, N., O'Dea, T., Pinkney, L., et al., 2000. Predictors of intussusception in young children. Arch. Pediatr. Adolesc. Med. 154 (3), 250–255.

Loening-Baucke, V., 1989. Factors determining outcome in children with chronic constipation and faecal soiling. Gut 30, 999–1006.

McGough, N., Cummings, J.H., 2005. Coeliac disease: a diverse clinical syndrome caused by intolerance of wheat, barley and rye. Proc. Nutr. Soc. 64 (4), 434–450.

McMillan, J.A., Nieberg, P.I., Oski, F.A., 1977. The Whole Paediatrician Catalogue: A Compendium of Clues to Diagnosis and Management. WB Saunders, Philadelphia, p. 278.

Martin, S., 2008. Against the grain: an overview of celiac disease. J. Am. Acad. Nurse Pract. 20 (5), 243–250.

Nilsson, N., 1985. Infantile colic and chiropractic. Eur. J. Chiropractic 33, 624–625.

Nolan, T., Debelle, G., Oberklaid, F., et al., 1991. Randomised trial of laxatives in treatment of childhood encopresis. Lancet 338, 523–527.

Partin, J.C., Hamill, R.N., Fischel, J., et al., 1992. Painful defecation and fecal soiling in children. Pediatrics 89, 1007–1009.

Roberton, D.M., South, M.J., 2007. Practical Paediatrics, sixth ed. Churchill Livingstone, Edinburgh.

Rodrigo, L., 2006. Celiac disease. World J. Gastroenterol. 12 (41), 6585–6593.

Sato, A., 1980. Physiological studies of the somatoautonomic reflexes. In: Haldemann, S. (Ed.), Modern Developments in the Principles and Practice of Chiropractic. Appleton Century Croft, New York.

Sato, A., Saot, Y., Shimada, F., et al., 1975. Changes in gastric motility produced by nociceptive stimulation of the skin in rats. Brain Res. 87, 151–159.

Scherer, J.R., 2008. Celiac disease. Drugs Today (Barc) 44 (1), 75–88.

Schuppan, D., Dennis, M.D., Kelly, C.P., 2005. Celiac disease: epidemiology, pathogenesis, diagnosis, and nutritional management. Nutr. Clin. Care 8 (2), 54–69.

See, J., Murray, J.A., 2006. Gluten-free diet: the medical and nutrition management of celiac disease. Nutr. Clin. Pract. 21 (1), 1–15.

Sherer, Y., 2008. Issues in rheumatology and autoimmunity. Preface. Isr. Med. Assoc. J. 10 (2), 138.

Sondheimer, J., 1997. Gastrointestinal tract. In: Hay, W.W., Groothius, J.R., Haywayd, A.R. et al. (Eds), Current Pediatric Diagnosis and Treatment, thirteenth ed. Appleton & Lange, Stamford.

Ulshen, M., 1996. Normal digestive tract phenomena. In: Behrman, R., Kliegman, R., Arvin, A. (Eds), Nelson Textbook of Pediatrics, fifteenth ed. WB Saunders, Philadelphia.

van Poecke, A.J., Cunliffe, C., 2009. Chiropractic treatment for primary nocturnal enuresis: a case series of 33 consecutive patients. J. Maip. Physiol. Therap. 32 (8), 675–681.

Weaver, L.T., Steiner, H., 1984. The bowel habit of young children. Arch. Dis. Child. 59, 649–652.

Pediatric neurology

7

Allan G. J. Terrett   Neil J. Davies

The pediatric neurological examination

The neurological examination is designed to establish the location of dysfunction in the nervous system. Owing to the local nature of many pathological and functional processes affecting the nervous system, an understanding of functional anatomy forms the foundation for diagnosis and, to an extent, management. In the neurological examination of the pediatric patient, at least two questions need to be answered:

• Is there any evidence to suggest a focal lesion?
• Has maturation and development appropriate for the child's age occurred?

This chapter will concentrate on the first 5 years of life, during which maturation of the nervous system is one of the major pediatric assessments. In conjunction with the phenomenon of lesion localization, maturational testing is a critical factor. As the child grows older, the maturational factors quickly become less significant and the examination of the nervous system more adult-like.

In the examination of very young children one needs to keep in mind that, while their responses are chiefly reflex in nature, they are closely dependent upon both maturity and current physical condition. The state of alertness, drowsiness, hunger or satiation at the time of examination will have marked effects upon the results. A child that has been recently fed is a poor candidate for neurological examination.

The neurological examination in the neonate and small child is, by necessity, based heavily on historical data provided by the parents, the process of observation and the normal symmetrical responses to tests. As such, the parents or caregiver accompanying the child should be carefully evaluated as to their reliability as historians before definite conclusions are drawn from historical data about neurological maturation.

A review of relevant functional and clinical neuroanatomy

Much of the nervous system is not functionally effective in infancy; patients are unable to cooperate with the examiner, nor can they respond to commands which are necessary in order to test aspects of the sensory examination (only pain and touch can be assessed in the newborn), cerebellum, sensorium, etc. Therefore the examiner has to deal largely with gross responses and attributes of lower levels of organization.

The somatic motor system

The major cortical units (but not all) of the corticospinal and corticobulbar systems are located in the posterior frontal lobe (precentral region, Brodmann area 4) and the premotor region (extrapyramidal cortex, Brodmann area 6). In the cortex there is a definite localization of function. Skeletal musculature is represented in reverse order upon the contralateral (precentral gyrus) motor area (Fig. 7.1).

The axons of the upper motor neurons pass caudally through the corona radiata, into the internal capsule, and down the ventral basis of the brainstem. Brainstem (cranial nerve) motor nuclei receive both crossed and uncrossed innervation (except the lower facial muscles) from the corticobulbar tracts. At the caudal portion of the medulla, the majority of the fibers destined for the spinal cord decussate (cross) to descend as the lateral corticospinal tracts (Fig. 7.2). These terminate at appropriate levels to supply the anterior motor horn cells in the spinal cord. The axons from the cranial nerve nuclei and anterior motor horn cells are the final common (efferent) pathway to the neuromuscular junction of striated muscles.

In the newborn infant the corticospinal system has little or no myelin sheathing. The process of myelination starts immediately after birth and is usually complete by the age of 2 years.

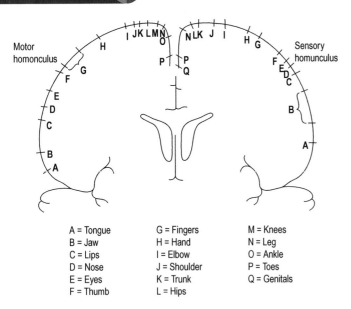

A = Tongue   G = Fingers   M = Knees
B = Jaw   H = Hand   N = Leg
C = Lips   I = Elbow   O = Ankle
D = Nose   J = Shoulder   P = Toes
E = Eyes   K = Trunk   Q = Genitals
F = Thumb   L = Hips

Figure 7.1 • The order in which the motor and sensory functions in the body are represented upon the contralateral cortex.

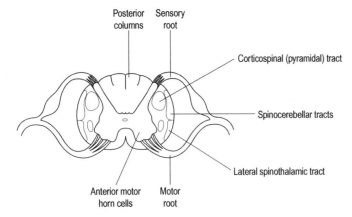

Figure 7.2 • Anatomy of the spinal cord in cross-sectional view.

Skilled movements of the upper limb and then walking are learned as the pathway matures and myelination progresses.

A lesion of the corticobulbar tracts produces little deficit, because of the bilateral cortical innervation to the brainstem nuclei (except for the muscles of the lower face).

A lesion of the corticospinal tracts causes weakness and spasticity.

A lesion of the anterior horn cells (lower motor neurons) produces weakness, muscle wasting, fasciculations and hyporeflexia or areflexia.

The somatic sensory system

In the newborn and infant, only pain and touch can be evaluated.

Impulses that carry superficial pain and temperature sensation arise in nociceptors, free or branched nerve endings. They travel along unmyelinated or thinly myelinated nerve endings to the dorsal root ganglion (the first cell body), then enter the dorsal spinal cord where they synapse in the substantia gelatinosa (the second cell body). They then cross the midline (anterior to the central canal) to ascend in the lateral spinothalamic tract (see Fig. 7.2) up the spinal cord, through the brainstem tegmentum (where they join the trigeminal pathways), to the ventral posterolateral (VPL) nucleus of the thalamus. The fibers then ascend to the parietal lobe, where the body is again represented in the reverse order, on the contralateral cortex, in the postcentral gyrus, so that the cortical area for right leg sensation abuts the cortical area for right leg movement.

Fibers that carry touch sensation have their origin in specialized end organs, Merkel's discs (general tactile sensibility) and Meissner's corpuscles (localized tactile sensibility). These travel to the dorsal root ganglion (the first cell body) and enter the dorsal spinal cord. Those fibers from Merkel's discs communicate with collaterals, cross the midline to the opposite ventral spinothalamic tract, and ascend to the thalamus. Those fibers from Meissner's corpuscles enter the dorsal spinal cord to enter the ipsilateral posterior column (fasciculus gracilis or cuneatus) (see Fig. 7.2), and ascend uncrossed and without synapse to the nuclei gracilis or cuneatus in the lower medulla, where they decussate as the arcuate fibers and ascend as the medial lemniscus to the thalamus. From the thalamus, touch fibers are carried (with those from the trigeminal nerve) to the same areas of the parietal cortex, as are those for pain and temperature.

The brainstem

The brainstem consists of three transverse subdivisions, the mesencephalon (midbrain), pons and medulla oblongata (Fig. 7.3), and three longitudinal unit subdivisions, the basis (anteriorly), the tegmentum and the tectum (Fig. 7.4). The structures found within these three subdivisions are shown in Table 7.1. The cerebellum is not part of the tectum, but evolved from the vestibular nuclei of the pontomedullary tegmentum.

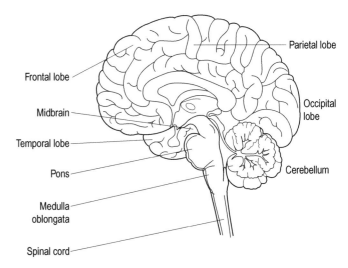

Figure 7.3 • The brainstem consists of three transverse subdivisions, namely the mesencephalon (midbrain), pons and medulla.

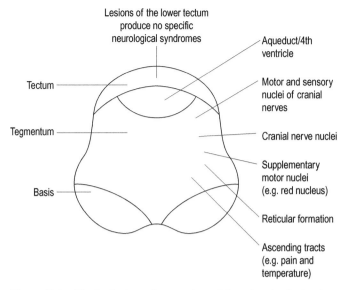

Figure 7.4 ● The brainstem also consists of three longitudinal unit subdivisions, namely the basis (anteriorly), the tegmentum and the tectum.

Table 7.1 Structures found with the three longitudinal unit subdivisions of the brainstem

Subdivision	Structure
The basis	Corticospinal and corticobulbar tracts
The tegmentum	Cranial nerve nuclei III–X and XII (motor and sensory)
	Supplementary motor nuclei (substantia nigra, red nucleus, inferior olivary nucleus)
	Ascending sensory tracts: medial longitudinal fasciculus, medial lemniscus (continuation of posterior columns), spinal and trigeminal lemniscus (pain and temperature sensation from the face and body), lateral lemniscus (hearing)
	Descending sympathetic pathway (between the descending tract of V and the ascending lateral spinothalamic tract)
	Reticular formation
The tectum	Quadrigeminal plate
	Medullary vela

The cranial nerves

Cranial nerves I and II are not true cranial nerves, but direct extensions of the brain.

The components, nuclei, and location of nuclei of the cranial nerves that convey motor function are summarized in Table 7.2.

The components, nuclei and location of nuclei of the cranial nerves that convey sensory function are summarized in Table 7.3.

Fig. 7.5 illustrates the anatomical arrangement of the visual pathway and visual deficits that are produced by lesions found in various positions along that pathway.

The neurological history and examination of the neonate, infant and toddler

The neurological examination of the newborn can be considered under three main headings:

- tonus
- primary or automatic reactions
- aspects common to older subjects, such as sensation and muscle reflexes.

The examination of the nervous system which should be performed by a chiropractor during the first year of a child's life is essentially a gross screening exercise, and is reliable for detecting extensive CNS disease. The examination is of little use, however, in pinpointing minute lesions or specific functional deficits because much of the nervous system is not yet functionally effective.

The central nervous system at birth lacks maturation and functions at subcortical levels. Cortical function develops slowly after birth and cannot be tested in its entirety until early childhood. Thus, in the newborn period and early infancy, findings of normal brainstem and spinal cord function do not ensure an intact cortical system. Abnormalities of the brainstem and spinal cord may exist without concomitant cortical abnormalities. There are a number of specific reflex activities (infantile automatisms) found in normal newborns that disappear in early infancy.

Important aspects of the clinical history

Pregnancy and birth details should be obtained. The duration of labor, the fetal presentation, drugs used during pregnancy and delivery, and any neonatal difficulties should be noted. Maternal history of alcohol use should be established, since measurable effects in reflexive behavior, delays in maturation of the motor system, muscle tone, the need for stimulation and tremulousness have been demonstrated in infants born to mothers who drink (Coles et al 1985). Tobacco, marijuana and drug abuse during pregnancy should also be noted. Neuromuscular signs such as convulsions, hypotonia, hypertonia, absence of the Moro reflex, and tremor seen in the perinatal period are associated with serious neurological disease which may not become evident until neurological maturation begins to occur (Saito et al 1983).

Familial history

A child who comes from a family that has any history at all of genetically transmitted neuromuscular disease should be carefully watched over a prolonged period for any abnormal signs or aberrations in developmental pattern, as they will not usually be apparent until further maturation of the nervous system occurs.

Medication schedule

If the patient is medicated at the time of presentation, a complete drug regimen is necessary. Some drugs may produce side-effects involving the neuromuscular system.

Table 7.2 Components, nuclei and nuclei locations of the cranial nerves that convey motor function

Cranial nerve	Somitic efferent nuclei	Branchial efferent nuclei	Visceral efferent nuclei	Location of nuclei
III	Oculomotor			Midbrain
			Edinger–Westphal	Midbrain
IV	Trochlear			Midbrain
V		Trigeminal nucleus		Pons
VI	Abducens			Pons
VII		Facial nucleus		Pons
			Superior salivatory nucleus	Pons
IX		Nucleus ambiguus		Medulla
			Inferior salivatory nucleus	Pons
X		Nucleus ambiguus		Medulla
			Dorsal motor nucleus	Medulla
XI (accessory)*		Nucleus ambiguus		Medulla
XII	Hypoglossal			Medulla

*The lower motor neurons of the spinal portion of cranial nerve XI are located at cervical levels 1–5

Table 7.3 Components, nuclei and nuclei locations of the cranial nerves that convey sensory function

Cranial nerve	Pain and temperature	Touch	Hearing	Taste	Location of nucleus
V	Spinal nucleus	Main sensory nucleus			Upper cervical spine Pons
VII				Nucleus solitarius	Medulla
VIII			Cochlear nucleus		Pontomedullary junction
IX				Nucleus solitarius	Medulla
X				Nucleus solitarius	Medulla

Developmental history

A general understanding of the child's development should be established and, in particular, language development may represent an early sign of mental retardation or depressed brain development.

Coordination

The parents should be questioned regarding the nature of the infant's movements. Are they spastic and/or jerky? Are they

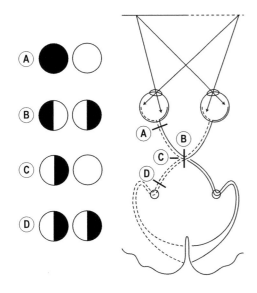

Figure 7.5 • Anatomical arrangement of the visual pathway and the visual deficits that are produced by lesions found in various positions along that pathway. (A) Blindness in one eye is due to damage of the retina, or one optic nerve, which may be due to a tumor or prolonged optic atrophy; (B) bitemporal hemianopsia is due to chiasmal lesions such as pituitary tumors or craniopharyngiomas; (C) nasal hemianopsia is due to a lesion lateral to the optic chiasm; and (D) lesions of the optic tract behind the lateral geniculate body produce homonymous hemianopsias. Lesions of the parietal lobe produce an inferior homonymous quadrantanopia, whereas lesions of the temporal lobe produce a superior homonymous quadrantanopia.

unilaterally depressed? Does the child assume a fixed posture? Even though the doctor will observe the child for these signs, the parents may have noticed something that will not occur during the course of the consultation.

Birthweight
Children with a very low birthweight have a high incidence of delayed motor development and persistent primitive reflexes (Marquis et al 1984).

Behavioral issues
Previously identified issues such as hyperkinesis, short attention span, impulsivity and depression should be noted and may need to be explored further.

Observation

Accurate detection of neurological pathology in young children frequently depends upon the observation of patterns of signs seen during history-taking and examination. The following observations are among the most common and important.

Posture

The normal child will not maintain a fixed posture. The following fixed postures should be considered to have clinical significance.

Fisting with thumb adduction
For the first 2 months of life the hands are shut most of the time with the thumb adducted across the palm. By the end of the second month, persistent 'fisting' (i.e. hand shut with the thumb adducted across the palm) may indicate a delay in motor development, and if one-sided may suggest hemiplegia. Children demonstrating persistent 'fisting' into and beyond the third month of life, especially if there are other signs of developmental delay or neurological deficit, should be referred for specialist investigation.

Scissoring of the legs
This is an early sign of hypertonicity (spasticity) and should be monitored for improvement as the infant receives chiropractic care. If this sign persists after successful management of the subluxation complex, the patient should be referred for specialist evaluation.

The 'frog-leg' position
This is a position in which the infant holds the arms in abduction, the hips in abduction and flexion, and the knees in flexion. This is a characteristic posture adopted by the hypotonic infant (Weiner et al 1981). It is important to assess whether the hypotonic baby is 'floppy and weak' or 'floppy and strong'. The infant who is both floppy and weak usually has a lower motor problem while the infant who is floppy but retains normal strength usually has an upper motor neuron cause or non-neurological cause such as Marfan syndrome (Harris et al 1992). The majority of children (75%) presenting with hypotonia between the ages of 6 months and 21 years have either perinatal encephalopathy (cerebral palsy) or idiopathic mental and motor retardation (Weiner et al 1981). Collective

chiropractic experience with idiopathic hypotonia has shown encouraging results, with some children having spontaneous remission with as little as one adjustment. There are many causes for hypotonia, however, and these are discussed later in this chapter.

The baby's cry characteristics

A baby that has a high-pitched piercing type of cry may have raised intracranial pressure and should be carefully assessed by fundoscopic inspection, measuring the head circumference and comparing the value to previous measurements on a standard percentile chart, checking the eyes for a setting sun sign, assessing the skull with transillumination and for Macewen's 'cracked pot' sign in children with a closed anterior fontanel (Barness 1981). Raised intracranial pressure is discussed more fully later in this chapter. A high-pitched cry has also been linked to maternal alcohol consumption and cigarette smoking (Nugent et al 1996).

A baby with a very hoarse type of cry may have cretinism, laryngeal abnormality referred to as a floppy larynx or glottal instability (Golub & Corwin 1982). If this infant has respiratory difficulty, sleeps excessively, is a poor sleeper and is generally sluggish, it should be immediately referred to a pediatrician for thyroid evaluation.

A 'floppy baby' with a feeble type of cry, physical evidence of hypotonia (frog-like posture when supine), dyspnea and feeding difficulties may reasonably be suspected of having Werdnig–Hoffmann disease (infantile spinal muscular atrophy) (Weiner et al 1981). The mother may suspect something was wrong during her pregnancy because of poor fetal movements late in the third trimester. This is a serious, inherited disease involving degeneration of the anterior horn cells which results in spinal muscular atrophy (the face is usually spared). This infant would also be areflexive, but fasciculations are not visible owing to the subcutaneous fat. Werdnig–Hoffmann disease (spinal muscular atrophy) has a very poor prognosis, usually resulting in death within the first year of life because of respiratory muscle paralysis.

Changes in the nature and duration of crying may be influenced by maternal substance abuse and drug addiction. In particular, babies of cocaine and marijuana abusers have been shown to have fewer cry utterances, shorter periods of crying, and less crying in the hyperphonation mode (Corwin et al 1992, Lester & Dreher 1989).

Ankle clonus

Brief ankle clonus may be normal in the first few weeks of life, but it exhausts itself after a few seconds. Sustained ankle clonus at any age is abnormal, and indicates corticospinal tract damage. Sustained ankle clonus, brought on by sharp dorsiflexion of the foot, may be indicative of a child who could suffer in the future from epileptic-type seizures. The child should be given chiropractic care and monitored for satisfactory change. Experience indicates that the upper cervical subluxation complex is capable of producing this clonic response. The patient should be thoroughly evaluated for any other signs of an upper motor neuron lesion (spasticity, hyperreflexia, Babinski response) which if found indicates the need for referral.

Rapid tremors

Rapid tremors may be caused by changes in blood calcium and glucose levels. Tetany and hypoglycemia are among the more common causes. However, rapid tremors may also occur without obvious cause (DeMyer 1994), making a short trial of chiropractic care an appropriate management strategy.

Asymmetrical spontaneous movement

The clinician should be aware that this may represent a focal lesion in the central or peripheral nervous system, but also be aware at the same time that it may be the result of an upper cervical subluxation complex or, if only one limb is involved, a local motion segment subluxation at the appropriate spinal level.

Facial ptosis

If the sign is associated with physical evidence of generalized hypotonia, the patient should be referred for specialist evaluation, as these are primary early signs of myasthenia gravis. This child would need pharmacological assessment (Tensilon test). If the ptosis exists as a single finding, VIIth cranial nerve inflammation (Bell's palsy) is the most likely diagnosis and the child should be given chiropractic care. Some facial neuropathies improve substantially within hours to days after the implementation of chiropractic care.

Sustained opisthotonos

Sustained opisthotonos (hyperextension of the cervical, thoracic and lumbar spines with flexion of the knees and elbows) is frequently seen in toxoplasmosis and meningitis, although not in the early stages of the infection. It is also seen in meningeal irritation, intracranial hemorrhage, kernicterus, tumors of the posterior fossa or cervical spine, decerebrate rigidity, tetanus and strychnine intoxication. A diagnosis of toxoplasmosis would be strengthened by the presence of urine smelling of maple syrup, persistent icterus neonatorum, poor feeding habits, microcephaly, microphthalmia, hydrocephalus, lymphadenopathy, fever or a maculopapular rash. This patient should be referred for specialist investigation and management.

Examination of the motor system

Tonus (active and passive)

Active tonus determines posture at rest, spontaneous and provoked movement.

Passive or permanent tonus has three aspects:

- consistency of muscles on palpation
- extensibility, i.e. the lengthening capacity of limb muscles when passively moved
- passivity, i.e. the degree of lack of reaction to passive stretching.

Traction response

In pulling the patient from a supine to a sitting position, the absence of response from the patient in maintaining head position relative to the trunk would indicate generalized hypotonia.

Range of motion

The joint ranges of motion should be evaluated, checking for muscular tone. This should be correlated with observations made of the patient's spontaneous movements.

The Babinski (extensor) response to the plantar reflex

The plantar surface of the foot is stimulated from the heel, forward along the lateral border, crossing over the distal ends of the metatarsals toward the base of the great toe with an instrument such as a key, a tongue depressor, or the examiner's thumbnail (Fig. 7.6). The normal response in the infant is the Babinski response, consisting of extension of the great toe and flaring of the other four (Fig. 7.7). In children who cannot tolerate

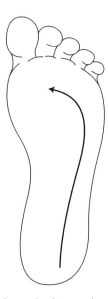

Figure 7.6 • Method of examination used to elicit the Babinski response in an infant.

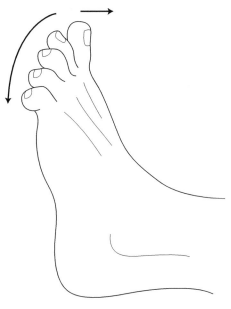

Figure 7.7 • Normal Babinski response in an infant. Note the upgoing great toe and the flaring of the other four toes.

the pressure on their sole, stimulation of the outer side of the foot is less objectionable, and the response the same. This sign is considered normal in the first 12 months of life and of equivocal clinical significance until age 18 months (when the child is walking and the corticospinal tract myelination is complete). Failure to elicit this sign before 12 months and persistence beyond 18 months is possibly abnormal (may be normal in some children up to 2 years of age). Asymmetry at any age is abnormal. If corticospinal tract pathology is suspected, then other signs such as sustained clonus, spasticity and hyperreflexia are evaluated.

Examination of the sensory system

Only pain and touch can be evaluated in the newborn and infant (Gamstorp 1985). Nerve root and peripheral nerve cutaneous distributions are the same as adults.

Evaluation of pain and touch is done by observing the infant's facial (grimacing, crying) and motor responses (withdrawal of the body part) to stimuli. Any of the above responses by the child indicates intactness of the pain and touch pathways. Withdrawal from a vibratory tuning fork placed on a bony prominence indicates at least touch perception, and suggests intactness of the posterior columns. An infant with a lesion of the sensory nerves and/or the spinal cord will consistently fail to show a response to the stimulus.

Abnormalities in skin temperature or the extent to which the infant perspires will indicate the level of a sensory deficit. This may be determined by slowly sliding the ulnar side of the palmar surface of the examiner's hand up the child's body.

Examination of the cranial nerves

As cranial nerve function is well advanced at birth, this examination is important and valuable. Owing to the inability of the patient to respond to verbal commands, the technique of the examination varies from that for an older child, adolescent or adult. Some cranial nerve functions cannot readily be tested in infancy. Cranial nerves can be assessed singularly or in groups according to the nature of the stimulus used. The following procedures are used to assess cranial nerve function in young children.

Cranial nerve I

The sense of smell, mediated by the first cranial nerve, is not functional in the newborn and as such never tested (Barness 1981), but is present by 5–7 months. Newborns will respond to irritating substances such as ammonia or vinegar but this is due to the irritation of the trigeminal (V) receptors in the nose and not cranial nerve I.

Cranial nerves II and VII

Flashing a bright red light in the child's eye produces a response mediated by both cranial nerve II and cranial nerve VII. The newborn infant will respond by blinking the eyelids and/or grimacing. This reaction indicates patency of cranial nerve II and that portion of cranial nerve VII involved in the response.

Cranial nerves II and III

A light shone into the infant's eye will normally result in pupillary constriction. This indicates intactness of cranial nerves II and III. In addition to loss of pupillary response to direct light stimulation, a significant III deficit may result in ptosis (Barness 1981).

Cranial nerve II

When one realizes the enormous territory needed for intact visual fields (from the eye, below the frontal lobes, through the temporal and parietal lobes, into the occipital lobes) it is obvious why visual field examination is a mandatory part of every neurological examination.

When held upright in a darkened room with a single source of light, the newborn will tend to turn the head so as to look towards the light. As the examiner moves the child's trunk away from the light, the child will tend to turn the head towards it. This reaction depends on the normal functioning of the visual cortex (this differs from most of the primitive reactions to be described later in this chapter, which are mediated at a subcortical level).

The blink response (closure of the eyelids when an object is suddenly moved toward the eyes) is used to determine functional vision is small infants (Barness 1981). The reflex is absent in the newborn, does not appear until 3–4 months, is present in about half of all 5-month-olds, and should be present in all 1-year-old infants.

In the infant, the visual fields can be tested by introducing objects (such as a favorite toy) from behind, above and below into the field of vision. Eye deviation in the direction of the object indicates that the child has seen it. For older children, ask them to look at your tongue, then wiggle a finger in the superior or inferior lateral field. If they see your finger move, they will automatically look at it.

Visual acuity can be assessed in toddlers by observing them at play, or by offering objects of varying sizes. In older children, acuity can be tested by special eye charts, with sharp objects commonly known to children. The ophthalmoscopic examination has been described in detail in Chapter 3.

Cranial nerves II, III, IV and VI

Note the position of the eyes at rest (III lesion causes eye abduction, VI lesion causes eye adduction, IV lesion is not usually noticeable at rest).

By 3 months, infants will follow an object (use a favorite toy) reasonably well with their eyes (Gamstorp 1985). The toy is moved through the six positions of gaze.

Alternative method

The examiner's face is placed about 25 cm from the patient's face and the baby's face is observed. The patient's head is taken into full rotation to both sides as well as flexion/extension. As the head is moved, the patient's gaze will usually remain, at least temporarily, fixed on the examiner and thus extrinsic eye muscles can be assessed.

Some parents will bring their children in for assessment because they are concerned that the child is 'cross-eyed'.

The child usually has no deviation from normal, but one is apparent because infants and young children have canthus dystopia, where the medial canthus is displaced laterally (thereby covering more of the medial conjunctiva than in adults), giving the appearance of inward deviation of the eyes, even though they are perfectly aligned. In children who can follow commands, focus on and follow a light source, the corneal light reflection or Hirschberg's test is useful. The practitioner positions a light source in the midline of the patient's head (i.e. in front of the nose), sits in front of the child, and shines the light into the child's eyes while asking them to look at the light. The practitioner notes the position of the corneal reflections, which should be symmetrical, and just medial to the centre of the pupil, and the child states that only one light is seen. The examiner then moves the patient's head with the light source, through the six positions of gaze; or the examiner can move the child's head from side to side, and up and down. The reflection should remain in exactly the same position on the pupil in all positions, and the child should see only one light in all positions. Ocular malalignment can be estimated by the location of the light reflection in relation to the center of the pupil. 'Deviation is approximately 15° if the reflection appears at the edge of the pupil, 30° if the reflection is half way between the edge of the pupil and the limbus (outer edge of the cornea) and 45° if the reflection is at the edge of the limbus' (Barness 1981).

A lesion of the medial longitudinal fasciculus (MLF) will produce an internuclear ophthalmoplegia (INO). Examination of conjugate gaze (moving the eyes to the right and left), will produce nystagmus of the leading eye, and failure of adduction of the following eye. Evidence that the medial rectus muscle, supplied by cranial nerve III, is not paralyzed is easily determined, because the eyes will still adduct on accommodation. Lesions of the superior colliculus (tectum of the mesencephalon) will produce difficulty with upward gaze which may be produced by lesions in the posterior fossa such as a pinealoma (Parinaud's syndrome).

Cranial nerve III and sympathetics

Note the size and symmetry of the pupils and their response to light. Observe for eyelid ptosis, which may be due to a cranial nerve III lesion (supplies levator palpebrae, which may be seen with pupil dilatation), a sympathetic lesion (supplies the superior tarsal, which will be seen with an ipsilateral pupil constriction).

Cranial nerve V

Observe and palpate the action of the temporalis and masseter muscles, and watch the jaw for any deviation on opening (unilateral V lesions result in jaw deviation to the side of the lesion).

Cranial nerves V$_{(1)}$ and VII

Observe the child for spontaneous blinking (Barness 1981). Is spontaneous blinking slower or less complete than would normally be expected? The corneal reflex is always present at birth and is readily tested by touching the cornea with a wisp of cotton (innervated by V), which should result in eyelid closure (innervated by VII).

Cranial nerves V$_{(3)}$, VII and upper cervical nerve roots

The rooting reflex is elicited by stimulating the cheek lateral to the mouth (V), which results in the child moving the head toward the stimulus (upper cervical nerve roots) while making sucking movements with the lips (VII).

Cranial nerves V, VII and XII

The sucking reflex is elicited by stroking the lips (V) of an infant which results in them making sucking movements with the lips (VII) and tongue (XII).

Cranial nerve VII

Observe for any facial asymmetry, such as normal wrinkling of the forehead, eye closure, depth of the nasolabial folds, etc. Any facial asymmetry is accentuated when the child laughs or cries.

The infant may respond to sugar or salt solutions applied to a previously dried and protruded tongue by a cotton-tipped applicator (VII supplies the anterior tongue) from the first day of life, reacting by smiling, grimacing or crying (the symmetry of the facial expression tests cranial nerve VII, and palatal elevation during crying tests cranial nerve X).

Cranial nerve VIII

Hearing is present from birth, but it may not be possible to elicit responses until the child is 7 weeks old. The aural palpebral reflex, in which the examiner makes a loud clapping noise with the hands outside the child's field of vision, may result in turning the eyes (by 7–8 weeks) or the head and eyes (by 12–16 weeks) in the direction of the sound (also tests cranial nerves III, IV, VI and the upper cervical nerves), blinking (VII), a Moro response (brachial and sacral plexuses) and/or crying (V, VII, IX and X). Any of the above responses indicates perception of sound (in at least one ear), but absence of a response is not diagnostic of deafness.

A child of 8 months or older should respond by turning the head (upper cervical nerves) to the sound of a bell, rattle, cellophane paper being crinkled, or a soft voice. The preschool age child is tested by asking him or her to repeat a very quietly spoken word or number.

Cranial nerves IX and X

The ability to swallow is sufficient evidence of IX and X being intact. The gag reflex is present from birth. Symmetry of the uvula and soft palate at rest should be observed as well as motility during crying.

Cranial nerve XI

Direct evaluation is difficult in the infant, but a measure of its functioning can be gained by eliciting the rooting, Landau and neck-righting reflexes. Patency may also be estimated by the response of the baby to having its head held in full forced rotation. In the older child, rotation of the head or shrugging

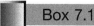

the shoulders against resistance provides an adequate assessment of cranial nerve XI.

Cranial nerve XII

Note the position of the tongue at rest. In the infant, the tongue is examined for signs of atrophy and fasciculations (seen as small depressions that appear and disappear quickly at irregular intervals more visibly on the under-surface of the tongue).

The tongue retrusion reflex is usually present from the first few weeks of life. It is tested by placing a firm object in the child's mouth, the response of the infant being to expel the object with the tongue.

The infantile automatisms

The normal newborn shows a repertoire of primary or automatic reactions, which normally exist for several months after birth. Most are mediated at a subcortical level (some are obtainable even in anencephalics). Their assessment is mandatory as it gives information related to not only the integrity of the brainstem and spinal cord, but also its degree of maturity. They also offer the opportunity for comparing one side of the body with the other, as most are bilateral reactions (Brett 1983). The evaluation of various primitive reflexes is an integral part of the neurological examination of the infant. Absence or asymmetry of these reflexes before certain ages, or persistence after certain ages, may indicate general developmental lag, because these reflexes, which develop during intrauterine life, are gradually suppressed as the higher cortical centers mature and become functional (Levine et al 1983). In very low birthweight infants, a clear relationship has been demonstrated between the strength of the primitive reflexes and early motor development as well as retention of primitive reflexes and delayed motor development (Marquis et al 1984). Alterations in retention time of primitive reflexes in neurologically high-risk infants has also been shown to be useful in the diagnostic identification of cerebral palsy, motor and mental retardation (Blasco 1994, Capute 1979, Futagi et al 1992, Zafeiriou et al 1995).

There are many primitive reflexes that may be evaluated in the first 2 years of a child's life. From the descriptions of tests which have been identified as important (McMillan et al 1977), those that lend themselves readily to successful performance in the chiropractic clinic environment have been selected for presentation here and have been classified as either being present at birth or appearing later, usually sometime during the first year of life (Box 7.1). The technique for eliciting these reflexes, the expected response from the child, and the clinical significance of variation in the age of disappearance are described in the following discussion.

Primitive reflexes which should form an integral part of the neurological examination in the neonate, infant and toddler are either present at birth or appear in the infancy/toddler period.

Box 7.1

Primitive reflexes that should form an integral part of the neurological examination in the neonate, infant and toddler are either present at birth or appear in the infancy/toddler period

Reflexes present at birth

- Galant reflex
- Moro reflex
- Palmar reflex
- Perez reflex
- Placing reflex
- Plantar reflex
- Sucking and rooting reflex
- Vertical suspension
- Walking reflex

Reflexes appearing after birth

- Landau reflex
- Parachute reflex
- Neck righting reflex

Reflexes that are present at birth and disappear

The Moro reflex

Technique
The Moro response is probably the most familiar of the neonatal primitive reflexes (Brett 1983) and is named after Dr Ernst Moro, 1874–1951 (Ignatius 1993). To obtain the Moro response, the infant is placed supine on an examination table or on the examiner's forearm with the head supported by the examiner's hand. The supporting hand is suddenly lowered to allow the head to fall backward 20–30°. The Moro response can be obtained in other ways including a loud noise to the child or a sudden blow to the surface on which the child is lying (Brett 1983, Gamstorp 1985).

Response
Extension of the trunk, symmetrical extension and abduction of the arms with extension of the fingers, followed by flexion and abduction of the arms.

Age of disappearance
The response begins to fade by 4–8 weeks, and disappears by 1–5 months (but can be reinforced by pressure on the knees, and then obtained at later ages) (Brett 1983, McMillan et al 1977).

Significance
It is extremely informative in children under 5 months of age. Its absence during the first few weeks of life or its persistence beyond 5 months indicates neurological dysfunction.

The Moro response indicates symmetrical intactness of multiple levels of the nervous system (cerebral cortex, corticospinal tracts, brachial plexus and peripheral nerves). Response will be diminished or absent unilaterally in hemiparesis, plexus, nerve, muscle, clavicle, humerus or shoulder injuries. It may also be absent in the neonate affected by drugs, sedation, hypoxia, infection or cerebral insult. It is possible that it may be affected by upper cervical subluxation complex. Persistence beyond the fifth month of life suggests diffuse central nervous system deficit.

The palmar grasp reflex

Technique
The examiner's finger is placed in the palm of the infant's hand.

Response
The infant's fingers close on the examiner's finger and hold even more tightly as the examiner attempts to withdraw the finger.

Age of disappearance
The response becomes weak by 2–3 months, at which time it will be covered by volitional action. It will have completely disappeared by 4 months (McMillan et al 1977).

Significance
Absence or asymmetry of the reflex prior to 2–3 months is suggestive of underlying neurological disease. Persistence beyond this time, or reappearance, indicates the possibility of a nervous system disorder. Asymmetrical responses should be viewed with caution as they are sometimes seen as an early sign in hemiparesis.

The plantar grasp reflex

Technique
The examiner applies pressure to the plantar surface of the foot close to the base of the toes.

Response
Flexion of the toes occurs to grasp the examiner's finger.

Age of disappearance
The plantar grasp reflex has usually disappeared by 8–15 months (McMillan et al 1977).

Significance
Absence or asymmetry of the reflex prior to 2–3 months of age is suggestive of underlying neurological disease. Persistence beyond the normal time of disappearance, or reappearance, indicates the possibility of a nervous system disorder.

The rooting and sucking reflexes

Technique
The examiner lightly strokes the face near the corner of the mouth. For the sucking reflex, the examiner lightly strokes the infant's lips.

Response
In the rooting reflex, the child turns the head towards the stimulus and begins a sucking action. For the sucking reflex, the child begins sucking when the lips are lightly stroked.

Age of disappearance
The age of disappearance of the rooting reflex is related to the waking state. It can be expected to persist until 7–8 months of

age in the sleeping child, but will have disappeared by 3–4 months in the child who is awake. The sucking reflex is only seen in the wakeful child and can be expected to disappear by the end of the first year of life (McMillan et al 1977).

Significance
The sensory limb of both responses is the trigeminal nerve. The sucking response of the lips tests the facial nerve (VII) and the tongue movement tests the hypoglossal nerve. The head turning in the rooting reflexes also tests the upper cervical nerve roots. Asymmetry in the sucking response suggests a lesion of cranial nerves V, VII or XII. The rooting response may persist in neurologically abnormal children or may reappear in those with progressive degenerative diseases.

The tonic neck reflex

Technique
The patient is placed supine and the head is rapidly rotated to one side and held there while the chest is maintained in a flat position.

Response
The expected response is for the child to extend the arm and leg on the side to which the head is turned and flex the arm and leg on the opposite side. This is referred to as the 'fencing posture'.

Age of disappearance
It will normally disappear by 6 months of age (McMillan et al 1977).

Significance
In a normal reflex, the fencing posture will only be momentarily maintained. Persistence of the posture, that is, one in which the infants are unable to extricate themselves, is referred to as an 'obligate reflex'. This infant will be unable to roll over. The obligate reflex should always be considered abnormal and the child referred for specialist investigation. Asymmetrical reflex may be an early sign of hemiparesis on the side of the increased response, but a subluxation complex at the upper cervical level should always be considered as a possible cause. Persistence beyond 6 months of age in the awakened state is a serious sign suggestive of a central motor lesion and may indicate spastic cerebral palsy. This child should be referred for specialist investigation. The reflex may persist as a momentary response during sleep up to 3 years of age.

The placing reflex

Technique
The patient is supported under the axillae while the dorsum of the foot is brought into contact with the edge of the examination table.

Response
The infant raises the stimulated foot as if to step up on to the table.

Age of disappearance
The reflex becomes less vigorous by 6 months of age.

Significance
The placing reflex is valuable in detecting asymmetrical responses of the two lower limbs. It serves as a good indicator of nervous system maturation when the expected response is present.

The walking reflex

Technique

The walking or stepping reflex is obtained by holding the infant upright over an examination table so that the soles of the feet are in contact with the surface.

Response

This technique initiates reciprocal flexion and extension of the legs, simulating walking. Owing to the action of the adductor muscles, one leg often gets caught behind the other. This must not be confused with adductor spasm.

Age of disappearance

The stepping response can be expected to persist as voluntary standing (Weiner et al 1981).

Significance

An intact response is a helpful indicator of nervous system maturation.

Reflexes which appear after birth

The Landau reflex

The Landau reflex is also known as 'posture in horizontal suspension' and is a test of head control and motor function (Weiner et al 1981).

Technique

The child is held by the examiner in a horizontal position.

Response

The child will attempt to arch the back and hold the head above the horizontal plane.

Age of appearance

The Landau response begins to be seen at 3 months and is consistently present by the end of the first year of life (McMillan et al 1977).

Age of disappearance

The Landau response is generally not seen after the end of the second year of life (McMillan et al 1977).

Significance

The Landau reflex is a general indication of maturing motor control, and infants with hypotonia, diplegia, tetraplegia or paraplegia will not exhibit the characteristic posture.

The parachute reaction

Technique

The examiner holds the patient firmly in midair in the horizontal position. The examiner then quickly lowers the child towards the surface of the examination table or the floor.

Response

The child will extend the arms, hands and fingers to protect themself from contact with the table or the floor.

Age of appearance

The parachute reaction will appear at 8–9 months (McMillan et al 1977).

Age of disappearance

There is no certain age at which this reaction will disappear.

Significance

The parachute reaction is an excellent test for the development of visual and vestibular sensory input, upper extremity pyramidal and peripheral nerve function. The response appears to be proportional to the size of any optic stimulus pattern on the examination table covering or the floor. An asymmetrical response suggests either an upper or a lower motor neuron lesion.

The neck righting reflex

Technique

The patient is placed supine on an examination table and the head is rotated 90° to one side and firmly held.

Response

The child tries to rotate the trunk and then the pelvis in order to bring the spine and pelvis into neutral alignment with the head and neck.

Age of appearance

The neck righting reflex is first noticed at 4–6 months of age (McMillan et al 1977).

Age of disappearance

The expected age of disappearance is between 1 and 2 years (McMillan et al 1977).

Significance

Persistence in older children may suggest spasticity or developmental retardation. It has, however, been seen in normal children as old as 9 years when the test is performed with the child on all fours (Brett 1983).

General developmental surveillance

As an integral part of all neurological examinations up to age 5, regular developmental screening assessments should be carried out. Developmental pediatrics and details of how to perform developmental screening assessments are covered in Chapter 8. In conjunction with the neurological examination and the developmental screening tests described earlier, it is useful to check the essential milestones of development shown in Table 2.3 (Chapter 2, p. 17). It should be pointed out, however, that these informal tables should never be relied upon as the sole method of conducting developmental surveillance as they have been shown to miss about two-thirds of all cases involving developmental delay (Brothers et al 2008). Indeed, even well-validated developmental screening as a surveillance tool needs to be performed longitudinally as the child grows, to reach acceptable standards of clinical accuracy (Rydz et al 2005).

Examination of the older child

Beyond infancy, once the automatisms have disappeared, the clinician should attempt to assess the neurological system using well-validated developmental screening tests, drawing ability, play skills, etc. Specific neurological testing is carried out in much the same way as in the adult as the child approaches school age. The sensory system may be assessed using pinprick and vibration as well as light touch in responsive patients.

Examination of the motor system

Observation of gait and posture

The child's posture can usually be discerned prior to the start of the examination. Walking and running gaits can be seen by playing with the patient, asking the patient to retrieve a ball and to run outside the examining room.

It is important to observe a child rise from the supine position for evidence of neurological deficits, muscular weakness and orthopedic defects. The 'Gower' pattern describes the way hypotonic children push themselves up their thighs when arising from the supine position (Fig. 7.8).

Muscle strength

By 5 years of age the motor system examination can be done in the adult manner. Muscle strength is graded 0–5:

0 = no evidence of muscle contraction

1 = evidence of slight contraction, no joint motion

2 = active movement, with gravity eliminated

3 = complete range of motion against gravity

4 = complete range of motion against gravity, with some resistance

5 = complete range of motion against gravity, with stronger resistance.

Muscle tone

Muscle tone is examined by manipulating major joints for hypotonia and for hypertonia (quickly for spasticity indicating corticospinal tract pathology, and slowly for rigidity indicating extrapyramidal pathology), and determining the degree of resistance. This can include elbow flexion–extension, forearm

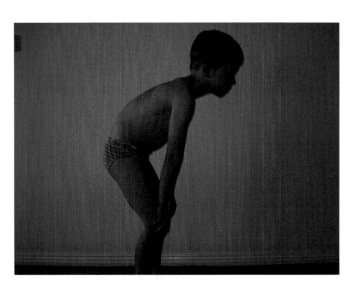

Figure 7.8 • A 'Gower' positive pattern. Note how the child walks up the thighs for support as she gets up from a supine position.

supination–pronation, wrist flexion–extension, and ankle dorsi-flexion–plantar flexion. A sensitive test for hypotonia in the upper limb is the pronator sign, where the patient is asked to raise the hands over the head with the palms facing each other (but not touching), and the involved forearm pronates.

Coordination

Tests for ataxia and tremors can be made by having the patient reach for and manipulate toys. In the older child the standard cerebellar finger-to-nose, heel to shin, dysdiadochokinesia tests (pronation–supination in the upper limb, and rapid toe-tapping in the lower limb) can be performed. These tests will be difficult with athetosis, choreiform or dystonic movements (extrapyramidal pathology).

Examination of the sensory system

Nerve root and peripheral nerve cutaneous distributions are the same as in adults.

An infant with a lesion of the sensory nerves and/or the spinal cord will consistently ignore the stimulus.

Abnormalities in skin temperature or in the amount of perspiration will indicate the level of a sensory deficit. This may be determined by slowly sliding the ulnar surface of the examiner's hand up the child's body.

Object discrimination can be determined in young children by using items well known to them such as a coin, pen or toy. This test should be done with the eyes closed.

Examination of the muscle stretch reflexes

The younger the child, the less informative are the muscle stretch reflexes. Reflex inequalities are common and less reliable than inequalities of muscle tone in ascertaining the presence of an upper motor neuron lesion. The muscle stretch reflexes are assessed in the child beyond infancy as in the adult. The routine examination should include:

• biceps (C5)
• brachioradialis (C6)
• triceps (C7)
• abdominal (T8–12)
• patella (L4)
• Achilles (S1)
• jaw jerk (motor and sensory portion of cranial nerve).

Examination of the cranial nerves

The difficulties encountered in the cranial nerve examination in infancy are not so apparent in this older age group. The only difference from the adult examination is in the VIIIth nerve. In the younger child a rattle and cellophane paper are used, while in the preschool-age child a selection of model farm animals is provided and they are asked to pick up the animal the examiner asks for. This simple test is referred to as the Kendall toy test (Bellman & Kennedy 2000). Techniques for assessment of hearing at different age levels have been presented in Chapter 3. Rinne's and Weber's tests, universally used in adult practice, are not usually able to be reliably performed until school age.

Important neurological syndromes encountered in children

There are many neurological conditions that affect children. This text intends to deal only with the more common conditions and those which, while less common, are serious and may possibly be encountered in general chiropractic practice. There is a wide range of known causes of headache in children and these are shown in Table 7.4.

Headache

Headache in children is common but usually short-lived. Most patients suffer from chronic or recurrent headache. It is the type of headache that causes much concern to parents, fearing their child may have a serious condition such as a tumor. Most recurrent headaches in older children and adolescents have a benign cause related to stress and tension (Gamstorp 1985). The probability of an organic cause in

children with headache is very low. It is important to alleviate the parent's fears, but only after a thorough history and examination of the child. Owing to the possibility of serious organic disease, in every child presenting with headache the clinician should take a careful clinical history and perform a full general and neurological examination, including ophthalmoscopy (Lindsay et al 1991). There is a wide range of causes of headache in children and these are summarized in Table 7.5.

Vascular headache

Vascular headache, when associated with fever, may arise from infection causing headache from generalized dilatation of cranial arteries. In non-febrile cases vascular headache may be caused by migraine (with or without aura), toxic exposure, hypertension, epilepsy and, rarely, intracerebral hemorrhage.

Infection

When fever is present, infection is the most likely cause of the child's headache. A search for the site of infection should be conducted and appropriate management implemented. Infection is a common cause of headache in children and in one study of 643 cases of pediatric headache more than half of the subjects had an infectious etiology, with the respiratory tract the most dominant site (van der Wouden et al 1999). Other infectious diseases associated with headache are acute, subacute and chronic meningitis, leukemic infiltration of the meninges, brain abscess and sinusitis (Gamstorp 1985, Moe & Seay 1997).

Patients with central nervous system infection, regardless of the organism, will present with similar symptom patterns. Neurological infections are usually bacterial or viral and structurally involve either the meninges or cerebral parenchyma. All patients, however, have some degree of involvement of both areas (Moe & Seay 1997). In infancy, the clinical features of meningitis are frequently non-specific, involving irritability, fever, cyanosis, lethargy, poor feeding and a high-pitched cry. There may also be bulging of the anterior fontanel and seizure activity that occurs in approximately one-third of all children with meningitis, principally those in whom *Haemophilus influenzae* is the infecting organism. In children over 12 months of age, signs consistent with meningeal irritation occur, principally a stiff neck, headache, and positive Kernig and Brudzinski signs (Weiner et al 1981). Such a presentation demands specialist referral for lumbar puncture.

While encephalitis and meningitis have very similar symptomatic presentations, brain abscess is more variable. 'In a child with an encapsulated abscess, headache is prominent. There may be no signs of infection; the child presents with a slowly evolving focal deficit, seizures or raised intracranial pressure. Other children are very ill and mimic the child with meningitis' (Weiner et al 1981). Brain abscess is more likely to occur in children who have congenital heart disease, a recent history of otitis media, head trauma or pulmonary infection.

Migraine

In children, migraine is a syndrome that may or may not involve headache. It is seen as early as 4 years of age and

Table 7.4 Suggested routine for the general physical examination of a child who presents with headache but no history of head trauma

Vital signs	Blood pressure, pulse rate, respiratory rate
Anthropometry	Head circumference, height, weight
Head and neck	Sutural palpation, lymphatic assessment, ear and eye examination, nasal inspection, oral examination including a careful inspection of the teeth, sinus assessment including transillumination, thyroid palpation, and auscultation of the carotid artery for bruits
Thorax	Respiratory and cardiovascular assessment
Abdomen	General evaluation looking carefully for organomegaly, signs of constipation/retained feces, lymphadenopathy or other masses, and renal artery for bruits
Musculoskeletal	General assessment of muscle tone and strength, posture, gait and range of motion including the chiropractic spinal assessment. Particular attention should be paid to any neck tension/stiffness, especially in children with recent-onset headache accompanied by fever
Neurological	Myotomes, dermatomes, muscle stretch reflexes, cranial nerves, cerebellar tests, automatisms (at appropriate ages), Babinski response, and assessment of posterior columns
Developmental	Age-appropriate assessment
Urinalysis	Chemical dipstick evaluation

Table 7.5 Differential diagnostic characteristics of headache in children (adapted from Lindsay et al 1991 with permission)

	Associated features which (if present) aid diagnosis	Recurrent attacks	Further investigations (if required)
Acute cause			
Sinusitis	Preceding 'cold' Nasal discharge	+	X-ray nasal sinuses
Migraine	Visual/neurological aura, nausea, vomiting	+	
Cluster headache	Lacrimation, rhinorrhea	+	
Post-traumatic	Preceding head injury Cervical spine whiplash	–	Skull X-ray, CT scan, motion palpation
Drugs/toxins	On vasodilator drugs		
Hemorrhage	Instantaneous-onset vomiting, neck stiffness, impaired consciousness level		CT scan Lumbar puncture
Infection (meningitis, encephalitis)	As above but more gradual onset with pyrexia	+ (if CSF fistula)	
Hydrocephalus	Impaired conscious level, leg weakness, impaired upward gaze	–	CT scan
Subluxation syndrome	Headache in various locations according to affected spinal level	++	X-ray, static and motion palpation, postural assessment, instrumentation
Subacute cause			
Infection (subacute, chronic meningitis, e.g. TB, cerebral abscess)	Impaired conscious level, pyrexia, neck stiffness, focal neurological signs	–	CT scan Lumbar puncture
Intracranial tumor Chronic subdural hematoma Hydrocephalus	Vomiting, papilledema, impaired conscious level ± focal neurological signs	+	CT scan
Benign intracranial hypertension	Vomiting, papilledema	+	CT scan CSF pressure monitoring
Subluxation syndrome	Headache in various locations according to affected spinal level	++	X-ray, static and motion palpation, postural assessment, instrumentation
Chronic causes			
Tension headache	Anxiety, depression	+	
Ocular 'eye strain'	Impaired visual acuity	+	Refractive errors
Drugs/toxins	On vasodilator drugs, neck, shoulder, arm pain	+	
Subluxation syndrome	Headache in various locations according to affected spinal level	++	X-ray, static and motion palpation, postural assessment, instrumentation

accounts for approximately 5% of all headaches in children (Weiner et al 1981). In the preschool-age child, migraine often presents as an episode of pallor and vomiting unassociated with recognizable illness (Weiner et al 1981), the so-called abdominal migraine syndrome, for which a complete diagnostic definition remains a little unclear. However, 'the presence of a well defined syndrome comprising episodes of midline abdominal pain of sufficient severity to interfere with normal activities and lasting for prolonged periods, frequently accompanied by pallor, headache, anorexia, nausea and vomiting is adequate to qualify a child for the diagnosis of abdominal migraine' (Symon & Russell 1986).

In children suffering from migraine in which headache is a feature, commonly referred to as 'children's migraine syndrome' (Knezevic-Pogancev 2008), the migraine may be classified as classic, common or complicated. In classic migraine, the child will describe an aura or visual prodrome preceding the onset of the headache which begins at the conclusion of the prodrome, whereas in common migraine there are no prodromal symptoms. The etiology of classic migraine is determined largely by genetic factors (Russell & Olesen 1995, Russell et al 1996), making the identification of migrainous symptoms in at least one first-degree relative a critical part of the clinical history. The etiology of common migraine seems to be determined by a combination of genetic and environmental factors (Russell & Olesen 1995, Russell et al 1996). Complicated migraine is so named owing to the association of other symptoms with the headache, such as difficulty talking, tingling of the face or extremities, hemiparesis or ophthalmoplegia (Weiner et al 1981).

The International Classification of Headache Disorders classification system, which was brought in by consensus in 1988 (ICHD-I) and last modified in September 2003 (ICDH-II), defines the parameters of the migraine syndromes in children. The characteristic symptom patterns encountered in children with the various migraine syndromes are presented in Table 7.6.

Toxic exposure to carbon monoxide

The early symptoms experienced by the child are diffuse, difficult-to-localize headache and vertigo. Continued exposure produces a bounding pulse, fixed dilatation of the pupils, vomiting, a dusky discoloration of the skin and, finally, convulsions.

Hypertension

Benign intracranial hypertension presents as headache and vomiting which has developed over a period of 48–72 hours. It is usually a consequence of infection, particularly otitis media. Papilledema is usually seen on examination and sometimes bilateral sixth nerve palsy and ataxia. This condition must be differentiated from brain abscess and meningitis.

Postictal

In children with epilepsy, headache following an attack is common and probably due to transient vascular dilatation.

Intracerebral hemorrhage

This condition is rare in childhood, but has a very high mortality rate. The most common causes of the hemorrhage are vascular malformation, bleeding into tumor, and coagulopathies (Livingstone & Brown 1986). Characteristic symptoms are usually quite non-specific but may include altered states of consciousness, headache, vomiting and focal neurological signs.

Muscular or tension-type headaches

In children, as in adults, tension-type headache is the most common form of headache that will be encountered in clinical practice. Characteristically, children with tension-type headache present with pain and tension in the suboccipital and neck muscles, which is usually accompanied by a feeling of heaviness or pressure. The pain tends to be worse during school hours when they are most active and ease again at the end of the day after they return home and have opportunity for food and rest. The tension-type headache is absent in the early morning and does not wake the child from sleep. There is often a positive family history of similar headaches in at least one first-degree relative. The child may have a concomitant clinical history of recurrent, non-specific abdominal pain and other gastrointestinal complaints.

Typically, there are no neurological signs present on examination and if electroencephalography has been performed it will invariably be negative. Refractive error is sometimes found

Table 7.6 Characteristic symptom patterns seen in children with migraine

Type of migraine	Characteristic symptom pattern
Classic migraine	Usually preceded by prodromal symptoms (scotomata) Nausea and vomiting common Pain usually, but not always, strictly one-sided Frequently no headache at all, especially in younger patients Scalp tenderness Photophobia Vegetative symptoms such as perspiration, pallor and diarrhea Sometimes associated with the passage of a pale stool Occasional neurological symptoms such as hemianopsia, localized paresthesia, hemiplegia and aphasia
Common migraine	Prodromal symptoms rare Sudden onset without warning Pain characteristics similar to classic migraine Frequently no headache at all, especially in younger patients Scalp tenderness Photophobia Sometimes associated with the passage of a pale stool
Abdominal migraine	Seen most commonly in younger children, but may persist in adult life Recurrent bouts of midline abdominal pain which is of sufficient severity to disrupt normal daily activities Pallor Headache variable Nausea and vomiting

on eye examination that will be normal in every other respect (Gamstorp 1985).

Non-organic headache

A thorough clinical history is the key to differentiating between an organic and a non-organic problem.

Depression

Other symptoms that may accompany the headache will be apparent from the clinical history and observation of the patient. These typically include loss of appetite, difficulty concentrating, sleep disturbances, and reluctance to participate in play and other activities. Depression sometimes results from an ongoing abusive situation at home or school.

Anxiety

A common cause of non-organic childhood headache is peer or social pressures experienced at school. The child may worry about schoolwork, difficulties with a teacher, bullies in the playground, toilet phobias, etc. Careful and sensitive clinical history-taking and sometimes consultation with the teacher will usually identify the anxious child. Anxiety may also be a result of an ongoing abusive situation at home. In one study of 634 children ranging in age from birth to 14 years, the incidence of idiopathic headache was 7.3 per 1000 person-years and the psychosocial factors most frequently identified as causative were problems in either the home environment or school (van der Wouden et al 1999).

Attention seeking

Headache is sometimes complained of by children under a variety of stressful circumstances (e.g. a new baby in the house, relocation, new school, etc.) to attract comforting and sympathetic attention to themselves.

Neurological causes of headache

There are a number of neurological causes of headache, principally the development of an intracranial tumor, neurological infection and raised intracranial pressure.

Intracranial tumors

Headache is a common presenting symptom in children with an intracranial tumor. Despite the proliferation of organ-imaging technology, misdiagnosis of intracranial tumor as a cause of headache remains a clinical problem. In one study of 74 children with brain tumors it was discovered that they had a mean duration of clinical history of nearly 6 months and had consulted their doctor between four and five times each before the diagnosis was made, despite the fact that the presenting symptoms were typical of children with intracranial tumor. Vomiting (65%), headache (64%) and personality change (47%) were the most common presenting symptoms (Edgeworth et al 1996). In addition to these three common features, headache associated with intracranial tumors may also be characterized by being woken from sleep by the headache, gait changes, increased pain with coughing or sneezing, changing position or otherwise increasing the intracranial pressure, macrocephaly, excessive rate of head growth, blurred or

double vision, paresis of cranial nerves III and/or IV, and papilledema (Moe & Seay 1997). In adult practice, brain tumors should always be considered as a differential diagnosis after a first seizure, since that relationship has an incidence of around 10%. In patients under the age of 20 years, however, the relationship between a first epileptic seizure and brain tumor is 0.02% (Patten 1996).

Raised intracranial pressure

Elevation of intracranial pressure (ICP) may result from the development of an expanding mass, increase in brain water content, an increase in the cerebral blood volume as a result of vasodilatation or obstruction of the venous outflow, or an increase in the total cerebrospinal fluid (CSF) volume. In addition to headache, raised ICP may produce nausea, vomiting and papilledema. Raised ICP, while it produces symptoms and signs, does not damage neuronal parenchyma provided that the cerebral blood flow is maintained. Damage does occur, however, in cases where the pressure has caused either tentorial or cerebellar tonsillar herniation (Lindsay et al 1991). The clinical effects of brain shift are shown in Table 7.7.

Hydrocephalus, which causes raised ICP, may result from obstructive conditions (non-communicating) such as the Arnold–Chiari and Dandy–Walker malformations, acquired disease such as aqueductal stenosis, development of a supratentorial mass and other tumors, hematoma and cyst formation. Communicating conditions include thickening of the leptomeninges, increased CSF viscosity, and excessive CSF production (Lindsay et al 1991).

In children, typical symptoms include an acceleration of the normal rate of head growth, tense anterior fontanel, positive Macewen's 'cracked pot' sign, eyelid retraction and impaired upward gaze referred to as the 'setting-sun' sign, thin scalp with dilated veins, mental retardation, failure to thrive, and sometimes an impaired conscious level. Untreated, non-communicating hydrocephalus results in death in around 50% of patients and many who survive have mental retardation (Laurence & Coates 1972).

Table 7.7 Common clinical effects of brain shift resulting from raised intracranial pressure

Type of brain shift	Clinical effects
Lateral tentorial herniation	Ipsilateral limb weakness Deterioration consciousness level Pupillary dilatation and failure to react to light
Central tentorial herniation	Loss of upward gaze followed by impaired eye movements Deteriorated consciousness level Pupils begin small and become moderately dilated Pupils fail to react to light Diabetes insipidus may develop
Cerebellar tonsillar herniation	Neck stiffness and head tilt Changes in respiratory control Depression of consciousness level

Children with hydrocephalus require urgent referral for neurological imaging studies and surgical treatment.

Extracranial disorders

There are a number of extracranial disorders that cause headache that must be considered. Principal among these are sinusitis, dental problems, ocular conditions, allergic reactions, hypoglycemia, prescribed medications, basilar impression syndrome and ear disease.

Sinusitis

Obviously, aeration of the sinus cavities is necessary before congestive disease can develop. As such, headache from sinusitis is not seen much before school age. Sinus headache may be due to either allergy or infection. The usual presentation is a child with frontal or retro-orbital headache that is often present on awakening but disappears shortly after rising, fever in patients with infection, rhinorrhea, and sometimes a positive family history of sinus disease.

Physical evidence that a child may have sinusitis includes increased local temperature and tenderness to palpation and percussion over the affected sinus. There may also be a failure of normal transillumination. Congestion will be clearly evident on X-ray. In children with sinus infection, resolution and prevention of recurrence is usually obtained by short-term antibiotic therapy used concurrently with chiropractic care and normal hygienic measures such as steam inhalation.

Dental problems

Unchecked dental caries or abscesses may cause headache. In some children, grinding of the teeth during sleep (bruxism) may also cause headache by increasing cranial muscle tension.

Disorders of the eye

Physical assessment of the child presenting with headache must include a careful evaluation of the eyes. Strabismus (squint), weakness of extraocular muscles, visual loss, poor pupillary response, papilledema, optic atrophy (which may arise from untreated hydrocephalus), and refractive errors must be ruled out (Lindsay et al 1991, Moe & Seay 1997). Apart from strabismus, children with eye pathology should be referred for specialist investigation. A trial of chiropractic care with strabismus is appropriate but referral is still necessary if the child shows no sign of improvement in the short term because uncorrected strabismus may lead to suppression amblyopia. Children with strabismus due to a functional neurological problem usually have subluxation of the upper cervical complex and disturbance of the craniosacral primary respiratory mechanism.

Allergy and hypoglycemia

A detailed discussion of these topics is found in Chapter 18.

Prescribed medication

Headache may sometimes result from the use of certain medications. Some of the drugs used commonly for children that have been shown to produce headache as a side-effect include antihistamine preparations, diazepam, phenytoin and the tetracyclines.

Basilar impression syndrome

Basilar impression syndrome results from softening of the basal cranial bones so they are no longer able to support the weight of the skull. As a result, the base of the skull becomes displaced upward into the cranial vault. The result of this upward displacement is compression of the structures of the brainstem by the odontoid process, the rim of the invaginated foramen magnum and the upper cervical vertebrae (Tachdjian 1972). Symptoms often seen in children with basilar impression syndrome are those that are consistent with brainstem compression: primarily persistent occipital headache, cranial nerve deficits, nystagmus, gait disturbance, spasticity, ocular disorders such as refractive errors, and astigmatism. Basilar impression syndrome is sometimes seen in children with Klippel–Feil syndrome and an obviously short neck.

The condition is best demonstrated by constructing McGregor's, Chamberlain's and McRae's lines on the lateral cervical radiograph. Affected children should be referred for corrective surgery.

Disorders of the ear

Acute otitis media, serous otitis media and mastoiditis can cause headache, but are likely to produce more local symptoms. The distribution of pain is typically from the suboccipital base, around the ear, and as far forward as the lateral canthus of the eye. Diagnosis and management of ear-related conditions are discussed in detail in Chapter 12.

Trauma-induced headache

Traumatic injury to the head in children may occur for a number of reasons, both accidental and non-accidental. In all cases where a child has suffered head trauma, a careful clinical history and full neurological examination are essential. The critical elements of history and examination are shown in Box 7.2. Children who have suffered mild head trauma need to be monitored for immediate short-term and long-term problems.

 Box 7.2

Critical elements of clinical history and examination in a child presenting with headache after closed head injury

- Assessment of the child's level of consciousness
- Evaluation of the child's ability to carry out age-appropriate tasks
- Tympanic membrane inspection for blood or CSF indicating basilar skull fracture
- Scalp inspection for evidence of localized areas of trauma (i.e. lacerations, bruises, etc.)
- Evaluation of pupillary size and reaction to light
- Determination of heart rate and blood pressure
- Assessment of respiratory pattern
- Muscle assessment to check for hemiparesis
- Gait evaluation
- Presence or absence of the Babinski response
- Measurement of head circumference

The most feared immediate problem following any head trauma in children is the development of a subdural or epidural hematoma with subsequent compression of the brainstem. Epidural hematoma is the result of venous bleeding, or arterial bleeding from a tear in the middle meningeal artery. The child with an epidural hematoma may slowly deteriorate after the injury, or go through periods of improvement only to deteriorate again later. Subdural hematoma is the result of venous or arterial bleeding. Symptoms characteristic of epidural and subdural hematoma formation are headache, a decreased level of consciousness, and fixed dilatation of the pupil on the same side as the hematoma, which is a late sign. When a subdural hematoma forms in the posterior fossa, disturbances of gait may be seen in older children (Weiner et al 1981).

Concussion is a common immediate effect of head trauma. The concussed patient will usually present with fixed pupillary dilatation, slowed reflexes, low blood pressure, a weak, thready pulse, eyes which appear glazed, and an inability to answer simple questions appropriate for age (e.g. 'What is your name?', 'How old are you?', 'When is your birthday?', 'Where do you live?'). Children showing signs of concussion should be sent immediately to hospital for observation and not adjusted until such time as all clinical evidence of concussion has resolved.

The short-term effects of mild to severe head trauma are well documented and commonly include symptoms such as headache, dizziness, fatigue and memory loss (Overweg-Plandsoen et al 1999). While it has been assumed that these symptoms have in the main arisen for cerebral edema, recent brain imaging studies have shown this not to be the case. Currently it is thought that the pathophysiological mechanisms for the short-term symptoms that follow mild head trauma include cortical spreading depression and trauma-triggered migraine. Research has demonstrated the involvement of the trigeminovascular pathways in both these disorders and shown that head trauma can be associated with non-congestive cerebral hyperemia (Sakas et al 1997).

The longer-term effect of mild head trauma in childhood has been the subject of much investigation. It has been found at 1-, 5- and 10-year-old follow-up that developmental status is almost completely unaffected (Bijur et al 1990, Farmer et al 1987, Jordan et al 1992). What has become clear, however, is that symptoms referable to the original head trauma are in evidence at 2-year follow-up; they include deterioration of school performance, development of hyperactive disorder, somatic complaints including headache, aggressiveness, problems socializing, thought and attention deficits, delinquency, dizziness, fatigue, and other behavioral problems (Asarnow et al 1991, Ong et al 1998, Overweg-Plandsoen et al 1999). Head trauma is discussed more fully later in this chapter.

Occasionally, after injury, a child may present with occipital neuralgia, which is head pain in the distribution of the second cervical dermatome arising from irritation of the greater occipital nerve. The pain will sometimes refer to the frontal and eye region. The symptoms associated with occipital neuralgia are commonly a result of the upper cervical subluxation complex and tend to resolve quickly after subluxation correction.

Diagnosis of headache

In children presenting with headache, diagnosis should only be made after carefully weighing the evidence from the history and physical examination. The diagnosis in headache cases is almost exclusively made clinically, investigations serving the purpose of confirming what the history and examination have shown. Very many cases of headache in children (and adults as well) are directly attributable to the subluxation complex and generally occur in predictable patterns. The neuroanatomical basis of this apparent patterning of cervicogenic headache is convergence in the trigeminocervical nucleus between nociceptive afferents from the field of the trigeminal nerve and the receptive fields of the first three cervical nerves. Only structures innervated by C1–C3 have been shown to be capable of causing headache. These structures include muscles, joints and ligaments of the upper three spinal motion segments, dura mater of the spinal cord and posterior cranial fossa, and the vertebral artery (Bogduk 1992). The role of craniosacral therapy in the treatment of patients with headache arising from these structures is obvious. This neuroanatomical model does not apply, however, in patients who describe their 'headache' as being at the base of the occiput and in the posterior neck muscles. The pathomechanics in this case usually involve the lower cervical motion segments or the lumbosacral junction. The relationship between anatomical location of headaches and the spinal level commonly affected by the chiropractic subluxation is shown in Table 7.8.

Management of the child with headache

Chiropractic management is guided by diagnosis in children presenting with headache. Once it can be confidently established that the child's headache is caused by the subluxation complex and is not due to pathology, chiropractic care can be implemented. To assist in the estimation of clinical progress, pain assessment evaluations and headache logs should be kept on the affected child (see Chapter 20). Failure of any child with headache to respond to some degree in the short term should always force a diagnostic re-evaluation, and a careful consideration of triggering factors such as bullying at school, allergy, food intolerance, other illness, etc.

Table 7.8 Common relationship between spinal levels of subluxation and the anatomical location of headache in children

Cranial location of headache	Spinal level of subluxation complex
Frontal region	Primarily occipitoatlantal, but may be axis/C3
Retro-orbital	Axis/C3
Temporosphenoidal	Atlantoaxial
Occipital (neuralgia)	Atlantoaxial
Suboccipital/neck	Lower cervical, lumbosacral, thoracolumbar junction

Neurocutaneous syndromes

There are a number of congenital conditions that have been classified as neurocutaneous syndromes (Gomez 1987). In this section, the three conditions most likely to be encountered in childhood will be discussed: neurofibromatosis, tuberous sclerosis and Sturge–Weber syndrome. Neurocutaneous syndromes, as the name implies, have both cutaneous and neurological features.

Neurofibromatosis

Neurofibromatosis (NF) is the most common of the neurocutaneous syndromes with an incidence of 1 in every 3000 people (Riccardi & Eichner 1986). Neurofibromatosis is an autosomal dominant disorder, the clinical presentation of which is highly variable (Huson et al 1988, Riccardi & Lewis 1988). There are the characteristic hyperpigmented skin lesions (café-au-lait spots) in addition to arterial and bony dysplastic lesions and tumors that primarily involve the nervous system (Blatt et al 1986, Yochum & Rowe 1996). The most common reason why a child with neurofibromatosis will present for chiropractic care is school learning difficulties. As many as 40% of children with NF have learning disabilities (Menkes 1995), making the diagnosis one which should be considered in all such children presenting for chiropractic care.

Neurofibromatosis divides readily into two subgroups. NF1 accounts for approximately half of all cases of neurofibromatosis (Carey et al 1979) and is characterized by multiple neurofibromas, café-au-lait spots, Lisch nodules, arterial or bony dysplasia, an increased incidence of optic nerve and other tumors (Roach 1992), and freckling in the axillary fossae and inguinal areas. NF1 is referred to as von Recklinghausen's disease. NF2, on the other hand, is characterized by bilateral acoustic neuromas and other intracranial and intraspinal tumors, but only infrequently are there café-au-lait spots or peripheral tumors (Eldridge 1981).

Café-au-lait spots are generally light brown and range in size from a few millimeters to several centimeters. They are usually present at birth and may increase in both size and number during the first 10 years of life (Whitehouse 1966). While one to three café-au-lait spots may be seen in normal children, a total of six or more having one diameter of at least 5 mm (pre-adolescent children) or 15 mm (adolescents) is considered diagnostic of neurofibromatosis (Behrman & Vaughan 1987, Moe & Seay 1997).

Neurofibromas, which arise from the peripheral nerves, are not commonly seen prior to puberty. Beyond puberty they frequently increase in both size and number until eventually several hundred lesions may be counted (Roach 1992). Neurofibromas are principally found on the trunk and, while they cause pain, progressive loss of function from nerve compression, and disfigurement, they seldom ever undergo malignant change. Tumors of the peripheral nerves may arise at any age and involve any of the major nerve trunks (Menkes 1995).

A small number of children with neurofibromatosis (NF1) will develop vascular complications, most often stenosis of the renal and carotid arteries (Roach 1992). There is also an increased incidence of pheochromocytoma causing hypertension, although this is found with a much greater frequency in the adult patient than in the child (Kalff et al 1982). The usual clinical presentation of children with cerebral vasculopathy is headache, seizures and focal neurological deficits (Levinsohn et al 1978). Cerebrovascular accidents may occur. These cause an abrupt evolution of neurological signs (Menkes 1995). A wide range of skeletal disorders may accompany neurofibromatosis, including sphenoid dysplasia, tibial pseudarthrosis (Holt & Kuhns 1976), scalloping of the vertebral bodies (Casselman & Mandell 1979, Yochum & Rowe 1996), shortness of stature (Riccardi 1981) and macrocephaly (Weichart et al 1973).

On ophthalmoscopy, Lisch nodules may be seen as pigmented hamartomas in the iris. Their clinical significance is akin to that of café-au-lait spots and some authors consider them pathognomonic of neurofibromatosis type 1 (Lubs et al 1991). Retinal hamartomas are also sometimes seen in association with neurofibromatosis. Whereas intraspinal tumors are rare in children, intracranial tumors may arise. These most commonly affect the optic nerve and produce generalized seizures in 7% of cases (Menkes 1995).

The diagnosis of neurofibromatosis is readily made when the typical characteristic features are all present. However, in younger children, it is common for several features to be absent, making confirmation of the diagnosis difficult if not impossible. For the chiropractic clinician faced with a child who has some of the signs of neurofibromatosis but not enough for diagnostic certainty, a referral to a pediatric specialist for evaluation is appropriate. Confirmation of the diagnosis is based on the demonstration of the café-au-lait spots, two or more neurofibromas, freckling in the axillary or inguinal areas, an optic glioma, two or more Lisch nodules, a dysplastic osseous lesion and a first-degree relative who meets the diagnostic criteria (Moe & Seay 1997).

Once the diagnosis is established, chiropractic management decisions revolve around safety issues. Before care is implemented, the chiropractor should be absolutely certain of the structural and histological integrity of the underlying tissues.

Tuberous sclerosis

Tuberous sclerosis is an autosomal dominant disorder that, like neurofibromatosis, may present with a wide range of symptoms (Moe & Seay 1997, Roach 1992). Tuberous sclerosis is an important cause of seizure activity and mental retardation. As many as 50% of all children with tuberous sclerosis are mentally retarded and 5% of all children with infantile spasms (a serious form of epilepsy) have tuberous sclerosis (Moe & Seay 1997). Seizure activity occurs in as many as 90% of tuberous sclerosis patients and, when seen in infants, it represents a poor prognostic sign for mental retardation later in childhood. Other lesions may be found in the brain, skin, eyes, kidneys, heart, bones and lungs (Yochum & Rowe 1996).

The most likely early signs which would prompt parents to bring their child for chiropractic care are seizures which may have a 'colic-like' appearance. The typical hypopigmented skin lesions will be seen on careful inspection during the routine physical assessment.

The characteristic appearance of the skin lesions is small, bright red or brownish nodules (adenoma sebaceum) extending across the nose and down toward the nasolabial folds, hypomelanotic macules (ash leaf spots), ungual fibromas (fleshy lesions arising from around the nail bed), or shagreen patches. While discreet early in life, these are usually present from birth (Moe & Seay 1997, Roach 1992).

Adenoma sebaceum will be present in 70–83% of patients with tuberous sclerosis (Gomez 1988), but the condition is not usually present at birth. It tends to appear between the fourth and tenth year of life (Roach 1992) when seizures may have already developed. Shagreen patches, slightly raised lesions with an irregular border and textured surface, are noted in 20–35% of post-pubertal patients but are not particularly helpful in confirming a diagnosis of tuberous sclerosis (Roach 1992). Café-au-lait spots are fairly common (Moe & Seay 1997), but their significance is unknown, since it is rare to see more than one or two in tuberous sclerosis patients. Ungual and gingival fibromas are present in only 15–20% of tuberous sclerosis patients and do not usually appear until adolescence (Roach 1992), making them of little value in the early diagnosis of this disorder.

White spots (leukoderma), rare in normal children, are seen in 78% of cases with tuberous sclerosis. These may be small white freckles measuring 2–3 mm or large (7–8 cm), but only 18% of white spots have the typical ash leaf shape. Parents of children with tuberous sclerosis uniformly comment that these white spots were present at birth. They neither increase in size and number as the child becomes older, nor do they disappear. Their detection is facilitated by the use of a Wood's lamp. The white spots of tuberous sclerosis need to be differentiated from vitiligo.

There are consistent ophthalmic features of tuberous sclerosis. In one case series, 87% of tuberous sclerosis patients had retinal abnormalities (Kiribuchi et al 1986). Abnormalities include the characteristic 'mulberry lesion' of retinal astrocytoma, plaque-like hamartomas, and achromic areas (Roach 1992).

The first sign of tuberous sclerosis in some children may be developmental delay, obviating the need to perform routine developmental screening on all pediatric patients.

The diagnosis of tuberous sclerosis is based on the demonstration of facial angiofibromas (adenoma sebaceum) or subungal fibromas, hypomelanotic macules, gingival fibromas, retinal hamartomas, cortical tubers or subependymal glial nodules, and renal angiomyolipomas (Moe & Seay 1997). Radiological imaging procedures are essential to confirm the diagnosis. Once the possibility of tuberous sclerosis is suspected, a pediatric referral in the first instance is appropriate, to have organ imaging procedures performed in order to document the extent of the disease. After this is accomplished, there is no reason why chiropractic treatment cannot be provided for these children, provided the usual spinal indications are present and no contraindications are demonstrable.

While the prognosis is variable, a good number of these children grow to have a full and productive adult life within the constraints of their degree of mental retardation.

Sturge–Weber syndrome

The Sturge–Weber syndrome consists of a port wine nevus seen over the first division of the Vth cranial nerve, a meningeal venous angioma and a choroidal angioma. The syndrome is sometimes seen without the facial nevus (Moe & Seay 1997). The only evidence of underlying neurological disease is often the facial nevus that may, on occasion, be more extensive than the first division of the Vth cranial nerve. Neurological symptoms and signs which may accompany the Sturge–Weber syndrome are focal seizures, hemiparesis and hemiatrophy of the limbs on the opposite side, intellectual impairment and occasionally glaucoma.

Only about 10% of all children with a facial cutaneous angioma actually have the typical brain lesion of Sturge–Weber syndrome (Roach 1992). Given that children with an intracranial angioma are initially normal, it is essential to arrange for a CT scan in all children who present with the typical facial nevus. Management of children with Sturge–Weber syndrome revolves around the need to control seizure activity. Chiropractic care is an integral part of the management of children with Sturge–Weber syndrome provided the usual clinical indications are present and no contraindications are demonstrated.

Head trauma

Head trauma is a common occurrence in childhood, both accidental (road trauma, schoolyard) and intentional (in the bosom of the family), and can readily result in bleeding into the epidural or subdural spaces, or into the cerebral substance itself.

The history of trauma may be lacking, or purposely suppressed, but the associated change in consciousness caused by direct damage to the brain should suggest what has happened. A skull and/or facial fracture and superficial signs of injury will strengthen the suspicion. Because of its flexibility, the infant and child's skull can sustain a greater degree of deformation than the adult skull before incurring a fracture.

Physical forces act on the head through acceleration, deceleration or deformation. The brain is injured through compression, tearing and/or shearing. Because of its elasticity and ability to undergo a greater degree of deformation, the skull of an infant absorbs the energy of the physical impact and protects the brain better than it does in older people. When the stationary head receives a blow, it is accelerated and the skull becomes deformed. Deformation that is both general and localized at the site of impact may produce a skull fracture. However, even fatal intracranial injuries may occur without fracture.

The forces described cause the brain to move differentially with respect to the skull, so that at the site of impact a momentary increase in pressure (compression) occurs, while negative pressures occur contralaterally. Differential movements of the brain and pressure changes are responsible for the contrecoup injury that may occur when the resting head is suddenly accelerated, so that an occipital blow may result in major injury to the frontal and/or temporal lobes. Conversely, when the brain is injured by sudden deceleration (as in falls), cerebral damage is generally greatest near the point of impact (Menkes 1995).

The most common effect of head trauma is concussion (a transient state of neuronal dysfunction, induced by trauma, and of instantaneous onset), which may be followed by lasting amnesia. Boys are more commonly involved than girls. The exact mechanisms of the neuronal dysfunction are not well understood. When the injury is mild, initial unconsciousness is brief, followed by confusion, somnolence and listlessness. Vomiting, pallor and irritability are common.

More severe head injuries induce gross and microscopic hemorrhages of the brain substance. Contusions are petechial hemorrhages along the superficial aspects of the brain, occurring at the site of impact (coup injuries) or at contrecoup areas. As a rule, contusions are less common in infants and small children than in adults subjected to comparable trauma.

An extradural hematoma is a localized accumulation of blood between the skull and the dura which develops at the point of impact. In children, extradural bleeding can be the consequence of even mild injury that has produced a tear in the dural veins or the meningeal arteries or veins. The severity of symptoms depends on the size of the hematoma, the speed of its evolution, and the development of transtentorial herniation. The child is usually stunned by the injury (or at worst has a brief period of unconsciousness), then, after a period of minutes to days (in general the younger the child the longer the latency), develops a delayed progressive loss of consciousness, and neurological signs appear (unequal pupils, hemiparesis, papilledema, cranial nerve paresis). The secondary effects of brain trauma develop as the result of cerebral edema and circulatory disorders. Cerebral edema induces vascular stasis, anoxia and vasodilatation. If the edema is of sufficient magnitude, and if the progression is not checked, a self-perpetuating sequence of events may develop which further increases cerebral swelling, causing brain herniations, resulting in occlusion of other vessels, further infarction and further herniation (Menkes 1995).

Cerebral lacerations are usually associated with penetrating or depressed skull fractures. These usually involve tears of the dura and tears of major blood vessels (resulting in thrombosis, hemorrhages and focal brain ischemia).

Traumatic thrombosis of the extracranial part of the carotid artery, from hyperextension and rotation injury to the neck, may cause hemiplegia. There is usually a latent period of up to 24 hours between the time of injury and onset of neurological signs. There may be emboli formed in the injured artery, which then enter the cerebral circulation. Another cause of internal carotid artery thrombosis is that of a child who has a pencil, lollipop or stick in the mouth and who falls forward, causing a non-penetrating injury to the peritonsillar area. Because of the latent period of up to 24 hours between the injury and the onset of neurological signs, the trauma may have been forgotten, or its significance overlooked. Symptoms include focal ischemia or a headache accompanied by an objective or subjective bruit and Horner syndrome (Menkes 1995).

Myasthenia gravis

Myasthenia gravis (MG) is rare in children. The variety of myasthenic syndromes seen in infancy and childhood is much more variable than that seen in adult life. Involvement of the eye muscles and ptosis occur in almost all, but weakness of the limbs is usually the presenting complaint.

There are three manifestations of MG in children. In neonatal MG, which may be seen in infants born to mothers with MG, symptoms appear within the first to third days of life, affecting the lower bulbar muscles, causing a weak cry and difficulty swallowing or sucking. This affects about 1 in 7 children born to myasthenic mothers. Generalized hypotonia is found in about half the infants. These children respond to anticholinesterase medication and, even if untreated, the manifestations of the disease usually last less than 5 weeks.

In congenital MG, where the mother does not have MG, the symptoms usually begin prior to 2 years of age, and one or more siblings may be affected. Fetal movements may have been noted to be reduced and there may be feeding difficulties and a weak cry. In childhood MG (2–20 years) the disease is often the sequel to acute febrile illness, and is two to six times more common in girls (Aicardi 1992, Brett 1983, Menkes 1995).

The diagnosis is often overlooked because of its rarity in childhood, and confusion with other diseases is easy. A variable ptosis may be attributed to ophthalmoplegic migraine, and it often seems to be precipitated by an infection or emotional disturbance. The very variability of the weakness and fatigability of muscles (which are the diagnostic features of the disease) may be misinterpreted as due to conversion hysteria or some other psychological disorder, especially if the symptoms begin soon after an emotional upset. The expressionless face may be attributed to depression. If the weakness comes on soon after an infection, a polyneuritis may be suspected.

Diagnosis is confirmed by rapid improvement after injection of Tensilon (edrophonium), electromyography before and after muscle stimulation and Tensilon injection, and the demonstration of acetylcholine receptor antibodies (Aicardi 1992).

Medication treatment of the myasthenic patient is by the use of anticholinesterase drugs. Patients may also have steroid medication, plasmaphoresis and thymectomy.

Spinal cord injury

Because of its protected location, a considerable amount of direct trauma is required to injure the spinal cord. In children, therefore, injuries to the spinal cord are most frequently the result of indirect trauma. This is seen in accidents marked by sudden hyperflexion, or hyperextension of the neck, or vertical compression of the spine by falls onto the head (diving into shallow water) or buttocks (fall from a height or athletic injuries) (Aicardi 1992).

Non-accidental injuries to the spinal cord may be induced by shaking the head, and may be responsible for some 'crib deaths'.

Pathological lesions include swelling of the cord with multiple punctate hemorrhages extending over several segments (hematomyelia); softening of the cord as a consequence of injuries to spinal arteries (myelomalacia); spinal epidural and subdural hematomas which may compress the cord; and direct trauma by bone or intervertebral disc material.

The clinical features of spinal cord injury vary with the location of the trauma, the structures affected, and the severity of the insult. Common sites for childhood spinal cord injuries are at the C2, T7, T10 and L1 vertebrae (Ruge et al 1988). Fracture dislocations of the vertebral column are the most frequent immediate causes of spinal cord injuries. Because of its mobility, the lower cervical spine is particularly prone to this type of injury. Fractures of T12 and L1 may produce a conus medullaris and cauda equina syndrome (Menkes 1995).

Direct violence along the axis of the vertebral column may produce fractures of the vertebral bodies and the spinal cord may be injured by fragments of bone entering the vertebral canal. Major spinal cord injuries (early paraplegia), without radiological evidence of either fracture or dislocation, are not unusual in children. Damage may be due to direct compression by bone and intervertebral disc, or from within by hematoma or interference with the spinal cord's vascular supply (Aicardi 1992).

In many patients who develop early paraplegia, the spinal cord shows no gross pathological abnormality. Such a picture has been termed spinal concussion and is characterized by transient loss of spinal cord function. The clinical picture depends on the severity of the injury and its location. Concussion can result from apparently minor falls on the back and is characterized by a temporary and completely reversible loss of function below the injured segment. Signs of recovery appear within hours to a few days.

With more extensive injuries, recovery is only partial, and permanent sequelae can be expected. When the cord is seriously compromised, the clinical picture is highlighted by spinal shock affecting the distal segments. Spinal shock is a transient decrease of synaptic excitability of neurons distal to the injury. It is caused by a loss of supraspinal impulses, which normally produce a background of partial depolarization of the spinal neurons. The first phase of spinal shock (flaccidity) is characterized by distal loss of motor, sensory, reflex and sphincter functions lasting 2–6 weeks. Gradually muscle tone returns. The earliest movements to occur in the legs are flexor. Muscle stretch reflexes (MSRs) then reappear and become hyperactive and the Babinski response to the plantar reflex can be elicited (Aicardi 1992, Menkes 1995).

Cord injury is rare in cephalic deliveries. Spinal cord injury in breech extractions has been long recognized as an important cause of fetal death and paraplegia; 75% of cases are related to breech deliveries. Hyperextension of the neck is an important factor and, if detected prenatally, cesarean section is indicated, which usually avoids cord damage or death. With improvements in obstetric techniques, such cases have become much rarer, and the spinal cord lesions less severe (Brett 1983, Menkes 1995). There are special problems in children with congenital anomalies of the spine, such as atlantoaxial instability as a consequence of Down syndrome, or of anomalies of the cervico-occipital articulation, or of the odontoid. Such children are prone to the development of quadriparesis or other deficits following minor trauma.

Examination of the child with spinal cord injury

The patient with suspected cervical spinal cord injury must be investigated with X-ray. Because movement may aggravate the cord injury, only the absolutely essential diagnostic studies are done.

In small children the clinician can best perform the sensory examination by demonstrating impairment of autonomic response. Shortly after the injury, the dermatomes below the lesion are dry. In general, sensory changes give a clearer indication of the level of the lesion than do motor changes. There are no reflex or motor responses seen during the acute phase of spinal shock. The severity of injury often cannot be determined immediately. An early return of reflex activity, particularly of extensor movements, is encouraging.

Management of the child with spinal cord injury

Spinal cord injuries are usually managed by using traction and/or surgery. Steroids are usually administered to prevent edematous swelling and resulting cord strangulation. Recovery may extend over 6–12 months. The long-term care of the paraplegic child is beyond the scope of this book.

Peripheral nerve injury in childhood

Peripheral nerve injuries are not common in childhood. The most common postnatal injuries are of the brachial plexus nerves caused by severe trauma to the shoulder or traction to the arm. Other nerve injuries in children include division of the median and ulnar nerves at the wrist owing to pushing the hand through a pane of glass; to the radial nerve following fracture of the mid-humerus; to the ulna nerve at the elbow owing to fracture or dislocation of the medial epicondyle; to the common peroneal nerve owing to fractures of the neck of the fibula; and to the sciatic nerve owing to misplaced injections in the buttock (Menkes 1995).

Symptoms similar to those seen in common peroneal neuropathy sometimes occur in children who have sustained an inversion injury to the ankle causing subluxation of the fibula at both its proximal and distal ends ('dropped fibula'). This subluxation complex is described in Chapter 27.

Tics and Tourette (Gilles de la Tourette) syndrome

Tics are involuntary contractions of related groups of skeletal muscles, involuntary noises, or involuntary utterances of words. Simple motor tics (blinking, nodding, shaking the head, shrugging the shoulders, repetitive throat clearing, snorting, shouting) are extremely common phenomena, occurring at some time during late preschool or early school years in at least 10% of all children.

Tourette syndrome is a genetically determined (autosomal dominant with greater penetrance in males) metabolic disorder. It has an incidence of 1% in school-age boys and 0.1% in school-age girls (Aicardi 1992). It is rare to find Tourette syndrome among black populations. Tourette syndrome tends to straddle the clinical disciplines of neurology and psychiatry. It is characterized by muscle twitching and the urgent need to say out loud obscene words, beginning in childhood (usually between the ages of 5 and 8 years). It occurs along a continuum of mild and transient tics at one end to the complete Tourette syndrome at the other (Aicardi 1992, Menkes 1995).

The first manifestation of the disease is the appearance of tics involving the face and neck. The movements increase with involvement of the shoulders and upper limbs, followed by the lower limbs. Respiration and phonation become involved, and the patient develops grunting or barking. The expulsion of air gives an explosive quality to the speech, with occasional hissing sounds. Some patients develop repetitive obscene sexual verbal expressions which they cannot control.

Tourette syndrome does not affect intelligence and, while it lasts for life, it does become less severe after adolescence (Aicardi 1992, Brett 1983, Menkes 1995). It may be associated with attention problems, difficulties with mathematics, conduct problems, fidgetiness, obsessiveness and compulsions (e.g. to touch things in passing), compulsive public exposure of the genitals, aggressive impulses and compulsive self-mutilation. Many psychiatric diagnoses may be considered before the correct diagnosis is established.

The majority of patients do not require specific treatment, and most can learn to live with the problem without too much embarrassment. The best approach is to make the correct diagnosis and inform the parents and child that there is not a primary psychological, psychiatric or neurological condition. The outcome with those who require medication is usually relatively good, but in many this is achieved at the price of some clouding of mental processes.

Neurological infection

The CNS responds to injury in a limited number of ways. Regardless of the nature of the invading organism, infectious diseases share a number of clinical and pathological features, with various unique symptom complexes being caused by virulence of the particular invading organism and variable expression of the host defense mechanisms.

These infections are a formidable challenge to clinicians who must recognize the conditions in the earliest stages for optimal results of treatment. With few exceptions, the many types of meningitis and encephalitis are clinically indistinguishable. The diagnosis requires radiology and laboratory studies, including the isolation and propagation of the suspected organism (Aicardi 1992, Brett 1983, Menkes 1995).

Despite major medical advances, infections of the nervous system remain common life-threatening conditions with great potential for permanent damage in survivors (mental retardation, seizures, hemi- or quadriparesis, deafness, vestibular disturbances, hydrocephalus, etc.). It has been estimated that, in the life of a cohort of 1000 newborns, bacterial meningitis will develop in at least six children, one of whom will die, and two will be left with serious permanent neurological defects (Brett 1983).

Box 7.3

Common symptoms associated with neurological infection

- Headache (often accompanied by photophobia)
- Fever
- Nausea
- Vomiting
- Lethargy
- Disorientation/alterations of sensorium
- Cranial nerve palsies (most commonly III, IV, VI, VII)
- Pupillary changes
- Hemiparesis (increased reflexes, Babinski response)
- Anorexia
- Seizures/convulsions
- Respiratory distress
- Irritability
- Jaundice
- Bulging or full fontanel
- Diarrhea
- Neck pain and stiffness
- Ataxia
- Papilledema

In the early phases of an acute infection of the brain and/or meninges the pathophysiological effects may undergo rapid changes and the clinician must be alert to recognize, and indeed should attempt to anticipate, these changes.

Signs and symptoms which should raise the suspicion of CNS infection (encephalitis, meningitis, abscess) are shown in Box 7.3.

Changes in muscle stretch reflex (MSR) response

The so-called 'deep tendon reflexes', which are not tendinous but more accurately termed muscle stretch reflexes, are of significant clinical use in pediatrics. They are sometimes not able to be elicited in smaller children and infants because of improper patient position. The muscle to be tested should be placed in a position midway between stretch and full contraction. The clinician should make sure that the tendinous fibers, rather than the muscle itself, are struck with the reflex hammer, as the latter would bring a response due to myostatic irritability.

The muscle stretch is a simple monosynaptic reflex arc originating in the muscle stretch receptors, moving along the afferent nerves to the dorsal root ganglion, over intermedullary fibers to the anterior horn and on to the terminal axonal structures at the muscle.

Review of functional anatomy

In the pediatric patient, four main reflexes are usually assessed during the neurological examination (Table 7.9). Children with changes in the muscle stretch reflexes may have other signs and symptoms suggestive of neurological disease and the clinician

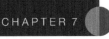

Table 7.9 The four principal reflexes in childhood

Reflex	Structure affected by reflex
S1	Achilles tendon
L4	Quadriceps muscle
C5	Biceps muscle
C7	Triceps muscle

should look carefully for these. When the median nerve is affected, changes may be seen in the thumb and thenar eminence, whereas the ulnar nerve affects the fifth finger and hypothenar eminence. When the radial nerve is affected, the child manifests wristdrop. In the lower extremity, weakness of hip flexion and knee extension result from involvement of the femoral nerve, footdrop results from involvement of the peroneal nerve, and pain in the lateral thigh with an absent Achilles reflex is seen in sciatic nerve involvement (Weiner et al 1981).

Grading and interpreting muscle stretch reflexes in children

Most chiropractors see a predominance of adult patients in day-to-day practice. For this reason, a brief discussion is needed on how to actually grade a muscle stretch reflex in a child. As a general rule, preschool-age children have a more brisk reflex response than do adolescents or adults. Tax (1985) suggests using an identical system of grading to that used for adults (0 to + 4), but with some variation in the interpretation. Using the suggested scale, + 4 would be considered very high or brisk, + 3 a normal response (which equates to + 2 in the adult), + 2 a slow or low response, + 1 a response obtainable only with muscle reinforcement, and 0 meaning no response at all, even with muscle reinforcement.

Clinical interpretation of the hyperreflexive response

Hyperreflexia from pathological causes suggests the presence of a lesion somewhere between the cerebral cortex and the anterior horn cells in the spinal cord. In a child with a reflex grade of +4, the presence of any of the clinical signs in Box 7.4 suggests such a neurological lesion and the child should be referred for specialist investigation.

Clinical interpretation of the hyporeflexive response

Hyporeflexia implies disease somewhere between the anterior horn cells and muscle. It may involve any part of that pathway (Box 7.5).

Abnormal growth of the head

The growth of the head of an infant depends on the growth of the mass inside the skull and the elasticity of the skull surrounding the mass. If the growth of the mass is abnormally

 Box 7.4

Clinical signs associated with hyperreflexia of pathological etiology

At history

- A perinatal history of any birth trauma
- Early development of handedness, particularly on the left. In children who favor the left hand, check the family history – if this is negative, the child may have left-sided brain damage
- History of neurological disease such as meningitis, head trauma, subdural hematoma, etc. which may have left the child with residual unilateral hyperreflexia

On examination

- An inappropriate for age Babinski response
- Sustained ankle clonus
- Contraction of the tensor fascia lata when the sole of the foot is stroked
- A symmetrical absence of the umbilical reflex – this suggests ipsilateral dysfunction of the pyramidal tract
- Asymmetry of limb size, fingers and toenails
- Persistence or absence of infantile automatisms

 Box 7.5

Structures which may be affected in the hyporeflexive child

- Peripheral nerve trunk
- Sensory nerve root
- Anterior horn cells in the cord
- Motor nerve root
- Myoneural junction
- Muscle

slow or the skull does not yield in a normal way, the head will remain abnormally small for age. This condition is called microcephaly (Gamstorp 1985). If the growth of the mass is abnormally fast, the skull will usually yield, and the head becomes large for age. This condition is called macrocephaly (Gamstorp 1985).

The determination of head growth is a fundamentally important aspect of clinical practice for all health care professionals entrusted with the care of children. Establishing the pattern of growth is a simple clinical exercise easily performed in a chiropractic office. The importance of making such measurements and plotting the values on standardized percentile charts is underscored by the fact that most conditions in which the growth of the head is affected are asymptomatic early in their course apart from the change they produce in the rate of growth of the head circumference.

Diagnosis of abnormal head growth

Abnormally large or small head circumferences cannot usually be determined by a single measurement, but require serial measurements to be made over several weeks to months. This is usually done during periodic well baby check-ups, a concept of health care which fits comfortably within the chiropractic paradigm of wellness maintenance. Normal head growth is determined when a child's head circumference consistently follows a given percentile (Fig. 7.9). It may also be normal, in the case of one or both parents having large heads, for there

to be a period of acceleration of the head circumference during the first few months of life followed by consistent growth around a percentile (Fig. 7.10). Abnormal growth is determined when the head circumference measurements either accelerate (Figs 7.11 and 7.12) or decelerate (Fig. 7.13) over time compared to the child's length and weight

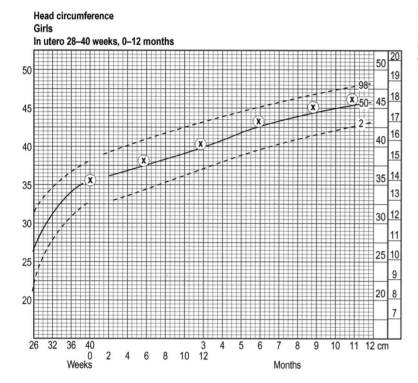

Figure 7.9 • Consistent head circumference measurements lying just above the 50th percentile in this child indicate normal rate of head growth over the first year of life.

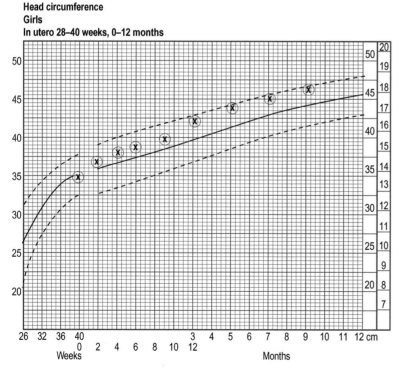

Figure 7.10 • Head circumference measurements which rise steadily from just above the 50th percentile at birth to the 97th percentile by 3 months of age and then stay at that level. This pattern is typically seen in a child whose same-sex parent has a large head circumference.

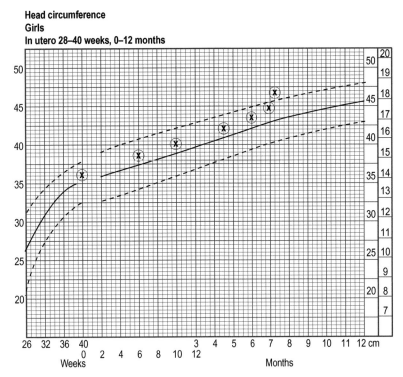

Head circumference
Girls
In utero 28–40 weeks, 0–12 months

Figure 7.11 • A head circumference that has consistently been just above the 50th percentile for the first 6 months of life and then suddenly accelerates. This is the pattern seen in a child with acquired macrocephaly from conditions such as non-communicating hydrocephalus.

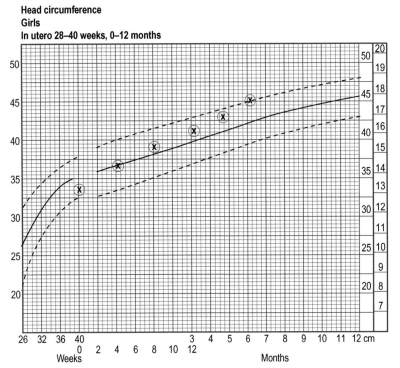

Head circumference
Girls
In utero 28–40 weeks, 0–12 months

Figure 7.12 • The head circumference is steadily accelerating over the first 9 months of life. This is reason for referral if the weight and length percentiles remain stable and therefore more and more out of proportion to the head circumference. Large-for-age anterior fontanel diameter would also be an issue in this case.

measurements. The parents' head size plays a significant role in determining the size of the child's head and should always be taken into account.

Changes in the diameter of the anterior fontanel play a significant role in physical diagnosis where the head is either rapidly enlarging or becoming microcephalic. In macrocephaly, the diameter of the fontanel enlarges as the skull expands. In addition, when the fontanel bulges because of raised intracranial pressure, there is a feeling of tightness in the membrane to palpation. Conversely, in a state of dehydration, the fontanel becomes depressed and feels very soft and 'empty' to palpation. In microcephaly, the fontanel tends to close early. Changes in

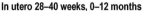

Head circumference
Girls
In utero 28–40 weeks, 0–12 months

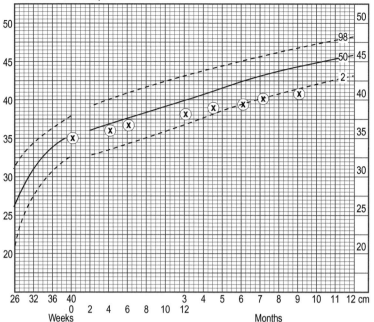

Figure 7.13 • A head circumference that starts at the 50th percentile and steadily decelerates over the first 9 months of life.

the anterior fontanel are a clinically useful and frequently sensitive sign of developing neurological pathology and should form a part of the routine examination of all infants.

Evaluation of the cranial sutures is essential in children manifesting changes in the rate of growth of the head. Ridging may be palpable at one or more of the sutures in children with microcephaly owing to stenosis, and widening may be seen on radiographic evaluation in macrocephaly, particularly when the cause is hydrocephalus. In hydrocephalic children, the sunset sign and Macewen's cracked pot sign are sometimes seen.

Changes in head growth patterns are frequently asymptomatic, particularly early in the course of the underlying condition which may be congenital or acquired.

Conditions which may be associated with microcephaly or abnormally shaped heads are shown in Table 7.10, while those which cause macrocephaly are shown in Table 7.11.

In addition to abnormalities in the velocity of head growth, it is common in the first year of life for the head to develop asymmetrically. The most common of these is plagiocephaly. This condition is commonly associated with impaired cervical spine function arising from the birth experience (Miller & Clarren 2000). Typically, the infant refuses to turn the head to one side, which dictates a fixed sleeping posture with subsequent asymmetrical development of the skull. Plagiocephaly is uncommonly caused by early closure and stenosis of the coronary suture on one side but it is usually functional and related to the birth process. In such non-stenotic, functional cases, surgical intervention is never required and early recognition and correction is essential if a satisfactory result is to be obtained in the short term by non-surgical means (Davies 2002, Kelly et al 1999, O'Broin et al 1999). Clinical experience in the Kiro Kids group of specialist pediatric clinics with a non-synostotic plagiocephaly diagnosed initially by a consultant pediatrician has shown that resolution with

chiropractic care and parental counseling in relation to sleep posture usually occurs before the end of the first year of life with only a minimal amount of care (Davies 2002).

Other conditions which may change the shape of the developing head include scaphocephaly, which is the most common form of pathological plagiocephaly, characterized by premature closure of the sagittal suture with subsequent lack of lateral development of the skull. Scaphocephaly is associated with neurocognitive deficits irrespective of the age at diagnosis (Virtanen et al 1999). Brachycephaly, oxycephaly, trigonocephaly and Crouzon's dysostosis craniofacialis are further rare causes of plagiocephaly (Gamstorp 1985).

Management of the child with abnormal head growth

For the chiropractor, management revolves around diagnostic recognition of a changing head circumference that should always be referred for appropriate diagnostic evaluation. There is little role for the chiropractor to play in either microcephaly, which is commonly due to craniosynostosis, or macrocephaly. In particular, children with macrocephaly due to hydrocephalus should not be adjusted in the upper cervical area owing to the increased kinking of the medullary–cord angle produced by the presence of the fluid. There have been some cases of infarction reported in such cases (Gatterman 1995).

Non-stenotic, functional plagiocephaly is readily managed with chiropractic care. Before care is given, however, the clinician must be sure that no sutural pathology exists, especially at the coronary suture (Gamstorp 1985). A number of studies have shown that when the ear on the flat side of the head is located anterior to its opposite pair, the pathology is almost universally non-stenotic and therefore safe for the chiropractor to manage.

Table 7.10 Symptoms, signs and differential diagnoses associated with an abnormally small head or an abnormally shaped head

Condition	Symptoms and signs
Craniosynostosis	Early closure of the sutures Sutural ridging Decelerating head growth Plagiocephaly
Scaphocephaly	Most common form of craniostenosis Premature closure of the sagittal suture Impaired growth in the width of the skull Normal head length Rarely, increased intracranial pressure Neurocognitive development frequently impaired
Brachycephaly	Premature closure of the coronary suture Skull is longitudinally short, narrow and tall Increased intracranial pressure Bulging fontanel Failure to thrive and vomiting in infants Vomiting and headache in older children Mental retardation, convulsions and optic atrophy may occur in some children in whom the elevated intracranial pressure develops slowly
Oxycephaly	Premature closure of the coronary suture and one other Presentation the same as brachycephaly
Plagiocephaly	Asymmetrical skull development Usually functional but may arise from asymmetrical closure of several sutures
Trigonocephaly	Usually apparent at birth Decreased intercanthal distance Triangular-shaped skull when viewed from above Impaired frontal lobe development Mental retardation
Crouzon's dysostosis	Oxycephaly Beaked nose Hypoplastic maxilla Exophthalmos Strabismus
Defective brain growth	Mental retardation from an early age May be due to prenatal damage from radiation or rubella infection Sometimes associated with dwarfism

Table 7.11 Symptoms, signs and differential diagnoses associated with an abnormally large head

Condition	Symptoms and signs
Physiological variants	Detected by serial head circumference measurement and comparison with parents
Abnormal increase in brain substance	Rare conditions which cause progressive mental, neurological and sometimes other system symptoms
Subdural hygroma	Failure to thrive Anorexia Vomiting Poor weight gain Delayed psychomotor development Convulsions
Hydrocephalus	Rapid increase in head circumference Bulging fontanel Widely separated sutures Engorged veins on the skull Positive sunset and Macewen's signs May be acquired or due to congenital malformation

The diagnosis of cerebral palsy is frequently difficult to make in the first few months of life, but by 8 months examination procedures become more consistently predictive of the diagnosis (Burns et al 1989). Other neurological symptoms and signs (Gamstorp 1985) may sometimes complicate cerebral palsy.

Etiology of cerebral palsy

Cerebral palsy is due to brain injury sustained during gestation, at birth, or acquired after the perinatal period that may have a multitude of causes (Table 7.12). Cerebral palsy most commonly presents as either spastic diplegia or spastic hemiplegia. In spastic diplegia the typical presentation involves adduction,

Table 7.12 Known causes of brain injury leading to cerebral palsy

Age period	Mechanism of brain injury
Prenatal	Infection Complications during pregnancy Autosomal recessive inheritance (rare)
Perinatal	Anoxia Intracranial hemorrhage Birth at <36 weeks of gestation Light-for-date infant Jaundice Meningitis Hydrocephalus
Postnatal	Trauma Infection Arteriovenous malformation

Cerebral palsy

This term is really a description of the presentation rather than a definitive diagnosis. Cerebral palsy has been defined as 'a fixed, non-progressive neurologic deficit acquired before, during or in the months after birth' (Weiner et al 1981). In any way it is defined, and many definitions have been formulated, cerebral palsy is characterized by the presence of a localized, non-progressive brain lesion, a clinical picture which changes with age, causes interference with normal development of the brain, and is dominated by disordered movement and posture.

extension and internal rotation of the legs, tightened Achilles tendons, increased muscle tone, brisk reflexes in the lower extremities, sometimes with sustained ankle clonus and upgoing toes, clumsiness and abnormal posturing in the upper extremities. Spastic hemiplegia, by comparison, is a result of a unilateral brain lesion and therefore involves an arm and a leg on the opposite side. Spastic hemiplegia is the most common form of cerebral palsy acquired after birth (Weiner et al 1981). The presenting symptoms and signs of spastic hemiplegia typically include hyporeflexia, flaccidity in the early months of life, with delay in attaining developmental milestones and, later, hypertonia and spasticity. Underdeveloped thumb and toenails on the affected side are common, as is strabismus. Some children with spastic hemiplegia develop seizure activity. Mental retardation has been found to be more common in these children. Persistent primitive reflexes and abnormal truncal muscle tone are not a part of the clinical picture in spastic hemiplegia (Yokochi et al 1995).

A further category of cerebral palsy is that caused by damage to the extrapyramidal system. The typical presentation of children with this form of the disease is retarded motor development, inability to sit, and persistent primitive reflexes. The infant is hypotonic and in the older child choreoathetosis and dystonia may be seen (Weiner et al 1981).

Diagnosis of cerebral palsy

A child with cerebral palsy may be brought to the chiropractor for any number of reasons. The diagnosis may already be made or the child may be brought because of clumsiness, failure to achieve developmental milestones or hypotonia. The responsibility of the chiropractor is first and foremost to recognize the symptoms and signs from the history and physical examination, and refer for specialist investigation (EEG, CT scan, CSF, hearing and vision). The key findings seen in the first year of life in a child with cerebral palsy are shown in Box 7.6.

Management of the child with cerebral palsy

Once the diagnosis has been firmly established, the management of a child with cerebral palsy becomes a team effort. The basic principles of management are maintenance of motor abilities, prevention of contractures, Achilles tendon lengthening and adductor myotomies (only in extreme cases of contracture), with psychological intervention to bring about a compatible school placement. Braces may be of assistance, and maintenance of spinal and large joint mechanics, especially in the lower extremities, is critical if the child's motor capabilities are to be optimized. Given the constant somatosomatic reflex input into the spinal cord arising from incompetent muscular action, regular spinal assessment and subluxation correction forms an essential part of the total management of children with cerebral palsy.

Parental counseling and support also form a helpful part of management. Parents should be shown how to apply muscle stretch techniques for use at home and advised to avoid baby walkers at all costs. These devices, apart from being dangerous, contribute to the development of common adverse sequelae of

---

Box 7.6

Key findings in clinical history and physical examination suggestive of a diagnosis of cerebral palsy

History

- Prematurity
- Light-for-date
- Low apgar score
- Blood group incompatibility
- Jaundice
- Respirator or oxygen needed at birth
- The child favors one hand
- A history of neurological infection
- The child has had a seizure
- Any other major illness during the first months of life

Examination

- Persistent automatisms
- Spasticity (increased muscle tone, hyperactive reflexes, Babinski response)
- Hypotonia (during first year of life only)
- Asymmetry of limb development, especially nails
- Disordered movement
- Congenital abnormalities
- Strabismus
- Changes to normal head growth
- Delayed developmental milestones

---

spastic cerebral palsy: heel cord contractures, dislocation of the hips, and pronation contractures of the upper extremities (Holm et al 1983).

Vertigo

Only occasionally do chiropractors see children suffering from vertigo. It is a very subjective symptom in which the affected individuals feel as though they, or the environment, are spinning. While adult vertigo can frequently be identified as disturbed proprioception from the cervical subluxation complex (Seifert 1990), most vertigo in children is a symptom associated with underlying disease. In a study of 50 cases of pediatric vertigo, Eviatar & Eviatar (1977) found that 50% were due to seizure activity, with other less common causes being post-infective (meningitis), post-traumatic (concussion), migraine, or vestibular disturbance associated with ear and upper respiratory infection; the remainder were identified as paroxysmal benign attacks or congenital sensorineural deafness. Other far less common causes in childhood include brainstem ischemia, other brainstem disease, vestibular neuronitis, labyrinthitis, postural change, vascular accidents, Ménière's disease, hypertension, hypoglycemia, tumors, drugs, and a variety of psychogenic causes including hyperventilation syndrome (Maran 1988, Tunnessen 1983).

Children with vertigo from middle ear disease describe a sudden sensation of spinning, either in the individual or of the surroundings. Evaluation of a child with vertigo should include: a detailed family and personal history with particular attention to a history of seizures, loss of consciousness, migraine headaches; ear, nose and throat examinations with a hearing evaluation; complete cardiovascular and neurological examination with particular emphasis on balance testing, audiometry, an EEG, and careful spinal assessment (Eviatar & Eviatar 1977, Maran 1988, Seifert 1990, Tunnessen 1983).

It is important in all vertigo cases to include a definitive diagnosis in order to make certain any underlying pathology is identified and addressed in the most appropriate manner. While it may be reasonable for the chiropractor to manage a given case of vertigo in childhood (e.g. in the case of otitis media, etc.), it should be remembered that proprioceptive dysfunction is not a common cause of vertigo in children.

Diagnosis and management of vertigo

Since all children presenting with vertigo require audiometry, EEG examination, and sometimes a CT scan, referral to a pediatric specialist should be made in the first instance. Once the diagnosis has been established, it is appropriate for chiropractors to manage benign cases. It has been established that the cervical spine plays an important role in vertiginous symptoms, particularly subluxation of the upper cervical complex (Seifert 1990). It is also often necessary to apply craniosacral therapy to such cases.

Generalized hypotonia ('floppy' infant)

An infant is considered 'floppy' when there is a diffuse, generalized decrease in the muscular tone. Hypotonia is a complex and difficult clinical problem. Weiner et al (1981) identify cerebral palsy and benign hypotonia (in which there is no pathology at all) as accounting for 75% of all cases. Of the remaining 25%, the lesion may be found anywhere within the neuromuscular system from the cortex to the muscle fibers and connective tissue surrounding the joints (McMillan et al 1977).

The clinical decision that a baby is hypotonic is aided by the following maneuvers:

- Note the head and leg position when the child is held in the prone horizontal position (Landau response). The floppy infant will literally fold around the examiner's hand, while the healthy child will follow the usual response described earlier in this chapter.
- Pull the supine child by the hands to a sitting position. Note the resistance developed in the arms, the strength of grasping with the fingers, and the position of the head, which will usually lag in a hypotonic child.
- With the infant supine, pick up each extremity individually, feel the muscular resistance as you do so, and then note how the limb falls to the examination table when it is released.
- Note the resistance of each of the joints of the extremities on range of motion assessment. In particular, note the response of the infant to rapid abduction of the flexed thighs as this is a common site for the first evidence of developing spasticity (McMillan et al 1977). The responsibility of the chiropractic clinician is to identify that

the presenting child is demonstrating symptoms and signs of hypotonia, not to define the cause.

Clinical history and physical examination are not decisively accurate when attempting to identify the cause of hypotonia and, in particular, the diagnostic conclusion of benign hypotonia can only be deduced from a lack of evidence of pathology on investigation. As such, all infants with generalized hypotonia require specialist referral for diagnostic investigation which may include any of the following: urine analysis, electrolyte evaluation, thyroid studies, amino acid screen, X-ray of the long bones and CT scan of the brain, measurement of creatine phosphokinase level, lumbar puncture, electroencephalography (EEG), nerve conduction tests, muscle biopsy, urinary screen and white blood cell enzyme assays, Tensilon test for myasthenia gravis, and stool culture for clostridia (Weiner et al 1981).

Once the diagnosis of benign hypotonia is established, the implementation of chiropractic care is appropriate. The natural history of hypotonia is for the infant eventually to regain normal tone and motor development. While it has been identified that some of these children have subtle histological variants in their skeletal muscle structure and therefore take additional time to develop fully (Hull & Johnston 1987), others seem to fit another category referred to by Weiner et al (1981) as idiopathic mental or motor retardation. Chiropractic care often provides this category of hypotonic children with a dramatically shortened natural history, some infants progressing from demonstrable weakness to normal motor function, graded on a standard developmental scale, in as little as a few weeks, suggesting a neurological effect caused by the subluxation complex.

Seizures

A seizure (or epileptic attack) is the consequence of a paroxysmal, uncontrolled discharge of neurons within the central nervous system. The clinical manifestations range from a major motor convulsion to a brief period of lack of awareness (Lindsay et al 1991). Some of the terms used in defining clinical effects associated with epilepsy are shown in Table 7.13.

Epilepsy is predominantly a disease of childhood and adolescence, but onset can occur at any age. Some 5% of the

Table 7.13 Terminology used to describe clinical phenomena associated with epilepsy

Term	Definition
Prodrome	Moods or behavior change which may precede the attack by several hours
Aura	The symptom immediately preceding loss of consciousness
Ictus	Refers to the attack itself
Postictal	The time period immediately following an attack during which the patient may be confused, disoriented and dominated by 'automatic' behavior

population suffer a single seizure at some time and 0.5% of the population have recurrent seizures. After a first non-febrile seizure, the chances of further seizure activity relate to the level of neurological impairment. In neurodevelopmentally normal children, 40% will experience further seizures; in children with mild neurological problems, the rate rises to 70%; and in those with severe neurological problems such as cerebral palsy, 90% will have further epileptic attacks (Harris et al 1992). In approximately 50% of all seizures, diagnosis defies description.

Some 90% of patients with recurrent seizures are 'pharmacologically controlled' and 6 years after diagnosis 40% of patients will experience remission, while after 20 years the figure rises to 75% (Lindsay et al 1991).

Classification of seizures

Seizures may be broadly classified as either epileptic or febrile/non-epileptic.

Epileptic seizures

The modern classification of seizures is based on the nature of the attack rather than the underlying cause. The classification of seizures has been aided by the use of EEG examination, which provides specific localization of the source or point of origin of the attack. Attacks are generally identified as focal, meaning they originate from a single location within one hemisphere, or as generalized, meaning they originate in deeper midline structures and project simultaneously to both hemispheres.

Partial seizures may be simple motor, simple sensory, or complex. Simple motor seizures arise from the frontal motor cortex and are seen as either tonic or clonic movement principally in the muscles of the face, trunk or limbs on the side opposite the point of origin. The affected muscles are often weak for a short period after the attack, a phenomenon referred to as Todd's paralysis (Lindsay et al 1991). Simple sensory seizures involve weakness of a limb without involuntary movement, but with associated paresthesia and tingling. Motor and sensory seizures imply the presence of brain disease and require investigation. Complex partial seizures are attacks which originate in the temporal lobe. They may produce a wide range of symptoms including visceral disturbances (hallucinations of taste and smell, epigastric fullness, a choking sensation, nausea, pallor, pupillary dilatation and tachycardia), memory disturbance (déjà vu, flashbacks, etc.), motor disturbance (fumbling movements, rubbing, chewing, semi-purposeful limb movements), and affective disturbance (displeasure, pleasure, depression, elation, fear) (Gamstorp 1985, Lindsay et al 1991).

A characteristic feature of seizure discharge is the capacity to spread from the original source to deeper structures such as the thalamus and upper reticular formation, which in turn discharges back to the whole cerebral cortex of both hemispheres. This progression can be seen on EEG examination and the patient subsequently experiences a tonic–clonic attack. These are referred to as partial seizures evolving to tonic–clonic convulsion. During the tonic phase there is loss of consciousness and the patient falls down with the eyes open,

the elbows flexed with the arms pronated, the legs extended, the teeth clenched, and the pupils dilated. Bowel or bladder function may be lost during this phase of the attack. The clonic phase is characterized initially by tremor which quickly gives way to violent generalized shaking. The eyes roll back and forth, the tongue may be bitten, and tachycardia develops. Tonic–clonic seizures usually result in sequelae characterized by a sense of confusion and headache (Gamstorp 1985, Lindsay et al 1991).

Generalized seizures arise from subcortical structures and involve discharge from the cerebral cortex of both hemispheres. Generalized seizures may be seen as absence attacks, myoclonic seizures, tonic seizures, tonic–clonic seizures, and atonic seizures. Absence attacks occur in children between 4 and 12 years of age and there is a strong familial occurrence. The patient tends to stare vacantly and may experience myoclonic jerking. Absence attacks may occur several times per day and have an average duration of 5–15 seconds. They may be induced by hyperventilation. Absence attacks are rarely seen in adolescents as they tend to progress to tonic–clonic seizure. Myoclonic seizures are characterized by sudden generalized muscle contraction of very short duration. Tonic seizures are seen as sudden-onset muscular contraction with immediate loss of consciousness. Tonic seizures occur as frequently as tonic–clonic seizures in childhood and may have an anoxic etiology. Atonic seizures, otherwise known as drop attacks, are characterized by a sudden loss of muscle tone which causes the patient to fall (Lindsay et al 1991). Tonic–clonic seizures have been described above.

Infantile spasms are an unclassified form of epilepsy. They occur in the first few months of life and are characterized by repetitive shock-like flexion of the neck and trunk with flexion of the knees, a phenomenon referred to as 'salaam attacks'. Some cases of infantile spasms are due to perinatal cerebral injury or a congenital abnormality. The remainder are of uncertain etiology and have a poor prognosis.

Febrile/non-epileptic seizures

These are termed benign febrile convulsions and are seen as a single lifetime entity in up to 3.5% of all children (Gamstorp 1985).

Fever decreases the threshold for fits in all children. Thus children who have afebrile fits may experience an increase in seizure frequency when they have febrile illness, a most important point to appreciate from the clinical history. The true benign febrile convulsion is provoked in an otherwise healthy child by the body temperature itself, not the underlying cause of the fever (i.e. infection). When conducting a clinical assessment of a child who has had a fit, the conditions necessary to establish the diagnosis of benign febrile convulsion include the age of onset, body temperature at the time of the seizure, the type and duration of the seizure, and lack of attendant neurological signs. Typically, the child will be between 6 months and 4 years of age, report concurrent fever, manifest a grand mal seizure type which may last for around 2 minutes but never exceed 10 minutes, and is not associated with any neurological signs, except in the immediate postictal period (Gamstorp 1985, McMillan et al 1977).

Diagnosis of epileptic and febrile/non-epileptic seizures

Unless a child who has had a seizure can be confidently fitted into the febrile/non-epileptic category, then chiropractic care should be delayed until specialist investigation can be carried out. This would include hematology, biochemistry assays, chest X-ray, CT scan in some cases, and EEG examination. Skull X-rays are often performed but have a very low positive return rate and are therefore of questionable clinical value. In children with seizures, the EEG is a most useful diagnostic aid. EEG examples demonstrate a range of normal tracings and some abnormal tracings associated with seizure activity (Fig. 7.14).

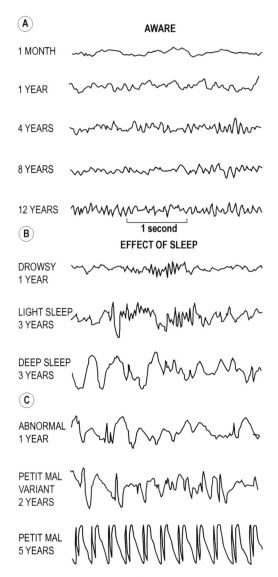

Management of the child with epileptic and febrile/non-epileptic seizures

Once the diagnosis is established, it is appropriate for chiropractors to provide regular care to children with both epileptic and non-epileptic seizures. Because of the nature of the muscular activity during a seizure, subluxation may be encountered anywhere in the axial skeleton. It is most commonly seen as craniosacral dysfunction and in the upper cervical and pelvic areas. Parents should be warned that some children may experience a temporary increase in their seizure frequency immediately following their adjustment, and informed consent should be obtained before proceeding with care. A close working relationship with the pediatrician managing the epileptic child is highly desirable. In the psychosocial area, the chiropractor is in a strong position to support the efforts of the pediatrician in counseling parents and patient about several common issues, such as fear of brain damage, discomfort with the stigmata of the term epilepsy or convulsion, the false belief that the child's condition is somehow related to them, the child's fear of dying or being injured during an attack, and overprotection of the child with inappropriate restrictions (Harris et al 1992).

A working knowledge of the names, actions and common side-effects of anticonvulsive medication may also be helpful when managing an epileptic child. This information is readily available in any drug compendium or on the internet.

Collective clinical experience in the Kiro Kids group of specialist pediatric clinics has demonstrated that when chiropractic care is given immediately after a tonic–clonic seizure there is a considerable shortening of the confusion and headache normally associated with the sequelae to that type of seizure. There is also sporadic evidence, both anecdotally from chiropractors involved in the care of children and in case studies reported in the literature, that epileptic patients who receive chiropractic care may experience a decrease in the frequency of seizures (Alcantara et al 1998).

Cerebral tumors

Cerebral tumor is the second most common malignancy in childhood. The subject is covered in detail in Chapter 17.

Ancillary neurodiagnostic procedures

After taking the patient's history and performing the physical examination, the practitioner then has to decide whether referral for further investigation is needed to assist in the assessment of the patient's complaint. Choice of procedure(s) should be determined by what is safest, least invasive and most economical, and what will most likely confirm or refute the current working diagnosis. A range of neurodiagnostic procedures may be ordered according to clinical presentation.

Cerebrospinal fluid (CSF) examination

CSF is a clear ultrafiltrate of blood produced by the choroid plexus of the lateral, third and fourth ventricles (about 500 ml/day), which provides a floatation layer around the brain and spinal cord that cushions them from trauma, aids in

Figure 7.14 • Encephalograms of infants and children. (A) Tracings from comparable areas of the scalp illustrating variations with age of electrical activity in the motor cortex; all were secured during a quiet phase just before sleep. (B) The effects of sleep – variations in patterns in normal children; compare these with the tracings in A and C. (C) Abnormal waves. (Reproduced with kind permission from Behrman & Vaughan 1987.)

regulation of pH and electrolytes, and allows the circulation of metabolites, electrolytes, hormones, antibodies, leukocytes, etc. Disease may increase or decrease intracranial pressure.

Increased CSF pressure may be due to expanding lesions, prolonged status epilepticus or hypoxia (which cause oedema), metabolic encephalopathies and obstructive lesions, and may be suspected by: bulging fontanel, split sutures, increasing occipitofrontal circumference, headaches, nausea and vomiting, dizziness, transient blurring of vision, mild obtundation.

Decreased CSF pressure may be due to medical procedures that pierce the meninges and cause a CSF leak, skull fractures causing CSF rhinorrhea or otorrhea, or severe dehydration, and may be suspected by: headache, vertigo, tinnitus, nausea, nausea and vomiting, especially when rising to a vertical position from a reclining position (may faint).

A needle is inserted into the CSF (subarachnoid) space. CSF pressure (depends on age) is measured by attaching a manometer to the needle (CSF pressure varies with age: 10–100 mmH$_2$O for infants). CSF should be 'sparkling clear' (cloudiness = increased WBCs, red = blood, yellow = free hemoglobin or bilirubin, or high protein). CSF glucose is normally about 66% of blood glucose (higher in preterm and term infants). High CSF glucose reflects high blood glucose; low CSF glucose implies diffuse meningeal disease (meningitis, encephalitis, neoplasia, etc.).

Plain film X-ray

Plain films serve little purpose if CT or MRI is required, but can be performed quickly and inexpensively, and demonstrate bone, teeth and air-filled cavities (contours, thickness, density, erosion, fracture, dislocation, malformation, foramina, sutures, calcification and calcified lesions), and can therefore screen for many conditions. *Risks*: negligible radiation exposure.

Computed tomography (CT)

CT is cheaper, more available, and has a shorter scanning time than MRI.

As well as showing the structures visualized by plain film X-ray, CT shows brain parenchyma and many parenchymal lesions, and the CSF spaces. CT can be viewed in three dimensions.

Intravenous injection of contrast material demonstrates larger brain vessels and many lesions that have abnormal blood vessels or blood–brain barrier disruption, but CT angiography with contrast material is inferior to magnetic resonance angiography (MRA) and direct angiography.

Order CT instead of MRI if the patient has magnetic metal or electronic devices in the body, if visualization of the vertebral column is a priority, or if time is critical (e.g. intracranial bleeding – CT often shows intracranial bleeding better than MRI). CT poorly visualizes lesions of the posterior fossa or base of the skull because the dense petrous bone degrades the image. CT shows calcifications whereas MRI does not. *Risks*: negligible radiation exposure; some patients may need to be sedated.

Myelography

Visualization of the spinal cord and vertebral lesions by CT or MRI has reduced the need for direct injection of contrast material into the subarachnoid space.

Magnetic resonance imaging (MRI)

Vastly superior specificity and sensitivity compared with CT. MRI is the procedure of choice for imaging the brain and spinal cord. There are a number of different MRI procedures: standard T1- and T2-weighted imaging, diffusion and perfusion weighted imaging, MRA, functional MRI, and spectroscopy (MRS – uses non-water protons). Ordered if there is suspected space-occupying lesion, cerebrovascular disease, demyelinating disease, primary or secondary neoplasia, trauma, acute infections, seizures, and for investigation of headache and the development of the brain.

Gadolinium enhancement shows blood vessels and sites of increased blood–brain barrier permeability (infarcts, contusions, neoplasms, demyelinating lesions). MRA is improved with injection of contrast material. *Risks*: no known adverse biological effects; cannot be used with implants of magnetic metals and certain electronic devices; some patients may become claustrophobic; some patients and infants require sedation to prevent movement during scanning.

Radionuclide scanning

This procedure includes SPECT (single-photon emission computed tomography) and PET (positron emission tomography). Injected (intravenous or into the subarachnoid space) or inhaled radioactive substances are detected by scanning. Studies metabolism of glucose and other metabolites, hyper- or hypoperfusion, localizing active epileptogenic focus, localizes brain activity during specific mental tasks, and brain death.

Doppler ultrasound

Demonstrates blood flow in the larger neck and some intracranial blood vessels.

Head ultrasound

Demonstrates gross cerebral lesions and hemorrhages in fetuses, newborn and young infants. Can be used to some extent until fontanel closure or until about 1 year of age. Can be done repeatedly prenatally, or at the bedside of a sick infant. *Risks*: no known risk.

Electroencephalography

Scalp electrodes record changes in electrical potentials in the underlying cerebrum (the EEG machine amplifies differences in voltage between pairs of electrodes and records them on paper or electronically). Pathology produces waves that are too high or too low in amplitude, too fast or too slow, or abnormal in configuration. Can be used in sleep disorders (combined with video-monitoring), changes in mental state, (confusion, syncope, coma), brain lesions, epilepsy, monitoring anticonvulsant treatment, and brain death.

Evoked responses

Electrodes are placed at various sites on the skin, over the brain or spinal cord, and the transmission through the sensory pathways to the brain is recorded. The studies consist of visual evoked responses, auditory evoked responses, brainstem evoked responses, somatic sensory evoked responses. Brainstem auditory evoked responses should be tested in infants who are late in speaking or who are suspected of deafness.

Electronystagmography

Records spontaneous nystagmus, or that elicited by caloric stimulation, positional change, or an optokinetic drum. Aids in diagnosis of patients with dizziness, brainstem or cranial VIIIth nerve disease.

Electromyography (EMG)

A needle electrode is inserted into a muscle and records the electrical potential when the muscle fibers depolarize and contract. Used to differentiate neurogenic and myopathic weakness.

Nerve conduction velocity

* *Motor*: a stimulating electrode is applied over a motor nerve trunk and the response is recorded by EMG.
* *Sensory*: the time between the passage of an electrical stimulus is measured at two points along a nerve to determine conduction velocity of sensory nerves.

Used in the diagnosis of peripheral neuropathies and nerve compression syndromes.

Nerve biopsy

Sensory nerves (usually the sural nerve) are biopsied. A few metabolic and heredofamilial neuropathies involve characteristic histological changes. The result is collated with muscle biopsy, electromyography and nerve conduction velocity studies.

Brain biopsy

To diagnose the histological type of neoplasms, Creutzfeldt–Jakob disease, rare degenerative diseases and herpes simplex encephalitis.

Sweat testing

For all sweat tests (hyper- or hypohidrosis), the patient is warmed so that sweating is more easily detected.

* *Finger drag method*: applying sufficient pressure to feel friction, the finger of the examiner is moved across the segment concerned while testing for a right–left difference.
* *Ophthalmoscopic method*: with a strong positive lens, pinpoints of reflection from sweat droplets are looked for.
* *Tinctorial method*: substances that change color when exposed to sweat are painted on the body.

References

Aicardi, J., 1992. Diseases of the Nervous System in Childhood. Blackwell Scientific Publications, Oxford.

Alcantara, J., Heschong, R., Plaugher, G., et al., 1998. Chiropractic management of a patient with subluxations, low back pain and epileptic seizures. J. Manipulative Physiol. Ther. 21 (6), 410–418.

Asarnow, R.F., Satz, P., Light, R., et al., 1991. Behavior problems and adaptive functioning in children with mild and severe closed head injury. J. Pediatr. Psychol. 16 (5), 543–555.

Barness, L.A., 1981. Manual of Pediatric Physical Diagnosis, fifth ed. Year Book Medical Publishers, Chicago.

Behrman, R., Vaughan, V. (Eds), 1987. Nelson Textbook of Pediatrics, thirteenth ed. WB Saunders, Philadelphia.

Bellman, M., Kennedy, N., 2000. Paediatrics and Child Health: A Textbook for the DCH. Elsevier Churchill Livingstone, Edinburgh.

Bijur, P.E., Haslum, M., Golding, J., 1990. Cognitive and behavioural sequelae of mild head injury in children. Pediatrics 86 (3), 337–344.

Blasco, P.A., 1994. Primitive reflexes: their contribution to early detection of cerebral palsy. Clin. Pediatr. (Phila) 33 (7), 388–397.

Blatt, J., Jaffe, R., Deutsch, M., et al., 1986. Neurofibromatosis and childhood tumours. Cancer 57, 1225–1229.

Bogduk, N., 1992. The anatomical basis for cervicogenic headache. J. Manipulative Physiol. Ther. 15, 67–70.

Brett, B.M., 1983. Paediatric Neurology. Churchill Livingstone, Edinburgh.

Brothers, K.B., Glascoe, F.P., Robertshaw, N.S., 2008. PEDS: developmental milestones – an accurate brief tool for surveillance and screening. Clin. Pediatr. (Phila) 47 (3), 271–279.

Burns, Y.R., O'Callaghan, M., Tudehope, D.I., 1989. Early identification of cerebral palsy in high risk infants. Aust. Paediatr. J. 25 (4), 215–219.

Capute, A.J., 1979. Identifying cerebral palsy in infancy through study of primitive reflex profiles. Pediatr. Ann. 8 (10), 589–595.

Carey, J.C., Laub, I.M., Hall, B.D., 1979. Penetrance and variability in neurofibromatosis: a genetic study of 60 families. Birth Defects 15 (SB), 271–281.

Casselman, E.S., Mandell, C.A., 1979. Vertebral scalloping in neurofibromatosis. Radiology 131, 89–94.

Coles, C.D., Smith, I., Fernhoff, P.M., et al., 1985. Neonatal neurobehavioural characteristics as correlates of maternal alcohol use during gestation. Alcohol. Clin. Exp. Res. 9 (5), 454–460.

Corwin, M.J., Lester, B.M., Sepkoski, C., et al., 1992. Effects of in utero cocaine exposure on newborn acoustical cry characteristics. Pediatrics 89 (6/2), 1199–1203.

Davies, N.J., 2002. Chiropractic management of deformational plagiocephaly in infants: an alternative to device-dependent therapy. Chiropractic J. Aust. 32 (2), 52–55.

DeMyer, W.E., 1994. Technique of the Neurological Examination: A Programmed Text, fourth ed. McGraw-Hill, New York.

Edgeworth, J., Bullock, P., Bailey, A., et al., 1996. Why are brain tumours still being missed? Arch. Dis. Child. 74 (2), 148–151.

Eldridge, R., 1981. Central neurofibromatosis with bilateral acoustic neuroma. Adv. Neurol. 29, 57–65.

Eviatar, L., Eviatar, A., 1977. Vertigo in children: differential diagnosis and treatment. Pediatrics 59, 833–838.

Farmer, M.Y., Singer, H.S., Mellits, E.D., et al., 1987. Neurobehavioural sequelae of minor head injuries in children. Pediatr. Neurosci. 13 (6), 304–308.

Futagi, Y., Tagawa, T., Otani, K., 1992. Primitive reflex profiles in infants: differences based on categories of neurological abnormality. Brain Dev. 14 (5), 294–298.

Gamstorp, I., 1985. Paediatric Neurology, second ed. Butterworth, London.

Gatterman, M.I., 1995. Foundations of Chiropractic: Subluxation. Mosby, St Louis.

Golub, H.L., Corwin, M.J., 1982. Infant cry: a clue to diagnosis. Pediatrics 69 (2), 197–201.

Gomez, M.R., 1987. Neurocutaneous Diseases. Butterworths, Boston.

Gomez, M.R., 1988. Neurologic and psychiatric features. In: Gomez, M.R. (Ed.), Tuberous Sclerosis. second ed. Raven Press, New York.

Harris, W., Choong, R., Timms, B., 1992. Examination Paediatrics. MacLennan & Petty, Sydney.

Holm, V.A., Harthun-Smith, L., Tada, W.L., 1983. Infant walkers and cerebral palsy. Am. J. Dis. Child 137 (12), 189–1190.

Holt, J.F., Kuhns, L.R., 1976. Macrocranium and macroencephaly in neurofibromatosis. Skeletal Radiol. 1, 25–29.

Hull, D., Johnston, D.I., 1987. Essential Paediatrics, second ed. Churchill Livingstone, Edinburgh.

Huson, S.M., Harper, P.S., Compston, D.A.S., 1988. Von Recklinghausen neurofibromatosis – a clinical and population study in south-east Wales. Brain 111, 1355.

Ignatius, J., 1993. 'Moro reflex' Ernst Moro 1874–1951. Duodecim 109 (9), 789–791.

Jordan, F.M., Cannon, A., Murdoch, B.E., 1992. Language abilities of mildly closed head injured (CHI) children 10 years post-injury. Brain Injury 6 (1), 39–44.

Kalff, V., Shapiro, B., Lloyd, R., et al., 1982. The spectrum of pheochromocytoma in hypertensive patients with neurofibromatosis. Arch. Intern. Med. 142 (12), 2092–2098.

Kelly, K.M., Littlefield, T.R., Pomatto, J.K., et al., 1999. Importance of early recognition and treatment of deformational plagiocephaly with orthotic cranioplasty. Cleft Palate Craniofac. J. 36 (2), 127–130.

Kiribuchi, K., Uchida, Y., Fukuyama, Y., et al., 1986. High incidence of fundus hamartomas and clinical significance of a fundus score in tuberous sclerosis. Brain Dev. 8 (5), 509–517.

Knezevic-Pogancev, M., 2008. Children migraine syndrome – definition and classification through the time [Article in Serbian]. Med. Pregl. 61 (3–4), 143–146.

Laurence, K.M., Coates, S., 1972. The natural history of hydrocephalus. Arch. Dis. Child. 61, 161–168.

Lester, B.M., Dreher, M., 1989. Effects of marijuana use during pregnancy on newborn cry. Child. Dev. 60 (4), 765–771.

Levine, M.D., Carey, W.B., Crocker, A.V., et al., 1983. Developmental Behavioural Pediatrics. WB Saunders, Philadelphia.

Levinsohn, P.M., Mikhael, K.A., Rothman, S.M., 1978. Cerebrovascular changes in neurofibromatosis. Dev. Med. Child Neurol. 20, 789–794.

Lindsay, K.W., Bone, I., Callander, R., 1991. Neurology and Neurosurgery Illustrated. Churchill Livingstone, Edinburgh.

Livingstone, I.H., Brown, I.K., 1986. Intracerebral haemorrhage after the neonatal period. Arch. Dis. Child. 61 (6), 538–544.

Lubs, M.E., Bauer, M.S., Formas, M.E., et al., 1991. Lisch nodules in neurofibromatosis type 1. N. Engl. J. Med. 324, 1264–1268.

McMillan, J.A., Nieburg, P.I., Oski, F.A., 1977. The Whole Pediatrician Catalogue: A Compendium of Clues to Diagnosis and Management. WB Saunders, Philadelphia.

Maran, A.C.D., 1988. Logan Turner's Diseases of the Nose, Throat and Ear, tenth ed. Wright, London.

Marquis, P.J., Ruiz, N.A., Lundy, M.S., et al., 1984. Retention of primitive reflexes and delayed motor development in very low birthweight infants. J. Dev. Behav. Pediatr. 5 (3), 124–126.

Menkes, I.H., 1995. Textbook of Child Neurology, fifth ed. Williams & Wilkins, Baltimore.

Miller, R.I., Clarren, S.K., 2000. Long term developmental outcomes in patients with deformational plagiocephaly. Pediatrics 105 (2), E26.

Moe, P.C., Seay, A.R., 1997. Neurologic and muscular disorders. In: Hay, W.W., Croothius, J.R., Hayward, A.R., et al. (Eds), Current Pediatric Diagnosis and Treatment. Appleton & Lange, Stamford.

Nugent, J.K., Lester, B.M., Creene, S.M., et al., 1996. The effects of maternal alcohol consumption and cigarette smoking during pregnancy on acoustic cry analysis. Child Dev. 67 (4), 1806–1815.

O'Broin, E.S., Allcutt, D., Earley, M.J., 1999. Posterior plagiocephaly: proactive conservative management. Br. J. Plast. Surg. 52 (1), 18–23.

Ong, L.C., Chandran, V., Zasmani, S., et al., 1998. Outcome of closed head injury in Malaysian children: neurocognitive and behavioural sequelae. J. Paediatr. Child Health 34 (4), 363–368.

Overweg-Plandsoen, W.C., Kodde, A., van Straaten, M., et al., 1999. Mild closed head injury in children compared to traumatic fractured bone: neurobehavioural sequelae in daily life 2 years after the accident. Eur. J. Pediatr. 158 (3), 249–252.

Patten, J., 1996. Neurological Differential Diagnosis, second ed. Springer, London.

Riccardi, V.M., 1981. Von Recklinghausen neurofibromatosis. N. Engl. J. Med. 305 (27), 1617–1627.

Riccardi, V.M., Eichner, J.E., 1986. Neurofibromatosis: Phenotype, Natural History and Pathogenesis. Johns Hopkins University Press, Baltimore.

Riccardi, V.M., Lewis, R.A., 1988. Penetrance of von Recklinghausen neurofibromatosis: a distinction between predecessors and descendants. Am. J. Hum. Genet. 42, 284–289.

Roach, E.S., 1992. Neurocutaneous syndromes. Pediatr. Clin. North Am. 39 (4), 591–620.

Ruge, J.R., Sinson, J.P., McClone, D.C., et al., 1988. Pediatric spinal injury: the very young. J. Neurosurg. 68, 25–30.

Russell, M.B., Olesen, J., 1995. Increased familial risk and evidence of genetic factor in migraine. Br. Med. J. 311 (7004), 541–544.

Russell, M.B., Iselius, L., Olesen, J., 1996. Migraine without aura and migraine with aura are inherited disorders. Cephalalgia 16 (5), 305–309.

Rydz, D., Shevell, M.I., Mainemer, A., et al., 2005. Developmental screening. J. Child Neurol. 20 (1), 4–21.

Saito, T., Fujti, T., Tango, T., 1983. Prediction of the development of cerebral palsy from perinatal risk factors. Brain Dev. 5 (1), 1–8.

Sakas, D.E., Whittaker, K.W., Whitwell, H.L., et al., 1997. Syndromes of posttraumatic neurological deterioration in children with no focal lesions revealed by cerebral imaging: evidence for a trigeminovascular pathophysiology. Neurosurgery 41 (3), 661–667.

Seifert, K., 1990. Differential diagnosis and therapy of vertigo of vertebral origin. Laryngorhinootologie 69 (7), 394–397.

Symon, D.N., Russell, C., 1986. Abdominal migraine: a childhood syndrome defined. Cephalalgia 6 (4), 223–228.

Tachdjian, M.O., 1972. Pediatric Orthopedics. WB Saunders, Philadelphia.

Tax, M., 1985. Podopaediatrics, second ed. Williams & Wilkins, London, p. 168.

Tunnessen, W.W., 1983. Signs and Symptoms in Pediatrics. JB Lippincott, Philadelphia.

Van der Wouden, I.C., van der Pas, P., Bruinjzeels, M.A., et al., 1999. Headache in children in Dutch general practice. Cephalalgia 19 (3), 147–150.

Virtanen, R., Korhonen, T., Fagerholm, I., et al., 1999. Neurocognitive sequelae of scaphocephaly. Pediatrics 103 (4/1), 791–795.

Weichart, K.A., Dine, M.S., Benton, C., et al., 1973. Macrocranium and neurofibromatosis. Radiology 107, 163–168.

Weiner, H.L., Bresnan, M.I., Levitt, L.P., 1981. Pediatric Neurology for the House Officer. Williams & Wilkins, Baltimore.

Whitehouse, D., 1966. Diagnostic value of the café-au-lait spot in children. Arch. Dis. Child. 41, 316–319.

Yochum, T.R., Rowe, L.R., 1996. Essentials of Skeletal Radiology, second ed. Williams & Wilkins, Baltimore.

Yokochi, K., Yokochi, M., Kodama, K., 1995. Motor function of infants with spastic hemiplegia. Brain Dev. 17 (1), 42–48.

Zafeiriou, D.I., Tsikoulos, I.C., Kremenopoulos, C.M., 1995. Prospective follow-up of primitive reflex profiles in high-risk infants: clues to an early diagnosis of cerebral palsy. Pediatr. Neurol. 13 (2), 148–215.

Developmental assessment, neuromaturational delay and school learning difficulties

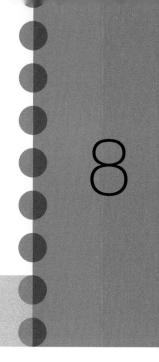

8

Neil J. Davies

Children are essentially 'developing anatomy' and, therefore, measuring the rate of developmental change over time offers the primary contact clinician a window of opportunity to identify normal from abnormal at the earliest possible age. The fact that many serious diseases commonly seen in the pediatric population affect this rate of developmental change makes such assessment an elemental clinical issue as chiropractors fit responsibly into the field of pediatrics.

As Illingworth (1983) notes:

> A thorough knowledge of the normal should be just as much the basis for the study of children as is physiology and anatomy for medicine in general: one needs to be fully conversant with the normal as a basis for the diagnosis and study of the abnormal. All those with responsibility for the care of children, whether clinical medical officers, family doctors, pediatricians or others, need a thorough knowledge of the normal, of the normal variations in development, and the reasons for those variations, almost every day of their work.

Every parent wants to know whether their child is developing normally, especially if with a previous pregnancy there had been a miscarriage, stillbirth or other condition impairing development, and especially if it will result in the child being mentally or physically handicapped. If there was an infection, toxemia or other illness in pregnancy, or some difficulty in delivery, it would be natural for parents to be particularly anxious. A family history of subnormality, cerebral palsy or other handicap will heighten their anxiety.

> Developmental paediatrics – this branch of the art and science of paediatrics, includes numerous clinical as well as social factors. It is concerned with maturational processes (from foetal viability to full growth), in structure and in function, of normal and abnormal children; second to ensure early diagnosis and effective treatment of handicapping conditions of body, mind and personality; and third to discover the cause and means of preventing such handicapping conditions.
>
> (Sheridan 1980)

Chiropractic has much to offer the pediatric patient, but many conditions exist in this age group, the symptoms of which simulate characteristic manifestations of cerebral dysafferentation. Given the place of developmental assessment in pediatric practice generally, it remains the responsibility of individual chiropractors to adequately screen pediatric patients in order to assist in the determination of their suitability for chiropractic care. This form of assessment fits neatly into the chiropractic paradigm of preventive health care, offering as it does a periodic well baby health check designed to document development and thus put the chiropractor in a position to identify variance at its earliest presentation. Unlike other forms of health care, however, chiropractic can offer the genuinely preventive step of correction of neurological dysafferentation which in turn will foster sustainably balanced neurological function and therefore give the best possible chance of the affected child attaining an optimal developmental outcome.

As much as the screening examination will be very helpful to the chiropractor, it must be remembered that it represents only the first step in the assessment process. The purpose of screening is to identify that a problem may exist, not necessarily what the problem is. Developmental screening, performed in a chiropractic clinic, is an examination procedure that has high sensitivity but very low specificity, meaning the procedure identifies the existence of a problem but does not make a diagnosis, a responsibility that remains the domain of the developmental pediatrician.

Theoretical models of developmental pediatrics

As mentioned earlier, developmental screening fits precisely into the chiropractic paradigm of health and wellness. Screening is that activity which has the express purpose of identifying deviant growth and development in its earliest phase, permitting a dynamic parent–clinician intervention in order to attain the most favorable developmental outcome for the child and therefore afford the child the best possible chance to compete in adult life.

© 2010, Elsevier Ltd, Inc, BV
DOI: 10.1016/B978-0-7020-3129-8.00008-6

The principle which underpins all efforts in pediatric health care is best summed up by Behrman et al (2007): 'The goal in the medical management of the child is to permit him to come into adulthood at his optimal state of development, physically, mentally and socially, so he can compete at his most effective level.' Commenting further along these lines, Oberklaid (1986) makes the following observations:

> In the first five years of life there is progression from a neonate who has relatively primitive ways of communicating and is capable of only brief periods of neurological organization so he can react to environmental stimuli, to a child starting school with the capability of sophisticated functioning in multiple domains. Many authors contend that the foundations for later cognitive performance and achievement are already firmly established by the time a child starts school. If there is deviation in development, it has usually become manifest during these years, at least for the more major disabilities. Many subtle developmental dysfunctions only become apparent as the child progresses through school.
>
> The rapid developmental changes occur in the first few years provide the opportunity for the accurate documentation of emerging skills and function, and the comparison of an individual child's progress with the expected. Despite the fact that there is considerable variability in the rate of development, there is consistency to allow the establishment of normal ranges of acquisition of developmental milestones, so that the development falling outside this range in a particular area gives rise to concerns.

Routine developmental screening of pediatric patients will allow the chiropractor to:

- identify developmental anomalies that can be adequately resolved by chiropractic care, parental stimulation and, sometimes, special care from teachers
- identify developmental deviance, the outcome of which will be enhanced if managed by a pediatric specialist, usually in conjunction with ongoing chiropractic care
- establish a developmental norm for each child that will offer a baseline for measurement of acute body weight loss and variations in other growth factors associated with rapid-onset infectious and febrile illness.

Like most new sciences, developmental pediatrics has evolved through a series of models. Early investigators based their observations on the main effect model, which then gave way to the interactional model, from which has now evolved the transactional model.

The main effect model

This model was proposed by Arnold Gessell, who founded the Clinic for Child Development at Yale in 1911 and was in fact the first person to attempt to evaluate childhood development over time using scientific methods. Gesell was of the Freudian viewpoint, studying development from the biological and behavioral perspective (Levine et al 1983).

The conceptual basis of the main effect model is very linear, suggesting a one-dimensional relationship between cause and effect (Fig. 8.1). The main effect model proposes that genetic factors and constitutional defects caused by pregnancy and delivery complications exert such strong influences that an understanding of these factors makes it

Figure 8.1 • The conceptual basis of the main effect model demonstrating the linear, one-dimensional relationship between effect and outcome.

possible to predict a child's later developmental status (Clements 1986).

The main effect model does not find support in any of the longitudinal studies that have been performed and as far back as 1956 Graham demonstrated minimal impairment of function by age 7 in children who had poor neonatal scores because of anoxia at birth (Levine et al 1983).

The interactional model

This model suggests that outcome may be predicted by a consideration of nature and factors related to nurture or the environment. This model asserts that the outcome of a child with constitutional problems will depend upon the degree of nurture inherent within the child's environment (Fig. 8.2). There is some support for this model, even today in the scientific literature, although it has largely given way to the transactional model. While the main effect model is decidedly one-dimensional, the interactional model is two-dimensional as shown in Fig. 8.3.

The transactional model

The transactional model proposes the more dynamic idea that constitution and environment constantly interact with each other to produce change over time (Fig. 8.4). This concept stresses the plasticity of the developing child and suggests that final outcome may remain obscure and unpredictable. Oberklaid (1986) makes the following observations about the transactional model of development:

> Development outcome is the end result of a complex, continuous transaction between constitutional or intrinsic factors in the child and environmental influences and life events. When the outcome is less

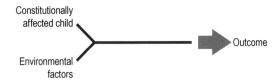

Figure 8.2 • The conceptual basis of the interactional model.

	Constitutional factors	
	Good	Bad
Environmental factors Good	Good	Medium
Environmental factors Bad	Medium	Good

Figure 8.3 • Conceptualization of the two-dimensional relationship between constitutional and environmental factors and outcome.

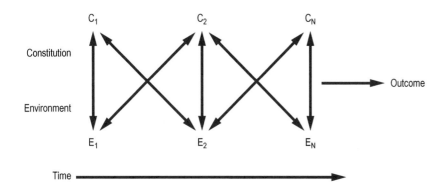

Figure 8.4 • Conceptualization of the transactional model demonstrating the dynamic, multidimensional effect of the sum of the constitutional and environmental factors on each other over time to produce the final outcome in adult life.

than optimal, and a child's development is abnormal, there may be responsible constitutional factors (genetic influences, metabolic disease, structural abnormalities) or factors arising from the environment or from outside the body (trauma, infection) which permanently affect the child's function. In addition to both these realms is the positive or negative effect that a child's environment provides in terms of learning experiences, stimulation, nutrition and other variables. There is evidence that a rich and nurturing environment can, in many instances, significantly ameliorate the effects of constitutional or early intervention programs, where attempts are made to prevent or minimize the subsequent effects of early developmental problems.

The lack of a nurturing environment may have profound effects on development. A child who is structurally intact, and who theoretically has the potential for normal development and cognitive achievement, may in fact be functionally retarded because of inadequate or inappropriate environmental input. This has been termed cultural/familial retardation and is more prevalent in lower socio-economic classes; the level of retardation is usually mild. Severe emotional conflict may similarly render a child developmentally delayed in a functional sense – she is prevented from functioning on a day to day level at her full potential because of these emotional problems. The type of insult to the brain will affect development in a different way, depending on the nature of the insult, the stage of neurological development at the time, and the site of the insult. Those areas of the brain that are undergoing the most rapid maturational changes are the most susceptible. The developing brain on the one hand is more susceptible to environmental insults, but on the other hand is more plastic in its ability to recover. Because of the variety of insults that may occur at various stages of development, there is a wide range of neurological impairments and a heterogeneity of developmental disabilities. It is dangerous to assume homogeneity in developmental delays. For example, a child with cerebral palsy and severe motor handicap, whilst at increased risk of problems in other areas of development, may in fact have normal cognitive functioning. Communication disorders may severely inhibit a child's ability to display intelligence. It is important, therefore, to define development in its very broadest sense, which includes motor, sensory, cognitive, language, social, behavioral and emotional development.

Clinical rationale for conducting periodic developmental screening

In order for developmental screening to be maximally effective, the tests themselves need to be reliable and should be repeated at regular intervals in order to assess development longitudinally against time. The general characteristics of a sound screening assessment instrument are as follows:

Reliability
Results should be consistent from one testing time to the next (test–retest reliability) and between two examiners observing or taking the same measurement (inter-rater reliability).

Validity
Accuracy should be achieved in separating affected from non-affected subjects with the final diagnosis giving confirmation to the test results. The test should offer a system of identifying the majority of subjects who will, if not treated, end up handicapped.

Suitability for mass testing
To facilitate the screening of a large number of subjects, tests should be acceptable to patients and caregivers, easy to administer, simple in format, and economical.

Appropriateness
Tests should be age-appropriate for each child screened. It would be useless, for example, to attempt a test that requires cognitive ability beyond that which would normally be found at a reliable, reproducible level in the subjects to be screened.

Screening the preschool-age child (birth to 4 years)

There are a great many instruments available for use in developmental screening. Some are simply an endless list of age-appropriate achievements which must be attained by the subject and yet others offer a visual or graphic picture of development. Of the latter, the most commonly used is the Denver Developmental Screening Test (DDST) which requires those who wish to employ it to undertake an extensive training program. The DDST instrument arose from a study of over 1000 children, the results of which were published in the early 1970s (Frankenburg et al 1971).

Another simple, questionnaire-based screening protocol, named the Parents Evaluation of Development Status (PEDS), has been proposed but does not compare well with the Denver II screening test (Theeranate & Cheungchitraks 2005) and was not found to be predictive of language, achievement and quality of life 2 years beyond school start when performed at school entry, with sensitivity and specificity values not supporting its use as a stand-alone screen to detect later problems (Wake et al 2005).

The Woodside developmental screening test was developed in Glasgow in the 1970s. This screening instrument, based around the early work of Sheridan, has been standardized against an Australian population sample (Eu 1986) and is the system recommended for use by chiropractors because it meets the criteria of a sound screening system, has a wide margin of safety, sits well within the broader definition of developmental assessment offered by Oberklaid (1986) and only requires minimal training for implementation. In fact, Gupta & Patel (1991) report favorably on a program conducted in India where nonprofessional health workers were trained to perform Woodside developmental screening assessments and did so with an acceptable level of competence following a basic training program.

The Woodside test utilizes a system of four charts, which together provide a visual summary of developmental progress from 6 weeks to 4 years of age. The test areas covered by the charts are social skills, hearing and language acquisition, vision and fine motor skills, and gross motor skills. The results of the assessment are recorded on the appropriate charts as shown in Fig. 8.5.

On the horizontal axis of each chart is shown the age of the child, with a range from 6 weeks to 4 years. The vertical axis contains a variety of tests set out in pairs with the pairs corresponding to appropriate ages and forming a step pattern across the chart. In each of the four charts the child's developmental ability is plotted against the age of the child. In practice there is a minimum total of eight test items to be applied for any individual child – that is, two test items for each of the four developmental areas.

With, for example, a 9-month-old child being assessed using the chart on 'Social' development, a mark is made on the upper level of the step if the child succeeds in both tests 11 and 12 and at the lower level of the steps if he or she only succeeds in one of them. If tests 11 and 12 are both failed, the child is assessed on tests 13 and 14, which are normally accomplished by a 6-month-old child. Success at one or both of tests 13 and 14 is scored at the appropriate level. Tests 15 and 16 are applied in the event of the child failing 13 and 14. For a bright child, tests 9 and 10 might be attempted, which are normally accomplished by a 12-year-old. This last procedure is not recommended routinely as the object is to identify delay rather than bright children.

The assessments recorded on the individual charts are interpreted as follows: if the marks on the chart fall on or above the step the child's development in the particular area is suspected to be normal; if the marks lie between the step and the dotted or 'threshold' line, development is considered to be doubtful; and if the marks fall on or below the dotted line development is considered to be abnormal/delayed.

When the assessment plot lies on or below the dotted line in the first year of life, the child's development is delayed by approximately 3 months; in the second year it is delayed 6 months; and in the third and fourth years it is delayed 12 months.

(Eu 1986)

It should be noted that those items marked H are assessed solely by asking parents or caregivers whether or not they have observed the child doing those things at home. All other items must be observed by the examiner during the course of the actual assessment.

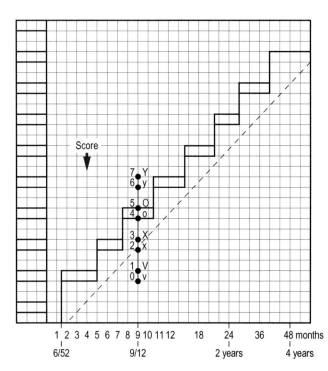

Emotional Reaction Check:

Mother/child interaction
Interest in surroundings/people
Activity, appropriate for age

Observation: Normal/Doubtul/Abnormal

Name:　　　　　　　　D.O.B.

Social

1. Able to dress – except laces and back buttons (H)
2. Dry at night (H)
3. Washes hands (H)
4. Pulls pants up and down (H)
5. Drinks and replaces cup (H)
6. Knows parts of the body (4)
7. Drinks from cup without spilling (H)
8. Indicates toilet needs (H)
9. Puts cubes into box after being shown
10. Finds toy under cup
11. Rings bell
12. Chews and swallows biscuit (observed)
    Copes with solid food
13. Puts objects into mouth (cubes)
14. Reaches for and shakes rattle
15. Responds to friendly face
16. Enjoys being handled by mother (H)
17. Smiles when spoken to
18. Some vocal sounds (H)

Figure 8.5 ● How to record the results of a Woodside developmental screening assessment on the test charts. H means that history of achievement is adequate evidence to mark the chart accordingly. (Reproduced with kind permission from Eu 1986.)

Social

1. Able to dress — except laces and back buttons (H)
2. Dry at night (H)
3. Washes hands (H)
4. Pulls pants up and down (H)
5. Drinks and replaces cup (H)
6. Knows parts of the body (4)
7. Drinks from cup without spilling (H)
8. Indicates toilet needs (H)
9. Puts cubes into box after being shown
10. Finds toy under cup
11. Rings bell
12. Chews and swallows biscuit (observed)
    Copes with solid food
13. Puts objects into mouth (cubes)
14. Reaches for and shakes rattle
15. Responds to friendly face
16. Enjoys being handled by mother (H)
17. Smiles when spoken to
18. Some vocal sounds (H)

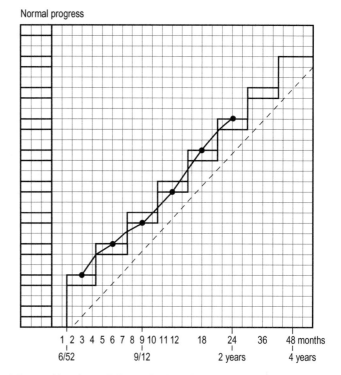

Figure 8.6 ● Normal developmental progress in the 'social' area. Note how all the marks fall either on the top or bottom of the age-appropriate step. (Reproduced with kind permission from Eu 1986.)

Examples of normal progress, doubtful progress, and abnormal progress are shown in Figs 8.6 to 8.9. In addition to the Woodside screening test, the development of each child should be checked against the 'essential milestones of development'. These milestones are shown in Table 8.1. The results of the Woodside screening assessment and the essential milestone checklist have considerable bearing on chiropractic management decisions. Table 8.2 gives suggested responses to common patterns of assessment outcome.

Screening the school-age child

While screening of infants, toddlers and preschool-age children has been the subject of intense research and attempts at age-specific standardization, the same is not true for the school-age child. Developmental delay in school-age children most commonly shows up as a learning deficit or inability with or without attendant behavioral problems. These children are often labeled as 'dyslexic', 'minimally brain damaged' or 'hyperactive', unhelpful terms which are neither diagnostically descriptive nor particularly helpful in management planning.

For the chiropractor, school-age screening and, in particular, school readiness testing should focus on neuromaturational status and the identification of genuine attention deficit and impulsivity problems that are discussed in Chapter 11. This current discussion will be limited to a presentation of how to identify and manage children with neuromaturational delay affecting their school performance.

That early identification of neuromaturational delays with implementation of appropriate interventional measures based on the transactional model of development is a worthwhile management strategy is eloquently attested to in the scientific literature. Multiple problems at 4 and 6 years of age, for example, have been shown to be strong predictors of later school problems (Glascoe 2002, Gottesman & Cerullo 1991, Rydell et al 1991), while children with a high (abnormal) neurodevelopmental score have been shown to have significantly higher rates of learning difficulty (Bax & Whitmore 1987, Huttenlocher et al 1990, Parry 2005), with the importance of the assessment of neurophysiological immaturity in a screening program clearly established as being of primary importance (Bayoglu et al 2007, Goldstein et al 1981, Gottesman & Cerullo 1989, Oberklaid & Efron 2005). It has also been established that school entry age in itself is not a good predictor of future academic risk (Morrison et al 1997).

The neurodevelopmental history

The vast majority of children brought to a chiropractor because of school-related problems do not have any demonstrable organic disease despite complaints of symptoms such as abdominal pain, headache, concentration difficulty, tiredness, aggressive behavior and hyperactivity. They are also frequently referred to by teachers as lazy and unmotivated (Green 1975). Nevertheless, a careful clinical history is essential in order to identify any evidence of organic disease and the multitudinous environmental and constitutional factors that may bear negatively on development and neuromaturation.

Hearing and Language

1. Two or more pronouns in conversation
2. Grammatical speech articulated correctly
3. Says first name
4. Knows own sex
5. Simple sentences (H)
6. Plays with miniature cup and saucer
7. Points to parts of body
8. Says five or more words (H)
9. Obeys simple commands, e.g. clap hands
10. Says fewer than five words including 'Mama', 'Dada', 'Baba' (if related to a person)
11. 'Mama', 'Dada', 'Baba'
12. Hearing tests above ear level
13. Unintelligible babble
14. Hearing tests at ear level
15. Turns eyes to sound
16. Looks round meaningfully when spoken to
17. Stills to bell
18. Stills to mother's voice

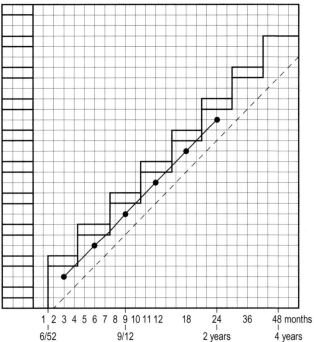

Doubtful progress

Figure 8.7 • Doubtful developmental progress in the 'hearing and language' area. Note how all the marks fall consistently between the bottom age-appropriate step and the dotted threshold line. (Reproduced with kind permission from Eu 1986.)

Vision and Fine Motor

1. Picks up and replaces very small objects, e.g. pins, with each eye covered separately
2. Copies a square
3. Copies a circle
4. Builds a bridge of three bricks when shown
5. Makes a vertical line when shown
6. Makes a tower of six bricks when shown
7. Makes a scribble on paper
8. Makes a tower of three bricks when shown
9. Pincer grasp using a small object, e.g. Smartie
10. Bangs bricks together when shown
11. Side of finger grasp using a small object, e.g. Smartie
12. Matches cubes
13. Picks up cube from table or hand
14. Transfers cube from one hand to another
15. Holds a pencil briefly
16. Follows a moving person with eyes
17. Follows a moving face with eyes

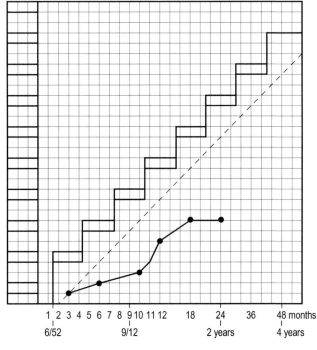

Abnormal progress

Figure 8.8 • Abnormal developmental progress in the 'vision and fine motor' area. Note how all the marks fall either on or below the dotted threshold line. (Reproduced with kind permission from Eu 1986.)

Gross Motor

1. Stands on one leg 3–5 seconds
2. Hops
3. Stands on leg momentarily
4. Walks on tiptoe (H)
5. Runs on whole of foot
6. Kicks ball
7. Picks objects from floor without overbalancing
8. Kneels without support (H)
9. Pulls to standing on furniture
10. 'Cruises' round furniture
11. Sits steadily on floor without support for few mins (H)
12. Stands holding on to furniture
13. Sits against wall or hand, no lateral support — 2/3 secs
14. Hold round waist and lower abruptly. Scissoring is a positive response
15. Pull from lying. Little or no head lag
16. Ventral suspension. Holds head above plane of body
17. Ventral suspension. Head in plane of body

(H) — History of achievement sufficient

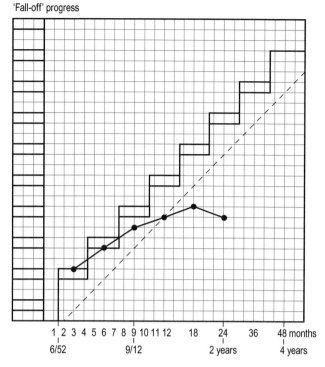

'Fall-off' progress

Figure 8.9 • Fall-off developmental progress in the 'gross motor' area. Note how all the marks fall progressively further from the dotted threshold line with time. (Reproduced with kind permission from Eu 1986.)

Table 8.1 Essential milestones of development (reproduced with kind permission from Illingworth 1983)

Birth	Prone – pelvis high, knees under abdomen Ventral suspension – elbows flex, hips partly extended
4–6 weeks	Smiles at mother Vocalizes 1–2 weeks later
6 weeks	Prone – pelvis flat
12–16 weeks	Turns head to sound Holds object placed in hand
12–20 weeks	Hand regard
20 weeks	Goes for objects and gets them without the object being placed in the hand
26 weeks	Transfers objects, one hand to another Chews Sits, hands forward for support Supine – lifts head up spontaneously Feeds self with biscuit

Table 8.2 Management protocols arising from combined results of the Woodside screening test and the essential developmental milestones

Developmental achievement	Chiropractic management decision
Failure to meet the essential milestones of development with normal Woodside test result	Full developmental history, physical and neurological examination
Two or more 'doubtful' marks on the Woodside test	Specialist referral for full developmental evaluation
Doubtful mark in the gross motor area only	Full developmental history, physical and neurological examination; begin chiropractic care, and monitor progress monthly
One or more abnormal/delayed marks with essential milestones reached	Full developmental history, physical and neurological examination; begin chiropractic care, and monitor progress monthly
One or more abnormal/delayed marks with essential milestones not reached	Specialist referral for full developmental evaluation
Fall-off pattern from normal to doubtful or abnormal/delayed over time	Specialist referral for full developmental evaluation

Environmental factors

The following paragraphs are quoted from Oberklaid (1984).

It is recognized that there are a number of factors pertaining to the child's environment which may contribute significantly to school problems. Children who come from depressed socioeconomic circumstances are often at major risk of poor school performance. The risk factors operating are often multiple, and include family disruptions, absence of appropriate role models, low parental education, lack of early stimulation and experience, suboptimal medical care and poor nutrition. Children who come from differing cultural backgrounds are at risk because they may have problems with language, coming from either multilingual backgrounds or families where English is not spoken. There may be conflict between differing cultures with the child attempting to meet the demands of parents and family on the one hand while at the same time attempting to conform with the peer group demands at school. Some children who reach school age have had very limited opportunity for socialization in the preschool period or may not have had any structured preschool experiences. There is a considerable body of evidence to suggest that a preschool and kindergarten experience is of considerable value to a child, and those children who have not had this stimulation or opportunity for peer socialization may be at a relative disadvantage when they commence formal schooling.

Other environmental factors have to do with the educational environment experienced by the child. For example, there is considerable variation between schools in terms of size and classes, availability of teaching resources, expectations of students, teaching methods, and so on. Children are also considerably influenced by their peer group, especially in preadolescence. All of these environmental factors need to be taken into account and may significantly influence the child's school performance, both positively and negatively.

Constitutional factors

It is obvious that factors intrinsic to the child may have a significant impact in contributing to a child's school problems. Some of these are outlined below.

Genetic factors

There is no doubt that cognitive ability and intelligence are inherited to a certain extent, although there continues to be controversy regarding the exact contributions of nature versus nurture. Some genetic aberrations are clearly responsible for mental retardation, and there is often a strong family history of learning problems in those children who present with school difficulties; however, there is no clear correspondence between genetic inheritance and school difficulties.

Perinatal factors

While it is true that children who have had any form of perinatal stress are at risk for the later development of school problems, the majority of children who present with learning difficulties do not have any such history. Many children of low birthweight or who suffer other perinatal insults do not subsequently have social problems. There is no one to one correspondence between the presence of perinatal stress and subsequent learning or behavioral problems. For a particular child, one can do no more than hypothesize a causal link between early life events and current academic difficulties. Clearly, environmental factors including family stability, social class and early life experiences modify the outcome in a particular child.

General health

Children with chronic disease are at major risk of subsequent school difficulties. This may be due to the condition itself, to the treatment prescribed, to frequent absences because of illness so that the child is unavailable for learning, to the child's lowered self esteem which may subsequently affect peer relationships and motivation, and to the altered perception of the child held by the parents, teachers and fellow students. On the other hand there are many children who have recurrent or chronic health problems who do very well at school. Ill health is thus another risk factor for school problems, with a direct casual relationship not always demonstrated.

Sensory handicaps

Children with problems of vision and hearing are predisposed to learning problems. Youngsters who have suboptimal visual acuity, strabismus and other visual handicaps have difficulty with a number of aspects of academic work. Children with any form of hearing loss may be at major risk of learning and behavioral problems. This not only applies to children with a significant sensorineural or conductive loss, but also to those children who have had repeated ear infections in the preschool period, leading to chronic ear problems and subsequent intermittent fluctuating conductive hearing loss. There is evidence that these children have subtle language problems and lower academic achievement than their peer group. Subtle hearing loss may also contribute to problems with attention and behavior, both in the classroom and at home.

Developmental weakness

Many children have school problems because of subtle weakness in one or more areas of development. A child needs to be competent or mature in each of the developmental areas described below in order to have a successful school learning experience. Conversely, it is hypothesized that children with learning problems have weaknesses in one or more of these developmental areas which contribute significantly to their difficulties. Thus, in addition to traditional history, physical, neurological and sensory examinations, it is useful to administer neurodevelopmental testing to children who present with school problems to elicit a profile of developmental strengths and weaknesses. Developmental areas that are assessed include the following:

Neuromaturation

The child is given tasks designed to elicit minor neurological signs. These include dysdiadochokinesia, synkinesia, motor impersistence, delayed laterality and choreiform movements. All of these are normal in younger children, but their continued presence beyond the age of 8 years gives clues to central nervous system immaturity or disorganization.

Gross motor

There is little direct link between gross motor dysfunction and subsequent learning problems, but proficiency in gross motor tasks is related to competence in sporting activities, self esteem and peer relationships. Children who are awkward and clumsy are often ostracized by their peer group and may become socially isolated. This in turn impinges on motivation and other aspects of classroom functioning.

Fine motor

Children with fine motor difficulties may present at various stages. Those with more severe problems in this area may present in the preschool period as having difficulty acquiring skills with pencils and puzzles, together with self help skills such as buttons, zippers and shoelaces. Subsequently they may have difficulty with handwriting and drawing. Their writing may be awkward, slow and labored, but sometimes these problems do not become apparent until later primary or even secondary school when the demands for written output increase.

Visual perceptual motor

Children may have weaknesses in visual perception, fine motor function, or in the integration of the two modalities. They may have difficulty in letter recognition, becoming confused between the letters b and d for example, as well as problems with copying letters, numbers or geometric shapes. These difficulties may continue when they begin reading, with ongoing confusion regarding spatial concepts and directionality, as well as difficulty with spelling and writing and problems organizing work neatly and efficiently on a page.

Sequencing

This is closely linked to short term memory. Children who have short term auditory or visual sequencing problems are at considerable risk of classroom dysfunction. They may have difficulty following instructions, and tend to become overloaded with a series of directions. Many have trouble with time concepts such as prepositions, month of the year, and telling time. Weakness in sequencing may impinge on all academic areas, because much instruction and retention in meaning depends on maintaining a serial order of things. Such children may develop secondary attentional and behavioral problems.

Receptive language

Children with subtle receptive language problems have difficulties with the processing of auditory commands, especially if these are complex or lengthy. They may be constantly asking the teacher to repeat things, may not be able to follow their meaning, and may not be able to integrate verbal instructions or explanations despite repeated explanations. They may increasingly tune out or exhibit secondary attentional or behavioral problems. Children with language problems have increasing difficulty in a number of academic areas, especially related to aspects of reading. As previously mentioned, difficulties can often be traced to recurrent ear infections and conductive hearing loss early in life.

Expressive language

Children with difficulties expressing themselves are at risk in both classroom and social situations. They may have problems in word finding so that they cannot express what they really want to, or have difficulty with articulation or organizing narrative. As they become older they may have increasing social difficulties because of their anxieties or self-consciousness about their expressive language. This may impair peer relationships and self esteem.

Attention

As children become older, their ability to focus on specific tasks becomes increasingly developed. A number of children have school problems because of difficulty in focusing attention. There may be related behaviors such as distractibility, motoric overactivity and impulsivity. Neurodevelopmental examination is important in these children in order to elicit any developmental weakness that may be primarily responsible. In some children these maladaptive behaviors may be secondary to underlying developmental weaknesses, such as difficulty with receptive language or auditory sequencing.

(Oberklaid 1984)

The clinical history taken on the child presenting to the chiropractor must address all of the above issues if an accurate description of the child's neuromaturational status is to be arrived at. The history is followed by a physical and neuro-developmental examination.

The physical examination

The physical examination in a child presenting with school learning difficulties should be thorough and as complete as possible in order to rule out the impingement of physical disease on neurodevelopment. The conduct of the physical examination of the school-age child is exhaustively covered in Chapter 3.

The neurodevelopmental assessment

The history is then augmented by a physical examination aimed at eliciting the presence of any so-called soft, or minor, neurological signs. There are, of course, no soft neurological signs per se. This term has been coined to describe a collection of neurological signs which are not normally related to imageable neuropathology and has been in use in the literature long enough to warrant its continued use provided what is implied by the term is clearly understood. Ideally, the examination should be conducted using the following order.

Anthropometry

Measure and plot head circumference, height and weight on standard growth charts for gender and age in order to identify any deviation from normal development. Perform a Tanner staging assessment of pubertal development (pubic hair and breasts in the female and pubic hair in the male) in order to identify precocious or delayed puberty. Measure the arm span between the outstretched fingertips on both sides with the arms at 90° abduction. The distance between outstretched fingertips should be the same as the standing height. Once again, significant differences should be investigated in an attempt to identify cause.

Assessment of hearing

In the school-age group, screening of hearing may be reliably assessed using Rinne's and Weber's tests. Any abnormality should result in the child being referred for full audiological assessment as hearing deficits are common and play a significant clinical role in learning dysfunction (Oberklaid 1989).

Assessment of vision

The three key aspects of vision should be routinely assessed. Far vision may be tested using a standard Snellen eye chart. Accommodation and near vision are assessed by asking the child to read a sentence of small print. Finally, peripheral vision is evaluated using the method described in Chapter 3.

In the event of a child reporting that the characters on the Snellen eye chart are unclear or have 'blurry edges', re-examination with the child looking at the eye chart through a pinhole in a piece of paper will help to determine if the reason for the visual difficulty is refractive error or pathology. In refractive error, the characters on the eye chart become crystal clear when looking through the pinhole. If this phenomenon persists after chiropractic care is administered, the child may need spectacles. If the characters remain blurred when the child looks through the pinhole, ocular pathology should be considered and the child referred for appropriate investigation.

Synkinetic movements

Synkinetic movement is evaluated by asking the child to perform a rapid, repetitive action with one hand while keeping the other hand still (Fig. 8.10). Involuntary mimicry on the opposite or non-tested side is considered a positive test. This is a normal finding in children up to 8 years of age. Persistence beyond that age has been shown to be associated with learning and behavioral dysfunction (Levine et al 1983).

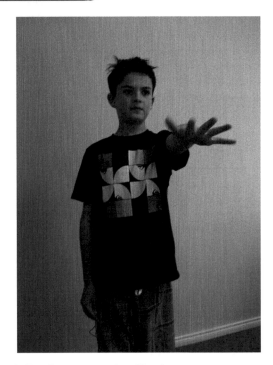

Figure 8.10 ● Assessment of synkinesis.

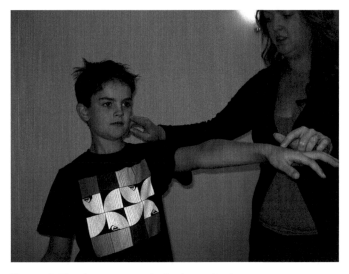

Figure 8.12 ● Assessment of stimulus extinction.

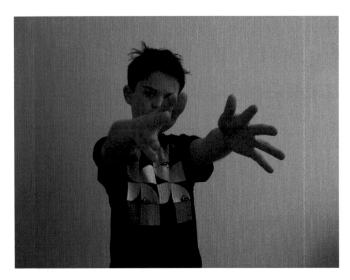

Figure 8.11 ● Assessment of diadochokinesia.

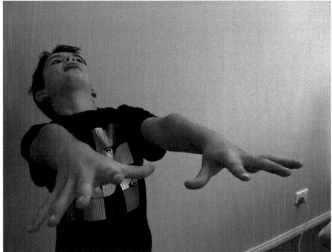

Figure 8.13 ● Assessment of motor impersistence.

Dysdiadochokinesia

Diadochokinesic function is tested by asking the child to rapidly supinate/pronate each hand simultaneously (Fig. 8.11). Incoordination or complete inability to perform the test implies developmental immaturity if this function cannot be successfully performed by 7 years of age (Levine et al 1983).

Stimulus extinction

Stimulus extinction is tested by simultaneously touching the child on the face and hand ipsilaterally and asking the child to identify where he or she has been touched (Fig. 8.12). Up to age 7 it is quite normal for the child to indicate only the proximal point, but persistence beyond this age is considered to be indicative of developmental dysfunction or immaturity (Levine et al 1983).

Motor impersistence

This test is performed with the child adopting a fixed stance with the arms extended, the mouth open, and the tongue protruding (Fig. 8.13). In children over 8 years of age, an inability to maintain this posture implies motoric impersistence and is commonly seen in children with attention deficits and learning problems (Oberklaid 1984).

Choreiform movements

Choreiform movement is normally noted in the outstretched fingers of young children (Fig. 8.14). Beyond the age of 8 years, it is indicative of neuromaturational delay and is associated with hyperactivity, impulsivity, poor frustration tolerance, emotional liability and learning difficulties (Levine et al 1983). Choreiform movement is identified by asking the child being examined to hold a fixed posture, standing with the arms extended, fingers spread, mouth open and tongue protruding while the examiner carefully watches the fingers.

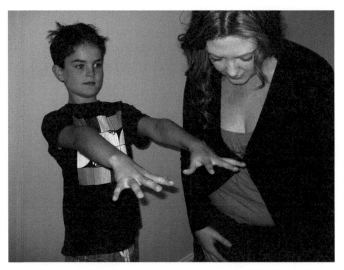

Figure 8.14 • Observation of a child holding fixed posture for the presence of choreiform movement. It may be normal for these movements to appear after 30 seconds or so.

School-age children should be able to hold this posture without developing choreiform movement for at least 30 seconds.

Left–right discrimination (laterality)

The school-age child should exhibit increasing ability to discriminate between the left and right sides of the body. The testing procedure is dependent upon age, as follows:

- Between 6 and 8 years: ask the child to identify left and right on their own body, using simple commands such as 'Show me your left hand', etc. (Fig. 8.15).
- Between 8 and 10 years: ask the child to identify left and right across the midline of their own body with commands such as 'Touch your right ear with your left hand', etc. (Fig. 8.16).
- Above 10 years: the child should be asked to identify left and right on the examiner, who should stand facing the child at a comfortable distance (Fig. 8.17).

Difficulties with left–right discrimination may result from a complex mixture of maturational, developmental, and basic

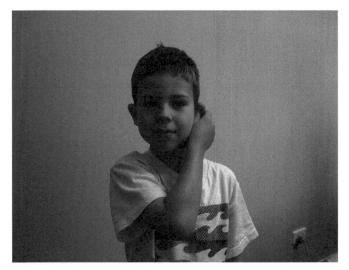

Figure 8.15 • Left–right discrimination testing in a 6-year-old.

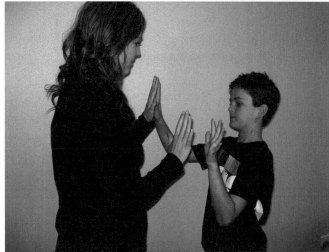

Figure 8.16 • Left–right discrimination testing in a 9-year-old.

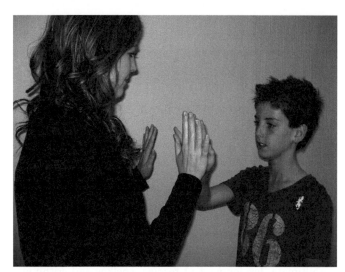

Figure 8.17 • Left–right discrimination testing in an 11-year-old.

processing functions (Levine et al 1983). It is commonly seen in children with poorly developed hemispherical coordination and neurological disorganization as inability to perform cross-crawl and a history of not having been able to do so (Walther 1988).

Gross motor evaluation

Assessment of gross motor function in the school-age period may be estimated by asking the child to perform a series of tasks which become progressively more difficult with age (Table 8.3). As the child performs these functions, the examiner should estimate the competence with which they are done, noting any clumsiness, jerky movements or complete inability to perform the tasks. Care should be taken to factor hemispherical dominance (i.e. handedness) into the assessment as this is well developed by school age.

Fine motor control

Competence in fine motor control may be estimated by watching a child use a pencil, as well as other tasks such as stringing beads, firstly with the eyes open and then with the

Table 8.3 Age-appropriate tasks for the assessment of gross motor function (adapted from Levine 1987, with permission)

Age (year)	Gross motor function tested
5–6	Skip, walk on heels, tandem gait forward, hop in place
6–7	Tandem gait backward, stand on one foot with eyes open (10 seconds)
7–8	Crouch on tiptoes with eyes closed (10 seconds), hop twice in place on each foot in succession (three cycles), stand in tandem gait position (heel–toe) with eyes closed (10 seconds)
9–10	Tandem gait sideways, catch tennis ball in air with one hand, throw tennis ball at target
10–12	Balance on tiptoes with eyes closed (15 seconds), jump in the air and clap heels together, jump in the air and clap hands three times

eyes closed, or picking up small objects such as paper clips from a desk top. As with gross motor function, the action of the child should be closely observed for eye–hand coordination, clumsiness, jerky movements, incompetence and frustration level.

Visual–perceptual–motor function

This function is tested by asking the child to copy geometric forms (Fig. 8.18). The examiner should show the age-appropriate shape to the child and allow them to look at it as long as they wish. The examiner should then provide the child with a clean sheet of paper and a pencil and ask them to draw the shape they have been shown or asked to copy.

Temporal–sequential organization

Since a child's appreciation of time and sequence is critical in the ultimate development of reading, spelling and arithmetic skills, temporal–sequential organization should form an integral part of neurodevelopmental testing in the school-age period. There are two forms of assessment of temporal–sequential organization, namely visual and auditory. These are assessed by testing sequencing function in both areas.

Children with deficits in sequential organization may have significant difficulty with short-term auditory memory resulting in maladaptive classroom behaviors as protective strategies or expression of frustration and anxiety (Levine 1987). Auditory sequencing may be evaluated either by asking the child to repeat a series of numbers spoken evenly at approximately 1-second intervals or by asking the child to perform a series of simple tasks in a given order. This function is referred to as short-term auditory memory. Expected capability for age is shown in Table 8.4. From this table it can be seen, for example, that a 7-year-old child should be able to repeat a set of five numbers in the same order in which they were given and perform a set of five simple tasks in the order in which they were verbally given. A 10-year-old child should be able either to perform the same function for a set of six numbers or repeat a set of four numbers in the reverse order to that in which they were given and perform a series of six simple tasks in the order

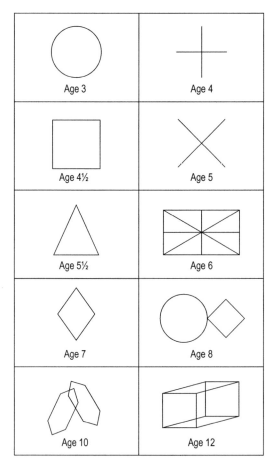

Figure 8.18 • Geometric shapes to copy for testing visual–perceptual–motor function. Impaired performance should not be automatically taken to imply that there is definitely a visual–perceptual–motor deficit as poor test performance may be due to fine motor delays, inattention or difficulties with conceptualization.
(Reproduced with permission from Weiner HL, Bresnan MJ, Levitt LP *Pediatric Neurology for the House Officer*, 2nd edn. Williams & Wilkins, Baltimore, 1982, p. 7.)

Table 8.4 Expected age-appropriate auditory discrimination capabilities for temporal–sequential organization, otherwise known as short-term auditory memory, for school-age children (adapted from Levine 1987, with permission)

Age (years)	Digits at approximately 1-second intervals	Serial commands
5–6	Repeats 4 digits forwards	3-step series
6–7	Repeats 4–5 digits forwards	4-step series
7–8	Repeats 5 digits forwards	5-step series
9–10	Repeats 6 digits forwards Repeats 4 digits backwards	5-step series
11–12 and over	Repeats 6 digits forwards Repeats 5 digits backwards	6-step series

Table 8.5 Expected age-appropriate visual discrimination capabilities for temporal–sequential organization in school-age children (adapted from Levine 1987, with permission)

Age (years)	Object span	Block tapping	Motor sequence
5–6	4 objects	4 squares	Simultaneously open and close both hands, arms extended
6–7	4 objects	4 squares	Imitative finger tapping (both hands, 3–4 steps)
7–8	5 objects	5 squares	Imitative finger–foot tapping (4–5 steps)
9–10	5 objects	5 squares	Alternate left and right, open and close fists, arms extended
11–12 and over	6 objects	6 squares	Imitate edge of hand on knee, then palm on knee, then clenched fist (4 cycles)

in which they were given. It is reasonable to give a child three attempts at each task before deciding that there is a deficit.

Visual sequencing can be simply evaluated using object span, block tapping and motor sequence (Table 8.5). Object span involves the examiner pointing to a number of objects and asking the child to point to the same objects in the same order. Similarly, block tapping involves the examiner pointing to a series of identically sized squares and asking the child to point to the same squares in the same order. Motor sequencing simply requires the child to mimic a series of motor activities performed by the examiner. The examiner should attempt to assess the child in both auditory and visual areas in order to come to a diagnostic conclusion about the stage of development of the child's temporal–sequential organization.

Intellectual development

Development of the child's intellect may be reasonably reliably estimated by using the Goodenough–Harris drawing test procedure. This test was originally designed and published by Florence Goodenough who spent a good portion of her professional life developing tools for assessing intelligence in young children. She hypothesized that IQ could be reliably measured with significant reproducibility for most preschool children.

Dr Goodenough first published her 'Draw-a-Man' test in the book *Measurement of Intelligence by Drawings* in 1926. Her protocol required the child being tested to draw a picture of a man. The test was non-verbal and intended for assessing children between the ages of 2 and 13 years. In the late 1940s the test was revised by Dale Harris, and is now commonly known as the Goodenough–Harris drawing test.

The child being examined is asked to draw a man and is carefully instructed to take their time and do it as well as possible. Care must be taken to see that parents and older siblings do not interfere by offering advice as to what should be drawn on the man. Box 8.1 contains the 51 individual items used for

Box 8.1

Items used to grade the Goodenough test (Reproduced with kind permission from Illingworth 1983)

Each item scores 1 point. Intellectual age is calculated by adding 1 year for each 4 points scored to the basal age of 3 years.

1. Head present
2. Legs present
3. Arms present
4. Trunk present
5. Length of trunk greater than breadth
6. Shoulders indicated
7. Both arms and legs attached to trunk
8. Legs attached to trunk; arms attached to trunk at correct point
9. Neck present
10. Neck outline continues with head, trunk, or both
11. Eyes present
12. Nose present
13. Mouth present
14. Nose and mouth in two dimensions; two lips shown
15. Nostrils indicated
16. Hair shown
17. Hair non-transparent, over more than circumference
18. Clothing present
19. Two articles of clothing non-transparent
20. No transparencies, both sleeves and trousers shown
21. Four or more articles of clothing definitely indicated
22. Costume complete, without incongruities
23. Fingers shown
24. Correct number of fingers shown
25. Fingers in two dimensions, length > breadth and angle >180°
26. Opposition of thumb shown
27. Hand shown distinct from fingers or arms
28. Arm joint shown, elbow, shoulder, or both
29. Leg joint shown, knee, hip, or both
30. Head in proportion
31. Arms in proportion
32. Legs in proportion
33. Feet in proportion
34. Both arms and legs in two dimensions
35. Heel shown
36. Firm lines without overlapping at junctions
37. Firm lines with correct joining
38. Head outline more than a circle
39. Trunk outline more than a circle
40. Outline of arms and legs without narrowing at junction with body
41. Features symmetrical and in correct position
42. Ears present
43. Ears in correct position and proportional
44. Eyebrows or eyelashes
45. Pupil of eye
46. Eye length > eye height
47. Eye glance direct to front in profile
48. Both chin and forehead shown
49. Projection of chin shown
50. Profile with not more than one error
51. Correct profile

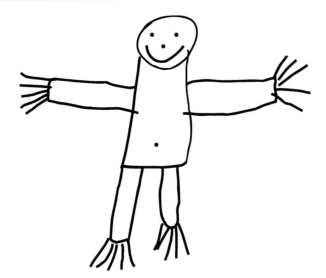

Figure 8.19 • Example of a drawing of a man for the Goodenough test by a child aged 8 years and 7 months. The raw test score for this drawing is 21, giving an estimated intellectual developmental age of 8 years and 3 months, well within reasonable limits for test validity.

assessing the drawing (Illingworth 1983). Intellectual age is estimated by applying one point for each of the 51 items found to be present in the finished drawing and adding 1 year for each 4 points scored to the base age of 3 years. Fig. 8.19 is a good example of a drawing made by a boy who was 8 years and 7 months old. His raw test score was 21, giving him and intellectual age of 8 years and 3 months.

Clinical decision-making and management

Clinical decision-making in this field of pediatrics is fraught with difficulty and frustration if one chooses to follow the typical medical model of disease. The object of the neuromaturational assessment in the child with learning problems, or indeed in the child about to enter school for whom you have been asked to perform a classroom evaluation, is simply to generate a profile of both strengths and weaknesses. There is almost never a reason for the chiropractor to refer these children for specialist investigation in the first instance unless significant pathology is identified during the conduct of the traditional physical examination. The process of identifying strengths and weakness allows the chiropractor to establish a benchmark of learning capability against which improvement can be measured. Such improvement should always be compared to educational achievement outcomes reported by the child's teachers. When managing the learning-impaired child, it will usually be best to network the assistance and cooperation of the child's teachers, parents, siblings, and in some cases the family general practitioner.

Role of the family general practitioner

The family GP should be consulted in the event of the physical examination identifying pathology. Consultation between the chiropractor and the GP should also characterize the management program for any child who is on long-term medication which may

affect the child's rate of neuromaturation, such as insulin for diabetes mellitus, ritalin (methylphenidate) for attention-deficit/hyperactivity disorder, anticonvulsants such as phenobarbital or Dilantin (phenytoin) among many others for epilepsy, or the various drugs used for asthma which may create irritability and increased motoric activity.

Role of the teacher

The teacher should always be a part of the management process as there is much consideration that can be offered the child at school if the teacher is made aware of the relative strengths and weaknesses identified during the neuromaturational assessment. For example, a child who has poor short-term memory may be given instructions in writing. Teachers are often helpful in assisting with management planning as their professional training gives the insights into how to assist learning-impaired children. Consultation with the teacher will also often help to avoid the psychological damage caused by labeling a child as naughty, hyperactive, unmotivated, lazy, etc. The teacher is also a wonderful ally to assist with periodic monitoring of the outcome of treatment protocols. Improvement in the strengths and weaknesses profile should be paralleled by improvement in the educational outcome. The teacher also plays a key role in identifying and controlling peer ridicule, bullying and harassment.

Role of the parents

The parent's role is usually a critical one, as many of the management protocols are carried out at home. Gaining the compliance of the parents is vital and for that reason sufficient time should be given to explaining the child's condition and the role the parents will play. Specific stimulation of areas of weakness is usually carried out by game- and role-playing activities at home, all of which require time and discipline.

Role of the educational kinesiologist

Educational kinesiology is a rapidly evolving practice that offers a very valuable service to the neuromaturationally delayed child. Where the service is available, referral for an assessment and implementation of management strategies, mainly carefully constructed integrative motor exercises, is well warranted.

Role of the dietician

In cases where poor dietary practices are likely to be impinging on optimal developmental outcome, referral to a professionally trained dietician is warranted.

Role of the chiropractor

The chiropractor, having generated a 'strengths and weaknesses' profile and identified the precise pattern of neurological dysafferentation, must now act as primary clinician, coach to the child, counselor to the parents, and care coordinator with other health care professionals. Imaginative games and role-playing exercises should be designed for parental implementation which address the specific weakness found on examination while accentuating the strengths. These exercises may include playing specific games like football, catch or basketball, involvement in 'around the house' projects, involvement in organized sport or other community-based activities, and deepening personal relationships between the child and parents. Parents should be counseled to constantly encourage and avoid criticism at all costs in order to raise the child's confidence level.

The chiropractor should contact the teacher to arrange a meeting in order to discuss the child's problem and cooperatively plan school-based strategies to help. The chiropractor must offer specific, corrective chiropractic care in order to eliminate the important role played by neurological dysafferentation in delaying neuromaturation and therefore the learning process. Commonly, children with such problems have patterns of dysafferentation seen at the upper cervical complex, sacral and cranial areas. Restoration and maintenance of normal neurological function is a critical aspect of the management program of children with neuromaturational delay and learning difficulties.

Finally, referral to an educational kinesiologist is warranted where such a service is available. In the event such a service is not available, prescription of exercises such as cross-crawl, star jumping, marching, etc. should be given in order to reinforce normal hemispherical coordination.

Specialist pediatric referral should be considered in children who fail to show response to the normal chiropractic management program.

References

Bax, M., Whitmore, K., 1987. The medical examination of children on entry to school. The results and use of neurodevelopmental assessment. Dev. Med. Child Neurol. 29 (1), 40–55.

Bayoglu, B.U., Bakar, E.E., Kutlu, M., et al., 2007. Can preschool developmental screening identify children at risk for school problems? Early Hum. Dev. 83 (9), 613–617.

Behrman, R.E., Jenson, H.B., Nelson, W.E., et al., 2007. Nelson Textbook of Pediatrics, eighteenth ed. WB Saunders, Philadelphia.

Clements, M. (Ed.), 1986. Infant and Family Health. Churchill Livingstone, Edinburgh.

Eu, B.S.L., 1986. Evaluation of a developmental screening system for use by child health nurses. Arch. Dis. Child. 61 (1), 34–41.

Frankenburg, W.K., Camp, B.W., van Natta, P.A., et al., 1971. Reliability and stability of the Denver Developmental Screening Test. Child Dev. 42 (5), 1315–1325.

Glascoe, F.P., 2002. Safety words inventory and literacy screener: standardization and validation. Clin. Pediatr. (Phila) 41 (9), 697–704.

Goldstein, P.K., O'Brien, J.D., Katz, G.M., 1981. A learning disability screening program in a public school. Am. J. Occup. Ther. 35 (7), 451–455.

Gottesman, R.L., Cerullo, F.M., 1989. The development and preliminary evaluation of a screening test to detect school learning problems. J. Dev. Behav. Pediatr. 10 (2), 68–74.

Gottesman, R.L., Cerullo, F.M., 1991. Validity of a screening test for school learning problems in a pediatric clinical setting. J. Pediatr. Psychol. 16 (3), 327–339.

Green, M., 1975. A developmental approach to symptoms based on age groups. Pediatr. Clin. North Am. 22, 571–581.

Gupta, R., Patel, N.V., 1991. Training of non-professional health workers in a simple technique of developmental screening of infants and young children. Indian Pediatr. 28 (8), 851–858.

Huttenlocher, P.R., Levine, S.C., Huttenlocher, J., et al., 1990. Discrimination of normal and at-risk preschool children on the basis of neurological tests. Dev. Med. Child Neurol. 32 (11), 1027.

Illingworth, R.S., 1983. The Development of the Infant and Young Child: Normal and Abnormal, eighth ed. Churchill Livingstone, Edinburgh.

Levine, M.D., 1987. Developmental pediatrics. In: Behrmann, R., Vaughan, V. (Eds), Nelson Textbook of Pediatrics. thirteenth ed. WB Saunders, Philadelphia.

Levine, M.D., Carey, W.B., Crocker, A.V., et al., 1983. Developmental Behavioural Pediatrics. WB Saunders, Philadelphia.

Morrison, F.J., Griffith, E.M., Alberts, D.M., 1997. Nature–nuture in the classroom: entrance age, school readiness and learning in children. Dev. Psychol. 33 (2), 254–262.

Oberklaid, F., 1984. Children with school problems – and expanding role for the paediatrician. Aust. Paediatr. J. 20, 271–275.

Oberklaid, F., 1986. Developmental observation and assessment. In: Clements, M. (Ed.), Infant and Family Health. Churchill Livingstone, Edinburgh.

Oberklaid, F., 1989. Auditory dysfunction in children with school problems. Clin. Pediatr. (Phila) 28 (9), 397–403.

Oberklaid, F., Efron, D., 2005. Developmental delay – identification and management. Aust. Fam. Physician 34 (9), 739–742.

Parry, T.S., 2005. Assessment of developmental learning and behavioural problems in children and young people. Med. J. Aust. 183 (1), 43–48.

Rydell, A.M., Bondestam, M., Hagelin, E., et al., 1991. Teacher rated problems and school ability tests in relation to preschool problems and parents' health information at school start. A study of first graders. Scand. J. Psychol. 32 (2), 177–190.

Sheridan, M.D., 1980. From Birth to Five Years: Children's Developmental Progress. NFER-Nelson, Windsor.

Theeranate, K., Cheungchitraks, S., 2005. Parents' evaluation of developmental status (PEDS) detects developmental problems compared to Denver II. J. Med. Assoc. Thailand 88 (Suppl. 3), S188–S192.

Wake, M., Gerner, B., Gallagher, S., 2005. Does parents' evaluation of developmental status at school entry predict language, achievement, and quality of life 2 years later? Ambul. Pediatr. 5 (3), 143–149.

Walther, D.S., 1988. Applied Kinesiology Synopsis. Systems DC, Pueblo, Colorado.

Weiner, H.L., Bresnan, M.J., Levitt, L.P., 1982. Pediatric Neurology for the House Officer, second ed. Williams & Wilkins, Baltimore.

Common infectious diseases of childhood

Neil J. Davies

Many of the infectious diseases commonly encountered by chiropractors in caring for children are associated with rashes. In some instances, the rash is diagnostic of the disease process, while other rashes are common to infections from a variety of organisms. Skin lesions associated with infectious disease in childhood may result from a number of mechanisms. The most common of these are shown in Box 9.1.

Diagnostic accuracy in infectious disease that is associated with a skin or mucous membrane lesion is challenging to say the least and requires a very careful clinical history and a detailed description of the lesion. Appropriate descriptive terms for skin lesions are found in Box 9.2. While it is certainly not possible to identify the class of etiological agent from the history and physical examination, one should attempt at least to try to assess whether an infection producing a skin lesion in children is likely to be viral, bacterial or rickettsial in origin.

The decision each chiropractor must make in children with infectious disorders is either to manage the child conservatively or to refer for laboratory investigation and possible specialist care. Conservative chiropractic management demands that the attending clinician have a firm understanding of the natural history of each of the common infections in addition

---

Box 9.1

Common mechanisms involved in skin rashes associated with infectious disease in childhood

- Direct inoculation of the skin (e.g. anthrax, tularemia)
- Hematogenous dissemination of microorganisms (e.g. meningococcemia)
- Contiguous spread from adjacent foci of infection (e.g. impetigo, herpes)
- The effect of toxins (e.g. scarlet fever)
- Antigen–antibody reactions (e.g. rheumatic fever)
- Delayed hypersensitivity to the infecting agent (e.g. erythema nodosum)

Box 9.2

Appropriate terms to be used when describing a skin lesion

- Erythematous
- Maculopapular
- Papulovesicular (also described as 'bullous')
- Petechial and/or hemorrhagic
- Ulcerative
- Nodular

---

to the clinical skills needed to monitor the child's physical condition and recognize parameters in each case that would identify disease progression and therefore demand specialist referral.

Measles (rubeola)

Measles is an acute communicable viral disease that is characterized, firstly, by an asymptomatic incubation stage; this is followed by a symptomatic prodromal stage and, finally, the appearance of the typical rash.

An infected child becomes infective to others approximately 9–10 days after exposure to the disease in another person (i.e. at the beginning of the prodromal phase). It is appropriate to advise parents and caregivers that a child with measles may remain an infective danger to other children for up to 5 days after the rash disappears. Given that children infected with measles may have temperatures as high as 102–104°F during the prodromal phase, careful observation of hydration is required.

A sudden rise in body temperature is usually the first sign to appear in the prodromal phase, closely followed by coryzal symptoms, conjunctivitis and cough. Koplik's spots, small lesions found on the buccal mucous membranes having a

© 2010, Elsevier Ltd, Inc, BV
DOI: 10.1016/B978-0-7020-3129-8.00009-8

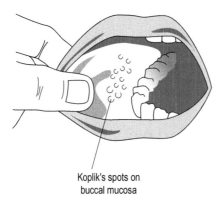

Koplik's spots on
buccal mucosa

Figure 9.1 • Koplik's spots, pathognomonic of measles (rubeola) are found on the buccal mucosa. Koplick's spots have been variously described as appearing like salt crystals, a grain of sugar, etc.

crystalline appearance like a grain of salt or sugar (Fig. 9.1), are pathognomonic of measles and generally appear 2–3 days after the initial symptoms. The typical confluent maculopapular rash (Fig. 9.2) follows a day or so later (Krugman et al 2004).

A sick, toxic child with a high fever will subluxate readily and during the height of the symptomatic period should be assessed two to three times a day and adjusted when necessary. Again, adequate fluid and electrolyte intake should be ensured and the child monitored for signs of physical deterioration or secondary infection, particularly otitis and pneumonia. Careful physical assessment at the daily visits should be adequate to identify such problems. Oral administration of calcium ascorbate and *Echinacea purpurea* is desirable. Quarantine is both ineffective and undesirable.

German measles (rubella)

This is a common communicable disease of childhood usually characterized by mild constitutional symptoms with a rash similar to that seen in scarlet fever. The child with rubella is infective to others for at least 7 days prior to the appearance of the rash and remains so until both the fever and the rash have resolved. A child infected in utero, however, remains infective to others for a period of up to 2 years.

The first symptoms are usually malaise with lymphadenopathy followed 2–3 days later by coryzal symptoms, conjunctivitis,

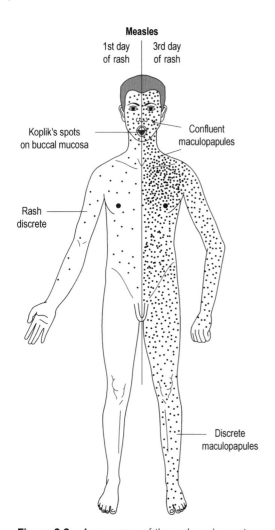

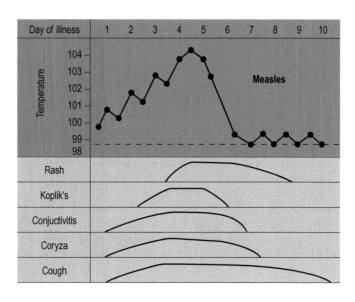

Figure 9.2 • Appearance of the rash and symptoms associated with measles (rubeola). (Reproduced with kind permission from Krugman & Ward 1958.)

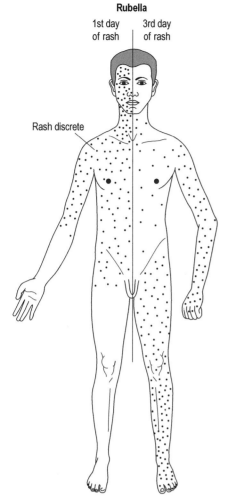

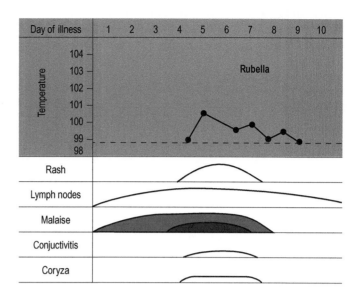

Figure 9.3 • Appearance of the rash and symptoms associated with German measles (rubella). (Reproduced with kind permission from Krugman & Ward 1958.)

the appearance of the typical discrete, evenly spread, fine rash (Fig. 9.3) and mild pyrexia, the child's temperature not usually exceeding 100–101°F (Krugman et al 2004). Once the rash disappears, the other symptoms quickly resolve, with the lymphadenopathy slowly disappearing over 7–10 days. The child with rubella infection is usually only mildly unwell and can be managed conservatively with chiropractic and hygienic care. Complications are uncommon.

Congenital rubella syndrome

An infant infected with rubella in utero may appear quite normal at birth despite recovery of the virus from the nasopharynx and urine. These infants are infectious to non-immune contacts and may remain so for up to 2 years. Box 9.3 lists the most common birth defects associated with congenital rubella syndrome. Box 9.4 lists the symptomatic manifestations which may appear several years after birth in children who are congenitally infected with rubella but had no obvious evidence at birth or in the immediate neonatal period.

Box 9.3

Defects commonly found in congenital rubella where symptoms are evident at birth (adapted from Overall 1981 with permission)

- Low birthweight (<2500 g)
- Hepatomegaly
- Splenomegaly
- Jaundice
- Petechiae
- Purpura
- Congenital heart disease
- Pneumonia
- Cataracts
- Micro-ophthalmia
- Bone lesions
- Anemia

Clinical manifestations of congenital rubella syndrome in children who have no physical evidence of the disease at birth*

- Hearing loss
- Psychomotor retardation
- Perceptual and motor impairment
- Diabetes mellitus

* It may take several years for these manifestations to appear.

Scarlet fever

Scarlet fever is a commonly occurring group A hemolytic streptococcal infection characterized by acute nasopharyngitis, tonsillitis, and a diffuse erythematous exanthem and enanthem. It is caused by production of erythrogenic exotoxins from a variety of streptococci and is rarely seen before age 3 and almost never after age 15.

Scarlet fever has an incubation period of between 2 and 5 days and a prodromal period of 1.5–2 days. Scarlet fever has a very low communicability, but infectivity lasts until all traces of the etiological organism have been eliminated.

The child with scarlet fever presents with the concurrent appearance of a sore throat, typical rash (Fig. 9.4) and fever. The fever may reach as high as 103°F during the prodromal period, after which it usually returns to normal within 3–4 days. The sore throat usually resolves without incident after 72 hours and the rash normally disappears after a week (Krugman et al 2004).

The child with scarlet fever has certain distinctive features on physical examination that will help to distinguish scarlet fever from other viral diseases associated with exanthem. The rash tends to be more dense in the neck, axilla and groin, there are often transverse hyperemic or petechial lines in the skin folds of the antecubital fossa, axilla and groin which fail to blanch on sustained pressure, there is a flushed-cheek appearance and the tongue is usually bright red (the so-called 'strawberry tongue'). A laboratory test known as the Schultz–Charlton test may be performed to confirm the diagnosis, but the typical features of the condition make a clinical diagnosis adequate (Krugman et al 2004).

Chiropractic management is the same as for measles (see above). In the event of secondary streptococcal infection, usually from the nasopharynx to the middle ears and sinus, the child should be referred for the administration of antibiotic therapy.

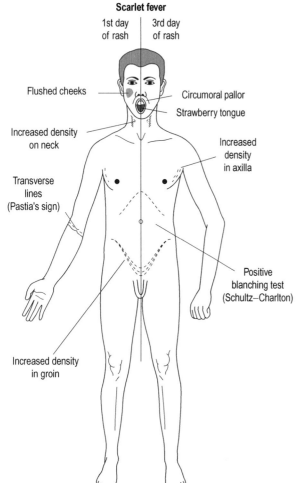

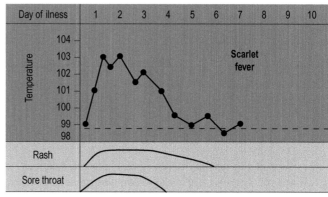

Figure 9.4 • Appearance of the rash and symptoms associated with scarlet fever. (Reproduced with kind permission from Krugman & Ward 1958.)

Chickenpox (varicella)

Chickenpox is an exanthem caused by infection with varicella zoster virus. The child typically becomes mildly ill with symptoms of fever, headache, anorexia and malaise with the typical skin lesions, arising in crops in their macular form, appearing very quickly (McMillan et al 1982). The lesions rapidly progress to their papular form, in which they lack central umbilication and become intensely painful and itchy. The papular lesions slowly become vesicular and finally encrusted. The skin lesions are profuse on the trunk but sparse on the extremities (Krugman et al 2004) (Fig. 9.5).

The incubation period for chickenpox is 12–16 days with a prodrome of only 1 day involving fever, anorexia and headache. Children with chickenpox are infective to others for a period beginning 2 days prior to the eruption of the first lesions until such time as all lesions have encrusted.

Management of the child with chickenpox is driven by the need to control pain and the intense itching and to watch carefully for the development of any complications. Aside from daily chiropractic care, the child with chickenpox should be given the homeopathic remedy nux vomica which assists in controlling

itching, calcium ascorbate to gut level tolerance, and *Echinacea purpurea* to stimulate immune function. Repeated bathing in antipruritic solutions such as pinetarsol and the use of lotions such as calamine are also helpful to reduce the intensity of the itching. Pediatric ibuprofen or other suitable analgesic/antipyretic agents may be used to reduce fever and pain if necessary. As with all episodes of infection, careful neurological examination and subluxation correction should be carried out after symptomatic resolution has occurred.

It is unnecessary to isolate the child with chickenpox, but exclusion from school for 1 week after the eruption of the first lesion is appropriate. Parents and caregivers should be counseled to disinfect articles of clothing soiled by discharges from the nose and throat routinely at home. The natural history of chickenpox is to run an uneventful course with complete resolution after 5–7 days in the great majority of children (Krugman et al 2004). Infrequently, complications may occur and these most commonly include: hemorrhagic skin lesions seen as purpura (Abdulmalik et al 2006, Becker & Buckley 1966, Maness & Rogers 1987); hepatitis (Feldman et al 1997, Garcia Aquilera et al 2008); neurological sequelae, especially cerebellar ataxia (Garg 1968, Guess et al 1986,

Chickenpox

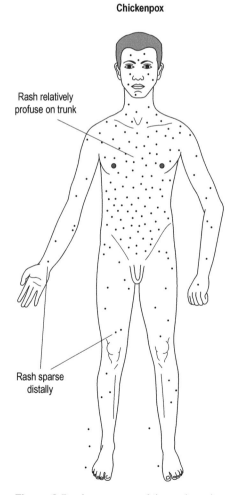

Rash relatively profuse on trunk

Rash sparse distally

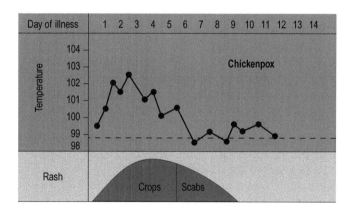

Figure 9.5 • Appearance of the rash and symptoms associated with chickenpox (varicella). (Reproduced with kind permission from Krugman & Ward 1958.)

Nussinovitch et al 2003) and encephalitis (Phuah et al 1998); Reye's syndrome; thrombocytopenia; cellulitis; and pneumonia (Jackson et al 1992, Reynolds et al 2008). The chiropractor should be alert to the development of complications in a child with chickenpox where the disease appears particularly severe or fails to follow the usual natural history. All cases of chickenpox in which complications occur should be referred for specialist assessment.

Roseola infantum (exanthem subitum)

Roseola is an acute disease seen in infants and toddlers. It is probably of viral origin and is quite unique in its presentation, as clinical improvement occurs simultaneously with the appearance of the diagnostic rash. The onset of roseola is sudden with temperatures as high as 104°F that may last for 3–4 days. As the temperature subsides, usually precipitously, the typical rash erupts, firstly over the trunk, then quickly spreading to the extremities, neck, hairline, and mildly to the face. The rash rarely lasts longer than 24 hours (Behrman et al 2007).

Individual lesions begin as brownish-red macules that progress to become papular, blotchy and confluent. Pressure held over the rash tends to produce blanching. In the laboratory, there will be a rise in the leukocyte level to as high as $16–20 \times 10^3/mm^3$ with an increase in the neutrophils in the first 24 hours of illness. After 48 hours, neutropenia becomes obvious with counts as high as $5 \times 10^3/mm^3$ occurring on the third and fourth day. On occasion a large number of lymphocytes may be present.

The most important diagnostic task for the chiropractor faced with a well-looking child with a high fever is to rule out other serious infections which commonly affect this age group, namely acute otitis media, acute pyelonephritis, pneumonia, meningitis and pneumococcal bacteremia (Behrman et al 2007). The cervical lymph nodes are only occasionally involved and the appearance of the typical rash as the temperature drops confirms the diagnosis.

Chiropractic management is the same as for the child with measles (see previous text). Oral administration of calcium ascorbate and *Echinacea purpurea* should be continued for at least 2–3 weeks after resolution of infection.

Glandular fever (infectious mononucleosis)

Glandular fever is a very common viral disease caused by the Epstein–Barr virus (Behrman et al 2007, Ernberg et al 1990, Schuster & Kreth 1992). In older children and adolescents this infection is characterized by fatigue, fever, cervical lymphadenopathy, hepatomegaly, splenomegaly, a maculopapular rash (McMillan et al 1982), and membranous tonsillitis with a sore throat (Endo et al 2001, Veltri et al 1975). In the young child, it usually presents with symptoms of fever, diarrhea, pharyngitis, tonsillitis, otitis media, pneumonia, cervical lymphadenopathy, hepatomegaly and splenomegaly. By the age of 4 years, between 30% and 70% of children will have acquired the antibodies to Epstein–Barr virus (Nystad & Myrmel

2007, Tamir et al 1974). Children with glandular fever may also occasionally present with jaundice (McMillan et al 1982). The frequency with which the symptoms and signs generally associated with glandular fever are seen is shown in Table 9.1.

Table 9.1 Frequency with which symptoms and signs related to glandular fever appear in young adults (reproduced with kind permission from McMillan et al 1982)

Symptom or sign	Percentage
Adenopathy	100
Malaise and fatigue	90–100
Fever	80–95
Sweats	80–95
Sore throat, dysphagia	80–95
Pharyngitis	65–85
Anorexia	50–80
Nausea	50–70
Splenomegaly	50–60
Headache	40–70
Chills	40–60
Bradycardia	35–50
Cough	30–50
Periorbital edema	25–40
Palatal enanthema	25–35
Hepatic or splenic tenderness	15–30
Myalgia	12–30
Hepatomegaly	15–25
Rhinitis	10–25
Ocular muscle pain	10–20
Chest pain	5–20
Jaundice	5–10
Arthralgia	5–10
Diarrhea or soft stools	5–10
Photophobia	5–10
Skin rash	3–10
Conjunctivitis	<5
Abdominal pain	<5
Gingivitis	<5
Pneumonitis	<5
Epistaxis	<5

Epstein–Barr virus was discovered during the 1960s when it was recovered in tumor cells from Burkitt's lymphoma. Today it is known to contribute to the pathogenesis of Burkitt's lymphoma, nasopharyngeal carcinoma (Ernberg et al 1990, Niedobitek et al 2001), Hodgkin's disease and other T cell lymphomas (Rezk & Weiss 2007, Schuster & Kreth 1992). The acute stage of glandular fever usually runs an uncomplicated course, ultimately leaving the child with an extended period of tiredness and lassitude. Children who are immunocompromised at the time of infection are at the greatest risk of experiencing complications that are known to include neurological, hepatic, cardiac and hematological conditions. Some of these are shown in Table 9.2. It should be noted, however, that while the symptoms associated with infectious mononucleosis can persist for many months, the notion of 'chronic mononucleosis' is essentially unsubstantiated (Jacobsen 1988).

The object of chiropractic management is to optimize the child's immune capabilities. Most children with glandular fever have poor muscle tone during the acute phase and are unable to exercise much. As a result, recurrent subluxation is a significant clinical problem. Neurological assessment twice weekly, and sometimes even more often than that, is required to maintain neurological balance. The child should also be given gut tolerance level calcium ascorbate, *Echinacea purpurea* and zinc as a basic measure to stimulate immune function. There is a school of thought which suggests that intravenous administration of sodium ascorbate in isotonic solution offers the best clinical outcome of glandular fever. Physicians at the forefront of this therapy are now admitting that this procedure is only marginally more effective than using orally administered calcium ascorbate at gut tolerance levels (Ng, personal communication, 1989). Electromagnetic field therapy is showing some encouraging signs of being helpful with immune stimulation in clinical conditions such as Epstein–Barr viral infection.

Table 9.2 Possible complications of Epstein–Barr viral infection in children (adapted from McMillan et al 1977 with permission)

System	Complication
Neurological	Guillain–Barré syndrome
	Meningitis
	Seizures
	Transverse myelitis
	Peripheral neuritis
	Optic neuritis
	Reye syndrome
Hepatic	Hepatitis
Cardiac	Pericarditis
	Myocarditis
Hematological	Anemia
	Thrombocytopenia
	Hemolytic uremic syndrome

Mucocutaneous lymph node syndrome (Kawasaki disease)

Kawasaki disease is a highly dangerous acute febrile illness seen most commonly in preschool-aged children. It mimics many other childhood diseases, especially measles and scarlet fever, and, because of this, initial misdiagnosis is common. Kawasaki disease was first described in Japan in 1967 and was initially called mucocutaneous lymph node syndrome. The etiology remains unclear and there is no specific diagnostic test. Eighty percent of patients are <5 years old (median age at diagnosis is 2 years) and the male to female ratio is 1.5 to 1. Kawasaki disease is the leading cause of acquired heart disease in children in the USA (Hay et al 2007).

Kawasaki disease is characterized by fever, conjunctival congestion (bilateral), strawberry tongue, erythema of the oral mucosa, sicca of the lips, indurative edema of the hands and feet followed by desquamation of the fingertips, polymorphous exanthema and cervical lymphadenopathy (Pinna et al 2008, Rubin & Cotton 1998, Terezhalmy 1979).

The only role the chiropractor has to play in the management of Kawasaki disease is diagnostic recognition and referral. Untreated, Kawasaki disease can lead to fatal cardiac complications, in particular coronary artery aneurysms (Pinna et al 2008, Rubin & Cotton 1998). It is critical to begin immunoglobulin (IVIG) and high-dose aspirin therapy before the ninth day of illness to offer the best prognosis in terms of the aortic aneurysms, given that these rarely form before the tenth day of illness. Not all the symptoms associated with Kawasaki disease appear at the same time and a clear understanding of when each one is likely to appear will assist with accurate diagnostic identification. The expected progression of symptoms over time is shown in Fig. 9.6.

Meningitis and meningococcemia

Meningococcemia is a very dangerous bacteremia which may result from meningococci colonizing in the nasopharynx and then penetrating the mucosa to become blood-borne. Meningococcemia is generally transmitted to children from adult carriers.

Meningococcemia has a 24-hour prodrome involving influenza-like illness with fever, malaise, myalgia, arthralgia, headache, and sometimes gastrointestinal symptoms (Behrman et al 2007, Wong et al 1989). Within hours to days of the onset of the prodromal symptoms, petechiae appear in areas of pressure, such as axillary folds, belt line and other skin folds, followed by purplish ecchymoses and maculopapular nodules which develop first on the trunk and then on the extensor surfaces of the thighs and forearms (McMillan et al 1977). Hypotension, disseminated intravascular coagulation, renal failure and coma may follow in unchecked disease. When meningitis follows hematogenous dissemination, symptoms usually include lethargy, photophobia, seizures, and other signs, which characterize meningeal irritation (Behrman et al 2007).

'Meningococcal meningitis may be complicated by deafness, ataxia, seizures, blindness, paresis of cranial nerves III, IV, VI,

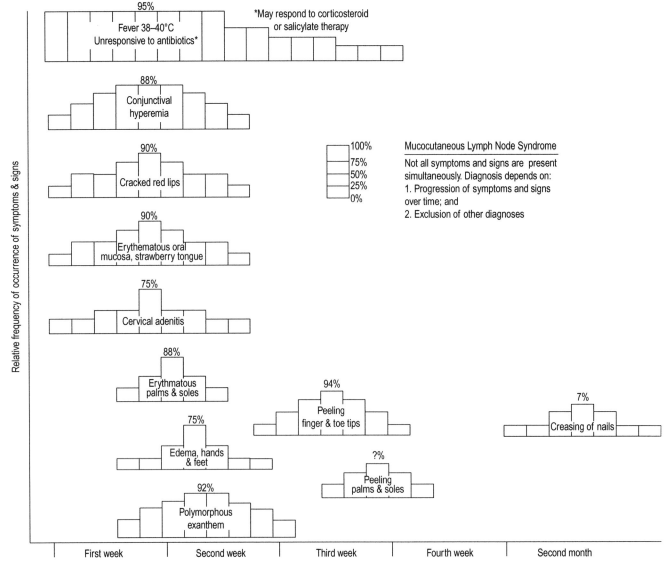

Figure 9.6 ● Expected progression of symptoms over time associated with Kawasaki disease (reproduced with kind permission from McMillan et al 1982).

and VII, hemiparesis, quadriparesis, spinal cord infarction or obstructive hydrocephalus. Meningococcemia may be complicated by adrenal hemorrhage, encephalitis, arthritis, myocarditis, pericarditis, pneumonia, lung abscess, peritonitis and disseminated intravascular coagulation' (Behrman et al 2007).

The prognosis for children with meningococcemia is good once they have survived the first 48 hours following symptomatic onset. Mortality may, however, be as high as 15–20% (Milonovich 2007).

The prognosis in meningococcemia can be reasonably estimated by the skin manifestations. These will take one of three forms: firstly, there may be no skin lesions at all (Wong et al 1989); secondly, there may be erythematous, macular and/or petechial lesions in a generalized distribution over the whole body; and thirdly, there may be large purpuric or ecchymotic lesions, mostly on the extremities, associated with petechial hemorrhaging. Patients who present without any skin manifestations have a much higher rate of concurrent meningitis than

is the case for those who have skin lesions. Patients in the third category have the worst prognosis with a higher rate of hyperpyrexia, coagulation abnormalities, shock and death than is the case in the other two (Nielsen et al 2001, Toews & Bass 1974).

The role of the chiropractor is clearly one of disease recognition followed by emergency hospital referral for investigation and crisis management. Time is a critical element owing to the fulminating nature of the infection. A more active role may be assumed for the chiropractor in the recovery and post-recovery period involving chiropractic care, craniosacral therapy and nutritional counseling to optimize immune system recovery.

Osteomyelitis

Osteomyelitis occurs predominantly in males and follows a history of trauma in about one-third of affected individuals. Most commonly, the affected child will present with fever and at the site of infection there will usually be swelling, tenderness and raised local temperature. False-negative results from the full blood evaluation are very high with as few as 30% of affected children showing a white cell count >15 000/mm^3. The ESR, however, rarely returns a false negative in the presence of osteomyelitis. Radiological demonstration of bone destruction is generally not seen in the first 10 days of infection (McMillan et al 1977).

The most common etiological agent in osteomyelitis in all age groups is *Staphylococcus aureus*. Streptococci are the next most commonly involved microorganisms, while *Haemophilus influenzae* is a common cause in children under 2 years of age (McMillan et al 1977). The bacterial etiology of osteomyelitis demands immediate parenteral antibiotic therapy. Clearly, the role of the chiropractor is to identify the diagnosis and make the appropriate referral immediately.

Urinary tract infection (UTI)

UTI is a common and important infectious problem in pediatrics. While it affects all age groups, diagnosis of infection of the urinary tract is very challenging as it presents differently at different ages. Generally speaking, during infancy the most common presenting symptoms are fever, weight loss, failure to thrive, nausea, vomiting, diarrhea and jaundice. Later in childhood, the more common signs are urinary frequency, abdominal pain and foul-smelling urine (Behrman et al 2007). UTI should always be excluded in children who present with fever of unknown origin (FUO) and daytime incontinence.

Involvement of the kidney (acute pyelonephritis) should be considered when the child presents with chills, fever, flank and/or abdominal pain. In this condition, the kidneys are often tender when palpated. The presenting symptoms of urinary tract infection by age are shown in Table 9.3.

Diagnosis can only be positively made by laboratory investigation. The definitive test for urinary tract infection is the demonstration of bacteriuria, provided adequate care has been taken to avoid specimen contamination during collection. In girls the labia should be manually separated, and in uncircumcised boys the prepuce should be retracted during sample collection. Pyuria is sometimes seen in the urine specimens of children with urinary tract infection, but not always. It is therefore not considered to be diagnostic but confirmatory once the diagnosis is established. Microscopic hematuria is common in acute cystitis and casts are frequently seen in the urinary sediment when there is renal involvement.

Clearly, since the etiology of urinary tract infection is bacterial, the role of the chiropractor is to recognize the range of symptoms associated with urinary tract infection, arrange for appropriate laboratory investigation, and refer for antibiotic therapy when it is confirmed. Concurrent chiropractic care aimed at normalizing neurological balance and immune function by nutritional supplementation is appropriate.

Acquired immune deficiency syndrome (AIDS)

AIDS has received wide publicity for the past 20–25 years. It is important to remember that the incidence of AIDS in children is very low, especially in countries such as Australia, the UK, USA, Canada, etc. There are, however, countries where the prevalence of AIDS among children and adolescents is high. Such countries include those on the African continent and some in south-east Asia. Almost all children with AIDS have acquired it from their mothers and therefore it represents a very low-priority diagnostic consideration in the chiropractic primary care setting. In the early to mid-1980s there was a risk of children acquiring AIDS through blood transfusion, but all blood products are so well screened now that this mode of transmission has for all practical purposes been eliminated.

Table 9.3 Presenting symptoms by age in children with urinary tract infection (adapted from McMillan et al 1982 with permission)

Presenting symptom	Percentage of patients with various symptoms by age			
	Birth–1 month	1 month–2 years	2–6 years	6–18 years
Failure to thrive, feeding problems	65	40	7	0
Diarrhea/vomiting	42	42	16	3
Unexplained fever	30	36	22	50
CNS symptoms such as convulsions, hypotonicity, irritability, sluggishness, etc.	29	7	9	5
'Sepsis', jaundice	47	0	0	0
Colic, irritability and screaming attacks	0	15	5	0
Discolored or malodorous urine	0	9	14	0
Urgency, frequency, dysuria	0	8	44	41
Abdominal or flank pain	0	0	10	66
Enuresis	0	0	38	29

The AIDS virus is spread by the exchange of human fluids such as blood or semen. It is not contracted via such actions as touching, cuddling or kissing. It is also extremely unlikely that the AIDS virus would be contracted via contact with saliva. Basically, there is no risk of a child developing AIDS from coming into contact with either another child or an adult who is infected unless there is an exchange of bodily fluids. There is no risk to you as a chiropractor treating a child with AIDS if you take the necessary precautions to avoid any contact with blood products from that child (Kaminsky & Oberklaid 1996).

References

Abdulmalik, A., Al-Ateeqi, W., Al-Khawari, M., et al., 2006. Varicella-associated purpura fulminans: chicken pox is not always benign. Med. Princ. Pract. 15 (3), 232–234.

Becker, F.T., Buckley, R.P., 1966. Purpura fulminans associated with varicella. Arch. Dermatol. 94 (5), 613–618.

Behrman, R.E., Jenson, H.B., Nelson, W.E., et al., 2007. Nelson Textbook of Pediatrics, eighteenth ed. WB Saunders, Philadelphia.

Endo, L.H., Ferreira, D., Montenegro, M.C., et al., 2001. Detection of Epstein–Barr virus in tonsillar tissue of children and the relationship with recurrent tonsillitis. Int. J. Pediatr. Otorhinolaryngol. 58 (1), 9–15.

Ernberg, I., Anderson, J., Linde, A., 1990. Epstein–Barr virus infection – clinical aspects and diagnosis. Nord. Med. 105 (1), 19–23.

Feldman, S., Crout, J.D., Andrew, M.E., 1997. Incidence and natural history of chemically defined varicella-zoster virus hepatitis in children and adolescents. Scand. J. Infect. Dis. 29 (1), 33–36.

Garcia Aquilera, X., Ledo Rodrigues, A., Teruel Canchez-Vegazo, C., et al., 2008. Acute hepatitis due to varicella zoster virus. Gastroenterol. Hepatol. 31 (3), 131.

Garg, B.K., 1968. Acute cerebellar ataxia following varicella. Indian Pediatr. 5 (5), 230–233.

Guess, H.A., Broughton, D.D., Melton 3rd., L.J., et al., 1986. Population-based studies of varicella complications. Pediatrics 78 (4/2), 723–727.

Hay, W.W., Levin, M.J., Sondheimer, J.M., et al., 2007. Current Diagnosis and Treatment in Pediatrics, eighteenth ed. Lange Medial Books/McGraw Hill, New York.

Jackson, M.A., Burry, V.F., Olson, L.C., 1992. Complications of varicella requiring hospitalization in previously healthy children. J. Pediatr. Infect. Dis. 11 (6), 441–445.

Jacobsen, E.J., 1988. Chronic mononucleosis – it almost never happens. Postgrad. Med. 83 (1), 56–57, 61–65.

Kaminsky, L., Oberklaid, F., 1996. From Baby to Child: The Australian Handbook. Mandarin, Port Melbourne.

Krugman, S., Ward, R., 1958. Infectious Diseases of Children. Mosby, St Louis.

Krugman, S., Katz, S., Gershon, A., et al., 2004. Krugman's Infectious Diseases of Children, eleventh ed. Mosby, St Louis.

McMillan, J.A., Neiberg, P.I., Oski, F.A., 1977. The Whole Pediatrician Catalogue: A Compendium of Clues to Diagnosis and Management. WB Saunders, Philadelphia.

McMillan, J.A., Stockman, J.A., Oski, F.A., 1982. The Whole Pediatrician Catalogue, vol. 3. WB Saunders, Philadelphia.

Maness, D.L., Rogers, D.Y., 1987. Hemorrhagic complications of varicella. Am. Fam. Physician 35 (2), 151–155.

Milonovich, L.M., 2007. Meningococcemia: epidemiology, pathophysiology, and management. J. Pediatr. Health Care 21 (2), 75–80.

Niedobitek, G., Meru, N., Delecluse, H.J., 2001. Epstein–Barr virus infection and human malignancies. Int. J. Exp. Pathol. 82 (3), 149–170.

Nielsen, H.E., Andersen, E.A., Andersen, J., et al., 2001. Diagnostic assessment of haemorrhagic rash and fever. Arch. Dis. Child. 85 (2), 160–165.

Nussinovitch, M., Prais, D., Volovitz, B., et al., 2003. Post-infectious acute cerebellar ataxia in children. Clin. Pediatr. (Phila) 42 (7), 581–584.

Nystad, T.W., Myrmel, H., 2007. Prevalence of primary versus reactivated Epstein–Barr infection in patients with VCA IgG-, VCA IgM- and EBNA-1-antibodies and suspected infectious mononucleosis. J. Clin. Virol. 38 (4), 292–297.

Overall Jr., J.C., 1981. Virus infections of the fetus and neonate. In: Feigin, R.D., Cherry, J.D. (Eds), Textbook of Pediatric Infectious Diseases. WB Saunders, Philadelphia.

Phuah, H.K., Chong, C.Y., Lim, K.W., et al., 1998. Complicated varicella zoster infection in 8 pediatric patients and review of literature. Singapore Med. J. 39 (3), 115–120.

Pinna, G.S., Kafetzis, D.A., Tselkas, O.L., et al., 2008. Kawasaki disease: an overview. Curr. Opin. Infect. Dis. 21 (3), 263–270.

Reynolds, M.A., Watson, B.M., Plott-Adams, K.K., et al., 2008. Epidemiology of varicella hospitalizations in the United States, 1995–2005. J. Infect. Dis. 197 (Suppl. 2), S120–S126.

Rezk, S.A., Weiss, L.M., 2007. Epstein–Barr virus-associated lymphoproliferative disorders. Hum. Pathol. 38 (9), 1293–1304.

Rubin, B., Cotton, D.M., 1998. Kawasaki disease: a dangerous acute childhood illness. Nurse Pract. 23 (2), 34, 37–38, 44–48.

Schuster, V., Kreth, H.W., 1992. Epstein–Barr virus infection and associated diseases in children. II. Diagnostic and therapeutic strategies. Eur. J. Pediatr. 151 (11), 794–798.

Tamir, D., Benderley, A., Levy, J., et al., 1974. Infectious mononucleosis and Epstein–Barr virus in childhood. Pediatrics 53 (3), 330–335.

Terezhalmy, G.T., 1979. Mucocutaneous lymph node syndrome. Review of a recently described disease complex. Oral Surg. Oral Med. Oral Pathol. 47 (1), 26–30.

Toews, W.H., Bass, J.W., 1974. Skin manifestations of meningococcal infection; an immediate indicator of prognosis. Am. J. Dis. Child. 127 (9), 552–556.

Veltri, R.W., Sprinkle, P.M., McClung, J.E., 1975. Epstein–Barr virus associated with episodes of recurrent tonsillitis. Arch. Otolaryngol. 101 (9), 552–556.

Wong, V.K., Hitchcock, W., Mason, W.H., 1989. Meningococcal infections in children: a review of 100 cases. Pediatr. Infect. Dis. J. 8 (4), 224–227.

Common respiratory illness in childhood

Neil J. Davies

The purpose of this chapter is to present, in detail, a discussion of those respiratory illnesses commonly suffered by children which are most likely to be encountered by a chiropractor in the primary care setting. It does not attempt to cover the whole spectrum of respiratory disease, but instead concentrates on those conditions which have either a significant prevalence and incidence or are of such importance in the diagnostic evaluation of a child with respiratory symptoms that safety considerations demand elucidation in a text of this nature.

Asthma

Asthma is the most common chronic respiratory disease of childhood, having a prevalence throughout the developed world of 12% (Hull & Johnston 1999).

Definition

Asthma is a disorder in which the airways demonstrate hyper-reactivity, which leads to paroxysms of luminal obstruction which, in turn, produce coughing, respiratory distress and wheezing.

Pathophysiology

Asthma is pre-eminently a multifactorial condition that has attracted several attempts at construction of a classification system. Attacks are known to result from exercise (exercise-induced asthma or EIA), IgE-modulated response to allergens such as the house dust mite (*Dermatophagoides pteronyssimus*), various seasonal pollens, animal fur, molds, drugs, some foodstuffs (e.g. dairy products), infection, neurotrophic disturbance, sudden change in weather, and psychological dysfunction. Generally, children with asthma may be graded into three groups:

1. The mild group includes children whose occasional attacks are usually precipitated by infection, but who have no symptoms between attacks. These children exhibit normal growth and pulmonary function tests apart from bronchoconstriction induced by exercise.

2. The intermediate or moderate group consists of those with severe, recurrent episodes of asthma, but who remain symptom-free between attacks apart, once again, from exercise-induced bronchoconstriction.

3. In the severe group, the asthmatic attacks may vary in severity but the child is never free of symptoms and the illness affects general growth and development. This child has abnormal lung function tests at all times with hyperinflation evident as chest wall deformity and on X-ray examination (Hull & Johnston 1999).

The relationship between asthma and the nervous system appears to be related to trophic disturbance of the respiratory sympathetic neuromeres (T2–T7) which results from sympathetic depletion or from facilitation of the respiratory parasympathetic neuromere (vagus nerve) resulting in parasympatheticotonia (Gatterman 1990). While there have been reports in recent chiropractic publications (Anrig & Plaugher 1998, Balon & Mior 2004, Gatterman 1990) of patients with asthmatic symptoms responding positively to adjustment or manipulation of the upper cervical complex, they also suggest, as does Beyeler (1965), that the influence of both the vagus nerve and reflexes from spinal centers together play the predominant role in the genesis of an asthmatic attack. This latter view generally concurs with the experience of the author in treating children with asthma.

Whether or not the subluxation is the instigating factor in an asthmatic attack, or the result of viscerosomatic reflex via sympathetic and/or vagal afferent irritation arising from mucus accumulation, inhaled debris such as dust, cigarette smoke or noxious fumes, all of which may cause bronchoconstriction (Gatterman 1990, Marieb 2009), is irrelevant since the chiropractic adjustment has the capacity to break the noxious cycle

© 2010, Elsevier Ltd, Inc, BV
DOI: 10.1016/B978-0-7020-3129-8.00010-4

and reduce the non-specific bronchial hyperreactivity (Balon & Mior 2004, Nielsen et al 1995), thus relieving the respiratory distress. It is virtually never possible unequivocally to determine the primacy of the subluxation and, therefore, the management planning for all asthmatic patients must necessarily address all the known etiological factors.

Natural history

The natural history of asthma is significantly influenced by the following five factors:

1. the age at which the child experienced the first episode of wheezing
2. the frequency of attacks in the first 12 months following the initial attack
3. evidence of airway obstruction between attacks
4. the development of chest deformity
5. impairment of growth.

The natural history for children with mild asthma is good, with attacks ceasing completely in most children somewhere between their 5th and 14th birthdays. Children with an early age of onset (usually in the first or second year of life), high frequency of attacks in the first 12 months, evident airway obstruction and hyperinflation between attacks, pigeon or barrel chest deformity, and impaired growth (Mcnicol et al 1973) have a much poorer outcome, with some children experiencing cessation of attacks in adolescence while others continue to have attacks into adulthood.

Clinical evaluation of the asthmatic child

Asthma is a result of a complex interaction of biochemical, autoimmune, immunological, infectious, endocrine, psychological (Behrman et al 2007) and biomechanical factors, all of which vary in degree in different individuals. Detail of these factors, which can be addressed when taking the case history, must be reflected in the clinical database of all children who suffer with this distressing condition if an optimal patient outcome is to be achieved.

Key aspects of the clinical history

In order to facilitate an appropriate, comprehensive management program for a child with asthma, it is critical that a very detailed clinical history be obtained.

Presenting complaint

Details of the characteristics of the child's symptoms should be sought. Important aspects include the presence of dyspnea, wheezing, cough; exercise tolerance (does the child always come last in races? etc.); nocturnal symptoms, especially significant if they wake the child; early morning tightness in the chest; history of use of bronchodilator medication; recurrent viral infection in the upper respiratory tract; cyanosis and syncope (Harris et al 2002).

The pattern of symptoms including the past history should also be established. Important information includes the time of day symptoms occur; seasonal, diurnal and geographic variation; severity; age of onset; course of previous episodes and the nature and success of previous treatment; obvious precipitants such as weather, infection, pollutants, allergy, environmental elements such as pollens and emotional lability (Harris et al 2002).

Finally, a thorough family and social history should be taken. This should include a three-generation family tree looking for any evidence of respiratory disease such as wheezing, recurrent bronchitis, allergies or cough. An attempt should also be made to ascertain the disease impact on the child and family.

In addition to the general information elicited from the presenting complaint, the following detailed information should also be sought.

Biochemical factors

A dietary survey should be undertaken in an attempt to identify any 'high-risk' food category that may be involved in any particular case. It is also wise to follow this up with a detailed dietary log that the parents keep for a week, which will help to quantify the foods and liquids consumed by the child. In one example, a completed dietary log showed that wheat products (e.g. Weetabix) were eaten to excess. This particular child, who was a severe asthmatic, almost fully resolved in the space of 3 weeks with chiropractic care and dietary manipulation in which the child was denied all foods containing or derived from wheat and encouraged to eat more fruit and vegetables. This case is an excellent illustration of the principle that children will crave the foods to which they are hypersensitive and which contribute to their illness.

Immunological factors

Enquiry should be made in relation to exposure to noxious substances such as hydrocarbons, cigarette smoke, airborne dust, pets (particularly cats, dogs and birds) which are allowed inside the home, feathers such as those found in duvets (doonas) and some pillows, and environmental irritants such as pollens and molds. A careful search for evidence of an asthmatic pattern associated with recurrent infection should be made. Asthmatic attacks concurrent with fever, runny nose, malaise, sore throat, sneezing or cough provide at least superficial evidence of an infectious trigger for that particular child's asthma. Viral agents, particularly respiratory syncytial virus (RSV) and parainfluenza virus (PV), are the most frequent offenders in this type of presentation, especially in younger children. In older children, rhinovirus is frequently involved, and with increasing age influenza virus assumes a greater degree of significance (Behrman et al 2007).

In addition, a history of hay fever, eczema and urticaria is significant. In a review of 315 children at their 14th birthday who had experienced wheezing to varying degrees, of those categorized as having severe asthma 80% had hay fever, 67% had eczema, and 57% had urticaria concomitant with their asthma (Mcnicol et al 1973).

Table 10.1 Clinical factors which assist the differentiation of bronchiolitis and asthma in an infant with a first episode of wheezing (reproduced with kind permission from McMillan et al 1982)

	Bronchiolitis	Asthma
Occurrence	Within the first 2 years, usually before 6 months	Any age
Frequency	Up to three episodes	More than three episodes
Season	Winter and spring	Any time
Etiology	Associated with epidemics of respiratory syncytial virus (RSV) and other respiratory viral infections	Allergy, infection, exercise, aspirin or pollutants
Signs	Fine crackles predominate Expiration = inspiration Shallow, rapid respirations	Wheezing predominant Expiration prolonged Tachypnea and hyperpnea
X-ray	Hyperinflation ± scattered infiltrates	Hyperinflation ± atelectasis
Response to sympathomimetics	Generally none	Some reversal of bronchospasm
Prognosis	Excellent	Variable, may become chronic

An attack of wheezing associated with hyperinflation of the lungs in the first year of life represents a diagnostic dilemma as to whether it represents the first attack of asthma or bronchiolitis of viral etiology as a result of infection of the lower respiratory tract. Table 10.1 provides a few clinical clues to assist the chiropractor in differentiating the two. The infant experiencing a first episode of wheezing who has a positive family history of allergy, nasal eosinophilia, eczema, elevated total serum IgE and whose symptoms are reversed with the administration of sympathomimetic drugs is more likely to have asthma than bronchiolitis (McMillan et al 1982).

Endocrine factors

Inquiry should be made in cases where the asthma has become suddenly or progressively worse in adolescent females whether there is a relationship between premenstrual tension and the asthmatic attacks. It is also known that thyrotoxicosis will exacerbate asthma. The onset of puberty improves asthma in some children (Mcnicol et al 1973).

Psychological factors

Asthma is strikingly affected by psychological incidents. An evaluation of the possible sources of psychological stress should be attempted, including the possibility of exposure to abusive episodes. Emotional or behavioral disturbances are, in the main, more related to poor control of the asthma generally than to the severity of any given attack, affecting the child's view of himself or herself and sometimes the parents' view of the child (Mcnicol et al 1973).

Biomechanical factors

During the review of systems, due consideration should be given to symptoms reported by the child which, while unrelated to the asthma, may indicate the presence of the chiropractic subluxation, particularly of the lumbosacral junction, upper thoracic region, and upper cervical complex. Symptoms such as headache, dizziness, blurred vision, nightmares, sleep disturbance, ear pain, shoulder or arm pain, back pain, leg pain, awkward gait and ambulation, knee pain, foot flare, enuresis, encopresis, attention deficit disorder, etc. are all suggestive of the presence of the chiropractic subluxation, which in turn may be bearing negatively on the asthma (Graham & Pistolese 1997).

The physical examination

The physical examination should not be discounted for any reason by the clinician entrusted with the responsibility of caring for children. In an asthmatic presentation, a full and complete physical examination is essential. The following discussion represents the key aspects of the physical examination likely to provide the chiropractor with valuable information about the patient, but in no way intends to suggest that other aspects of examination not mentioned should be omitted.

Inspection
The fully disrobed patient should be inspected from both the anterior and posterior. Box 10.1 identifies various findings on inspection that may be related to asthma.

Anthropometry
Head circumference, height, weight, arm span, upper and lower body ratios, and sitting height should all be measured, the values obtained being plotted on appropriate anthropometric charts where available. Shortness of stature or underweight for age values in children with asthma represents a poor prognosis indicator (McMillan et al 1977). Tanner staging for pubertal status is important since delayed puberty may be precipitated by asthma (Harris et al 2002).

Box 10.1

Clinical findings on inspection of the disrobed patient which may be associated with asthma

- Pigeon breast is characterized by protrusion of the sternum
- Barrel chest is characterized by persisting equality of the anteroposterior and transverse diameters
- Flaring is seen at the lower lateral margins of the rib cage, immediately below what would be described as a depression
- The angle formed by the lower rib margin with the sternum may exceed 45°
- Evidence of hyperinflation
- Harrison's sulci may be seen as transverse lines on the anterior chest wall at the inferior border of the pectoralis muscle bulk
- Allergic shiners or dark rings under the eyes may be seen in atopic children
- A transverse line across the nose sometimes accompanies atopic disease in which the nose is irritated, causing the child to rub it constantly (allergic salute)
- Tanner staging. Delayed puberty may be precipitated by asthma
- Tachypnea at rest and use of accessory muscles of respiration
- Dry skin and patches of atopic eczema at the knees and elbows

Vital signs

These should include temperature (as evidence of infection), pulse rate, respiratory rate, blood pressure, and peak respiratory flow measured both before and after the administration of bronchodilators where possible.

Ear, nose and throat

Pneumatic otoscopy should be carried out in order to demonstrate functional adequacy of the middle ear and Eustachian tube. The nasal membranes should be inspected for any evidence of allergic rhinitis (pale, swollen nasal mucosa with a clear to greenish discharge) or enlargement of the inferior turbinates which may be providing a mechanical obstruction causing recurrent infection. In the throat, redness or the presence of any exudate or postnasal drip should be noted. The cervical lymph nodes should also be palpated.

The chest

In addition to observation described earlier, the chest should be palpated, percussed and auscultated. On auscultation,

asthma may be evidenced by expiratory wheezing and is sometimes complicated by the presence of crackles in both late inspiration and expiration. Peak flow measurements should be taken, preferably both before and after the administration of bronchodilators, since peak flow meters provide an estimate of large airway patency. While there is some dispute over the reliability of peak flow measurement as a means of estimating large airway patency (Frischer et al 1995, Sly 1993, Uwyyed et al 1996), it remains a widely used and useful tool in the overall assessment and office-based chiropractic management of a child with asthma (Harris et al 2002).

Clinical investigations

It is appropriate, when an allergic etiology is suggested by the history and physical examination, to order specific testing procedures in an attempt to identify those foodstuffs which may be provoking bronchial hyperreactivity. A chest X-ray is also appropriate in a first episode of wheezing in order to rule out other diagnoses such as an inhaled foreign body, pneumothorax, etc.

Chiropractic management strategies

The chiropractic management plan for a child with asthma involves the careful application of chiropractic adjusting, implementation of home-based support strategies, reinforcement of minimal allopathic intervention/prevention measures, and parent/child/teacher education.

Chiropractic care

The asthmatic child should be provided with chiropractic care and carefully monitored using the home symptom recording sheet (Fig. 10.1). Should the caregiver notice a shift in severity of symptoms, particularly those occurring at night or in the early morning, necessitating an increased use of bronchodilator medication, the chiropractor should be notified and an unscheduled assessment carried out. An increase in night symptoms is particularly significant to the chiropractor since it has been shown that, when this occurs, peak expiratory flow usually remains constant, suggesting that mechanisms other than impairment of lung function are responsible for increased

Figure 10.1 • Clinical factors for caregivers of asthmatic children to facilitate home monitoring of symptoms.

Name:	Age:	Date of observation:

Aspect monitored	Record by caregiver:		
Coughing	☐ None ☐ Daytime	☐ Moderate ☐ Night	☐ Severe ☐ Early morning
Wheezing	☐ None ☐ Daytime	☐ Moderate ☐ Night	☐ Severe ☐ Early morning
Difficulty breathing	☐ None ☐ Daytime	☐ Moderate ☐ Night	☐ Severe ☐ Early morning
Medication frequency	☐ Increased	☐ As prescribed	

symptoms in the supine position (Chugh et al 2006, Greenough et al 1991). Neurological dysafferentation should always be presumed to be one of those mechanisms and corrected accordingly.

Home support strategies

Management of asthmatic symptoms at home should include the following advice to parents:

- Keep smoking cigarettes, cigars, etc. outside the house only.
- Avoid vacuuming carpets late in the day. This should be done in the morning, preferably when the child is at school or otherwise out of the house.
- Keep pets, especially cats and birds, outside.
- Keep the child away from vehicle emissions in closed places such as garages, sheds, etc.
- Use blankets instead of duvets and place pillows in a plastic bag.
- Limit physical activity during times when exercise tolerance is likely to be severely affected, such as when there is very cold or windy weather.
- Avoid foods which have been shown by allergy testing to provoke symptoms. Referral to a naturopathic practitioner is often helpful in controlling allergic responses in asthmatic children.

Reinforcement of the medical management program

Asthma can and does account for pediatric deaths in every country of the world. These deaths are largely preventable by bronchodilator medication, or, in an emergency, corticosteroid administration in a hospital-based setting. The chiropractor, in constructing a management plan, should have on record the name of the family physician responsible for the child's medication schedule. Every attempt should be made to encourage the caregivers and child to adhere to the medication schedule and the physician should be requested to monitor carefully the need for such medication as the child is given chiropractic care.

In addition, it is essential that the caregiver has a written crisis management plan, which, if not provided by the physician, should be provided by the chiropractor. This plan should include the following:

1. Is there a nebulizer available for emergency situations?
2. Is transport available to take the child to the local physician at all times of the day?
3. Is transport available to take the child to your office at all times of the day?
4. Is transport available to take the child to a hospital at all times of the day?
5. Has a contingency plan been identified to obtain transport if none is available at home?
6. Are caregivers and teachers adequately educated to know when to stop using the nebulizer and seek professional assistance?

The chiropractor should always be a part of emergency care. While it is recognized that adjusting has little effect on objective lung function, it does have a considerable effect on non-specific bronchial hyperreactivity, patient-rated asthma (Graham & Pistolese 1997, Nielsen et al 1995) and frequency of recurrence (Graham & Pistolese 1997). Adjusting children in asthmatic crisis often modulates the need for pharmacological intervention strategies.

Education of the child, caregiver and teachers

As part of the management plan, the chiropractor should endeavor to gain an estimate of the knowledge the child has of the disease and the awareness of appropriate measures to be taken by the caregiver or teachers involved with the child. This includes education related to the following (Harris et al 2002):

1. the child (e.g. knowing to take aerosol before exercise, etc.)
2. the caregiver (e.g. understanding the necessity for, and mechanisms involved in, treatment; knowing how to monitor the child's condition; knowing not to have the child avoid sport at school; being aware of the prognosis)
3. the teacher (e.g. allowing the child to have the inhaler on hand at all times; appreciating the need for treatment; not inappropriately excluding the child from games, sports, etc.).

Bronchiolitis

Definition

Bronchiolitis is an acute lower airway infection encountered primarily during the first year of life. Respiratory syncytial virus (RSV) is the etiological agent in 60–90% of cases (Boeck 1996, Lugo & Nahata 1993). Parainfluenza 3 virus, mycoplasma and adenoviruses account for the balance of cases not produced by RSV (Behrman et al 2007). Occasionally, bronchiolitis is confused clinically with bacterial bronchopneumonia (Behrman et al 2007).

Pathophysiology

Bronchiolitis results from bronchiolar obstruction from edema, accumulation of mucus and cellular debris from epithelial necrosis (Carvalho et al 2007, Horst 1994), which may result from hyperresponsiveness to bronchoprovocation (Behrman et al 2007, Leung et al 2005), as well as invasion of the bronchial tree by virus. Since resistance to airflow in a tube is directly proportional to the fourth power of the radius of that tube, even a minor obstruction to the airway can produce profound changes in total airflow (Behrman et al 2007). The pathophysiological process impairs normal gaseous exchange in the lung, often resulting in hypoxemia early in the course of the disease. Retained carbon dioxide (hypercapnia) is infrequent. When it does occur, it is evidenced by a respiratory rate in excess of 60 breaths per minute (Behrman et al 2007). Hypercapnia represents one of the most urgent indications for hospital referral in cases of acute bronchiolitis.

Natural history

Acute bronchiolitis usually follows exposure to a source of respiratory infection in the week prior to the onset of symptoms. In cases not affected by complication, the infected infant is likely to appear very ill for 48–72 hours, after which time improvement rapidly occurs. Recovery is complete within a few days.

Clinical evaluation of the infant with bronchiolitis

A history of exposure to individuals with upper respiratory infection within 7 days of the onset of symptoms provides a basis for considering bronchiolitis as the diagnosis in an infant who presents with sudden-onset fever, lassitude, loss of appetite, nasal discharge, sneezing, wheezy cough, irritability and dyspnea. The physical examination should seek to identify the presence of wheeze, crackles that are usually widespread throughout the chest, short inspiration, tachypnea and fever (usually within the range 38.5–39°C).

Symptoms encountered in acute bronchiolitis vary from mild wheezing to severe respiratory distress (American Academy of Pediatrics 2006, Nahata et al 1985), and therefore careful observation of the patient throughout the conduct of the physical examination is essential in order to identify the cardinal physical signs which would mandate hospital referral (Behrman et al 2007, Everard 1995, Mai et al 1995, Nahata et al 1985). A summary of the key findings is shown in Box 10.2. It is virtually never necessary to conduct laboratory investigations in children with acute bronchiolitis as the white cell count is usually within normal limits (McMillan et al 1982) and lymphopenia, commonly found in other viral disease, is not seen in bronchiolitis (Behrman et al 2007). Demonstration of RSV by immunofluorescence in recovered nasal secretions can be performed but carries little clinical significance. The demonstration of RSV in nasal discharge has been shown to have no predictive value of the need for hospitalization for ventilatory and supportive therapy (Gavin et al 1996).

Chiropractic management of children with bronchiolitis

Acute bronchiolitis is a common childhood infection affecting 6–10% of the population (American Academy of Pediatrics

---

Box 10.2

Cardinal physical signs which identify the need for hospital referral in infants presenting with acute bronchiolitis

- Respiratory rate >60 breaths/min
- Cyanosis
- Intercostal recession
- Sternal retraction
- Nasal flaring
- Acute bodyweight loss >7.5%

2006, Nahata et al 1985). Although infants with this condition, can appear desperately ill, particularly in the first 2 days, even among those who meet the criteria for hospitalization only 3% will require ventilatory support and intensive care (Dawson et al 1993). Despite these figures, and the amenability of patients with this condition to be conservatively home managed, the keystone of the chiropractic management plan rests on the ability of the chiropractor to identify the clinical indicators for hospital referral. Once it has been determined that it is safe and appropriate to manage the infant in a home-care setting, the following strategies should be considered:

- Begin chiropractic adjusting as soon as possible. This usually involves the upper cervical spine, the sacrum, and the craniosacral primary respiratory mechanism.
- In breastfed infants, prescribe vitamin C for the mother to gut level tolerance. In non-breastfed infants, advise the parents or caregiver to administer 250–500 mg of vitamin C per day in several small doses. Rosehip syrup may be a convenient form in which to administer it.
- Maintain fluid level according to the formula set out in Chapter 4 to guard against dehydration. If the child demonstrates an acute body weight loss exceeding 5% or clinical signs of dehydration appear, the child should be referred for hospital admission so fluid therapy can be started.
- Ask the parents or caregiver to take and record the infant's temperature at 2-hourly intervals. Any sudden change upward should be reported immediately since spiking fever may represent serious neurological or other infection.
- Instruct the parents and caregiver to handle the infant as little as possible (Dawson et al 1993).
- Until the symptoms begin to subside, examine the child's vital signs, lungs and upper respiratory system, including the ears, each morning and evening to check for signs of disease progression. Adjust the infant as required on these visits since subluxation recurrence is highly likely because of active viscerosomatic reflexes from the bronchial tree, which is richly supplied with chemoreceptors and therefore vulnerable to toxic input from the pathological process accompanying the disease.
- Prescribe *Echinacea purpurea* extract for mothers who are breastfeeding. Echinacea extract (*Echinacea purpurea* in particular) has a well-documented immunostimulatory effect (Bukovsky et al 1993, 1995; Melchart et al 1995) and is considered to have virtually no toxicity, even when used in doses well above that recommended for human consumption (Mengs et al 1991).

Acute bronchitis

Definition

Much about acute bronchitis in children is uncertain, even its definition. It is usually diagnosed on the basis of a presentation involving cough, sputum production, rales and/or rhonchi on auscultation, and a clinical history of lower airway disease over the preceding 12 months (Braman 2006, Vinson 1991). Despite this being the case in general clinical practice, the definition of acute bronchitis and its clinical parameters remain obscure and uncertain (Braman 2006, Dunlay & Reinhardt 1984).

If this be so for acute bronchitis, the situation is even more obscure for chronic bronchitis, a term which should be considered more a description of a symptom complex that may or may not involve identifiable pathology of either the upper or lower airway than a diagnosis in itself. Chronic bronchitis should rarely be accepted as a final diagnosis. A clear definition, identification of pathology, description of natural history, delineation of appropriate therapy and prognosis have not been described for the chronic bronchitis complex in childhood (Morgan & Taussig 1984).

A chronic or frequently recurring productive cough usually indicates an underlying pulmonic or systemic disease; affected patients should be examined for immune deficiency, allergic disorders, environmental disease, upper airway infection with postnasal discharge, cystic fibrosis, immotile cilia syndrome and bronchiectasis. Cough and wheezing are common, often suggesting an allergic basis. Rarely, bronchial irritation may be secondary to the chronic inhalation of dust or noxious fumes (Behrman et al 2007).

Neurological dysafferentation affecting the upper cervical complex, with its suppressive effects on the respiratory centers in the brainstem and susceptibility to chronic recurrence via neural pathways accommodating the viscerosomatic reflex (Gatterman 1995, Homewood 1977, Plaugher 1993) from the sensory-rich bronchial tree, affords a sound reason why chronic bronchitis continues to baffle medical scientists trying to build a paradigm based on a reductionist model.

Pathophysiology

Acute bronchitis is almost always associated with viral airway disease causing inflammation of the bronchial tree (Hueston & Mainous 1998), accumulation of mucus, and bronchial spasm which provokes coughing and may easily be mistaken for asthma (Behrman et al 2007). During the course of acute bronchitis, pneumococci, streptococci, *Haemophilus influenzae* and a variety of hemolytic streptococci may be recovered from the patient's sputum, but this does not imply a bacterial etiology and antibiotic therapy does not alter the course of the disease. Only rarely is acute bronchitis the result of bacterial disease.

Natural history

In the vast majority of children with acute bronchitis, resolution occurs uneventfully 5–10 days after the onset of respiratory symptoms. The natural history remains unaffected by antibiotic therapy (Behrman et al 2007; Hueston 1991, 1997; King et al 1996), antihistamines or expectorants (Behrman et al 2007).

The natural history of chronic bronchitis has not been adequately defined, although Mellis (1984) suggests that recurrent acute viral bronchitis shows progressive improvement throughout childhood.

Clinical evaluation of the child with bronchitis

Acute bronchitis is usually preceded by evidence of upper respiratory tract infection that is typically mild. These symptoms are followed by the development of a frequent, dry, unproductive, hacking cough of gradual onset beginning some 3–4 days after the initial appearance of rhinitis (Behrman et al 2007). A burning quality substernal pain usually accompanies the coughing. Patients often describe whistling sounds as they breathe which are almost certainly rhonchi, soreness in the chest, presumably muscle pain from exertion during coughing, and shortness of breath. The cough becomes productive after several days with purulent sputum being expelled from the bronchial tree. The child with acute bronchitis generally demonstrates considerable malaise that may persist for several days to a week after the disappearance of overt symptoms (Behrman et al 2007).

On physical examination, there will usually be signs of nasopharyngitis, rhinitis and conjunctivitis. Breath sounds will be harsh throughout both inspiration and expiration with the respiratory rate within normal limits. Both coarse and fine moist-sounding crackles can be heard, usually during late inspiration and early expiration, and high-pitched rhonchi which can easily be mistaken for the wheeze associated with asthma. The moist sounds can be cleared with a bout of coughing, after which breath sounds become normal again for a short period of time. Fever is variable and usually low grade when it is a feature of the disease.

Dehydration from insensible fluid loss over several days is always a consideration. Acute body weight loss should be determined where possible and the clinical signs of dehydration evaluated regularly throughout the duration of the acute symptoms.

Chiropractic management of children with acute bronchitis

Acute bronchitis is a common childhood infection that produces distressing symptoms but seldom has complications. Antibiotics are completely inappropriate in the first instance and should be advised against in favor of chiropractic and supportive care at home. The keystone of the chiropractic management plan rests on the ability of the chiropractor to identify the clinical indicators for hospital referral that may develop days after symptomatic onset. In the first instance, the following strategies should be considered:

- Begin chiropractic care as soon as possible. This will often involve adjusting of the upper cervical complex, sacrum and the craniosacral respiratory mechanism, although frequent coughing makes it essential to assess the ribs, thoracic levels and lumbosacral area.
- Maintain fluid level according to the formula set out in Chapter 4 to guard against dehydration. If the child demonstrates an acute body weight loss exceeding 5% or clinical signs of dehydration appear, the child should be referred for hospital admission so fluid therapy can be started.

- Ask the parents or caregiver to take and record the infant's temperature at 2-hourly intervals and to report any sudden upward change immediately.
- Until the symptoms begin to subside, examine the child's vital signs, lungs and upper respiratory system, including the ears, each morning and evening to check for signs of disease progression. Adjust the child as required on these visits.
- The use of *Echinacea purpurea* extract for mothers who are breastfeeding may confer some benefit to the child.

Although complications from acute bronchitis are rare in otherwise healthy children, in undernourished children and those with a history of poor health, progression to conditions such as otitis media, sinusitis and pneumonia are more frequently encountered. Such 'at-risk' children need very careful monitoring throughout the course of the disease. Children who present with recurrent bouts of bronchitis with concomitant sinusitis and otitis media in whom there is a positive family history of bronchiectasis and/or male infertility should be referred to a pediatrician for evaluation for immotile cilia syndrome (Behrman et al 2007).

The management of chronic bronchitis revolves around efforts to establish the definite absence of primary airway disease. Chiropractic management will then be governed by the diagnosis. For example, in the likely event that the condition is liked to an allergic response, chiropractic management will be directed at control of the allergic condition (see Chapter 18).

The child with chronic bronchitis and cough

Although adult chronic bronchitis is defined as 3 or more months of productive cough each year for 2 or more consecutive years, such is not the case for children. In fact, there is considerable doubt that chronic bronchitis is a valid diagnosis in the pediatric age group.

A child with a chronic or recurrent productive cough usually has underlying pulmonary or systemic disease. Affected patients should be investigated for immune deficiency, anatomical abnormalities, allergic disorders, environmental disease, upper airway infection with postnasal discharge, cystic fibrosis, immotile cilia syndrome and bronchiectasis. Cough and wheezing are common symptoms in children, often resulting from allergic disease. Rarely, bronchial irritation may result from chronic inhalation of noxious fumes, dust, tobacco, marijuana smoke, industrial fumes or vehicle exhaust fumes (Behrman et al 2007).

After history-taking and examination, such patients should be appropriately investigated and a management plan implemented by the diagnosis.

Pneumonia

Definition

Pneumonia is an acute pulmonary infection of either viral or bacterial etiology. It is usually a result of aspiration into the lungs of secretions from the oropharynx and nasopharynx that contain bacteria (Moore 1992). The bacteria in turn cause areas of lung to become inflamed, followed by collapse and consolidation. Pneumonia is usually classified by the anatomical region of the lung affected (e.g. bronchopneumonia, lobar pneumonia, etc.) or the etiological agent (e.g. viral pneumonia, pneumococcal pneumonia, etc.). In childhood, the peak incidence occurs in the first 4 years of life and is seasonally oriented toward winter and early spring (Behrman et al 2007).

Pathophysiology

Pneumonia in childhood is primarily a phenomenon related to secondary bacterial infection. Aside from children with impaired immune function or cystic fibrosis, primary infection of lung parenchyma is rare (Behrman et al 2007, Hull & Johnston 1999). Pneumonia generally results from a non-specific viral infection of the upper respiratory tract or acute viral bronchitis which has caused altered immune conditions in the lung including inhibition of phagocytosis, modification of the normal bacterial flora, and temporary disruption of the normal epithelial layer of the respiratory tree (Behrman et al 2007). Aspiration of secretions containing bacteria (Moore 1992) is the usual route of microbial entry to the immune-compromised lung tissue.

Natural history

The natural history of pneumonia depends to a large extent on the infecting organism, host susceptibility and the patient's age. In the pre-antibiotic era, pneumonia progressed to death in up to 50% of all cases. Today, complete resolution can be expected provided adequate antimicrobial therapy with penicillin is implemented early in the disease process and adequate nursing and hygienic care is provided. Mortality from pneumonia is now approximately 1% (Behrman et al 2007).

While viral pneumonia has historically been, and remains, less dangerous than bacterial pneumonia, immune-compromised children, especially infants, can rapidly develop complications that can only be adequately managed in the hospital environment. Among those complications are bronchiolitis obliterans, unilateral hyperlucent lung and fatal acute fulminant pneumonia (Behrman et al 2007).

Evaluation of the patient with pneumonia

Chiropractic has no role to play in the management of children with either viral or bacterial pneumonia while it is in its acute phase. Therefore the evaluation of children with pneumonia revolves around recognition of the disease process in order to identify the need to effect an appropriate referral. For the chiropractic clinician, pneumonia is a dreaded complication of viral respiratory tract infection such as croup, the common cold, bronchitis or bronchiolitis for which chiropractic care may have initially been the clinical management of choice.

The key diagnostic features of pneumonia developing in an infant or toddler are shown in Box 10.3.

Box 10.3

Key diagnostic signs of developing pneumonia in an infant or toddler

- History of respiratory tract infection for a few days preceding sudden onset of fever
- Restlessness and apprehension
- Occasionally central cyanosis
- Respiratory distress with flared nostrils, suprasternal and intercostal retractions
- Tachypnea
- A dull percussive note, particularly over the middle lobe or bases of the lower lobes
- Fine crackles heard on auscultation of the affected lobe
- Tachycardia is sometimes associated with pneumonia
- Chills, cough and fever are usually only seen in older children and adolescents

If, in the course of rendering chiropractic care to a child with viral respiratory disease, symptoms and signs begin to appear which suggest the development of pneumonia, a hospital or pediatric specialist referral should be made without delay. Once the acute stage of the infection is controlled, the child should be returned to chiropractic care in order to optimize immune function and afford the highest possible level of protection against recurrence or the development of postinfective sequelae.

Croup

Definition

Viral croup is the most common form of airway obstruction in children between 6 months and 6 years of age. It typically presents in the late autumn and winter, is often preceded by an upper respiratory infection, and is characterized by a low-grade fever, barking cough and inspiratory stridor (Sholnik 1993).

Pathophysiology

Croup is an upper airway infection that may cause varying degrees of obstruction due to inflammation. The principal microbial organisms responsible for croup at all ages are the parainfluenza viruses. Respiratory syncytial virus is seen in children <5 years of age, while *Mycoplasma pneumoniae* is a significant cause of croup only in children >5 years of age (Denny et al 1983).

As the airway becomes compromised by inflammation, air hunger and restlessness occur briefly followed by severe hypoxemia and weakness, accompanied by decreased air exchange and stridor, increasing pulse, and eventual death from hypoventilation (Behrman et al 2007).

The incidence of croup is related to allergic disease (Laufer 1986, Nafstad et al 2005, Pearlman 1989) and environmental stresses, particularly low temperatures (Cohen & Hunt 1988). Some children with croup also show an increased

non-specific bronchial hyperresponsiveness and tend to produce a higher level of IgE than children without croup, suggesting a relationship between the incidence of asthma and croup (Konig 1978, Nafstad et al 2005, Pearlman 1989). This fact needs to be carefully accommodated when constructing a chiropractic management plan for children who have had more than one episode of croup.

Clinical evaluation of a child with croup

At history, the typical picture is the onset of fever, a brassy cough, and intermittent stridor following an upper respiratory tract infection. As the airway obstruction becomes more severe, the stridor becomes constant and associated with signs of dyspnea such as nasal flaring and retractions of the suprasternal, infrasternal and intercostal areas. Agitation and crying greatly exacerbate the symptoms and the child shows a preference for the sitting position (Behrman et al 2007). As the airway compromise becomes more severe, the stridor actually becomes quieter, with dyspnea at rest the dominant symptom, a critical clinical point to appreciate when managing a child who has been sick for some time.

For the chiropractor, the physical examination is driven by the need to identify the degree of airway obstruction in order to determine if immediate hospitalization is necessary. Objective evaluation is sometimes difficult and arterial blood gas determinations are often relied upon when making clinical decisions. The use of a clinical croup scoring system (Table 10.2) which has been proposed by Downes & Raphaely (1975) will permit the chiropractor to make a determination of the severity of the respiratory distress without the need for an arterial blood gas determination.

A score of 4 or more indicates moderate airway obstruction and demands a specialist pediatric referral. A score of 7 indicates impending respiratory failure and represents an extreme emergency for which immediate hospital referral is essential. These children will most likely require an artificial

Table 10.2 Clinical croup scoring system for determining the severity of respiratory distress without employing arterial blood gas determinations (Reproduced with kind permission from McMillan et al 1982)

	0	1	2
Inspiratory breath sounds	Normal	Harsh with rhonchi	Delayed
Stridor	None	Inspiratory	Inspiratory and expiratory
Cough	None	Hoarse cry	Bark
Retractions and flaring	None	Flaring and suprasternal retractions	As under 1, plus subcostal/intercostal retractions
Cyanosis	None	In air	In 40% oxygen

tracheal airway (Downes & Raphaely 1975). In children who have a score of less than 4, conservative chiropractic management is appropriate. Clinical experience with such children suggests that the natural history can be significantly shortened.

Chiropractic management of children with viral croup

The keystone of the chiropractic management plan rests on the ability of the chiropractor to identify the clinical indicators for hospital referral based on the clinical croup score. In children whose score is greater than 4, the following strategies should be considered:

- Begin chiropractic care as soon as possible. This will often involve adjusting of the upper cervical complex, the sacrum and the craniosacral respiratory mechanism, although frequent coughing makes it essential to assess the ribs, thoracic levels and lumbosacral area.
- Maintain fluid level according to the formula set out in Chapter 4 to guard against dehydration. If the child demonstrates an acute body weight loss exceeding 5% or clinical signs of dehydration appear, the child should be referred for hospital admission so fluid therapy can be started.
- Ask the parents or caregiver to take and record the infant's temperature at 2-hourly intervals and to note any excessive drooling or pooling of the saliva with apparent swallowing difficulty. A sudden increase in temperature or the development of drooling and pooling with swallowing difficulty may indicate acute epiglottitis.
- Until the symptoms begin to subside, re-evaluate the clinical croup score three times per day in order to identify disease progression. If the score exceeds 4 at any time, make a specialist pediatric referral immediately.

- The use of *Echinacea purpurea* extract for mothers who are breastfeeding may confer some benefit to the child.

Acute epiglottitis

This is a dramatic, potentially fatal condition in which viral infection causes inflammation and edema of the epiglottis, primarily in children 2–7 years of age. It is characterized by a fulminating course of fever, sore throat, dyspnea, and rapidly progressive respiratory obstruction. It is common for the child to be completely well at bedtime, only to awaken later in the evening with a high fever, aphonia, drooling, and moderate to severe respiratory distress with stridor (Behrman et al 2007).

Confronted with such a presentation, the chiropractor must not attempt any examination, but refer for immediate hospital admission.

Conclusion

Chiropractic has a key role to play in the management of children with airway disease. The appropriateness of chiropractic care will always depend upon accurate diagnosis and a keen understanding of both complicating factors and the natural history of the particular condition encountered. While referral is always an option for the chiropractor confronted by a child with airway disease, it remains that in about 80% of such cases an accurate diagnosis can be arrived at by the use of a pertinent clinical history, careful observation of the child, and a thorough physical examination without recourse to laboratory or radiological investigation (McMillan et al 1982). Table 10.3 may prove helpful in concluding a diagnosis in respiratory tract disease from history, observation and examination.

Table 10.3 Differentiation of respiratory disease on the basis of history, observation and physical examination (reproduced with kind permission from McMillan et al 1982)

Ages	Croup 3 months–3 years	Epiglottitis 3–6 years	Bronchitis 3 years and older	Bronchiolitis 1 month–2 years	Pneumonia All ages	Asthma 3 years and older
Etiology	Parainfluenza 1,2,3* Influenza A Adenovirus Rhinovirus Respiratory syncytial virus	H. influenzae, type B* Occasionally diphtheria	Viruses* Myxovirus Respiratory syncytial Adenovirus Bacteria	Respiratory syncytial virus*	Viruses* S. pneumoniae Mycoplasma	Respiratory tract
Pathogenesis	Subglottic	Supraglottic	Major bronchi	Bronchioles	Alveoli	Respiratory tract
Rapid onset	No (0), except spasmodic	Yes (+)	No (0)	No (0)	No (0)	Yes–No
Stridor	++	+++	0	+	0	(+ – ++)
Dysphonia	+++	+++	0	0	0	0
Fever	0 – +	+++	0 – +	+ – 0	+ – +++	0
Prostration	0 – +++	0	0 – +++	0	0	0 – +
Family history	0	0	0	0	0	+++
Response to epinephrine (adrenaline)	0	0	0	0	0	+++
Wheezing	0	0	0	+++	0	+++
Rhonchi	0	0	++	+	++	++
Influenced by weather	++(?)	0	0	0	0	0 – ++
Stridor	+ – +++	+++	0	0	0	0
Expiratory effort	0	0	0	+ – +++	0	+ – +++
Productive cough	0	0	0 – ++	0	+ – +++	0
Cyanosis	0	0	0	0 – +++	0 – +++	0 – ++
Retractions	+ – +++	+++	0	+ – +++	0 – ++	0 – +++
Rales	0	0	0	+++ (I & E)	+++ (I)	0
Hyperinflated lungs	0	0	0	+++	0	+++
Elevated WBC	0	++	0	0	0 – +++	0 – +
Complications	Pneumothorax Mediastinal emphysema	Pneumothorax Mediastinal emphysema Pyarthrosis Meningitis	Pneumonia	Bacterial infection Pneumothorax Mediastinal atelectasis	Otitis media Sinusitis Empyema Atelectasis	Atelectasis Pneumothorax Pneumomediastinum Pneumonia

Key: 0 = absent; + = slightly present; ++ = moderately present; +++ = always present, marked.
*Organism most commonly found.

References

American Academy of Pediatrics Subcommittee on Diagnosis and Management of Bronchiolitis, 2006. Diagnosis and management of bronchiolitis. Pediatrics 118 (4), 1774–1793.

Anrig, C.A, Plaugher, G. (Eds), 1998. Pediatric Chiropractic. Williams & Wilkins, Baltimore.

Balon, J.W., Mior, S.A., 2004. Chiropractic care in asthma and allergy. Ann. Allergy Asthma Immunol. 93 (2 Suppl. 1), S55–S60.

Behrman, R.E., Jenson, H.B., Nelson, W.E., et al., 2007. Nelson Textbook of Pediatrics, eighteenth ed. WB Saunders, Philadelphia.

Beyeler, W., 1965. Experiences in the management of asthma. Ann. Swiss Chiropr. Assoc. 3, 111–117.

Boeck, K.D., 1996. Respiratory syncytial virus bronchiolitis: clinical aspects and epidemiology. Monaldi Arch. Chest Dis. 51 (3), 210–213.

Braman, S.S., 2006. Chronic cough due to acute bronchitis: ACCP evidence-based clinical practice guidelines. Chest 129 (Suppl), S95–S103.

Bukovsky, M., Kostalova, D., Magnusova, R., et al., 1993. Testing for immunomodulating effects of ethanol-water extracts of the above ground parts of the plants *Echinacea* (Moench) and *Rudbeckia* L. Cesk. Farm. 42 (5), 228–231.

Bukovsky, M., Vaverkova, S., Kostalova, D., 1995. Immunomodulating activity of *Echinacea gloriosa, Echinacea angustifolia* DC and *Rubeckia speciosa* Wenderoth ethanol-water extracts. Pol. J. Pharmacol. 47 (2), 175–177.

Carvalho, W.B., Johnston, C., Fonseca, M.C., 2007. Acute bronchitis, an updated review. Rev. Assoc. Med. Bras. 53 (2), 182–188.

Chugh, I.M., Khanna, P., Shah, A., 2006. Nocturnal symptoms and sleep disturbances in clinically stable asthmatic children. Asian Pac. J. Allergy Immunol. 24 (2–3), 135–142.

Cohen, B., Hunt, D., 1988. Recurrent and non-recurrent croup: an epidemiological study. Aust. Pediatr. J. 24 (6), 339–342.

Dawson, K., Kennedy, D., Asher, I., et al., 1993. The management of acute bronchiolitis. Thoracic Society of Australia and New Zealand. J. Paediatr. Child Health 29 (5), 335–337.

Denny, F.W., Murphy, T.F., Clyde Jr., W.A., et al., 1983. Croup: an 11-year study in pediatric practice. Pediatrics 71 (6), 871–876.

Downes, J.J., Raphaely, R.C., 1975. Clinical croup score. Anesthesiology 43, 238–250.

Dunlay, J., Reinhardt, R., 1984. Clinical features and treatment of acute bronchitis. J. Fam. Pract. 18 (5), 719–722.

Everard, M.L., 1995. Bronchiolitis: origins and optimal management. Drugs 49 (6), 885–896.

Frischer, T., Meinert, R., Urbanek, R., et al., 1995. Variability of peak expiratory flow rate in children: short and long term reproducibility. Thorax 50 (1), 35–39.

Gatterman, M.I., 1990. Chiropractic Management of Spine Related Disorders. Williams & Wilkins, Baltimore.

Gatterman, M., 1995. Foundations of Chiropractic: Subluxation. Mosby, St Louis.

Gavin, R., Anderson, B., Percival, T., 1996. Management of severe bronchiolitis: indications for ventilator support. N. Z. Med. J. 109 (1020), 137–139.

Graham, R.L., Pistolese, R.A., 1997. An impairment rating analysis of asthmatic children under chiropractic care. J. Vertebral Subluxation Res. 1 (4), 41–48.

Greenough, A., Everett, L., Pool, J., et al., 1991. Relation between nocturnal symptoms and changes in lung function on lying down in asthmatic children. Thorax 46 (3), 193–196.

Harris, W., Choong, R., Timms, B., 2002. Examination Paediatrics, second ed. MacLennan & Petty, Sydney.

Homewood, A.E., 1977. The Neurodynamics of the Vertebral Subluxation. Valkyrie Press, St Petersburg, Florida.

Horst, P.S., 1994. Bronchiolitis. Am. Fam. Physician 49 (6), 1449–1453.

Hueston, W.J., 1991. A comparison of albuterol and erythromycin for the treatment of acute bronchitis. J. Fam. Pract. 33 (5), 476–480.

Hueston, W.J., 1997. Antibiotics: neither cost effective nor 'cough' effective. J. Fam. Pract. 44 (3), 261–265.

Hueston, W.J., Mainous III., A.G., 1998. Acute bronchitis. Am. Fam. Physician 57 (6), 1270–1276.

Hull, D., Johnston, D., 1999. Essential Paediatrics, fourth ed. Churchill Livingstone, Edinburgh.

King, D.E., Williams, W.C., Bishop, L., et al., 1996. Effectiveness of erythromycin in the treatment of acute bronchitis. J. Fam. Pract. 42 (6), 601–605.

Konig, P., 1978. The relationship between croup and asthma. Ann. Allergy 41 (4), 227–231.

Laufer, P., 1986. The relationship of respiratory allergies to croup. J. Asthma 23 (1), 9–10.

Leung, A.K., Kellner, J.D., Davies, H.D., 2005. Respiratory syncytial virus bronchiolitis. J. Natl. Med. Assoc. 97 (12), 1708–1713.

Lugo, R.A., Nahata, M.C., 1993. Pathogenesis and treatment of bronchiolitis. Clin. Pharmacol. 12 (2), 95–116.

McMillan, J.A., Neiberg, P.I., Oski, F.A., 1977. The Whole Pediatrician Catalogue: A Compendium of Clues to Diagnosis and Management. WB Saunders, Philadelphia.

McMillan, J.A., Stockman, J.A., Oski, F.A., 1982. The Whole Pediatrician Catalogue, vol. 3. WB Saunders, Philadelphia.

Mcnicol, K.N., Macnicol, K.N., Williams, H.B., 1973. Spectrum of asthma in children. I. Clinical and physiological components. Br. Med. J. 6 (4), 7–11.

Mai, T.V., Selby, A.M., Simpson, J.M., et al., 1995. Use of simple clinical parameters to assess severity of bronchiolitis. J. Pediatr. Child Health 31 (5), 465–468.

Marieb, E., 2009. Essentials of Human Anatomy and Physiology, nineth ed. Pearson/Benjamin Cummings, San Francisco.

Melchart, D., Linde, K., Worku, R., et al., 1995. Results of five randomized studies on the immunomodulatory activity of preparations of *Echinacea*. J. Altern. Complement. Med. 1 (2), 145–160.

Mellis, C., 1984. Children with cough. Aust. Fam. Physician 13 (2), 122–123.

Mengs, U., Clare, C., Poiley, J., 1991. Toxicity of *Echinacea purpurea*: acute, subacute and genotoxicity studies. Arzneimittelforschung 41 (10), 1076–1081.

Moore, K.L., 1992. Clinically Oriented Anatomy, third ed. Williams & Wilkins, Baltimore.

Morgan, W.J., Taussig, L.M., 1984. The chronic bronchitis complex in children. Pediatr. Clin. North Am. 31 (4), 851–864.

Nafstad, P., Brunekreef, B., Skrondal, A., et al., 2005. Early respiratory infections, asthma, and allergy: 10-year follow-up of the Oslo Birth Cohort. Pediatrics 116 (2), e255–e262.

Nahata, M.C., Johnson, J.A., Powell, D.A., 1985. Management of bronchiolitis. Clin. Pharmacol. 4 (3), 297–303.

Nielsen, N., Bronfort, G., Bendix, T., et al., 1995. Chronic asthma and chiropractic spinal manipulation: a randomized clinical trial. J. Clin. Exp. Allergy 25 (1), 80–88.

Pearlman, D.S., 1989. The relationship between allergy and croup. Allergy Proc. 10 (3), 227–231.

Plaugher, G., 1993. Textbook of Clinical Chiropractic: Biomechanical Approach. Williams & Wilkins, Baltimore.

Sholnik, N., 1993. Croup. J. Fam. Pract. 37 (2), 165–170.

Sly, P.D., 1993. Peak flow monitoring in children. Monaldi Arch. Chest Dis. 48 (6), 662–667.

Uwyyed, K., Springer, C., Avital, A., et al., 1996. Home recording of PEF in young asthmatics: does it contribute to management? Eur. Respir. J. 9 (5), 872–879.

Vinson, D.C., 1991. Acute bronchitis in children: building a clinical definition. Fam. Pract. Respir. J. 11 (1), 75–81.

Attention-deficit/hyperactivity disorder

Thelma Buchanan   Neil J. Davies

Attention-deficit/hyperactivity disorder (AD/HD) is the current name given to a common but complex biological disorder characterized by excessive inattentiveness, impulsiveness or hyperactivity that significantly impairs a child's functioning in a number of environments, including home and school (in the classroom, in the playground and sports field).

The disorder changed names a number of times during the 20th century as research has refined the criteria for diagnosing the condition and attempted to determine the possible causes of the disorder.

Attention-deficit/hyperactivity disorder is characterized by the behavioral sets and subsets described in the fourth edition of the *Diagnostic and Statistical Manual of Mental Disorder* (DSM-IV), a publication of the American Psychiatric Association (1994). The disorder is classified as having three possible types:

- attention-deficit/hyperactivity disorder, predominantly hyperactive–impulsive type
- attention-deficit/hyperactivity disorder, predominantly inattentive type
- attention-deficit/hyperactivity disorder, combined type.

Assessment and diagnosis are best conducted in a multi-method mode by relevant practitioners, who, following best practice, will involve the various people with whom the child has contact such as the child's parents, teachers and carers. The mainstay of treatment among the medical community for children with AD/HD has been stimulant medication. A cooperative team approach to treatment, however, is believed to yield a more effective long-term management of the disorder. Contrary to former theories of the disorder, adolescents do continue with many of the symptoms of AD/HD into adulthood.

Definition

As research has refined an understanding of neurological disorders, the definition of AD/HD has undergone subtle changes (Table 11.1). One cannot assume that the final definition has been achieved even now, as research into this disorder continues. The criteria for attention-deficit/hyperactivity disorder are listed in the widely available DSM-IV (APA 1994). In the UK, diagnosis is generally done on the basis of the International Classification of Diseases, or ICD-10 (WHO 1992), which includes hyperactivity as a key criterion. Kewley (1998) and Cosgrove (1997) believe, therefore, that AD/HD is underdiagnosed in the UK.

Children with AD/HD display behaviors which may be seen in other children. However, children with AD/HD display inattentive, impulsive or hyperactive behaviors more frequently and to a more severe degree than is typically observed in children at a comparable age level. These behaviors, shown in Box 11.1, are described as the core behaviors of AD/HD by Green & Chee (1994). The fundamental criteria for a child to be diagnosed as having AD/HD are that these behaviors must have been present before the child reached the age of 7 years, persisted for at least 6 months, and be exhibited in a variety of settings.

Gordon (1994) includes variability of performance as a feature of the behaviors exhibited by children with AD/HD, predominantly combined type. Teachers often report that one day a child can perform a task that he or she was unable to even attempt the day before or the following day. While this variability of performance is certainly a feature of the learning style of children with AD/HD, it is not considered a diagnostic criterion.

Prevalence

While it is estimated that 3–5% of the childhood population has been diagnosed with AD/HD, many more boys than girls are affected, particularly when the figures are taken from clinic-based samples. Boys are generally referred to clinics for the secondary characteristics of AD/HD such as aggression, oppositional defiance disorder and conduct disorder.

Children who are predominantly inattentive will usually present as restless, lethargic and dreamy. They will be referred for help with their poor academic achievement rather than

© 2010, Elsevier Ltd, Inc, BV
DOI: 10.1016/B978-0-7020-3129-8.00011-6

Table 11.1 An historical overview of attention-deficit/hyperactivity disorder (adapted from Lerner & Lerner 1991 with permission)

Date	Diagnostic terminology	Source	Characteristic
1902	Defects in moral control	Still	
1941	Brain damage syndrome	Strauss & Werner	Hyperactivity, distractibility, impulsivity, emotionally unstable presentation V
1947			
1962	Minimal brain dysfunction (MBD)	Clements & Peters	Soft neurological indicators, specific learning deficits, hyperkinesis, impulsivity, short attention span
1968	Hyperkinetic reaction of childhood	DSM-II	Hyperactivity
1980	Attention deficit disorder with hyperactivity (ADDH)	DSM-III	Onset before age 7, duration of at least 6 months, inattention, impulsivity, motor hyperactivity
	Attention deficit disorder (ADD)		Inattention, impulsivity, disorganization, difficulty completing tasks
1987	Attention-deficit hyperactivity disorder (ADHD)	DSM-III-R	Any 8 of a set of 14 symptoms, onset before age 7, duration of at least 6 months
	Undifferentiated attention deficit disorder (U-ADD)		Developmentally inappropriate and marked inattention
1994	Attention deficit/hyperactivity disorder (AD/HD) DSM-IV	DSM-IV	Onset before age 7, present in two or more locations (e.g. at school and at home), duration of at least 6 months
	Three types:		
	Predominantly inattentive type		6 or more of 9 listed symptoms of inattention
	Predominantly hyperactive–impulsive type		6 or more of 9 listed symptoms of hyperactivity and impulsivity
	Combined type		Criteria for both types met
	Possible change:		
	Attention deficit disorder		6 or more of 9 listed symptoms of inattention from DSM-IV
	Behavior inhibition disorder	Barkley 1997a	Problems with self-control and executive function, poor perception of time

---

Box 11.1

Behaviors associated with AD/HD (adapted from Green & Chee 1994 with permission)

Core behaviors

- Inattention: the child is easily distracted, forgets instructions, flits from task to task, and is best with one-to-one supervision
- Impulsiveness: the child speaks and acts without thinking, and has a short fuse
- Overactivity: the child is restless, fidgety and has 'rump hyperactivity'

Additional behaviors

- Insatiability: the child is never satisfied, nags, never lets a matter drop
- Social clumsiness: the child is 'out of tune' socially, acts silly in a crowd, misreads social cues
- Poor coordination: the child is clumsy, has poor flow of movement, has difficulty doing two actions at the one time
- Disorganization: the child is blind to mess, is compelled to touch everything, has problems structuring work
- Variability: the child suffers from mood swings, and has good and bad days to the extreme
- Specific learning disabilities – examples are: dyslexia, language problems, difficulties with handwriting and mathematics

difficult behaviors. Those with the predominantly inattentive type AD/HD tend most often to be girls and are more frequently underdiagnosed and therefore undertreated (Aust 1994; Barkley 1992, 1998; Reif 1993). Barkley (1992) suggests that AD/HD occurs in a ratio of 1 girl for every 3 boys. Gordon (1994) suggests that 60–90% of children classified as AD/HD are boys.

Diagnosis

Diagnosis of AD/HD, based on the DSM-IV or ICD-10 criteria, is generally achieved through a collaborative approach as described by Burnley (1993) and recommended in the Position Paper of the Australian Psychological Society (1997) as well as the clinical guidelines published by National Institute for Health and Clinical Excellence (NICE) in the United Kingdom (2008) and the American Academy of Pediatrics (2000, 2001). While restless, hyperactive behavior is often evident by the age of 3 or 4 years, inattention is often not raised as an issue until the child's first years at school.

The pediatrician, to whom the child has been referred by the general practitioner, will then conduct interviews with the child and the parents to determine the health status of the child and to explore any other possible explanations for the child's behavior, such as a physical, emotional or mood problem.

The pediatrician may ask the school counselor or a child psychologist for an opinion of the child's behavior and level of intellectual ability. The role of the psychologist is to assess the child's intellectual ability using one of the standardized instruments such as the Wechsler Preschool and Primary Scale of Intelligence – Third Edition (WPPSI-III) (for children aged 4–7 years), the Wechsler Intelligence Scale for Children – Fourth Edition (WISC-IV) (for children aged 6–16 years) or the Stanford–Binet – Fifth Edition (SB-V) (for all ages from 2 to older adult).

Parents and the teachers may then be requested to complete some rating scales which obtain data from parents/carers and teachers in a standardized format that facilitates comparison with other children (Achenbach 1987). Among such rating scales are the Strengths and Difficulties Questionnaire (Goodman 1997), Conners Teacher and Parent Rating Scales – Third Edition (Conners 3) (2008), AD/HD Rating Scale (DuPaul 1991, DuPaul et al 2008), the SWAN Rating Scale (Swanson et al 1983, 1992) and the Home and School Questionnaires (Barkley 1997a). The Achenbach Child Behaviour Checklist (Achenbach & Edelbrock 1983) can be electronically scored and profiled to reveal whether the child is presenting behaviors that are of clinical significance in relation to other disorders as well as AD/HD.

For the chiropractor faced with a child who is suspected or reported to be hyperactive, there are several 'user-friendly' questionnaires which may be employed to determine if a child should be referred to a pediatric specialist and psychologist for evaluation. These questionnaires are gender specific and have standardized age-related norms. These scales enable the practitioner to determine whether the number of behaviors recorded for each of the symptoms of inattention, hyperactivity, impulsivity, and disorders in peer relationships are developmentally appropriate for the child or in the excessive range. These questionnaires are known as the SWAN Rating Scale (Swanson et al 1983, 1992) (Fig. 11.1), the Home Situations Questionnaire (Fig. 11.2 and Table 11.2) and the School Situations Questionnaire (Fig. 11.3 and Table 11.3) (Barkley 1997a).

Generally, the definitive diagnosis of AD/HD is made by the pediatric specialist based on the information gathered from interviews with the child and the parents/carers as well as information gained from the psychological assessment and rating scales completed by the parents/carers and teachers. An interesting study by Landau et al (1991) found that children with AD/HD did not admit to as many of the symptoms of the disorder as their mothers had attributed to them. This unawareness or denial of symptoms by the children with AD/HD has implications for both diagnosis and treatment of the condition.

Etiology

No single cause for AD/HD has been discovered although many have been suggested. Initially it was believed that children with AD/HD actually had a brain trauma of some description. While some children do develop inattentiveness and impulsivity, most children with AD/HD do not have diagnosable injury, hence the evolution of the term 'minimal brain dysfunction'. Sophisticated technologies such as computed tomography (CT) and magnetic resonance imaging (MRI) have not revealed findings consistent with specific structural abnormalities of the brain. Regional blood flow/computed tomography (rCBF/CT) has, however, detected low metabolic activity in the central and frontal regions of the brain (Lou et al 1984). Anderson (1997) states that the positron emission tomography (PET) research by Zametkin et al (1990), which found a significant reduction in glucose metabolism when comparing adults with and without attentional deficits, provides the most compelling evidence that the deficiency of AD/HD children may be at a functional, neurochemical level rather than the result of discrete neuropathology or neurodevelopmental abnormalities.

Neurochemical factors are thought to be involved. There is a lowered effective rate of transmission of signals across the synapse of connecting nerves in the brain, resulting in incomplete or jumbled messages (Serfontein 1990). Part of the justification for this theory is based on the improved neurological functioning of children diagnosed as AD/HD who are taking stimulant medication (Anderson 1997). Animal studies suggest that methylphenidate (MPH; Ritalin) and dexamfetamine act via the monoaminergic system to (1) inhibit uptake, (2) increase release of amines, and (3) inhibit monamine oxidase activity – all actions that serve to increase concentration of catecholamines at the synaptic cleft, thus enhancing efficient transmission of neural impulses.

The most convincing cause of AD/HD is hereditary. There is a strong family history of learning difficulties and AD/HD for children with AD/HD. Parents often recognize their own undiagnosed learning difficulties when they describe their child's learning and behavioral difficulties. No specific chromosomal abnormality has yet been identified to explain the genetic connection.

In the 1970s Feingold (1975) suggested that specific food preservatives and colorings as well as some natural salicylates were related to hyperactivity, claims which have not been substantiated by ongoing clinical research. Goldstein & Goldstein (1998) and Green & Chee (1994) recognize that there are some children who are particularly sensitive to some foods, which may result in some behaviors similar to AD/HD. If eliminating the offending foods controls the behavior, then it is reasonable to conclude that the clinical problem was one of food intolerance and not AD/HD.

Educational factors and associated problems

Some children present with a 'pure' AD/HD whereas others have associated problems such as a learning disability (LD), behavior disorder (BD) oppositional defiance disorder (ODD), conduct disorder (CD), or a combination of all three. Anderson (1997) described the quantification of four subgroups and found that the percentages of each group were 28% for pure AD/HD, 35% for AD/HD + LD, 26% for AD/HD + BD and 13% for AD/HD + BD + LD.

The SWAN Rating Scale for ADHD

Child's name: _____ Gender: M/F _____ d.o.b. _____

Completed by: _____ Parent/Teacher/Professional (circle one)

Date completed: _____

Children differ in their abilities to focus attention, control activity and inhibit impulses. For each item, how does this child compare to other children of the same age? Select the best rating based on your observations over the past 3 months. Compared to other children, how does this child do the following?

	Not at all	Just a little	Pretty much	Very much
1. Give close attention to detail and avoid careless mistakes	___	___	___	___
2. Sustain attention on tasks or play activities	___	___	___	___
3. Listen when spoken to directly	___	___	___	___
4. Follow through on instructions and finish school work and chores	___	___	___	___
5. Organize tasks and activities	___	___	___	___
6. Engage in tasks that require sustained mental effort	___	___	___	___
7. Keep track of things necessary for activities (doesn't lose them)	___	___	___	___
8. Ignore extraneous stimuli	___	___	___	___
9. Remember daily activities	___	___	___	___
10. Sit still (control movement of hands or feet or control squirming)	___	___	___	___
11. Stay seated (when required by class rules or social conventions)	___	___	___	___
12. Modulate motor activity (inhibit inappropriate running or climbing)	___	___	___	___
13. Play quietly (keep noise level reasonable)	___	___	___	___
14. Settle down and rest (control constant activity)	___	___	___	___
15. Modulate verbal activity (control excessive talking)	___	___	___	___
16. Reflect on questions (control blurting out answers)	___	___	___	___
17. Await turn (stand in line and take turns)	___	___	___	___
18. Enter into conversation and games without interrupting or intruding	___	___	___	___

Scoring section: For each question, place a 1 next to the question number if the response is 'not at all' or 'just a little', and a 0 if the response is 'quite a bit' or 'very much'.

1. ___
2. ___
3. ___
4. ___
5. ___
6. ___
7. ___
8. ___
9. ___

10. ___
11. ___
12. ___
13. ___
14. ___
15. ___
16. ___
17. ___
18. ___

1. If the sum of 1–9 is 6 or greater, the child is likely ADHD-inattentive type. Consider referral to pediatrician or mental health worker
2. If the sum of 10–18 is 6 or greater, the child is likely ADHD-hyperactive/impulsive type. Consider referral to pediatrician or mental health worker
3. If both the sums of 1–9 and 10–18 are 6 or greater, the child is likely ADHD-combined type. Consider referral to pediatrician or mental health worker
4. If either sum is 5 or less, the child likely does not have ADHD or symptoms are under control with current treatment.

Sum nos 1–9 ___ nos 10–18 ___

Figure 11.1 • SWAN rating scale.

HOME SITUATIONS QUESTIONNAIRE

Child's Name _____ Date _____

Name of Person Completing This Form _____

Instructions: Does your child present any problems with compliance to instructions, commands, or rules for you in any of these situations? If so, please circle the word Yes and then circle a number beside that situation that describes how severe the problem is for you. If your child is not a problem in a situation, circle No and go to the next situation on the form.

Situations	Yes/No (Circle one)		Mild	If yes, how severe? (Circle one)							Severe
While playing alone	Yes	No	1	2	3	4	5	6	7	8	9
While playing with other children	Yes	No	1	2	3	4	5	6	7	8	9
At mealtimes	Yes	No	1	2	3	4	5	6	7	8	9
Getting dressed	Yes	No	1	2	3	4	5	6	7	8	9
Washing and bathing	Yes	No	1	2	3	4	5	6	7	8	9
While you are on the telephone	Yes	No	1	2	3	4	5	6	7	8	9
While watching television	Yes	No	1	2	3	4	5	6	7	8	9
When visitors are in your home	Yes	No	1	2	3	4	5	6	7	8	9
When you are visiting someone's home	Yes	No	1	2	3	4	5	6	7	8	9
In public places (restaurants, stores, church, etc.)	Yes	No	1	2	3	4	5	6	7	8	9
When father is home	Yes	No	1	2	3	4	5	6	7	8	9
When asked to do chores	Yes	No	1	2	3	4	5	6	7	8	9
When asked to do homework	Yes	No	1	2	3	4	5	6	7	8	9
At bedtime	Yes	No	1	2	3	4	5	6	7	8	9
While in the car	Yes	No	1	2	3	4	5	6	7	8	9
When with a babysitter	Yes	No	1	2	3	4	5	6	7	8	9

For Office Use Only

Total number of problem settings _____ Mean severity score _____

Figure 11.2 ● Home Situations Questionnaire for children with AD/HD (from *Defiant Children: A Clinician's Manual for Assessment and Parent Training*, 2nd edn, by Russell A. Barkley. Copyright 1997 by The Guilford Press).

Table 11.2 Normative data for the Home Situations Questionnaire for children with AD/HD (reproduced with permission from Breen MJ, Altpeter TS 1991 *Factor Structures of the Home Situations Questionnaire (HSQ) and School Situations Questionnaire (SSQ)*. Plenum Press, New York)

Age group (in years)	*N*	Number of problem settings			Mean severity		
		Mean	**SD**	**+1.5 SD**	**Mean**	**SD**	**+1.5 SD**
Boys							
4–5	162	3.1	2.8	7.3	1.7	1.4	3.8
6–8	205	4.1	3.3	9.1	2.0	1.4	4.1
9–11	138	3.6	3.3	8.6	1.9	1.5	4.2
Girls							
4–5	146	2.2	2.6	6.1	1.3	1.4	3.4
6–8	202	3.4	3.5	8.7	1.6	1.5	3.9
9–11	142	2.7	3.2	7.5	1.4	1.4	3.5

Key: *N*, sample size at this age for this gender; SD, standard deviation; +1.5 SD, score at the threshold of standard deviations above the mean (approximately the 93rd percentile).

SCHOOL SITUATIONS QUESTIONNAIRE

Child's Name _____ Date _____

Name of Person Completing This Form _____

Instructions: Does this child present any problems with compliance to instructions, commands, or rules for you in any of these situations? If so, please circle the word Yes and then circle a number beside that situation that describes how severe the problem is for you. If this child is not a problem in a situation, circle No and go to the next situation on the form.

Situations	Yes/No (Circle one)		Mild	If yes, how severe? (Circle one)							Severe
While arriving at school	Yes	No	1	2	3	4	5	6	7	8	9
During individual deskwork	Yes	No	1	2	3	4	5	6	7	8	9
During small-group activities	Yes	No	1	2	3	4	5	6	7	8	9
During free playtime in class	Yes	No	1	2	3	4	5	6	7	8	9
During lectures to the class	Yes	No	1	2	3	4	5	6	7	8	9
At recess	Yes	No	1	2	3	4	5	6	7	8	9
At lunch	Yes	No	1	2	3	4	5	6	7	8	9
In the hallways	Yes	No	1	2	3	4	5	6	7	8	9
In the toilets	Yes	No	1	2	3	4	5	6	7	8	9
On field trips	Yes	No	1	2	3	4	5	6	7	8	9
During special assemblies	Yes	No	1	2	3	4	5	6	7	8	9
On the bus	Yes	No	1	2	3	4	5	6	7	8	9

For Office Use Only

Total number of problem settings _____ Mean severity score _____

Figure 11.3 ● School Situations Questionnaire for children with AD/HD (from *Defiant Children: A Clinician's Manual for Assessment and Parent Training*, 2nd edn, by Russell A. Barkley. Copyright 1997 by The Guilford Press).

Table 11.3 Normative data for the School Situations Questionnaire for children with AD/HD (reproduced with permission from Breen MJ, Altpeter TS 1991 *Factor Structures of the Home Situations Questionnaire (HSQ) and School Situations Questionnaire (SSQ)*. Plenum Press, New York)

Age group (in years)	N	Number of problem settings			Mean severity		
		Mean	SD	+1.5 SD	Mean	SD	+1.5 SD
Boys							
6–8	170	2.4	3.3	7.4	1.5	2.0	4.5
9–11	123	2.8	3.2	7.6	1.9	2.1	5.1
Girls							
6–8	180	1.0	2.0	4.0	0.8	1.5	3.1
9–11	126	1.3	2.1	4.5	0.8	1.2	2.6

Key: *N*, sample size at this age for this gender; SD, standard deviation; +1.5 SD, score at the threshold of standard deviations above the mean (approximately the 93rd percentile).

Many children with AD/HD have associated learning difficulties. Hutchins (1990) states that learning and attention problems usually coexist. Their variability of performance results in children who can do what is required of them one day but not the next. Their restless behavior, impulsivity and inattention create problems within the classroom for both their own and other children's learning. However, not all children with learning difficulties have AD/HD. Neuromaturational delay, for example, is a very common cause of learning difficulty and may lead to behavioral dysfunction which is completely unrelated to AD/HD. This subject has been explored in detail in Chapter 8.

The New South Wales Department of Education in Australia has recognized that in order for the child with AD/HD to learn efficiently in the classroom, the teacher and parents need to work together with the help of educational and behavioral professionals in order to provide a structure for the child to operate within. The Department has published a workbook entitled *Talk Time Teamwork* (1995) detailing strategies for teachers and parents to use in order to assist the child with AD/HD in the school.

In an epidemiological study of 100 children with AD/HD attending a specialist clinic in the UK, comorbidity of AD/HD with dyslexia, dyspraxia, attention-deficit disorder, attention-deficit/hyperactivity disorder, obsessive-compulsive disorder and Tourette syndrome was found to be at a prevalence of 95% (Pauc 2005). The astute diagnostician will bear this in mind as the AD/HD child is clinically assessed, treated and monitored. In children with AD/HD who also have Tourette syndrome there is ongoing research into the safety and effectiveness of treatment for those who have both disorders.

About half of the children with AD/HD, mostly boys, tend to develop oppositional defiance disorder (ODD). Such children tend to be stubborn, have outbursts of temper, or act belligerently or defiantly. Sometimes, this can progress to the more serious conduct disorders where children with this combination of problems are at risk of getting into trouble at school and even with the police. They tend to take unsafe risks and break laws, such as stealing, starting fires, destroying property and driving recklessly.

Some of the younger boys may also experience the emotional disorders of anxiety and depression. Those who are anxious tend to feel tremendous worry, tension or uneasiness even when there is nothing to fear. Those who feel depressed are so down that their sleep, appetite and ability to think are seriously disrupted (NIMH 1996).

Family factors

In his book, *Your and Your ADD Child*, Wallace (1996) stresses that 'the first problem is the child's ADD condition. The problem begins with the ADD child's demanding and difficult behavior, not with poor parenting'. The intention of this book is to educate parents about ADD and how to implement effective management strategies. Throughout his book Wallace reassures parents that 'while ADD kids are difficult, many turn out to be delightful and successful adults'.

Often the parents of a child with AD/HD wonder why they are unable to manage their child's behavior with the techniques which have proven successful with other children. The disruption that children with AD/HD bring to family life creates stress for all family members. Parents who have participated in parenting programs that are specifically tailored to meet the needs of those families with children with disruptive behaviors (Barkley 1990) are better able to manage their child's behavior. Once the parents feel in control again, relationships between the child and the parents, particularly the mother, and the rest of the family also generally improve.

The confusing factor is that children who are brought up in families that are described as dysfunctional often display a behavior pattern that is similar to that of children with AD/HD. Green & Chee (1994) comment that it is much more difficult to bring about positive changes for such children than it is for children with AD/HD.

Management

The management program that appears to have the best chance of producing a positive long-term effect is that which uses a combination of therapeutic approaches. However, as Baker (1994) and Jarman (1996), among many others, point out, no two children with AD/HD are the same and decisions need to be made about the most appropriate treatments for each child as there are no single best therapy or intervention. It is important, in the initial patient assessment, to identify any pathological, emotional or environmental conditions that may be contributing to the child's behavioral dysfunction and to treat it accordingly. A child who finds work difficult may tend to act out in class rather than ask for help. Such a child may find it less harmful to be the class clown than to be identified as someone who is struggling to keep up.

The role of the chiropractor

The role of the chiropractor in the management of AD/HD is to identify neurological dysafferentation and any factor which may be bearing on neurological function such as poor dietary practices, hypersensitivity reactions to foods or environmental conditions such as pollution, etc. It is usual for AD/HD children to have multiple patterns of dysafferentation which emerge over time as corrective procedures are implemented. Cranial adjusting will almost always follow extracranial neurological correction in AD/HD children. Recurrence of previously subdued patterns of dysafferentation is common and often frustrating for both the parents and the chiropractor. For this reason alone, an adequate schedule of visits is essential if lasting effects are to be produced. It is important for the chiropractor, as an integral part of the health care team, to be proactive in supporting both the family of the AD/HD child and the strategies employed by the other health care professionals involved in the child's management. Occasionally, case conferences with all the health care professionals involved in the care of a child suffering with AD/HD may prove fruitful. Parents should be invited to these conferences to provide feedback on the child's progress. Such conferences serve to keep all the practitioners aware of total management strategy being employed and the clinical reasons for their use.

The role of the pediatric specialist

It is the role of the pediatric specialist to make the definitive diagnosis. Once the AD/HD diagnosis is established, the management strategy most commonly used by the pediatrician is stimulant medication, either methylphenidate or dexamfetamine. It has been demonstrated that about 70% of children with AD/HD will respond positively to at least one of these medications. For the 30% that do not respond positively, other medications are usually trialed. These are summarized in Table 11.4.

Methylphenidate or dexamfetamine effectively treats the symptoms of AD/HD but only while they are active. If taking the short-release version the child takes one dose in the morning after breakfast and another in the middle of the day. The medications provide only short-term relief from the symptoms and have no capacity to cure the disorder in the long term.

There is a slow-release form of Ritalin called Concerta, which is taken in the morning before school and the effect should last through the day, wearing off before bedtime. The benefits of the slow-release drug is that the child or adolescent does not need to remember to leave the classroom to go and get the midday dose. Medication is kept in the home and the child is more settled in the afternoon and more able to engage in after-school activities. (Pelham et al 2001, Watkins & Byrne 2008).

Werry comments that 'stimulant medications help children to show what they know but are unlikely to alter children's knowledge of what needs to be done' (Barkley 1998).

It is believed that these drugs stimulate the neurotransmitters to relay messages smoothly across the synapses so that the children are better able to focus, concentrate, and inhibit their behavior. As stimulant medications, that is, not sedatives, they make the child more focused and alert and not more withdrawn and/or sleepy.

In most states of Australia, pediatricians require specific authority to prescribe stimulant medication to children, and in New South Wales a register is kept of all children receiving these drugs. The doses given to the children are relatively small and if taken as prescribed will not lead to addiction. Only methylphenidate and dexamfetamine are restricted medications and doctors may tend to prescribe some of the others that are not restricted rather than seek permission for methylphenidate or dexamfetamine (Hutchins 1997).

Table 11.4 Names, major actions and side-effects of medications commonly used in the management of children with AD/HD

Drug name	Major action in AD/HD	Side-effects
Methylphenidate (Ritalin) 　Stimulant 　Short-acting: 30–60 minutes after 　　administration for 3–4 hours Dexamfetamine 　Stimulant 　Short-acting: 30–60 minutes after 　　administration for 3–4 hours	Releases dopamine from storage vesicles Reduces restlessness, increases concentration Inhibits reuptake of dopamine Reduces restlessness, increases concentration	Initially: loss of appetite, loss of weight Sleeping problems Teariness, headaches, over-subdued May worsen tics. Contraindicated for children 　with a family history of tics
Pemoline (Cylert) 　Stimulant 　Long-acting: given once a day	Improves attention, decreases distractibility and level of restlessness	Can take 2–4 weeks for clinical response May worsen tics. Regular blood tests required to 　check liver function
Imipramine (Tofranil) 　Tricyclic antidepressant 　Long-acting: 8-hour half-life 　Given 7 days a week to build up steady 　　level in the blood 　Withdraw over 2 weeks	Inhibits re-uptake of norepinephrine (noradrenaline) Improves concentration Decreases impulsivity Reduces oppositional behavior	Uncommon Sleepiness, tiredness Slight dryness of the mouth, constipation, excessive 　perspiration Development of tolerance to the drug
Clonidine (Catapres, Dixarit) 　Alpha-noradrenergic antagonist 　Used in combination with Ritalin or 　　dexamfetamine 　Long-acting: given every day to maintain 　　constant level in bloodstream	Blocks norepinephrine (noradrenaline) autoreceptors Extremely effective in children with oppositional or 　aggressive behavior, and comorbid Tourette 　syndrome Counteracts insomnia	Free of any significant side-effects Can be taken from 10 days to 2–3 months before 　maximal benefit apparent with behavior getting worse 　initially Withdrawal needs to be monitored by a medical 　practitioner to prevent rebound hypertension
Moclobemide (Aurorix) 　Long-acting: given daily to maintain 　　constant level in bloodstream	Inhibits breakdown of dopamine and norepinephrine 　(noradrenaline) by monoamine oxidase Used to treat depression in children	Free of side-effects Rarely, difficulty falling asleep and decrease 　in appetite
Thioridazine (Mellaril) 　Antipsychotic 　Long-acting: given 2–3 times a day for 　　7 days a week	Blocks dopamine autoreceptors Used in children with oppositional or aggressive 　behavior	Negative effect on academic attainments Stiffness. Sleepiness Appetite increase Increased sensitivity of the skin to sunburn Parkinsonian symptoms – even after stopping the 　medication

The effects of the drugs often last only 3–4 hours and the second dose usually needs to be taken at school. This is sometimes embarrassing for the child who has to go to a member of school staff to receive the medication. In the USA, both drugs are available in a long-acting form but research has demonstrated that children prefer the short-acting form. (Neither of the long-acting versions is available in Australia.)

An alternative to stimulant medication is Strattera®, which is an atomoxetine. Following extensive research, this medication was approved for use for people with AD/HD in the USA in 2002 and in Australia in 2007. It claims to be most beneficial for those children and adolescents who cannot tolerate stimulant medication or have comorbid conditions (Lilly 2009, Michelson et al 2001).

There are many sites on the Internet suggesting non-drug treatments of AD/HD and these need to be treated with caution as they are rarely based on sound scientific research validating their claims. Methylphenidate is the most heavily researched pediatric medication and the results indicate that for most children it is effective in controlling the symptoms of AD/HD. Unwanted reactions to the use of AD/HD medication include effects in the cardiovascular system (e.g. palpitations, tachycardia, increased blood pressure, etc.), the central nervous system (e.g. psychotic episodes at recommended doses, overstimulation, restlessness, dizziness, insomnia, dyskinesia, tremors, headache, etc.), the gastrointestinal system (e.g. mouth dryness, unpleasant taste, diarrhea, constipation, etc.) and the endocrine system in adolescents and adults (e.g. impotence, decreased libido, etc.). In addition, anorexia and weight loss have been reported in some cases. These adverse reactions and the potential for drug interaction which has been widely reported in the scientific literature need to be kept in mind by the chiropractor when participating in comprehensive management strategies of affected children.

The use of medication in children with AD/HD is summarized in Box 11.2.

Home/individual interventions

Barkley (1987, 1997b, 1998), Goldstein & Goldstein (1998), and Wallace (1996), among many other researchers in the field

of AD/HD, recommend the education of parents regarding firstly AD/HD and then about the most effective methods of managing the child's behaviors. Sheridan & Sanders (1996) state that an effective family intervention for ADHD should 'aim to empower families to manage their child's disorder by teaching parents active problem-solving skills and to be advocates for their child's needs'. The key features of such an intervention involve a collaborative approach between the clinicians and parents working as a team, psychoeducation about AD/HD, positive parenting and child-management skills, stress coping skills, anger management for the parents, advocacy skills, partner and social support, and helping their children with schoolwork.

Wells (1987) has found that combining stimulants with behavior therapy has helped many more children achieve normal levels of functioning on many symptom measures than using either stimulants or behavior therapy as a single treatment. Cognitive behavior therapy emphasizes the need for children to be aware of their behavior and to develop strategies to self-manage the behavior. Whalen & Henker (1987) believe that while cognitive behavior has been found to be not directly useful in controlling the symptoms of AD/HD, the cognitive therapy approach has at least ensured that the child is included in decisions about the proposed treatment and the evaluation of its effectiveness.

There are support groups for parents/carers of children with AD/HD that provide advice and support to the parents. There are many books written directly for the parents as well as for children. The books for children use stories or direct explanation of what AD/HD is and how it affects the child who suffers from the disorder. They help the children realize that they are not alone with this problem and that many other children in their own or other schools are learning to cope with similar problems.

School

It is important for good communication to be established between the parents, the treating doctors and the school for the child to have the best chance of success at school. Education of the teachers regarding AD/HD and how it affects each particular child in the classroom is the first important step.

Box 11.2

Summary points in the use of medication for children with AD/HD

- There are long-acting versions of Ritalin and dexamfetamine. One tablet is administered daily but there is slow uptake of action (1–2 hours) with the same precautions and side-effects as for the short-acting versions
- 70% of children with AD/HD are effectively treated with a single medication such as Ritalin or dexamfetamine
- AD/HD children are given stimulant medications. They are not given sedatives
- Although related, Ritalin and dexamfetamine have different actions. Some children respond better to one than to the other and, if one does not help, the other should be trialed

- The child should take the smallest effective dose of a medicine. Finding the most effective dose may involve trialing the medication at gradually increasing doses and measuring the beneficial effects
- All medicines can have side-effects. The safety and efficiency of Ritalin, especially, has been extremely well researched for years
- Clonidine is effective in children with oppositional and aggressive behavior. It works well in combination with Ritalin or dexamfetamine
- Children with tics, or a family history of tics, are better treated with clonidine, or Tofranil, than with either Ritalin or dexamfetamine

However, it is a whole school issue because many of the child's problems may occur in the playground where each member of staff is rostered for duty at some time during the school week.

Children with AD/HD often have difficulty making and keeping friends because of their lack of age-appropriate social skills. These social skills need to be specifically taught, preferably in a group setting at school. It has been found that the most effective teaching of social skills is that which happens in the environment in which they are needed. Learning such skills in a clinic may not lead to the child generalizing those skills to other environments.

Other interventions

EEG biofeedback, EEG neurofeedback, or neurotherapy is a form of treatment in which subjects learn to pay attention to their own brain activity and then learn how to change and control their own brainwave activity. High-speed computers provide immediate feedback for the subject. This treatment is claimed to be useful with a variety of disorders including depression, migraine headaches and bedwetting. The length of treatment can vary between 20 and 40 sessions of 30 minutes each. Rossiter & La Vaque (1995) suggest that the EEG biofeedback program may be effective when medication is ineffective or when compliance with taking medications is low. Goldstein & Goldstein (1998) contend that the application of EEG biofeedback technology in the treatment of AD/HD is still unproven and controversial.

Some authors recommend medical, psychological and educational methods of treatment for children with AD/HD (Nash 1994). Various other treatments have been suggested but Nash (1994) specifically does not recommend them. Examples of these other treatments include hypnotherapy, diet therapy, megavitamin therapy and long-term psychotherapy. These treatments have generally been found to address coexisting or secondary symptoms rather than the three main symptoms of AD/HD, namely inattention, hyperactivity and impulsivity.

Feingold (1975) suggested that hyperactivity could be controlled by eliminating food additives such as preservatives, colorings and salicylates from the diet of children with AD/HD. An abundance of research since then has investigated suboptimal levels of nutrients and sensitivities to certain foods and food additives as possible causes of AD/HD or contributive factors to the constellation of symptoms associated with it. Sinn (2008) conducted a review of this research and provides an up-to-date account of clinical trials that have been conducted with zinc, iron, magnesium, Pycnogenol, omega-3 fatty acids, and food sensitivities. Although further research is required, the current evidence supports indications of nutritional and dietary influences on behavior and learning in these children, with the strongest support to date reported for omega-3 fatty acids and behavioral food reactions. It is always recommended that parents who wish to trial an elimination diet do so under the guidance of their chiropractor, general practitioner or a qualified dietician.

Guidelines

In the past decade there has been a worldwide movement towards developing guidelines for practitioners regarding the diagnosis, management and treatment of ADHD. The National Institute for Health and Clinical Excellence (NICE) in the UK has published guidelines covering children, young people and adults. These guidelines recommend that all treatment plans be comprehensive and include psychological counseling, behavioral and educational advice and intervention, and drug therapy in children of school age (NICE 2008). Drug therapy has not been recommended for preschool-age children.

The American Academy of Pediatrics (2000, 2001) has developed clinical practice guidelines for the 'assessment and diagnosis of school-aged children with attention-deficit/hyperactivity disorder'. These guidelines are intended for the use of primary care clinicians working in primary care settings. They include diagnosis based on the DSM-IV criteria, and the recommended treatments encompass both medication and behavior management.

The Royal Australian College of Physicians released a media statement in June 2007 that it is involved in managing the review and development of a new set of guidelines for the management of AD/HD. The College has been commissioned to develop these guidelines by the Australian National Health and Medical Research Council.

Prognosis

While there is general consensus that stimulant medication is effective for controlling the symptoms of AD/HD and improving academic performance in the short term, there is no clear indication of the long-term effect on overall scholastic achievement. About 70% of children with AD/HD continue to have the symptoms, mainly of impulsivity and inattention, into adolescence and in 25–30% the symptoms continue into adulthood.

References

Achenbach, T.M., 1987. How is a parent rating scale used in the diagnosis of attention deficit disorder? In: Loney, J. (Ed.), The Young Hyperactive Child: Answers to Questions about Diagnosis, Prognosis, and Treatment. Haworth Press, New York.

Achenbach, T.M., Edelbrock, C.S., 1983. Child Behaviour Checklist – Teacher's Report. University Associates in Psychiatry, Burlington.

American Academy of Pediatrics, 2000. Clinical practice guideline: diagnosis and evaluation of the child with attention-deficit/hyperactivity disorder. Pediatrics 105 (5), 1158–1170.

American Academy of Pediatrics, 2001. Clinical practice guideline: treatment of the school-aged child with attention-deficit/hyperactivity disorder. Pediatrics 108 (4), 1033–1044.

American Psychiatric Association, 1994. Diagnostic and Statistical Manual of Mental Disorders, fourth ed. American Psychiatric Press, Washington, DC.

Anderson, V., 1997. Attention deficit-hyperactivity disorder: neuropsychological theory and practice. In: Bailey, J.G., Rice, D.N. (Eds), Attention Deficit/ Hyperactivity Disorder: Medical, Psychological and Behavioural Perspectives. Australian Association of Special Education, Sefton, New South Wales.

Aust, P.H., 1994. When the problem is not the problem: understanding attention deficit disorder with and without hyperactivity. Child Welfare 73 (3), 215–227.

Australian Psychological Society, 1997. Attention Deficit Hyperactivity Disorder: A Guide to Best Practice for Psychologists. A position paper. Australian Psychological Society, Canton, Victoria.

Baker, J., 1994. Attention deficit disorder: a creation of the medical profession? Aust. J. Guid. Couns. 4 (1), 65–80.

Barkley, R.A., 1987. What is the role of group parent training in the treatment of ADD children? In: Loney, J. (Ed.), The Young Hyperactive Child: Answers to Questions About Diagnosis, Prognosis and Treatment. Haworth Press, New York.

Barkley, R.A., 1990. Attention Deficit Hyperactivity Disorder: A Handbook for Diagnosis and Treatment. Guilford Press, New York.

Barkley, R.A., 1992. ADHD: What Do We Know? Program Manual for Video. Guilford Publications, New York.

Barkley, R.A., 1997a. AD/HD and The Nature of Self-Control. Guilford Publications, New York.

Barkley, R.A., 1997b. Defiant Children: A Clinician's Manual for Assessment and Parent Training, second ed. Guilford Press, New York.

Barkley, R.A., 1998. Attention-deficit hyperactivity disorder. Sci. Am. 279 (3), 66–71.

Breen, M.J., Altpeter, T.S., 1991. Factor Structures of the Home Situations Questionnaire (HSQ) and School Situations Questionnaire (SSQ). Plenum Press, New York.

Burnley, G.D., 1993. A team approach for identification of an attention deficit hyperactivity disorder child. Sch. Couns. 40, 228–231.

Clements, S.D., Peters, J.E., 1962. Minimal brain dysfunction in the school age child: diagnosis and treatment. Arch. Gen. Psychiatry 6, 185–197.

Conners, K.C., 2008. Conners, third ed. Multi-Health Systems, Newbury.

Cosgrove, P.V.F., 1997. Attention deficit hyperactivity disorder: a UK review. Primary Care Psychiatry (3), 101–113.

DuPaul, G.J., 1991. Parent and teacher ratings of ADHD symptoms: psychometric properties in a community-based sample. J. Clin. Child Psychol. 20, 245–353.

DuPaul, G.J., Power, T.J., Anastopoulos, A.D., et al., 2008. ADHD Rating Scale-IV: Checklists, Norms, and Clinical Interpretation. Available at http://www.guilford.com/excerpts/dupaul2EX.html (accessed 2 April 2008).

Feingold, B.F., 1975. Why Your Child is Hyperactive. Random House, New York.

Goldstein, S., Goldstein, M., 1998. Managing Attention Deficit Hyperactivity Disorder in Children: A Guide for Practitioners. John Wiley, New York.

Goodman, R., 1997. The strengths and weaknesses questionnaire: a research note. J. Child Psychol. Psychiatry 38, 581–586.

Gordon, C., 1994. Attention deficit hyperactive disorder: issues for special educators. Australas. J. Spec. Educ. 18 (2), 36–49.

Green, C., Chee, K., 1994. Management of attention deficit disorder: a personal perspective. Mod. Med. Aust. 37 (2), 38–50.

Hutchins, P., 1990. Biological perspectives on behaviour problems: an essential consideration for practical resolution. In: Richardson, S., Izard, J. (Eds) Practical Approaches to Resolving Behaviour Problems. ACER, Melbourne.

Hutchins, P., 1997. Attention deficit-hyperactivity disorder: collaboration between teacher and doctor – tuning teaching, management and medication. In: Bailey, I.C., Rice, D.N. (Eds), Attention Deficit/ Hyperactivity Disorder: Medical, Psychological and Behavioural Perspectives. Australian Association of Special Education, Sefton, New South Wales.

Jarman, F.C., 1996. Current approaches to management of attention deficit hyperactivity disorder. Aust. Educ. Dev. Psychol. 13 (1), 46–55.

Kewley, C.D., 1998. Attention (hyperactivity) disorder is underdiagnosed and undertreated in Britain: a personal paper. Br. Med. J. 316, 1594–1596.

Landau, S., Milich, R., Widiger, T.A., 1991. Conditional probabilities of child interview symptoms in the diagnosis of attention deficit disorder. J. Child Psychol. Psychiatry 32 (3), 501–513.

Lerner, J.W., Lerner, S.R., 1991. Attention deficit disorder: issues and questions. Focus Except. Child. 24 (3), 1–17.

Lilly, 2009. Strattera atomoxetine HCI advice sheet. Available at http://strattera.com/index.jsp (accessed 31 August 2009).

Lou, H.C., Hennicksen, L., Bruhn, K., 1984. Focal cerebral dysfunction in developmental learning disabilities. Lancet 335, 8–11.

Michelson, D., Faries, D., Wernicke, J., et al., Atomoxetine ADHA Study Group; 2001. Atomoxetine in the treatment of children and adolescents with attention-deficit/ hyperactivity disorder: a randomized, placebo-controlled, dose–response study. Pediatrics 108 (5), e83.

Nash, H., 1994. Kids, Families and Chaos: Living with ADD. Ed-Med Publications, Sydney.

National Institute of Mental Health (NIMH), 1996. Attention Deficit Hyperactivity Disorder: Decade of the Brain. Online: http://www.nimh.nih.gov/publicat/adhd.htm. NIH Publication No. 96–3572. US Government Printing Office, Washington, DC.

New South Wales Department of School Education, 1995. Talk Time Teamwork: Collaborative Management of Students with ADHD. Special Education Directorate, Sydney.

NICE, 2008. Guideline CG72. Attention Deficit Hyperactivity Disorder (ADHD). Online: www.nice.org.uk/Guidance/CG72 (accessed January 2009).

Pauc, R., 2005. Comorbidity of dyslexia, dyspraxia, attention deficit disorder (ADD), attention deficit hyperactive disorder (ADHD), obsessive compulsive disorder (OCD) and Tourette's syndrome in children: a prospective epidemiological study. J. Clin. Chiropractic 8 (4), 189–198.

Pelham, W.E., Gnagy, E.M., Burrows-Maclean, L., et al., 2001. Once-a-day Concerta methylphenidate versus three-times-daily methylphenidate in laboratory and natural settings. Pediatrics 107 (6), e105.

Reif, S., 1993. How to Reach and Teach ADD/ ADHD Children. Center for Applied Research in Education, West Nyack, New York.

Rossiter, T.R., La Vaque, T.J., 1995. A comparison of EEC biofeedback and psychostimulants in treating attention deficit hyperactivity disorders. J. Neurother. (Summer) 48–59.

Royal Australasian College of Physicians media statement, (12.06.2007). Online: www.racp.edu.au (accessed February 2009).

Serfontein, C., 1990. The Hidden Handicap: Dyslexia and Hyperactivity in Children. David Bateman, Buderim, Queensland.

Sheridan, J., Sanders, M.R., 1996. The need for effective early behavioural family interventions for children with attention deficit hyperactivity disorder. Aust. Educ. Dev. Psychol. 13 (1), 29–39.

Sinn, N., 2008. Nutritional and dietary influences on attention deficit hyperactive disorder. Nutr. Rev. 66 (10), 558–568.

Still, G.F., 1902. Some abnormal psychical conditions in children. Lancet 1, 1008–1012.

Strauss, A.A., Werner, H., 1941. The mental organization of the brain injured mentally defective child. Am. J. Psychiatry 97, 1194–1203.

Swanson, J.M., Sandman, C.A., Deutsch, C., et al., 1983. Methylphenidate hydrochloride given with or before breakfast: I. behavioral, cognitive, and electrophysiologic effects. Pediatrics 72 (1), 49–55.

Swanson, J., Schuck, S., Mann, M., et al., 1992. Categorical and dimensional definitions and evaluations of symptoms of ADHD: the SNAP and SWAN Ratings Scales. Online http://www.adhd.net (accessed August 2009).

Wallace, I., 1996. You and Your ADD Child: Practical Strategies for Coping with Everyday Problems. Harper Collins, Sydney.

Watkins, C., Byrne, G., 2008. Available at: http://www.baltimorepsych.com and e.g. http://www.ncpamd.com/Stimulants.htm (accessed 29 August 2009).

Wells, K.C., 1987. What do we know about the use and effects of behaviour therapies in the treatment of ADD? In: Loney, J. (Ed.), The Young Hyperactive Child: Answers to

Questions About Diagnosis, Prognosis and Treatment. Haworth Press, New York.

Whalen, C.K., Henker, B., 1987. Cognitive behavior therapy for hyperactive children: what do we know? In: Loney, J. (Ed.), The Young Hyperactive Child: Answers to Questions about Diagnosis, Prognosis and Treatment. Haworth Press, New York.

World Health Organization, 1992. The ICD-10 Classification of Mental and Behavioural Disorders: Clinical Descriptions and Diagnostic Guidelines. World Health Organization, Geneva.

Zametkin, A., Notdahl, T., Gross, M., et al., 1990. Cerebral glucose metabolism in adults with hyperactivity of childhood onset. N. Engl. J. Med. 20, 1361–1366.

Pediatric otolaryngology

12

Neil J. Davies

Ear, nose and throat conditions are so common in children that otitis media alone will affect two-thirds of all children in the USA by their second birthday (Anrig & Plaugher 1998). Otitis media is the most common cause of hearing loss in children and is the most common childhood disease that requires the care of a physician (Agency for Health Care Policy and Research 1994, Bluestone 1994, Fireman 1997a,b). The cost of medical care alone is huge and becoming greater each year (Agency for Health Care Policy and Research 1994), and estimates fail to take into account resultant cost factors such as time taken off work by carers at the time of illness. Added to all this is the mounting body of scientific evidence that treatment by antibiotic and surgical intervention is not nearly as successful as first thought (Schmidt 1996) and may in fact lead to recurrent infection and chronic disease rather than cure (Maran 1988).

Chiropractic care of children with conditions of the ears, nose and throat is demonstrably safe, effective, and free of the unwanted gastrointestinal and immunological side-effects of antibiotics (Davidson 1988, Gutmann 1987, La Francis 1990).

The chiropractor has a central role to play as a 'portal of entry' primary care provider for children suffering from common diseases of the ear, nose and throat. Chiropractic care will reduce the burden of cost currently borne by parents paying for inappropriate treatment in addition to reducing the duration of suffering for individual children by shortening the natural history of the disease and minimizing recurrence. Chiropractic management strategies for children with common ear, nose and throat complaints requires careful history-taking, physical examination, and recognition of pathology requiring medical intervention.

The ear

The anatomy of the ear

The ear can be readily divided into three parts, namely the outer ear, the middle ear and the inner ear. The outer ear is made up of the pinna and external ear canal, the middle ear includes the tympanic cavity, ossicle and Eustachian tube, and the inner ear the membranous labyrinth with its vestibular and auditory components. The outer and middle ear compartments are primarily involved with hearing via air conduction, while the inner ear is concerned with neurosensory hearing and balance.

A review of gross anatomy of the ear and temporal bone is shown in Figs 12.1 and 12.2.

Box 12.1 lists the examination procedures available to the chiropractor to assist in assessment of the function of the ear. The technique of the ear examination has been described in detail in Chapter 3.

Common outer ear complaints

The outer ear refers to the external auditory canal and the pinna.

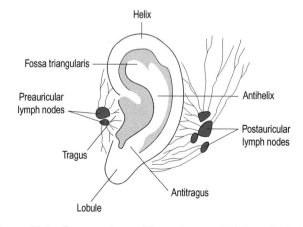

Figure 12.1 • Gross anatomy of the outer ear which is available to the clinician for direct inspection, palpation and percussion.

© 2010, Elsevier Ltd, Inc, BV
DOI: 10.1016/B978-0-7020-3129-8.00012-8

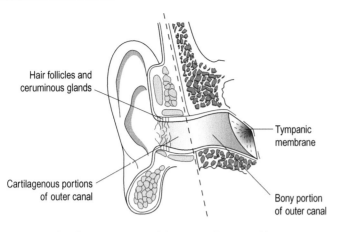

Figure 12.2 ● Gross anatomy of the ear and temporal bone as seen on coronal section.

Box 12.1

Examination procedures used in an office-based practice to assess the function of the outer, middle and inner ear

Outer ear

- Direct inspection of pinna
- Palpation of pinna, tragus and mastoid
- Palpation of pre- and postauricular lymph nodes
- Percussion of mastoid
- Otoscopic inspection of outer canal

Middle ear

- Otoscopic inspection of tympanic membrane
- Pneumatic otoscopy
- Gross hearing tests
- Audiometry

Inner ear

- Balance testing
- Vestibular testing
- Gross hearing test
- Audiometry

Congenital anomalies of the pinna

The most common congenital anomaly of the pinna is the accessory auricle. This is actually a developmental anomaly involving the growth of normal tissue, usually found immediately over or anterior to the tragus. It is of no clinical significance and is not associated with underlying abnormality.

Hematoma or seroma of the auricle

Both hematoma and seroma of the auricle usually result from trauma but may on occasion arise spontaneously. Auricular perichondritis may follow hematoma or result from extension of infection from a furuncle on the posterior meatal wall. The usual causal organism is *Pseudomonas pyocyanea* which tends to produce pus that has a bluish tinge to it. The auricle becomes very swollen and disfigured and the infection may

finally cause cartilaginous necrosis with shriveling of the auricle (Maran 1988).

Hematoma, seroma and auricular perichondritis require immediate referral to an ear, nose and throat (ENT) specialist for management.

Foreign bodies and impacted wax

Children, especially toddlers and preschoolers, are well renowned for putting objects into body cavities. The ears do not escape their attention. Careful direct inspection followed by otoscopy in which the examiner very slowly inserts the speculum into the outer canal will always demonstrate the presence of a foreign body. Extraction is exclusively the realm of the medical specialist and under no circumstances should a chiropractor attempt such a maneuver, regardless of where in the outer canal the foreign body may be located.

Frequently, otoscopic inspection of the tympanic membrane will be impossible to perform because of impacted wax, which usually results from an accumulation of desquamated skin cells and secretions produced by the sebaceous and ceruminous glands. No attempt should be made to dislodge this wax. If it is imperative to visualize the tympanic membrane, the patient should be referred to an ENT specialist for wax removal and clinical opinion of the membrane. Patients should be actively discouraged from attempting to remove the wax themselves with items such as hairpins or cotton buds. Syringing ears with warm water is also unadvisable as the tympanic membrane may be perforated.

Osteoma

Osteoma is a benign exostosis of the bony canal usually arising as a physiological response to repeated cold exposure such as that experienced by swimmers, surfers and divers. These tumors seldom cause any symptoms in the patient and are usually of no clinical consequence.

Furunculosis

A furuncle is an inflammatory skin lesion that results from obstruction of either an apocrine or a sebaceous gland. *Staphylococcus aureus* is the most common cause of furunculosis in the outer ear. Furuncles cause severe ear pain, itching, and sometimes decreased hearing. Signs elicited by physical examination include localized swelling, erythema and palpatory tenderness at the external auditory meatus. A patient with a furuncle can often be given considerable pain relief by using local measures such as the application of heat using hot water bottle in addition to analgesics, which should always be offered to assist with pain control until the furuncle ruptures or resolves. Children with furunculosis should be routinely referred for topical and oral antibiotic therapy. In some patients, where the abscess is large, surgical drainage may be required.

While medical referral is essential, concomitant chiropractic care may also be helpful if the child is to mount an optimal immune response to the infection. In cases where a less than optimal immunological response can be demonstrated to be an issue, short-term nutritional and supplemental therapy in the form of vitamins A and C as well as liquid echinacea extract and omega-3 (fish oil) is indicated. Once a furuncle ruptures,

Table 12.1 Distinguishing features of furunculosis of the external meatus with edema and otitis media with mastoiditis

Furunculosis	Otitis media
Recent staphylococcal infection	Head cold or influenza
Boil seen on shallow otoscopy	Typical tympanic appearance
Hearing is not usually affected	Conductive hearing loss
Continuous dull throbbing pain	Sharp, piercing pain
Pain when the auricle is moved or tragus compressed	No pain on movement of the auricle or on tragal compression
Maximal tenderness is over the tragus and against the mastoid in the postauricular sulcus	Maximal tenderness is over the posterior surface of the mastoid and mastoidal antrum

Table 12.2 Clinical characteristics of mastoiditis and otitis externa

Mastoiditis	Otitis externa
Tenderness over mastoidal antrum	Diffuse tenderness
Loss of the posterior auricular sulcus	Posterior auricular sulcus preserved
No lymphadenopathy	Pre- and postauricular lymphadenopathy
No tragal tenderness	Tragal tenderness commonly noted
Bony change on X-ray common	No radiological change demonstrated
Mucopurulent discharge	Discharge containing a large amount of epithelial debris

it is appropriate to instruct the parents to keep the area clean and adequately disinfected.

It is sometimes difficult to differentiate furunculosis from otitis media with mastoiditis. A diagnostic checklist is shown in Table 12.1 that will assist in making the correct diagnosis. Mastoiditis will necessitate urgent medical referral.

Recurrence of furuncles in a child's ear should lead the chiropractor on a search for other signs of poor immunological function or evidence of diabetes mellitus. Children with diabetes may create an optimal environment for infection by picking their noses and then scratching their ear canals, thus transmitting infection.

Otitis externa

This condition is not common in childhood. It may be bacterial (*Pseudomonas aeruginosa*, *Staphylococcus aureus*), fungal (*Candida albicans*, *Asperigillus fumigatus*), or viral (*Herpes zoster*) (Roland & Stroman 2002). Herpes zoster oticus, otherwise known as Ramsay Hunt syndrome, presents as facial paralysis, hearing loss and vertigo with characteristic vesicular eruptions in the external canal (Wetmore 2007).

Otitis externa may present in either an acute or a chronic stage. In acute otitis externa, the patient usually presents with a feeling of heat in the affected ear that soon gives way to pain that is exacerbated by mandibular movement and manipulation of the pinna and tragus, and ear discharge. Conductive hearing loss is also common, resulting from an accumulation of debris in the canal. Physical examination will usually reveal swelling and erythema, and debris within the external canal, in addition to periauricular lymphadenopathy.

The outstanding feature of chronic otitis externa is itching which becomes unbearable at night. There is usually intermittent deafness for the reason outlined above. It is not uncommon to be confronted with the clinical task of differentiating otitis externa, a relatively easy condition for a chiropractor to manage, from mastoiditis that requires immediate specialist referral. Differentiating characteristics of these two conditions are shown in Table 12.2.

Otitis externa requires local antibiotic therapy as the mainstay of management as opposed to oral antibiotics. Because locally applied antibiotics directly target the infected site, a high antibiotic concentration is achieved exactly where it is required; this contains bacterial overgrowth and avoids the unwanted side-effects of oral antibiotics (Langford & Benrimoj 1996).

Otomycosis

Fungal infection in the outer ear canals of children is common. It is especially common in tropical and subtropical regions of the world. By far the most common infection is with *Candida albicans* which often follows antibiotic therapy for otitis externa. Children presenting with this problem tend to have irritation in their ears and a mass of debris in the outer canal that quickly re-forms after cleansing. On otoscopy, *Candida albicans* appears whitish to silver and is commonly seen on the margins of the tympanic membrane. Children with *Candida albicans* infection tend to have chronic upper cervical subluxations, the correction of which remains elusive until the otomycosis is cleared up. This appears to be due to an activated viscerosomatic reflex (Gatterman 1995, Homewood 1981, Plaugher 1993).

Another less commonly found fungal infection is with *Aspergillus niger*. This fungus appears dark brown to black on otoscopy and leaves dark specks in the epithelial debris. Treatment of both *Candida albicans* and *Aspergillus niger* requires the application of antifungal preparations. A referral to a natural therapist for treatment may also be appropriate. Once the infection is cleared up and the upper cervical subluxation is corrected, there is no reason to expect recurrence since it is reasonable to suggest that the integrity of local tissue immunity is at least to some extent dependent upon the absence of the subluxation (Gatterman 1995).

Common middle ear complaints in children

Without question, the great majority of ear complaints in children for which health care professionals are consulted involve infection and its sequelae in the middle ear. The US Department of Health and Human Services has estimated that there are approximately 5.2 million acute otitis media episodes occurring annually (Marcy et al 2000).

These conditions are categorized using descriptive terms such as chronic serous otitis media, otitis media with effusion, chronic suppurative otitis media, acute otitis media, etc. While spontaneous recovery from acute otitis media is common (Alho et al 1996), and the administration of chiropractic care may be effective in both shortening the natural history and reducing the severity of symptoms (Froehle 1996, Hawk et al 2007), it remains an imperative to take a thorough patient history and conduct an extensive physical examination in order to establish a clinical benchmark against which to evaluate patient progress. A thorough knowledge of the symptoms, signs, and natural history of disease associated with middle ear infection and progression of the infectious process itself is a critical safety feature in chiropractic management planning.

The physical examination of the child who presents with middle ear infection should begin with the pinna, temporal bone and outer ear, as shown in Box 12.1, before proceeding to the following:

- otoscopic inspection of the tympanic membrane
- pneumatic otoscopy
- gross hearing tests
- audiometry.

The technique of otoscopy in the infant and small child has been described in detail in Chapter 3. The largest diameter speculum that can be comfortably inserted into the external canal should always be used in order to obtain the widest field of view possible. On otoscopic inspection, the tympanic membrane should be systematically assessed for color, contour changes, evidence of any discharge, polyposis, granulation or perforation. The clinical significance of each of these is identified in Table 12.3. The appearance of the normal healthy tympanic membrane is shown in Fig. 12.3.

Pneumatic otoscopy is routinely performed after inspection. The examination is performed by inserting a speculum of the largest possible size into the outer canal in such a way that it forms an airtight seal. The examiner then puffs air into the outer canal by gently but quickly squeezing the insufflator. Pneumatic otoscopy is based on the physiological principle that in a normally aerated ear the pressure is at standard atmospheric pressure (atm) on either side of the drum. When the air pressure is momentarily elevated in the outer canal by sharply squeezing the pneumatic bulb, the tympanic membrane moves first inwardly, and then as the air rushes out, temporarily reducing the pressure in the outer canal below standard atmospheric pressure (atm), the membrane moves outwardly before returning to the neutral or resting position. Observation of this phenomenon permits the examiner to deduce that normal aeration of the middle ear is present and therefore no effusion or adhesive disease such as chronic serous otitis media is present. Possible reasons for failure of the tympanic membrane to move appropriately under pneumatic investigation are given in Box 12.2.

It is also necessary to assess quantitative and qualitative hearing. This requires a series of gross hearing tests that can be easily performed by the chiropractor in addition to an audiometric assessment that can be obtained by referring the child to an audiology clinic.

Table 12.3 Clinical significance of the characteristic appearance of the tympanic membrane in middle ear disease

Appearance	Significance
Color	
Red	Associated with acute otitis media and other infection
Dull	Usual appearance in chronic serous otitis media
Blue	Implies blood behind the tympanic membrane
Contour	
Bulging	Acute otitis media and other less common causes
Retracted	Negative middle ear pressure associated with chronic serous otitis media and Eustachian tube dysfunction
Discharge	
Mucoid	Usually associated with benign middle ear disease
Squamous debris	Frequently associated with cholesteatoma
Polyposis	Frequently associated with cholesteatoma or local tissue reaction to surgical intubation
Granulation	Frequently associated with cholesteatoma
Perforation	
Central	Discrete central perforations are usually associated with benign middle ear disease
Marginal	Associated with cholesteatoma

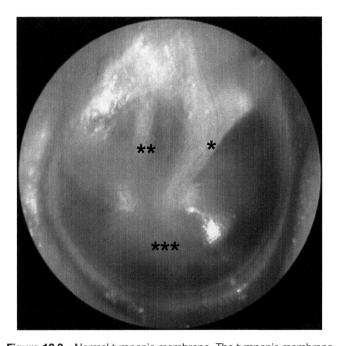

Figure 12.3 • Normal tympanic membrane. The tympanic membrane is translucent, allowing visualization of the middle ear structures, including the short and long processes of the malleus (*), incudostapedial joint (**), promontory and round window niche (***). (Adapted from Wetmore 2007 with permission.)

Box 12.2

Common reasons why a tympanic membrane may fail to move or demonstrate diminished movement on pneumatic otoscopy

- Perforation
- Middle ear effusion
- Negative middle ear pressure
- Middle ear mass such as cholesteatoma
- Tympanostomy tube in situ

In the school-age child and adolescent, gross hearing is assessed using Schwabach's, Rinne's and Weber's tests, all of which rely for their accuracy on the ability of the patient to make cognitive decisions about the relative loudness of sound produced by a tuning fork. These, as well as age-specific tests for the neonate, infant, toddler and preschool-age child, have been described in detail in Chapter 3.

Chiropractic management of acute otitis media

Acute otitis media is a common childhood complaint and is heralded by a sudden onset of fever and ear pain. The tympanic membrane will usually appear reddened, bulging under the pressure of pus in the middle ear, and in some cases the squamous epithelium will appear macerated. The tympanic membrane will usually be non-motile under these circumstances. Pain originating from pathology in the middle ear may be described by the child as being 'inside the ear itself' or in the vicinity of the ear in a pattern as shown in Fig. 12.4. Ear pain in this pattern is often due to middle ear pathology in children and the diagnosis provided by careful otoscopy is usually unmistakable. There are, however, several other important causes of

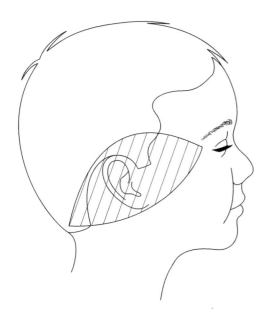

Figure 12.4 • Possible pattern of head pain produced by middle ear pathology.

Box 12.3

Conditions which may cause pain in a pattern similar to that seen with middle ear pathology

- Dental caries
- Teething in infants
- Tonsillitis
- Acute pharyngitis
- Nasopharyngeal fibroma
- Acute stomatitis or glossitis
- Postauricular lymphadenopathy
- Sinusitis
- Postsurgical (adenoidectomy)
- Acute mastoiditis
- Upper cervical subluxation complex
- Cranial faults (especially temporal dysfunction)

pain occurring in this pattern that the chiropractor should be aware of. These have been identified in Box 12.3.

The natural history of acute otitis media in children is short and usually explosive, frequently terminating with tympanic perforation followed by expulsion of mucopus and blood. The pain is generally relieved once tympanic perforation occurs. Chiropractic management is based on adjusting the child in order to enhance the natural immune response, keeping the child as comfortable as possible by using systematic analgesia and local treatments, then observing the child closely throughout the resolution phase to ensure there are no unwanted sequelae such as the development of chronic serous otitis media or mastoiditis, or the formation of cholesteatoma, etc.

The diagnosis of acute otitis media requires three clinical components (Wetmore 2007):
- a history of acute onset within 48 hours of presentation
- presence of middle ear effusion
- symptoms or signs of middle ear inflammation.

Once the diagnosis of acute otitis media has been established beyond a reasonable doubt, an appropriate chiropractic management plan would be as follows:

- Begin chiropractic adjusting as soon as possible. This usually involves the upper cervical spine and the craniosacral respiratory mechanism.
- Prescribe analgesia, preferably from the ibuprofen family because of their superior antipyretic qualities, especially in cases involving fever >38.5°C.
- Prescribe echinacea in liquid form to assist with immune modulation and anti-inflammatory action.
- Prescribe naturopathic or herbal preparations for ear pain (Sarrell et al 2003).
- Insert two drops of warm olive oil into the affected ear and apply a heating pad such as a hot water bottle over the ear to provide additional pain relief (Mendelsohn 1990).
- Counsel parents to expect perforation, in which case they may find mucopus and blood on the child's pillow or dripping from the ear.
- Carry out otoscopic evaluation and hearing tests, including audiometry, until resolution is complete. If no signs of

resolution are seen after 72 hours following onset of the symptoms, it would be appropriate to refer the child for treatment with antibiotics. The reason for this is related to studies that demonstrate both the presence of bacterial organisms such as *Streptococcus pneumoniae*, *Haemophilus influenzae*, *Moraxella catarrhalis* and *Staphylococcus* with concurrent bronchiolitis and respiratory syncytial virus (Andrade et al 1998). Given the plethora of studies that have shown that antibiotics confer limited benefit in the management of acute otitis media (Wetmore 2007), it is unreasonable and clinically unwise to arrange for provision of these medications at the first sign of disease. This policy of later rather than earlier provision of antibiotics has been very successfully implemented among otolaryngologists in countries such as the Netherlands and Sweden but remains somewhat controversial in countries such as Australia and the USA.

• Continue chiropractic care and encourage parents to keep up a prophylactic level of liquid echinacea for several weeks in order to afford the child the best chance of avoiding recurrence, which is common.

Echinacea extract is a powerful antiviral and antibacterial compound. It has a synergistic immunopharmacological effect (Sharma et al 2008), and is an anti-inflammatory and antioxidative agent, its action being to alleviate or reverse the effects of virus-induced stimulation of the proinflammatory cytokines (Barcz et al 2007, Chicca et al 2009). It has no known toxicity in children, even in the event that they are taking antibiotics or other prescribed medications (Freeman & Spelman 2008). One case reported in the literature by Mullins (1998), however, needs comment. Mullins suggested there may be a relationship between echinacea ingestion and allergic reactions in atopic patients, but his research was confined to a single case, an adult female, and there have been no further reports in the literature of such reactions.

Chiropractic management of chronic otitis media with effusion

Chronic otitis media with effusion is otherwise known as *chronic serous otitis media* (CSOM), *'glue ear'*, *secretory otitis media*, *seromucinous otitis media*, *exudative otitis media* or *non-supportive otitis media*, the myriad of names reflecting the lack of understanding of this common and troublesome complaint. Some common causes of CSOM are changes in the antibody immune response, chronic viral infection, large adenoids and allergy.

Clinically, CSOM presents as a conductive hearing loss, usually bilateral, which may be associated with delayed speech development, occasional mild ear discomfort, vertigo and recurrent infection. The clinician should remember, however, that glue ear is frequently asymptomatic, a good reason to routinely screen gross hearing and perform otoscopic examination of all pre-adolescent patients.

The clinical findings in CSOM include evidence of tympanic retraction and reduced or absent membrane motility with a dull blue, gray or deep reddish color, often associated with what appear to be bubbles or spots seen on otoscopic inspection. Impedance tympanometry shows a typical *'flat*

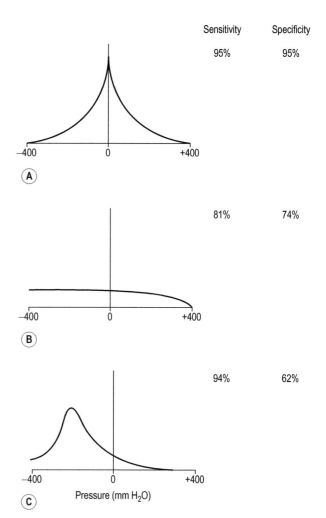

Figure 12.5 • Impedance tympanograms (with their specificity and sensitivity relative to findings on tympanocentesis) showing: (A) normal response indicating a healthy, aerated middle ear; (B) fluid in the middle ear; (C) reduced middle ear pressure due to Eustachian tube dysfunction. (Adapted from Wetmore 2007 with permission.)

tympanogram' (Fig. 12.5) and will assist in differentiating this condition from otosclerosis and Eustachian obstruction (Wetmore 2007). The long-term sequelae of chronic otitis media with effusion include temporary air conductive hearing loss and cholesteatoma, a benign mass which arises from retraction pockets in the tympanic membrane. Congenital cholesteatoma is evident on otoscopic examination as a pearly cyst located anterior to the handle of the malleus (Fig. 12.6), while the attic cholesteatoma appears as a marginal attic perforation with keratin accumulation, evidence of chronic infection, and tympanic membrane collapse. Patients with cholesteatoma frequently have a scanty, malodorous discharge that has been described as smelling something like the fur of a wet cat. Cholesteatoma invariably requires surgical intervention.

Once the diagnosis of chronic otitis media with effusion has been established beyond reasonable doubt, it is appropriate to begin a comprehensive chiropractic management plan. Management is based on the following principles:

• improve Eustachian tube function in order to produce drainage and aeration of the middle ear, and

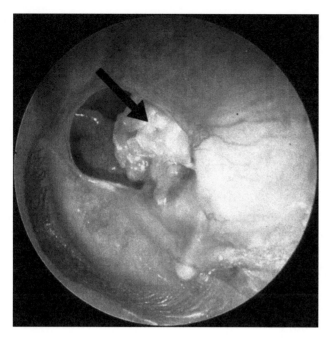

Figure 12.6 • Cholesteatoma (arrow) seen through a posterior superior tympanic membrane perforation. (Adapted from Wetmore 2007 with permission.)

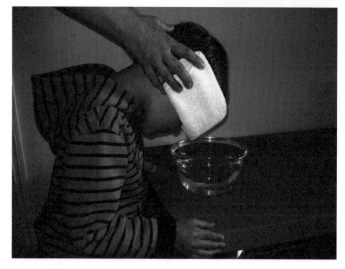

Figure 12.7 • The use of steam inhalation to assist with Eustachian tube drainage. Care must be taken not to hold the child too close to the source of the steam and the eyes must be protected with a towel, as shown.

- improve the immune response to optimal levels.

  The chiropractic management plan is carried out as follows:

- Begin chiropractic adjusting as soon as possible. This usually involves the upper cervical spine and the craniosacral respiratory mechanism. There is a growing body of evidence linking craniosacral treatment and resolution of this condition. Children with chronic otitis media with effusion should by all means have craniosacral treatment as an integral part of their management program.

- Prescribe prophylactic levels of vitamin C and *Echinacea purpurea* extract.

- Have the child undergo steam inhalation morning and night until otoscopy demonstrates that the middle ears have drained. Steam inhalation is prepared by placing 5 ml of inhalant oil in 600 ml of boiling water and having the child inhale the steam produced for a period of 1–2 minutes. Care must be taken not to hold the child too close to the source of the steam and the child's eyes must be protected by covering them with a towel (Fig. 12.7). It is preferable to use inhalant oil that contains a mixture of pine, menthol and camphor rather than eucalyptus. Inhalation should not be used with children below school age as it may produce laryngeal edema (Maran 1988).

- At the very beginning of the chiropractic management program, it is useful to give the child pediatric strength nose drops containing epinephrine (adrenaline) for use after the steam inhalation. The drops are used to attempt to reduce the edema in the epithelial lining of the Eustachian tube in order to promote drainage. In order to accomplish this, the child is placed supine with the head held in extension. Two drops are placed in each nostril and the jaw is worked gently from side to side. This has the effect of stretching the nasopharyngeal opening of the Eustachian tubes which allows the epinephrine in the drops to penetrate. The use of nose drops should be restricted to a maximum of 3 days.

- An exclusion diet for dairy products should be recommended for the first 21 days of the management program. If the child has responded well after this time, a brief challenge with dairy foods should be undertaken with careful otoscopic monitoring of the middle ear to check for the reappearance of any effusion. If the challenge causes recurrence of either the middle ear effusion or the child's subluxation pattern, then the child must be kept on a dairy-free diet and appropriately supplemented. If the child fails to show resolution of the middle ear effusion after 21 days then an exclusion trial for products containing wheat should be undertaken.

- Counsel parents to keep their house free of cigarette smoke, the expectant mother not to smoke at all (Ely et al 1995), and to maintain the home-based strategies.

Poor parent/patient compliance is by far the most common reason why the above management program fails.

The use of antibiotics is not to be encouraged. Repeated courses or long-term use of antibiotics has not been shown to change the natural history of chronic otitis media with effusion, and when their immunosuppressive effects are taken into account it is best simply to avoid them altogether. Maran (1988) states that antibiotics have no role to play in the treatment of chronic otitis media with effusion and reports that, in studies where they have been given, they cannot be recovered from fluid aspirated from the middle ear, indicating a complete lack of penetration at the target organ.

Myringotomy surgery to aspirate middle ear fluid and place grommet drainage tubes into the tympanic membrane in order to keep the middle ear dry is a commonly employed surgical strategy in the treatment of chronic otitis media with effusion. There is no question that this procedure produces immediate changes to hearing levels (Maran 1988, Wetmore 2007) and from the perspective of the parents this is a most desirable outcome. Repeated studies, however, have not only failed to demonstrate substantial difference in long-term (12 months) outcome in both hearing and language acquisition, but have identified that children who have undergone myringotomy are at a significantly higher risk of developing tympanosclerosis and other disorders of the tympanic membrane than children who did not (Lous et al 2005, Slack et al 1984). On the other side of the ledger is the short-term benefit to hearing (Maran 1988) and, therefore, in cases where it may be an issue, the acquisition of language skills and the resolution of middle ear effusion-related vertigo (Golz et al 1997). The decision on the part of the individual chiropractor as to what advice to give to parents about this issue will always come down to an assessment, on balance, of the cost–benefit ratio in each case, but recommendation for ENT surgery is probably best reserved for the most severe cases.

The role of allergy as an etiology in chronic otitis media with effusion remains somewhat controversial owing to the fact the IgE levels remain unaffected in many cases where a child has allergic symptoms. Bernstein et al (1981), however, reported that IgE reactions were significant in as many as 15% of children presenting with earaches that were described as allergic on the basis of clinical and laboratory evidence.

In trying to bring this whole issue into a sensible, balanced focus, Schmidt (1996) correctly identifies so-called allergic reactions as either true allergy or hypersensitivity reactions. He then goes on to outline an allergy control program in his excellent text *Healing Childhood Ear Infections*.

The nose and sinuses

There are two forms of examination available to the chiropractor to assist with assessment of the nose and sinuses, these being sinus radiography and direct nasal inspection via the otoscope (described in Chapter 3).

Acute upper respiratory tract infection

The nasal examination is of particular use to the chiropractor when confronted by children with acute upper respiratory tract infection. In the acute presentation, evidence of infection in the nose that is found to be accompanying infection of other areas of the upper and lower respiratory system, including the ears, is strongly suggestive that the infection is of viral etiology rather than bacterial. Conversely, if the child with tonsillitis, for example, has little evidence of infection in the ears, nose or lower respiratory tree, then the etiological agent is most likely to be bacterial and should be treated accordingly.

In managing children with viral infection in the upper respiratory tract, the key elements are the chiropractic adjustment and complementary medicines (e.g. *Echinacea purpurea*, vitamin C, etc.) to optimize the immune response, implementation of pain control measures, frequent use of steam inhalation to prevent coughing from dry mucous membranes, and daily clinical re-evaluation. After 72 hours, if active viral infection is still in evidence, the possibility of secondary bacterial infection

developing grows exponentially and the child should be referred for protective antibiotic therapy. Restoration of gastrointestinal flora by the use of *Lactobacillus acidophilus* or *Lactobacillus bulgaricus* supplementation should be provided as a matter of course for all children who undergo antibiotic therapy. It is advisable to continue the immune-stimulating complementary medicines and the *Lactobacillus* supplementation for at least 30 days after all evidence of infection has cleared and the antibiotic therapy has been withdrawn (Schmidt 1996).

Chronic catarrh

The child with chronic catarrh presents a difficult clinical problem for health care providers, including chiropractors. Chronic catarrh is a common health problem in children and is usually multifactorial in nature. Some of the predisposing factors that must be considered when formulating the chiropractic management program are the child's home environment, recurrent viral infection from immunosuppression or immune incompetence, allergy, mechanical obstruction, and what is referred to as the 'snuffly baby' syndrome (Maran 1988).

The typical clinical features of chronic catarrh are a combination of nasal congestion, recurrent upper respiratory tract infection, sore throats, recurring otalgia, anorexia, pallor, a non-productive cough, and delayed growth and development factors. Eczema also commonly occurs in children with chronic catarrh, some of whom eventually 'grow out of it' but continue to have catarrhal symptoms, and some of whom develop asthma. The clinician should be aware of this pattern of progression when planning and implementing maintenance care in children who initially present with eczema and catarrhal symptoms. Uncommonly, recurrent upper respiratory tract infection in children will be due to hypothyroidism or hypogammaglobulinemia.

The socioeconomic status of the parents and their 'all round knowledge' of parenting often affect the home environment in which a child lives. At interview, discreet inquiry should be made into such matters as smoking in the house, domestic hygiene, personal hygiene, knowledge of nutrition, contact with pets, and factors which may negatively affect air quality such as proximity to a busy road, local factories, etc.

Recurrent viral infection may be the result of immune incompetence or may be the result of repeated or long-term use of antibiotics. In either case, the clinical effect is the same and must be addressed accordingly.

Allergy is a frequent predisposing factor to chronic catarrh that is known to be hereditary. If both parents have atopic disease, their offspring stand a 75% chance of developing symptoms of nasal allergy (Maran 1988). The allergy, or hypersensitivity, is usually to a food substance, commonly of diary origin.

A mechanical obstruction, produced by polyposis or hypertrophy of the inferior turbinate (Neskey et al 2009), may become a site for chronic infection. Though rare, polyps may be seen as a visible swelling behind the soft palate. Hypertrophy of the inferior turbinate is much more commonly encountered and is seen as an obstruction to the airway on inspection with the otoscope. Both conditions require surgical intervention.

The so-called 'snuffly baby' syndrome is seen in children who simply produce nasal secretion at a greater rate than most. This causes some distress during feeding where nasal breathing is difficult. The nose must be inspected for evidence of choanal atresia; otherwise there is usually no other evidence of sickness and the parents should be counseled accordingly. Mechanical removal of the mucus using gentle suction immediately prior to, and perhaps during, feeding may be of some assistance.

The chiropractic management plan for the child with chronic catarrh is carried out as follows:

- Begin chiropractic adjusting as soon as possible. This usually involves the upper cervical spine and the craniosacral respiratory mechanism. There is a growing body of evidence linking craniosacral treatment and resolution of this condition. Children with chronic otitis media with effusion should by all means have craniosacral treatment as an integral part of their management program.

- Prescribe prophylactic levels of vitamin C and *Echinacea purpurea* extract.

- Have the child undergo steam inhalation morning and night until otoscopy demonstrates that the middle ears have drained. Steam inhalation is prepared by placing 5 ml of inhalant oil in 600 ml of boiling water and having the child inhale the steam produced for a period of 1–2 minutes. Care must be taken not to hold the child too close to the source of the steam and the child's eyes must be protected by covering them with a towel (see Fig. 12.7). It is preferable to use inhalant oil that contains a mixture of pine, menthol and camphor rather than eucalyptus. Inhalation should not be used with children below school age as it may produce laryngeal edema (Maran 1988).

- At the very beginning of the chiropractic management program, it is useful to give the child pediatric strength nose drops containing epinephrine (adrenaline) for use after the steam inhalation. The drops are used to attempt to reduce the edema in the epithelial lining of the Eustachian tube in order to promote drainage. In order to accomplish this, the child is placed supine with the head held in extension. Two drops are placed in each nostril and the jaw is worked gently from side to side. This has the effect of stretching the nasopharyngeal opening of the Eustachian tubes which allows the epinephrine in the drops to penetrate. The use of nose drops should be restricted to a maximum of 3 days.

- An exclusion diet for dairy products should be recommended for the first 21 days of the management program. If the child has responded well after this time, a brief challenge with dairy foods should be undertaken with careful otoscopic monitoring of the middle ear to check for the reappearance of any effusion. If the challenge causes recurrence of either the middle ear effusion or the child's subluxation pattern, then the child must be kept on a dairy-free diet and appropriately supplemented. If the child fails to show resolution of the middle ear effusion after 21 days then an exclusion trial for products containing wheat should be undertaken.

- Counsel parents to keep their house free of cigarette smoke, the expectant mother not to smoke at all (Ely et al 1995), and to maintain the home-based strategies.

Poor parent/patient compliance is by far the most common reason why the above management program fails.

Sinusitis

Acute and chronic infection of the sinuses is sometimes seen in the catarrhal child. While this may be identified on transillumination, sinus radiography is mandatory. The sinus most frequently affected in young children (from 4 years old) is the ethmoid and, as they get older (from 8 years old), the maxillary and frontal. All children suspected of having sinus infection should be referred to an ENT specialist for concomitant management, since sinus infection involving the ethmoid can spread via the lamina papyracea to cause orbital cellulitis and intracranial infection (Maran 1988, Ong & Tan 2002, Ouraishi & Zevallos 2006).

The oral cavity

The examination procedure for the oral cavity has been extensively described in Chapter 3. Much information can be gleaned from inspection of the oral cavity, principally in relation to infection, but also to changes to lymphoid tissue and evidence of blood dyscrasias.

Herpes infection

Stomatitis derived from herpetic infection is obvious on the lips. In addition to maintenance chiropractic care, patients with recurrent outbreaks of infection should be given lysine prophylactically as well as C and B complex vitamins. Foods containing arginine should be eliminated from the diet.

Oral ulcers

Ulceration of the oral mucosa is less common in children than in adults. The ulcers may be aphthous ulcers that tend to form multiple lesions but are most likely to be those classified as non-specific recurrent oral ulceration. These lesions are painful, interfere with normal feeding, and have a natural history of healing without scarring in 7–10 days. Children with recurrent ulceration should be assessed for vitamin B_{12}, iron and folic acid deficiency as part of their chiropractic management program. There is no evidence to blame herpes simplex virus as an etiological agent for these lesions (Maran 1988). In addition to chiropractic care and complementary medicine, it is appropriate to suggest the use of commercially available local anesthetic preparations and an antimicrobial mouthwash during the course of the illness to assist with pain control. Systemic analgesia such as paracetamol appears to offer only minimal relief from painful mouth ulcers.

Candidiasis

This appears as white, multiple, plaque-like lesions that can be readily scraped off with an instrument such as a tongue depressor. Candidiasis looks so much like patches of milk curd that attempting to move it with a spatula is necessary to establish the diagnosis. When the plaque-like structure is due to candidiasis, scraping it off usually causes local bleeding, an effect which never occurs with milk curd.

In infants with candida infection, it is an essential part of the chiropractic management program to carefully counsel the nursing mother to treat her nipple and areolar areas, because the offending organism tends to survive very well in a warm, dark and frequently wet environment. Failure on the mother's part to treat her nipples will result in a great deal of frustration as the child experiences constant reinfection. Babies with candidiasis should be routinely treated with a local fungicide, many of which are available commercially without a prescription. Candidiasis commonly follows antibiotic use.

In children with oral candidiasis, it is not uncommon to see intercurrent infection of the perianal area. Inspection of the anus should be routinely carried out in all children who have evidence of oral infection. Treatment of older children who are on solid food should include administration of *Lactobacillus acidophilus* or *Lactobacillus bulgaricus* in addition to the local fungicide.

Koplik's spots

These are clusters of tiny yellow to whitish spots on the buccal mucosa which are pathognomonic of measles (rubeola). Koplik's spots are often likened in appearance to tiny crystals of sugar or salt against the red background of the buccal mucosa. Koplik's spots are a very early sign of measles infection and may be seen during the infectious stage up to 4 days prior to the appearance of general symptoms and/or the characteristic skin rash (Bhaskar 1986).

Petechiae

Petechiae may sometimes be seen on the soft palate. Petechial hemorrhaging is a result of either a decrease in the total number of platelets or dysfunctional platelets. While infection commonly causes a transient decrease in the total number of platelets, iron deficiency anemia, idiopathic thrombocytopenic purpura (ITP) and leukemia also produce the same effect. When petechiae are seen on the soft palate area, a Hess test should be carried out and, if positive, a full blood evaluation. The Hess test is performed using the sphygmomanometer. Firstly, the child's blood pressure is established and a circle 2.5 cm in diameter is drawn in the antecubital fossa. Secondly, a constant pressure is held with the sphygmomanometer at a value half-way between systole and diastole for a period of 3 minutes. In the presence of low platelet numbers, petechial hemorrhages will appear in the antecubital fossa. The Hess test would be considered positive when 6–10 hemorrhages appear in the defined circle after the completion of the 3-minute period, an outcome known as the Rumpel–Leede phenomenon (Wetmore 2007).

Lymphoma

Malignant changes in lymphoid tissue are sometimes seen in the oral cavity. While it is usual in these cases to see a mass in the floor of the mouth, lymphoma may manifest as one palatine tonsil enlarged to the midline of the oropharynx. In such a case, enlarged lymph nodes may also be seen in the submandibular area with floor of the mouth lesions and at the angle of the mandible (tonsillar node) with palatine tonsil lesions.

Pharyngitis

The pharynx is a common site of infection in children, the classic 'sore throat' with difficulty swallowing. It is often associated with swollen palatine tonsils which occasions mouth breathing. The infectious agent will be either bacterial or viral. Diagnostic differentiation of the type is critical to sound chiropractic management.

Bacterial infection

When the infection is bacterial, the most common pathogen is *Streptococcus pyogenes*, a Gram-positive organism that exhibits beta-hemolysis of blood agar by culture and a group A cell wall carbohydrate antigen. It is therefore referred to as a group A beta-hemolytic streptococcus (GABHS). Other organisms which may be involved are *Corynebacterium diptheriae*, *Neisseria gonorrhoeae*, *Arcanobacterium haemolyticium*, *Haemophilus influenzae*, *Streptococcus pneumoniae*, *Streptococcus viridians*, *Staphylococcus aureus*, *Staphylococcus epidermidis* and *Moraxella catarrhalis*.

The diagnosis of bacterial pharyngitis or tonsillitis can usually be made by careful observation of the symptoms and signs. The clinical presentation is usually a sudden onset of sore throat, fever, headache, abdominal pain, nausea and vomiting. On inspection of the oral cavity there will be erythema and exudates on the tonsils and pharynx, soft palate petechiae (doughnut lesions), uvular swelling and erythema, anterior cervical adenitis, and a scarletiniform rash (Wetmore 2007). Since bacterial infection is typically unifocal, cough, rhinitis, stridor, hoarseness, conjunctivitis and diarrhea are absent.

From the perspective of the chiropractor, while it is appropriate to provide supportive care, bacterial pharyngitis cases universally require antimicrobial therapy, making a medical referral a necessity.

Viral infection

When the cause of the pharyngotonsillitis is viral, in addition to the local signs described above the child will demonstrate multifocal signs of infection such as cough, rhinitis, stridor, hoarseness, conjunctivitis and diarrhea. Epstein–Barr virus infection is the most important causative agent of viral tonsillitis. The tonsillar area appears reddened and covered with a yellow to white membrane. The child has a very sore throat, breathes loudly, and has difficulty swallowing. The swelling of the tonsil in some cases is so severe that they may actually touch in the midline. In such cases, breathing may be obstructed to the point where oxygen perfusion may be seriously decreased and hospital management is essential to ensure the best clinical outcome. The child with Epstein–Barr virus infection will also usually have lymphadenopathy, hepatomegaly and splenomegaly, with the diagnosis being confirmed by laboratory evaluation of the blood.

The medical management of viral tonsillitis is largely supportive, focusing on maintenance of hydration, pain control, and preservation of caloric intake. The chiropractic management is as follows:

- Begin chiropractic adjusting as soon as possible. This usually involves the upper cervical spine and the craniosacral respiratory mechanism. There is a growing body of evidence linking craniosacral treatment and resolution of this condition.
- Prescribe prophylactic levels of vitamin C and *Echinacea purpurea* extract.
- Have the child undergo steam inhalation morning and night if high acceleration coughing is a feature of the condition. Steam inhalation is prepared by placing 5 ml of inhalant oil in 600 ml of boiling water and having the child inhale the steam produced for a period of 1–2 minutes. Care must be taken not to hold the child too close to the source of the steam and the child's eyes must be protected by covering them with a towel (see Fig. 12.7). It is preferable to use inhalant oil that contains a mixture of pine, menthol and camphor rather than eucalyptus. Inhalation should not be used with children below school age as it may produce laryngeal edema (Maran 1988).
- A constant watch must be kept on the child's level of hydration.

- Implementation of pain control measures will usually be a significant clinical issue in tonsillitis cases, as it can be very painful condition. Methods of pain control are discussed in detail in Chapter 20.
- In cases where improvement is not evident 72 hours after the onset of symptoms, or where there has been a sudden sustained rise in the core body temperature, secondary bacterial infection should be considered and a referral for antibiotic prescription made.

In cases of viral tonsillitis in which the child has tested positive for Epstein–Barr virus infection, the recruitment of a natural therapist well versed in the use of the whole range of complementary medicines is recommended. Coupled with maintenance chiropractic care, the complementary medicine approach offers the child the best chance of recovery free of debilitating postviral sequelae. Before the decision to manage a child with a diagnosis of viral tonsillitis using chiropractic and complementary medicine is made, careful assessment is needed to ensure that initial hospital-based care to ensure an adequate airway is not required.

References

Agency for Health Care Policy and Research, 1994. Clinical Practice Guideline #12: Otitis Media with Effusion in Young Children. US Department of Health and Human Services, Rockville, MD.

Alho, O., Laara, E., Oja, H., 1996. What is the natural history of recurrent otitis media in infancy? J. Fam. Pract. 43 (3), 258–264.

Andrade, M., Hoeberman, A., Glustein, J., et al., 1998. Acute otitis media in children with bronchiolitis. Pediatrics 101 (4/1), 617–619.

Anrig, C., Plaugher, G., 1998. Pediatric Chiropractic. Williams & Wilkins, Baltimore.

Barcz, E., Sommer, E., Nartowska, J., et al., 2007. Influence of *Echinacea purpurea* intake during pregnancy on fetal growth and angiogenic activity. Folia Histochem. Cytobiol. 45 (Suppl. 1), S35–S39.

Bernstein, J., Ellis, E., Li, P., 1981. The role of IgE mediated hypersensitivity in otitis media with effusion. J. Otolaryngol. Head Neck Surg. 89 (5), 874–878.

Bhaskar, S.N., 1986. Synopsis of Oral Pathology. Mosby, St Louis.

Bluestone, C., 1994. Otitis media with effusion in young children. Abstracts of Clinical Care Guidelines 6 (10), 1–6.

Chicca, A., Raduner, S., Pellati, F., et al., 2009. Synergistic immunopharmacological effects of N-alkylamides in *Echinacea purpurea* herbal extracts. Int. Immunopharmacol. 9 (7–8), 850–858.

Davidson, R.G., 1988. Atlantoaxial instability in individuals with Down syndrome: a fresh look at the evidence. Pediatrics 81 (6), 857–865.

Ely, J., Holberg, C., Aldous, M., et al., 1995. Passive smoke exposure and otitis media in the first year of life. Pediatrics 95 (5), 670–677.

Fireman, P., 1997a. Otitis media and eustachian tube dysfunction: connection to allergic rhinitis. J. Allergy Clin. Immunol. 99 (2), S787–S797.

Fireman, P., 1997b. Otitis media and its relation to allergic rhinitis. Allergy Asthma Proc. 18 (3), 135–143.

Freeman, C., Spelman, K., 2008. A critical evaluation of drug interactions with *Echinacea* spp. Mol. Nutr. Food Res. 52 (7), 789–798.

Froehle, R., 1996. Ear infection: a retrospective study examination improvement from chiropractic care and analysing for influencing factors. J. Manipulative Physiol. Ther. 19 (3), 169–177.

Gatterman, M., 1995. Foundations of Chiropractic: Subluxation. Mosby, St Louis, p. 157, 182.

Golz, A., Angel-Yeger, B., Joachims, H., et al., 1997. Balance disturbances in children with middle ear effusions. Harefuah 133 (11), 518–521.

Gutmann, G., 1987. Blocked atlantal nerve syndrome in babies and infants. Man. Med. 25, 5–10.

Hawk, C., Khorsan, R., Lisi, A.J., et al., 2007. Chiropractic care for nonmusculoskeletal conditions: a systematic review with implications for whole systems research. J. Altern. Complement. Med. 13 (5), 491–512.

Homewood, A.E., 1981. The Neurodynamics of the Vertebral Subluxation. Valkrie Press, St Petersburg, Florida.

La Francis, M., 1990. A chiropractic perspective on atlantoaxial instability in Down's syndrome. J. Manipulative Physiol. Ther. 13 (3), 157–160.

Langford, J.H., Benrimoj, S.I., 1996. Clinical rationale for topical antimicrobial preparations. J. Antimicrob. Chemother. 37, 399–402.

Lous, J., Burton, M.J., Felding, J.U., et al., 2005. Grommets (ventilation tubes) for hearing loss associated with otitis media with effusion in children. Cochrane Database Syst. Rev. 25 (1): CD001801.

Maran, A.G.D, 1988. Logan Turner's Diseases of the Nose, Throat and Ear, tenth ed. John Wright, London.

Marcy, M., Takata, G., Shekelle, P., et al., 2000. Management of Acute Otitis Media: Evidence Report/Technology Assessment No. 15 (AHRQ Publication No. 01-E010). US Department of Health and Human Services, Rockville, MD.

Mendelsohn, R., 1990. How to Raise a Healthy Child in Spite of Your Doctor. Ballantine Books, Chicago.

Mullins, R., 1998. *Echinacea*-associated anaphylaxis. Med. J. Aust. 168 (4), 170–171.

Neskey, D., Elov, J.A., Casiano, R.R., 2009. Nasal, septal and turbinate anatomy and embryology. Otolaryngol. Clin. North Am. 42 (2), 193–205.

Ong, Y.K., Tan, H.K., 2002. Suppurative intracranial complications of sinusitis in children. Int. J. Pediatr. Otorhinolaryngol. 66 (1), 49.

Ouraishi, H., Zevallos, J.P., 2006. Subdural empyema as a complication of sinusitis in the pediatric population. Int. J. Pediatr. Otorhinolaryngol. 70 (9), 1581–1586.

Plaugher, G., 1993. Textbook of Clinical Chiropractic: A Specific Biomechanical Approach. Williams & Wilkins, Baltimore.

Roland, P.S., Stroman, D.W., 2002. Microbiology of acute otitis externa. Laryngoscope 112, 1166–1177.

Sarrell, E.M., Cohen, H.A., Kahan, E., 2003. Naturopathic treatment for ear pain in children. Pediatrics 111 (5/1), e574–e579.

Schmidt, M., 1996. Healing Childhood Ear Infections. North Atlantic Books, Berkeley.

Sharma, M., Schoop, R., Hudson, J.B., 2008. Echinacea as an antiinflammatory agent: the influence of physiologically relevant parameters. Phytother. Res. 23 (6), 863–867.

Slack, R., Maw, A., Capper, J., et al., 1984. Prospective study of tympanosclerosis developing after grommet insertion. J. Laryngol. Otol. 98 (8), 771–774.

Wetmore, R.F., 2007. Pediatric Otolaryngology: The Requisites in Pediatrics. Mosby Elsevier, Philadelphia.

Zitelli, B.J., Davis, H.W 1997. Atlas of Pediatric Physical Diagnosis, third ed. Mosby-Wolfe, St Louis.

The enuretic child

Neil J. Davies   Ailsa van Poecke

Primary nocturnal enuresis (PNE), or bedwetting as it is commonly referred to, can be a distressing complaint for both the child and the parents. This socially difficult condition causes many children to feel embarrassed and to avoid talking about the condition (Ng & Wong 2004), preventing their participation in sleepovers, school camps and other activities. Additionally the parents are faced with the added tasks of caring for a child who wets the bed. Not all families handle this situation well and it remains an all too common occurrence for frustrated parents to be critical of their bedwetting child and to implement punitive procedures to 'correct' perceived laziness.

Bedwetting not only frustrates the child and parents, but its cause and 'best treatment' remain obscure to health care providers. This has resulted in the development of the plethora of traditional treatments currently available, most of which concentrate on behavioral therapies and medication regimens (Nijman et al 2002). Box 13.1 details some commonly used methods of treatment for bedwetting. While some of these treatment protocols are successful some of the time, much discussion has ensued as to why some children respond and others do not, and yet others show considerable rates of relapse (Bath et al 1996, Rombis et al 2005, van Poecke & Cunliffe 2009). The heterogeneous nature of study inclusion parameters often makes clarification of the wide-ranging response rates difficult (Butler & Gasson 2005). Responses to alarm treatment have been reported as between 30% and 87% (Butler & Gasson 2005) and are thought to be greatly reliant on the ability of the child to be aroused by the alarm (Butler & Robinson 2002). Additionally, the efficacy of treatment with desmopressin has been questioned (Bath et al 1996, Devitt et al 1999, Hunsballe et al 1998, Lee et al 2005, Medel et al 1998, Neveus et al 2005, Radvanska et al 2006, Rombis et al 2005). Furthermore, some treatments rely at least to some extent on family compliance, a notoriously negative factor in management planning. It is important to note that the collection of epidemiological data on any population sample that, at any given point in time, is variably affected by neurological dysafferentation may produce flawed or misleading information to a greater or lesser extent, especially when it can be demonstrated that the natural history of the condition being studied can be significantly changed in a percentage of that population by the provision of chiropractic care.

The natural history of nocturnal enuresis

When do children normally stop wetting their bed? In order to understand the problem of nocturnal enuresis, an appreciation of the normal developmental range is necessary. It has been reported in the literature (Dodge et al 1970) that by age 4–5, 85% of boys and 90% of girls are dry at night. There were no racial differences between Caucasian and black children identified in this study of American children. However, Kanaheswari (2003), in a study of 3371 urban-dwelling primary school children in Kuala Lumpur, Malaysia, noted that primary enuresis was reported in only 6.2% of children and secondary enuresis in 1.8%, figures that were reflective of the situation in both Korea and Taiwan. It was further noted in this study that these figures are generally lower than those reported in first world countries. Illingworth (1987), however, indicates that being mainly dry at night by 3 years for both boys and girls is an essential milestone of development, an assessment for which he finds support from Hull & Johnston (1999). Behrman et al (2007), on the other hand, claim that bladder control may not be established until age 4 years and therefore no child should be deemed enuretic until at least that age. Touchette et al (2005) conclude that children who do not attain the developmental milestones may be demonstrating delayed development of the CNS and an increased risk for PNE. While it may be the case that children of 3 years of age should be mainly dry at night, some report that treatment is rarely undertaken before the age of 6 years, even though only 5% of 4-year-olds who continue to be wet at night achieve spontaneous resolution (Lissauer & Clayden 2003)

© 2010, Elsevier Ltd, Inc, BV
DOI: 10.1016/B978-0-7020-3129-8.00013-X

Box 13.1

Some of the commonly employed methods for treating primary nocturnal enuresis

Bell and pad

A pad which is connected to a loud bell is placed on the child's bed. When wetting begins, the bell sounds, waking the child, who is then expected to void in the toilet. This method has had some degree of success in converting nocturnal enuresis into nocturia.

Imipramine

This medication, also known as Tofranil, is an antidepressant medication normally prescribed for patients with a major depressive disorder, anxiety or attention deficit disorder which is unresponsive to stimulants such as Ritalin. Tofranil is only briefly effective in controlling bedwetting, the response seldom outlasting the administration period. There are several serious side-effects such as hypotension, hypertension, tachycardia, restlessness, nightmares, dry mouth, and occasionally blood dyscrasias.

Voiding exercises

This treatment requires the child to force fluids during the day and hold the urine as long as possible in order to stretch the bladder. When the child urinates, the urine is caught in a glass measuring cup in order to determine the urinary output. This process is continued for 3–6 months and requires considerable cooperation and persistence by the parents and patient.

Rewards

This is not so much a system of treatment as a form of encouragement for having a dry night. A daily chart is devised and stars or another symbol are placed on the days following a dry night. After an agreed number of consecutive dry nights, the child is rewarded with a small gift, an outing, or a treat of some kind.

From the chiropractic perspective, it seems reasonable to follow the guideline established by Illingworth (1987), who is widely regarded as having produced the standard reference volume on developmental pediatrics, that children should be mainly dry by 3 years of age. Any child who wets consistently beyond that age should be considered for chiropractic management.

Familial, social and congenital factors in nocturnal enuresis

Given that Illingworth's guideline of mainly dry by 3 years of age is an acceptable benchmark for establishing a diagnosis of nocturnal enuresis, the chiropractic clinician needs to bear in mind that genetic (von Gontard et al 2001) and congenital factors have been suggested as important etiological aspects in the development of bladder control. McMillan et al (1982) reported enuresis at the age of 4–5 years in up to 43.5% of children who had one parent (either mother or father) who was enuretic at the same age. Similarly, Jarvelin et al (1988) found that a child with a father who had been enuretic after 4 years of age had a 7.1 times greater risk of having nocturnal enuresis; with a mother who had been enuretic, the risk was 5 times greater. McMillan et al (1982)

further reported enuresis in 77.3% of children aged 4–5 years from families where both parents were enuretic at the same age. There is also a high correlation in monozygotic twins. By contrast, only 15% of children from a family where neither parent had been enuretic were enuretic at age 4–5 years. More recent studies have also found particular chromosomal associations. Linkage had been found to markers on chromosome 22 (Loeys et al 2002, von Gontard et al 1999) and also to marker sites on chromosomes 12 and 13 (Eiberg et al 1995, Loeys et al 2002). It has also been suggested that children with a family history of PNE may demonstrate functional cortical differences (Freitag et al 2006). In addition to the familial nature of enuresis a male dominance has also been noted. Some variance exists as to the precise ratio but male preponderance is consistently reported (Butler & Gasson 2005, Chiozza et al 1998, Rawashdeh et al 2002, Wen et al 2006, Yeung et al 2006).

Taking a careful family history will enable the chiropractor to properly advise the family of a child with nocturnal enuresis in order to avoid making the mistake of raising expectations unnecessarily. Family pedigrees involving a presentation where there is no familial factor and a second case where there is no strong male-related factor for three generations are shown in Figs 13.1 and 13.2 respectively.

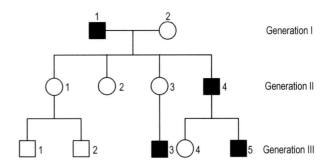

Figure 13.1 ● Pedigree table for a child (generation III, number 3) presenting with primary enuresis. There is no suggestion of familial predisposition to enuresis. This child has the best possible chance of a positive response to chiropractic care provided there is no evidence of pathology or congenital abnormality.

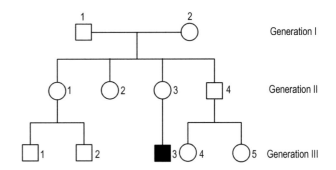

Figure 13.2 ● Pedigree table for a child (generation III, number 3) presenting with primary enuresis. There is a strongly positive family history extending over three generations and also involving a male cousin. This child has the most limited possible chance of a good response to chiropractic care.

A number of psychosocial aspects have also been recognized. Large family size (Cher et al 2002, Oge et al 2001) poses an increased risk for nocturnal enuresis, as does the parental educational level and low parental socioeconomic class (Cher et al 2002, Devlin 1991, Gumus et al 1999, Oge et al 2001, Ozkan et al 2004). Other psychosocial factors that have been recognized include an increased risk for those children whose mothers smoke at least 10 cigarettes per day and who were aged less than 20 at the child's birth (Rona et al 1997). Finally, but by no means exclusively, when considering the plethora of psychosocial factors (Butler 2004) which may play a role in the enuretic etiology, the impact that breastfeeding may have on PNE should be considered. The most recent study on this topic performed by Barone et al (2006) suggests that breastfeeding for longer than 3 months may protect against bedwetting during childhood.

In addition to familial and social factors, a number of congenital anomalies can cause a child to wet well beyond the normal age of bladder control. Chief among these are spina bifida, ureteric stricture and myelomeningocele. A careful history and physical examination are required in order to identify these conditions. It should be noted that psychological problems have been reported in the literature (Cher et al 2002, Devlin 1991, Gumus et al 1999, Oge et al 2001, Ozkan et al 2004) to be linked to PNE and need to be taken into account in any proposed management plan.

Pathological and other factors in nocturnal enuresis

A number of significant pathologies also contribute to the etiology of nocturnal enuresis (Gür et al 2004). Their prevalence is small, but awareness of such conditions is nevertheless vital in correctly assessing the enuretic child. Urinary tract infection must always be excluded, although it represents an exceedingly low etiological rate of 0.25% (Gür et al 2004). Box 13.2 identifies a list of potential clinical conditions that may be encountered by a chiropractor consulting enuretic children in the primary care setting. Clearly, a detailed history and thorough physical examination are required in order to identify these uncommon but important conditions. The clinical history should seek to identify symptoms of infection such as fever, flank and other abdominal pain, and other symptoms such as headache, edema, failure to thrive, convulsions, or a known history of hypertension. The frequency with which the child urinates (Table 13.1) should be recorded (Green 1998) in addition to the volume of urine (Behrman et al 2007) (Table 13.2). Where possible, an estimation of the child's fluid intake should also be recorded. Any known history of congenital or developmental anomalies should be noted, as detailed earlier in this chapter. Sleep pattern is important since consistently disturbed sleep suggests chronic anxiety that may be related to the child's bedwetting.

A search of the family history should be made for any evidence of renal disease, deafness, hypertension, renal calculi, anomalies of renal tract development or syndromes known to be associated with renal disease such as polycystic kidney disease. A psychological and psychosocial profile of both the

Box 13.2

Organic conditions that may be found to cause bedwetting in children beyond the age when bladder control would normally be expected to develop

Obstructive lesions
- Urethral valves
- Ectopic ureters
- Urethral stricture
- Meatal stenosis
- Contraction of the neck of the bladder
- Labial atresia
- Phimosis

Neurogenic disorders
- Occult neuropathic bladder
- Seizures
- Spinal cord injuries
- Spinal cord tumors

Infection
- Urinary tract infection
- Vertebral body osteomyelitis
- Genital infection from sexual abuse in females

Metabolic
- Diabetes insipidus
- Diabetes mellitus

Table 13.1 Frequency with which children usually urinate at different ages

Age	Number of times to void/day
Infancy	6–30
1–2 years	May remain dry for up to 2 hours
3–5 years	8–14
5–8 years	6–12
8–14 years	The child slowly approaches the adult pattern of 6–8

Table 13.2 Expected average daily urinary output according to age (adapted from Forfar & Arneil 1973 with permission)

Age	Average daily urinary output
1–3 years	500–600 ml
3–4 years	800–700 ml
5–7 years	650–1000 ml
8–14 years	800–1400 ml

child and the family is helpful; in particular, details of the child's progress at school and interaction with peers may provide information critical to the final diagnosis. Finally, any evidence at either history-taking or examination of non-accidental injury, sexual or deprivational abuse should be identified.

Constipation

It has been recognized that the enuretic child also frequently suffers from constipation (Foreman & Thambirajah 1996, Kalo & Bella 1996, O'Regan et al 1986). Constipation has also been recognized as a risk factor for PNE (O'Regan et al 1986) and it has additionally been suggested that constipation should be treated before treatment for PNE can occur (Hirasing 1994). Recognizing through history and physical examination that the child may be suffering from constipation is therefore of significant clinical importance in planning a management strategy.

Secondary or regressive bedwetting

Secondary or regressive bedwetting describes a child who has demonstrated a period of nighttime control of at least 6 months and suddenly begins wetting again (Caldwell et al 2005). The wetting is usually episodic, but may be every night. The great majority of patients who exhibit this pattern of enuresis do so as a result of environmental stressors causing psychological problems or the development of organic pathology (Caldwell et al 2005, Petermann et al 2004). It is never due to congenital abnormality. A careful history and physical examination are essential when confronted with a secondary bedwetter as this will usually reveal the etiology, most of which will need to be considered by the chiropractor. The most common psychological and pathological causes of regressive bedwetting are shown in Table 13.3.

While the chiropractic subluxation may be solely responsible for regressive bedwetting, it would be dangerous simply to make this assumption and implement care before conducting a wider search for other possible causes. It is critical to

Table 13.3 Causes of secondary or regressive enuresis likely to be encountered by the chiropractor at the primary care interface

Category	Cause
Psychological	Most common cause of secondary bedwetting
	Domestic and marital disharmony
	Child abuse and excessive discipline
	School-related stress
	Chronic anxiety, depression, etc.
Neurogenic disorders	Seizures
	Spinal cord injuries
	Spinal cord tumors
Infection	Urinary tract infection
	Vertebral body osteomyelitis
	Genital infection from sexual abuse in females
Metabolic	Diabetes insipidus
	Diabetes mellitus
Neoplastic	Wilms' tumor
	Neuroblastoma
Trauma	Physical trauma resulting in subluxation, particularly of S2/3, the lumbosacral junction and the upper cervical complex

Case study 13.1

Regressive bedwetting

A 10-year-old male child presents with episodic bedwetting over a 2-year period after having previously been dry at night for approximately 3 years. On careful questioning, the patient's father was able to identify a particularly stressful event which, in his opinion, precipitated the wetting. The child, then 8 years old, unexpectedly came home from school because of illness and witnessed his mother having sexual intercourse with a man he did not know. The subsequent breakdown of the marriage and parental separation became increasingly acrimonious until the mother finally moved to a city at some distance from the family home. The episodes of wetting, most of which lasted between 3 and 10 days, invariably followed phone conversations with the mother who apparently called every 2–3 weeks.

The child was referred to a pediatric psychologist and on her advice the father monitored the next phone call from the mother who told the child he was 'not wanted in the first place' and is the 'reason for all the trouble now'. The child also exhibited craniosacral subluxation, the correction of which, along with a parental blockade of the abusive phone calls, quickly resolved the problem.

remember, however, that even in the event of a psychological or pathological etiology being identified, the subluxation will almost always be a coexistent factor, demanding concurrent care in order to produce an optimal patient outcome. In any event, it remains that recruitment of other health care providers, particularly child psychologists, in the management of regressive bedwetting is axiomatic to good management.

The dominant role of psychological stress in the pathogenesis of regressive enuresis is clearly demonstrated in Case study 13.1.

Evaluation of the enuretic child

After completing the clinical history, physical examination and investigation of the urine, radiographic evaluation should be carried out when indicated. The essential elements of the physical examination that should form a routine part of the chiropractic evaluation include the following:

Inspection

The whole of the child's body should be carefully inspected in order to identify pallor associated with renal infection, skin lesions or hair patches suggestive of underlying neurological disease (Alexander 2005), and any non-accidental injury or other forms of child abuse. If it is possible, male children should be observed urinating to check the force of the urinary stream. Obstructive lesions significantly diminish the force with which a child can urinate.

Anthropometry

Head circumference, height, weight, arm span, upper and lower body ratios, and sitting height should all be measured, the values obtained being plotted on appropriate percentile charts where available. Shortness of stature or deviations from normal body ratios are consistent with chronic renal disease (Derakhshan et al 2007, Habel 1982, Lewy & New 1975, Pasqualini & Ferraris 2003, Qayyum et al 2003, Rocchini 1984, Stickler 1976) in addition to being underweight for age in failure-to-thrive syndrome (Tunnessen 1983).

Blood pressure

Elevated systole is strongly suggestive of renal hypertension (Swinford & Portman 2004). A variety of studies also reported by Rocchini (1984) demonstrate that between 60% and 80% of all children with hypertension also have renal disease. Other authors have suggested that 38% of children with chronic kidney disease are having concomitant treatment for hypertension (Swinford & Portman 2004). Measured values should be plotted on appropriate normal distribution graphs in order to identify shifts up or down in either systole or diastole. In a child free of overt signs of disease, however, a diagnosis of systolic hypertension can only be made after three measurements over a 6–12-month period all show an elevated systole (Rocchini 1984, Salgado & Cavalhaes 2003).

Pulse and respiratory rates

In the presence of renal infection, it is common to see an elevated pulse rate and less commonly an elevated respiratory rate or increased depth of respiration (Tunnessen 1983).

Temperature

The core body temperature is routinely measured in enuretic children and the parents or caregiver asked if any elevation has been observed. Infection in the urinary tract may cause the onset of bedwetting in a previously dry child. Elevated temperature may, of course, be present in children with urinary tract infections (Shaikh et al 2007).

Neurological

The patient should be neurologically examined from the waist down. The extent of the examination is shown in Table 13.4.

Table 13.4 The extent of the neurological examination required in all children presenting with primary nocturnal enuresis

Aspect of examination	Observation/response
Muscle stretch reflexes	Patella (L4) and Achilles (S1)
Other reflexes	Babinski, cremasteric, perianal, and umbilical
Motor	Each muscle group in the pelvis and lower extremity should be assessed for tone and graded for strength (0–5)
Sensory	Each dermatome from T12 downwards should be evaluated
Vibration	Comparison bilaterally over bony prominences at the hips, knees, and ankles

Table 13.5 Orthopedic tests that should ideally be carried out in all children presenting with primary nocturnal enuresis

Patient position	Name or description of test
Sitting	Slump test
	Sitting straight leg raise
	Kemp's test
Supine	Straight leg raise
Prone	Lumbar springing test

Orthopedic

Tests that suggest dysfunction of the lumbar spine and pelvis should be routinely carried out and correlated with the neurological examination. While there are many tests that may be performed, those shown in Table 13.5 are adequate to demonstrate a significant orthopedic problem. It may occasionally be necessary to perform other tests in order to clarify a situation where the principal orthopedic problem is outside the lumbar spine, such as would be seen in hip pathology, etc. The principal reason for performing the orthopedic examination and correlating it to the neurological assessment is to identify concomitant pathology and the need for further investigation.

Abdominal

A careful abdominal examination is essential in order to identify palpable lesions of the kidneys, masses in the lower abdominal quadrants, emptying deficits of the bladder, and malformations in the external genitalia of male patients. Palpation of the left lower quadrant should identify any fecal masses which may be suggestive of constipation.

Spinal

The usual thorough chiropractic spinal assessment to identify both the level and directional vectors involved in the subluxation complex will obviously form a major part of the physical examination.

In addition to the physical examination, the following investigations are appropriate:

Radiological

The X-ray examination will only be necessary in young children when a neurological deficit has been demonstrated suggesting the possibility of a congenital malformation or other acquired lesion of the lumbar spine or pelvic area.

Urine analysis

The urine should be evaluated in all cases of enuresis in both males and females. The chemical evaluation is used to identify the presence of glycosuria, pus cells, protein or blood, and to measure urinary osmolality (specific gravity). A low osmolality in the presence of glycosuria raises the possibility of diabetes as a diagnosis, while pus cells, protein or blood all suggest infection. All females who present with enuresis should also have a microscopic urinary assessment that would include an attempt to culture bacteria (Bagga 2001, Green 1998). It is worthy of note that 1–4% of school-age girls and up to 0.2% of school-age boys (Green 1998, Hull & Johnston 1999) have asymptomatic bacteriuria which was once considered a manifestation of active infection. It is now thought to be of questionable clinical significance in school-age children and definitely not a cause of enuresis (Hull & Johnston 1999).

Clinical decision-making in primary nocturnal enuresis

The decision to implement chiropractic care in a child presenting with primary nocturnal enuresis is driven by the need first to demonstrate the absence of clinical factors which would demand either further diagnostic investigation such as voiding cystourethrography, excretory urography or CT scanning, or referral for concomitant treatment such as antibiotic therapy or psychological counseling. The courses of action necessitated by various examination and investigation outcomes of children with nocturnal enuresis are shown in Box 13.3.

Box 13.3

Outcomes of clinical history, physical examination and diagnostic investigations that would imply the need for referral to a pediatric specialist for further investigation or concomitant management

Clinical history

- Diurnal enuresis (daytime incontinence)
- Evidence of child abuse
- Parental report of polydipsia
- Evidence of psychological etiology (regressive enuresis)
- Night terrors, nightmares and sleep disorders

Physical examination

- Hypertension (elevated systole)
- Widened pulse pressure
- Polyuria
- Evidence of child abuse
- Weak urinary stream in male patients
- Abdominal mass
- Shortness of stature with no previous family history

Diagnostic investigations

- Evidence of infection on urinalysis
- Low urinary osmolality (specific gravity = 1.000 to 1.002)
- Glycosuria
- Gross structural malformation of lumbar spine on X-ray
- Evidence of spinal pathology

Chiropractic management of primary nocturnal enuresis

Once the diagnosis of primary nocturnal enuresis, not complicated by any of the clinical symptoms or signs shown in Box 13.3, has been established, a chiropractic management plan may be safely and carefully implemented. While adjusting the subluxation alone will occasionally produce excellent clinical outcomes, consistent results are more likely when the parents and child are encouraged to adopt a number of home-based strategies in addition to the child's chiropractic visits.

The first step in implementing a broad-based care program for an enuretic child is to establish the degree to which the patient is voiding urine during waking hours. The volume measured is then compared to the expected daily output derived on an age basis using the data in Table 13.2. It is usually best to measure daily urinary output on a weekend when both the child and parents are at home. On each visit to the toilet the child is asked to void into a glass measuring container and the total for each urination recorded. The total at the end of the day is then compared to expected urinary output as per Table 13.2 and entered into the clinical record as a percentage.

After the last urination for the day, the child is put to bed. Between 60 and 90 minutes after the onset of sleep, the child should be awakened and, provided they are not already wet, encouraged to void into the measuring container again. These measurements provide the basis for calculating the percentage of expected daily urinary output after as little as 60 minutes of REM sleep, making the protocol of waking them to void a very useful one when combined with adjusting and other home-based strategies to be discussed later in this chapter. Box 13.4 gives an example calculation for daily urinary output for such a patient.

In the child with constipation, it is ideal to attempt to resolve it prior to initiating treatment for nocturnal enuresis (Hirasing et al 2004).

Box 13.4

Example calculation for daily urinary output in primary nocturnal enuresis

Patient characteristics: age = 6 years; weight = 24 kg

Expected daily urinary output: 50 ml/kg body weight = 1200 ml

Actual waking hours output:

7.00	=	102 ml
9.30	=	100 ml
13.00	=	86 ml
15.30	=	75 ml
17.30	=	105 ml
20.30	=	108 ml
Total	=	576 ml (48%)

Output after 90 minutes of REM sleep: 444 ml (37%)

This patient has such a significant level of urinary output on awakening that implementing the protocol of waking to void each evening in an attempt to modify a behavioral pattern is an appropriate management strategy when combined with adjusting the subluxation. Taken alone, waking a child after 90 minutes of sleep to void is seldom successful in the long term.

The next step, prior to giving the first chiropractic adjustment, is to provide basic counseling to the parents or caregivers in relation to the etiology and natural history of primary nocturnal enuresis. This aspect of the management strategy is critical. The three-generation family pedigree charts should be carefully explained to the parents, making sure that they understand the significance of the family history in terms of probable clinical outcome for their child. Unreal patient and parent expectations are very difficult to manage should they perceive the treatment program to be failing and may become the cause of a great deal of unnecessary frustration. A clear understanding of the factors that are known to have a bearing on clinical outcome will go a long way toward averting such a reaction should the child not respond to treatment.

Poor parental response to a child's bedwetting can result in serious psychological problems later on. The psychosocial etiology of bedwetting necessarily requires that these issues should be addressed before treatment can be effective (Cher et al 2002, Devlin 1991, Gumus et al 1999, Oge et al 2001, Ozkan et al 2004). Clearly this may require a very tactful approach in educating parents who may be struggling with what they perceive to be a difficult social problem. This is especially true in a family where there may be several siblings and one is a bedwetter (Cher et al 2002, Oge et al 2001). Furthermore, obscurities and contradictory information have been recognized when analyzing the self-reports of enuretic children regarding anxiety/depression and being withdrawn, with parents perceiving their children as internalizing problems to a greater degree than do the children themselves (van Hoecke et al 2004). Parents should be carefully counseled to avoid, at all costs, making comments to their child such as:

'You are lazy and would rather urinate in your bed than get up and go to the toilet.'

'You are just dirty and you smell really bad – why don't you just stop wetting.'

'You are a big nuisance and you just make more work for your mother.'

'If you don't stop wetting I will smack you hard.'

In place of these groundless, inappropriate comments, parents should be encouraged to positively affirm the child for each dry night and to positively console the child after a wet night. Parents should also be encouraged to identify exacerbating factors and attempt to limit their effect on the child. Getting to bed very late, drinking just before bedtime, television programs and video games which overstimulate the child immediately before going to bed are all examples of exacerbating factors which parents can help the child to avoid. In the 15 minutes or so before bedtime, it is wise to keep the child calm and quiet. It is usually helpful to read a favorite story in bed, pray with the child or just have a quiet cuddle. This all helps to produce a sense of acquiescence in preparation for sleep. These bedtime strategies are particularly important in children who have anxieties about the night, darkness or dreams they may anticipate having. It is always appropriate to leave the door open or a nightlight burning if that brings comfort.

Having the parents implement the strategy of keeping a daily star chart where the child sticks a star against each day

Monday	Tuesday	Wednesday	Thursday	Friday	Saturday	Sunday
★	★	Wet (x1)	Wet (x1)	★	Wet (x2) Party	Wet (x1)
Wet (x1)	Wet (x1)	★	Wet (x1)	Wet (x1)	★	Wet (x1)
Wet (x1)	Wet (x2) School upset	Wet (x1)	Wet (x1)	Wet (x1)	Wet (x1)	Wet (x1)
Wet (x1)	★	★	Wet (x1)	Wet (x1)	Wet (x1)	Wet (x1)
Wet (x1)	Wet (x1)	★				

Figure 13.3 • A star chart kept by the parents of an enuretic child for a continuous period of 1 month.

on which he or she was dry can enhance positive affirmation (Glazener & Evans 2004) for a dry night. Fig. 13.3 is an example of a star chart that has been kept for a month.

In addition to providing positive affirmation for the achievement of a dry night, the star chart record provides the chiropractor with a means of determining percentage change from wet to dry nights on a month-to-month basis. It also provides a visual means of identifying patterns of wetting which may have some influence on management planning or counseling. For example, the child represented by the star chart in Fig. 13.4 is wetting because of being subject to bullying at school.

Monday	Tuesday	Wednesday	Thursday	Friday	Saturday	Sunday
★	Wet (x1)	Wet (x1)	Wet (x1)	Wet (x1)	★	★
Wet (x1)	Wet (x1)	Wet (x1)	Wet (x1)	★	★	★
Wet (x1)	Wet (x2) School upset	Wet (x1)	Wet (x1)	Wet (x1)	★	★
Wet (x1)	Wet (x1)	Wet (x1)	Wet (x1)	★	★	★
Wet (x1)	Wet (x1)	Wet (x1)				

Figure 13.4 • A star chart kept on an enuretic child who is receiving chiropractic care. The obvious pattern shown by this chart indicates that there may be some stress during the week that causes the child to wet that is not present on the weekend. Subsequent enquiry identified that this child was the subject of constant schoolground bullying.

In addition to the child placing stars on it, the chart also provides parents with an opportunity to make brief notes of what they may consider to be of importance or think may have influenced the pattern of wetting. Such comments as 'late to bed', 'attended friend's party' or 'upset because mother in hospital' would represent appropriate comments which could possibly help the chiropractor to interpret the pattern of wetting and plan future management.

Finally, the star chart may be used in conjunction with another positive affirmation protocol, that of providing rewards when an agreed number of consecutive dry nights have been achieved. Parents should be encouraged to negotiate a reward of, say, five consecutive dry nights. When the star chart has five consecutive entries, the child then duly receives the agreed reward. Rewards and star charts are an excellent way to gain maximum family compliance in the management of the enuretic child in addition to helping create a positive and affirming environment at home.

Lastly, after all the above strategies have been put in place, the pattern of neurological dysafferentation must be identified and corrected. By far the most common area of the body to have a direct cause–effect relationship with enuresis is that involving the sacral segments. Occasionally, dysafferentation affecting the upper cervical complex and less commonly the thoracolumbar and lumbosacral junction areas may also be involved as a cause of the child's wetting (Davies 1997). Clear understanding of the principle 'less is better' is critical to producing consistently good outcomes in enuretic children. The first adjustment carries by far the most potency to correct the dysafferentation (Himes, personal communication, 1975) and, after it is given, the chiropractor should be loath to attempt any further intrusions for several weeks to several months. Only in the event that a child has stopped wetting and started again, or has experienced some sort of trauma which could reasonably make the subluxation recur, should further correction be attempted inside this period of time. Overadjusting probably represents the most common reason for failure in enuretic children who have a negative family history. Recent research (van Poecke 2007) has suggested that children who respond to chiropractic treatment for enuresis using the Neuro Impulse Protocol (NIP) received only 2.04 ± 1.32 adjustments with a 12-month period. Cranial

subluxations and dysfunction of the craniosacral primary respiratory mechanism in general are frequently identified as existing secondary to the primary subluxation complex. These cranial problems should be corrected using respiratory assisted procedures concurrently with the subluxation or they tend to cause primary subluxation recurrence, presumably via the mechanism of somatosomatic reflex.

It is recommended that review visits for children with enuresis should generally be scheduled at 2-weekly intervals for the first month, monthly for the next 3 months, then 3-monthly until resolution occurs. This pattern would obviously be affected by clinical factors demanding a greater frequency such as trauma, infection that involved a lot of coughing, etc.

It is not uncommon to see resolution of bedwetting in as little as 2–4 weeks with recurrences due to subluxation resolving within days (Blomerth 1994). Certainly in those children who respond to chiropractic treatment, 80% will have shown a change in their wet night frequency 1 month after the delivery of the first adjustment (van Poecke & Cunliffe 2009).

Chiropractic management of secondary enuresis

Once a child has been identified as a secondary bedwetter, it becomes the responsibility of the chiropractor to network other health care providers as required by the underlying diagnosis. The two most frequently needed practitioners to assist in the management of secondary enuresis will be the child psychologist and the pediatric physician. At the psychological level, counseling will usually be of great benefit in aiding the child to cope with whatever stress is causing the bedwetting and, as a direct result, will assist the chiropractor to maintain correction of the subluxation complex. The range of organic pathologies known to cause secondary bedwetting will, of course, need to be managed by the pediatric physician. In particular, treatment of urinary tract infection which has caused regressive wetting, especially where proteinuria has been demonstrated, requires the care of a pediatric specialist (Lerner 1994). Concurrent chiropractic care remains an imperative if optimal clinical outcome is to be achieved.

References

Alexander, M.A., 2005. Spina Bifida. KidsHealth, Nemours Foundation, Wilmington.

Bagga, A., 2001. Urinary tract infections: evaluation and treatment. Indian J. Pediatr. 69 (Suppl. 3), S40–S45.

Barone, J.G., Ramasamy, R., Farkas, A., et al., 2006. Breastfeeding during pregnancy may protect against bed-wetting during childhood. Pediatrics 118 (1), 254–259.

Bath, R., Morton, R., Uing, A., et al., 1996. Nocturnal enuresis and the use of desmopressin – is it helpful? Child Care Health Dev. 22 (2), 73–84.

Behrman, R.E., Jenson, H.B., Nelson, W.E., et al., 2007. Nelson Textbook of Pediatrics, eighteenth ed. WB Saunders, Philadelphia.

Blomerth, P.R., 1994. Functional nocturnal enuresis. J. Manipulative Physiol. Ther. 17 (5), 335–338.

Butler, R.J., 2004. Childhood nocturnal enuresis: developing a conceptual framework. Clin. Psychol. Rev. 24, 909–931.

Butler, R.J., Gasson, S.I., 2005. Enuresis alarm treatment. Scand. J. Urol. Nephrol. 39 (5), 349–357.

Butler, R.J., Robinson, J.C., 2002. Alarm treatment for childhood nocturnal enuresis: an investigation of within-treatment variables. Scand. J. Urol. Nephrol. 36 (4), 268–272.

Caldwell, P.H.Y., Edgar, D., Hodson, E., et al., 2005. Bedwetting and toileting problems

in children. Med. J. Aust. 182 (4), 190–195.

Cher, T.W., Lin, G.J., Hsu, K.H., 2002. Prevalence of nocturnal enuresis and associated familial factors in primary school children in Taiwan. J. Urol. 168 (3), 1142–1146.

Chiozza, M.L., Bernardinelli, L., Caione, P., et al., 1998. An Italian epidemiological multicentre study of nocturnal enuresis. Br. J. Urol. 81 (Suppl. 3), 86–89.

Davies, N.J., 1997. Case Study Manual as Part of the Master of Chiropractic Science (Paedatrics) Degree Course, RMIT University, Melbourne.

Derakhshan, A., Karamifar, H., Razavi Nejad, S.M., et al., 2007. Evaluation of insulin like growth factor-1(IGF-1) in children with different stages of chronic renal failure. Saudi J. Kidney Dis. Transpl. 18 (2), 173–176.

Devitt, H., Holland, P., Butler, R., et al., 1999. Plasma vasopressin and response to treatment in primary nocturnal enuresis. Arch. Dis. Child. 80 (5), 448–451.

Devlin, J.B., 1991. Prevalence and risk factors for childhood nocturnal enuresis. Ir. Med. J. 84 (4), 118–120.

Dodge, W.F., West, E.F., Bridgforth, E.B., et al., 1970. Nocturnal enuresis in 6- to 10- year-old children. Correlation with bacteriuria, proteinuria and dysuria. Am. J. Dis. Child. 120 (1), 32–35.

Eiberg, H., Berendt, I., Mohr, J., 1995. Assignment of dominant inherited nocturnal enuresis (ENUR1) to chromosome 13q. Nat. Genet. 10 (3), 354–356.

Foreman, D.M., Thambirajah, M.A., 1996. Conduct disorder, enuresis and specific developmental delays in two types of encopresis: a case-note study of 63 boys. Eur. Child Adolesc. Psychiatry 5 (1), 33–37.

Forfar, J., Arneil, G., 1973. Textbook of Paediatrics. Churchill Livingstone, Edinburgh, p. 1967.

Freitag, C.M., Rohling, D., Seifen, S., et al., 2006. Neurophysiology of nocturnal enuresis: evoked potentials and prepulse inhibition of the startle reflex. Dev. Med. Child Neurol. 48 (4), 278–284.

Glazener, C.M., Evans, J.H., 2004. Simple behavioural and physical interventions for nocturnal enuresis in children. Cochrane Database Syst. Rev. 2, CD003637.

Green, M., 1998. Pediatric Diagnosis: Interpretation of Symptoms and Signs in Children and Adolescent, sixth ed. WB Saunders, Philadelphia.

Gumus, B., Vurgun, N., Lekili, M., et al., 1999. Prevalence of nocturnal enuresis and accompanying factors in children aged 7–11 years in Turkey. Acta Paediatr. 88 (12), 1369–1372.

Gür, E., Turhan, P., Can, G., et al., 2004. Enuresis: prevalence, risk factors, and urinary pathology among school children in Istanbul, Turkey. Pediatr. Int. 46, 58–63.

Habel, A., 1982. Aids to Paediatrics. Churchill Livingstone, Edinburgh.

Hirasing, R.A., 1994. [Guideline nocturnal enuresis.] Ned. Tijdschr. Geneeskd. 138 (7), 1360–1366.

Hirasing, R.A., van Leerdam, F.J., Bolk-Bennink, L.F., et al., 2004. Effect of dry bed training on behavioural problems in enuretic children. Acta Paediatr. 91 (8), 960–964.

Hull, D., Johnston, D., 1999. Essential Paediatrics, fourth ed. Churchill Livingstone, Edinburgh.

Hunsballe, J.M., Hansen, T.K., Rittig, S., et al., 1998. The efficacy of DDAVP is related to the circadian rhythm of urine output in patients with persisting nocturnal enuresis. Clin. Endocrinol. (Oxf) 49 (6), 793–801.

Illingworth, R.S., 1987. The Development of the Infant and Young Child: Normal and Abnormal, nineth ed. Churchill Livingstone, Edinburgh.

Jarvelin, M.R., Vikevainen-Tervonen, L., Moilanen, I., et al., 1988. Enuresis in seven-year-old children. Acta Paediatr. Scand. 77 (1), 148–153.

Kalo, B.B., Bella, H., 1996. Enuresis: prevalence and associated factors among primary school children in Saudi Arabia. Acta Paediatr. 85, 1217–1222.

Kanaheswari, Y., 2003. Epidemiology of childhood nocturnal enuresis in Malaysia. J. Paediatr. Child Health 39 (2), 118–123.

Lee, T., Suh, H.J., Lee, H.J., 2005. Comparison of effects of treatment of primary nocturnal enuresis with oxybutynin plus desmopressin, desmopressin alone or imipramine alone: a randomized controlled clinical trial. J. Urol. 174 (3), 1084–1087.

Lerner, G.R., 1994. Urinary tract infections in children. Pediatr. Ann. 23 (9), 463 466–473.

Lewy, J.E., New, M.I., 1975. Growth in children with renal failure. Am. J. Med. 58 (1), 65–68.

Lissauer, T., Clayden, G., 2003. Illustrated Textbook of Paediatrics, second ed. Mosby, London.

Loeys, B., Hoebeke, P., Raes, A., et al., 2002. Does monosymptomatic enuresis exist? A molecular genetic exploration of 32 families with enuresis/incontinence. Br. J. Urol. 90 (1), 76–83.

McMillan, J.A., Stockman, J.A., Oski, F.A., 1982. The Whole Paediatrician Catalogue, vol. 3. WB Saunders, Philadelphia.

Medel, R., Dieguez, S., Brindo, M., et al., 1998. Monosymptomatic primary enuresis: differences between patients responding or not responding to desmopressin. Br. J. Urol. 81 (Suppl. 3), 46–49.

Neveus, T., Johansson, E., Nydahl-Persson, K., et al., 2005. Diuretic treatment of nocturnal enuresis. Scand. J. Urol. Nephrol. 39 (6), 474–478.

Ng, C.F.N., Wong, S.N., 2004. Primary nocturnal enuresis: patient attitudes and parental perceptions. Hong Kong J. Paediatr. 9, 54–58.

Nijman, R.J.M., Butler, R., van Gool, J., et al., 2002. The conservative management of urinary incontinence in childhood. Incontinence, second ed. Proceedings of the 2nd International Consultation on Incontinence. Heath Publications, Plymbridge Distributors, Plymouth.

Oge, O., Kocak, I., Gemalmaz, H., 2001. Enuresis: point prevalence and associated factors among Turkish children. Turk. J. Pediatr. 43 (1), 38–43.

O'Regan, S., Yazbeck, S., Hamberger, B., et al., 1986. Constipation a commonly unrecognised cause of enuresis. Am. J. Dis. Child. 140, 260–261.

Ozkan, K.U., Garipardic, M., Toktamis, A., et al., 2004. Enuresis prevalence and accompanying factors in schoolchildren: a questionnaire study from southeast Anatolia. Urol. Int. 73 (2), 149–155.

Pasqualini, T., Ferraris, J., 2003. Chronic renal insufficiency and growth. Medicina 63 (6), 731–736.

Petermann, F., Hampel, P., Stauber, T., 2004. Enuresis: pathogenesis, diagnostics and interventions. Prax. Kinderpsychol. Kinderpsychiatr. 53 (4), 237–255.

Qayyum, N., Alcocer, L., Maxwell, H., et al., 2003. Skeletal disproportion in children with chronic renal disease. Horm. Res. 60 (5), 221–226.

Radvanska, E., Kovacs, L., Rittig, S., 2006. The role of bladder capacity in antidiuretic and anticholinergic treatment for nocturnal enuresis. J. Urol. 176 (2), 764–768.

Rawashdeh, Y.F., Hvistendahl, G.M., Kamperis, K., et al., 2002. Demographics of enuresis patients attending a referral centre. Scand. J. Urol. Nephrol. 36 (5), 348–353.

Rocchini, A.O., 1984. Childhood hypertension: etiology, diagnosis and treatment. Pediatr. Clin. North Am. 31 (6), 1259–1273.

Rombis, V., Triantafyllidis, A., Balaxis, E., et al., 2005. Nocturnal enuresis in children: a four year experience in outpatient clinics of pediatric urology. Folia Med. (Plovdiv) 47 (2), 24–28.

Rona, R.J., Li, L., Chinn, S., 1997. Determinants of nocturnal enuresis in England and Scotland in the '90s. Dev. Med. Child Neurol. 39 (10), 677–681.

Salgado, C.M., Cavalhaes, J.T., 2003. Arterial hypertension in childhood. J. Pediatr. (Rio J.) 79 (Suppl. 1), S115–S124.

Shaikh, N., Morone, N.E., Lopez, J., et al., 2007. Does this child have a urinary tract infection? J. Am. Med. Assoc. 298 (24), 2895–2904.

Stickler, G.B., 1976. Growth failure in renal disease. Pediatr. Clin. North Am. 23, 885–894.

Swinford, R.D., Portman, R.J., 2004. Measurement and treatment of elevated blood pressure in the pediatric patient with chronic kidney disease. Adv. Chronic Kidney Dis. 11 (2), 143–161.

Touchette, E., Petit, D., Paquet, J., et al., 2005. Bed-wetting and its association with developmental milestones in childhood. Arch. Pediatr. Adolesc. Med. 159 (12), 1129–1134.

Tunnessen, W., 1983. Signs and Symptoms in Pediatrics. JB Lippincott, Philadelphia.

van Hoecke, E., Hoebeke, P., Braet, C., et al., 2004. An assessment of internalizing problems in children with enuresis. J. Urol. 171 (6/2), 2580–2583.

van Poecke, A.J., Cunliffe, C., 2009. Chiropractic Treatment for Primary Nocturnal Enuresis: A case series of 33 consecutive patients. J. Manip. Physiol. Therap. 32 (8), 675–681. Chiropractic (Paediatrics), McTimoney College of Chiropractic, University of Wales.

von Gontard, A., Eiberg, H., Hollmann, E., et al., 1999. Molecular genetics of nocturnal enuresis: linkage to a locus on chromosome 22. Scand. J. Urol Nephrol. Suppl. 202, 76–80.

von Gontard, A., Schaumburg, H., Hollmann, E., et al., 2001. The genetics of enuresis: a review. J. Urol. 166 (6), 2438–2443.

Wen, J.G., Wang, Q.W., Chen, Y., et al., 2006. An epidemiological study of primary nocturnal enuresis in Chinese children and adolescents. Eur. Urol. 49 (6), 1107–1113.

Yeung, C.K., Sreedhar, B., Sihoe, J.D., et al., 2006. Differences in characteristics of nocturnal enuresis between children and adolescents: a critical appraisal from a large epidemiological study. BJU Int. 97 (5), 1069–1073.

Common orthopedic syndromes in childhood

Allan G. J. Terrett   Neil J. Davies

14

This chapter presents a group of orthopedic syndromes that could be encountered in chiropractic pediatric practice (up to the age of 15 years). It cannot cover every orthopedic eventuality encountered by chiropractors seeing children. This presentation is based on the best available evidence and is structured to assist the practitioner to be able to accurately identify a number of orthopedic syndromes and implement safe and effective chiropractic management programs.

Musculoskeletal pain in children is a very common presentation to chiropractors. Many clinical conditions in children occur within a very narrow age range which greatly assists the practitioner in making a list of differential diagnoses (Table 14.1). Careful history and examination are needed to determine the anatomical tissue(s) involved, and then the process involved to determine a working hypothesis/diagnosis for the child's complaint.

Fractures and dislocations in the growing years

The key issue for the chiropractor lies in the ability to identify the characteristic features of bony fracture so that the appropriate medical care is not delayed and/or inappropriate care rendered.

The characteristic features of fracture are a history of very recent trauma, localized tenderness, swelling and reluctance to use the area. Definitive diagnosis is dependent on imaging.

Just as in other clinical conditions, children cannot be considered as 'little adults', as reactions of children's tissues differ greatly from those of adults. The differences between children and adults which become less striking as the child approaches adulthood are:

- Fractures are more common in children due to the combination of slender bones and their carefree capers.
- Crack, buckle, hairline and greenstick fractures are not serious, while intra-articular and epiphyseal fractures are very serious.

- In a child who is not yet walking but who has a fracture, the possibility of child abuse must be considered.
- In children the periosteum is stronger, less readily torn, and more osteogenic.
- The rate of bone healing is much faster in children.
- Non-union of fractures in children is rare.
- The appearance of the epiphyseal plates may be mistaken for fracture lines so careful radiographic comparison with the uninjured limb is important.
- Extensive remodeling can correct the deformity of a malunited fracture.
- Disturbance of the epiphyseal growth plate causes growth disturbances.
- Osteomyelitis secondary to open fracture, or open reduction of a closed fracture, tends to be more extensive, and may destroy the epiphyseal growth plate.
- Volkmann's ischemic contracture and myositis ossificans are more common complications in children.
- Children's ligaments are strong and resilient, and therefore a sudden powerful traction on a ligament is more likely to cause separation of the epiphyseal plate than tear the ligament.
- The total blood volume in children is proportionally smaller (in a 20 kg child a loss of 500 ml represents 33% of total blood volume, whereas in an adult it represents only 10%), and so blood loss is a common cause of shock and death.

Inflammatory and infectious disease

Pyogenic (septic) arthritis

Pyogenic arthritis is seen across all pediatric age groups, the source of infection varying with the age of a child. The likely source of infection in the infant is spread from adjacent osteomyelitis. In the older child it is usually seen as an isolated

© 2010, Elsevier Ltd, Inc, BV
DOI: 10.1016/B978-0-7020-3129-8.00014-1

Table 14.1 Age-related common orthopedic syndromes in pediatrics

Age group (years)	Orthopedic syndromes
Hip	
0+	Congenital hip dislocation (CHD)
3–10	Transient synovitis (TS, observation hip)
5–10	Perthes' disease (LCP)
10–16	Slipped upper femoral epiphysis (SUFE)
Knee	
1–3	Benign genu varum of toddlers
3–5	Benign genu valgum of childhood
10–14	Osgood–Schlatter's disease (OSD)
10–14	Sinding–Larsen–Johansson's disease (SLJ)
8–20	Osteochondritis dissecans (OD)
Older child–adolescent	Patella dislocation
Foot–ankle	
10–14	Sever's disease
3–5	Köhler's disease
13–18	Freiberg's disease
Intoeing	
0–2	Metatarsus adductus
1–4	Internal tibial torsion
0–8	Femoral anteversion
Shoulder	
0+	Clavicle fracture
0+	Sprengel's deformity
Elbow	
2–6	Pulled elbow
5–10	Panner's disease
Wrist and hand	
0+	Infantile trigger thumb
Cervical spine	
0+	Congenital–infantile torticollis
Thoracic spine	
10+	Adolescent idiopathic scoliosis
13–19	Scheuermann's disease
Lumbar spine	
5+	Pediatric low back pain (PLBP)

infection, normally without any bony involvement, and in the adolescent it is generally secondary to systemic disease involving organisms with an affinity for joints. The initial joint effusion becomes rapidly purulent with an associated white cell count exceeding $100\ 000/\mu L$ and an elevated erythrocyte sedimentation rate (Hay et al 1997).

The clinical presentation of pyogenic arthritis also varies with the age of the patient. In infancy, the patient is generally irritable and feeding poorly. Paralysis of the affected limb may be in evidence and, when the hip joint is involved, there will usually be a decrease in the normal range of abduction. Fever is a poor indicator of disease at this age and many infants with pyogenic arthritis do not have an elevated temperature.

In the older child and adolescent the symptoms are striking, with fever, malaise, vomiting and restriction of motion in all directions of the affected joint (Hay et al 1997). Refusal to walk is also characteristic (Fysh 1998). Immediate medical referral is mandatory for investigation (imaging, joint aspiration) and medical treatment must be begun without delay.

Optimal clinical outcome is dependent upon early surgical drainage of the joint to prevent destruction of the articular cartilage, and fibrosis and arthrosis of the affected joint (Renshaw 1986). Damage to the growth plate may also occur, particularly when the infection is in the hip joint (Betz 1990).

Once the child is out of hospital and taking oral antibiotics, corrective chiropractic care should be given, followed by maintenance care. Particular attention should be paid to the state of the child's immune system and appropriate supportive nutrition prescribed when necessary.

Osteomyelitis

Approximately 85% of all cases of osteomyelitis occur in children under the age of 16 years, which makes this serious condition very much a part of pediatric practice and one which every chiropractor who regularly treats children should be acutely aware of. It results from hematogenous spread in most cases, in which it arises from an open wound or an adjacent infected focus. In the majority of cases, the organism involved is *Staphylococcus aureus* (Renshaw 1986).

> The pathology of osteomyelitis of the proximal femur depends upon the vascular anatomy, which in turn is related to the age of the child. At any age, however, the infection usually begins in the metaphyseal region. During the first 12–18 months of life, the growth plate is traversed by vascular channels of communication between the epiphysis and metaphysis. This means that there is little resistance to the extension of infection across the physis into the proximal femur. For this reason, osteomyelitis in the infantile period can rapidly destroy the femoral head, and it often extends into the hip joint to become septic arthritis. After infancy, the growth plate acts as a barrier since the vascular channels traversing it have dropped out. Infections that are initially localized to the metaphyseal region may reach the hip joint by erosion through the thinned metaphyseal cortex, which is intracapsular. The metaphyseal region of a bone is the most common site of osteomyelitis because the arteriolar loops feed into a relatively large venous capillary bed, where blood flow is slow and oxygen tension is low. This predisposes the area to seeding with pathological bacteria.
>
> The diagnostic picture of osteomyelitis of the proximal femur is quite variable depending on the age of the patient. In the infant, fever and signs of systemic toxicity are usually absent, the most common clinical signs being irritability, poor feeding, localized limb edema and pseudoparalysis (muscle guarding and unwillingness to move the affected limb). In the older child, signs of sepsis are the rule. Localized signs of inflammation are present, and protective reflex myospasm is seen. Clearly, the time it takes to examine the motion of a child's hip gently and to compare it with the other side may well be worthwhile if the cause of a child's lethargy, irritability, poor feeding or fever is osteomyelitis of the proximal femur. Whenever there is any question of possible septic arthritis or osteomyelitis, the hip joint must be aspirated.

(from Renshaw 1986, with permission)

The role of the chiropractor is the same as that outlined earlier for septic arthritis. Early disease recognition and referral is critical to obtain optimal clinical outcome. While the typical signs of sepsis would be likely to persuade parents to take the affected child to a medical physician in the first instance, the same cannot be said for the infant whose probable presentation will be irritability, poor feeding and possibly fever, a presentation which is commonly seen first by the family chiropractor. This places a heavy burden of responsibility on the chiropractor to ensure a thorough examination is carried out with irritable infants who have suddenly stopped feeding normally.

Once the child is out of the hospital and taking oral antibiotics, corrective chiropractic care should be given followed by maintenance care. Particular attention should be paid to the state of the child's immune system, and appropriate supportive nutrition should be prescribed when necessary.

Juvenile chronic arthritis

Juvenile chronic arthritis (JCA) is the preferred term for a group of non-infective inflammatory joint diseases causing pain, swelling and stiffness of more than 3 months' duration in children under 16 years of age, occurring in about 1 per 1000 children (Apley & Solomon 1993).

The pathology of JCA is like that of rheumatoid arthritis (RA) in that there is synovial inflammation leading to fibrosis and ankylosis. There are four subtypes:

1. systemic (Still's disease) – 15% where the patient (usually under 3) has a systemic illness (almost daily fever, rashes, malaise, and appears ill), and the arthritis (joint swelling) develops later
2. pauciarticular – 60–70% (usually under 6, more common in girls) which affects a few larger joints (knees, elbows, ankles, wrists) and is complicated by iridocyclitis in about 50%
3. polyarticular – (10%) seen in older children and closely resembles RA
4. seronegative spondyloarthritis – 5–10%, seen in older children (usually boys) and may take the form of sacroiliitis and spondylitis, sometimes involving the hips and knees (HLA-B27 is often positive and may be a 'juvenile ankylosing spondylitis').

The lower limb

Lower limb pain in children is due to pathology far more often than is the case in adult practice and therefore demands of the chiropractor a great deal of care when making clinical management decisions. Pain syndromes in the lower limb arise principally from subluxation of the lumbar spine/pelvis or pathology of the hip or knee areas. Bone tumors in the lower extremity in children are among the less common but very important causes of pain presentations to chiropractors. A full discussion of this important subject is given in Chapter 17.

The hip region

Developmental dysplasia of the hip

Developmental dysplasia of the hip (DDH) is a spontaneous dislocation occurring before, during or shortly after birth in the neonatal period. It was formerly called congenital dislocation of the hip (CDH) but recent research has shown that it is not necessarily congenital and in some cases can take some months

to become clinically identifiable. It may be bilateral in almost half the children affected. One infant in 60 is born with instability of one or both hips, with 88% of those recovering spontaneously in the first 2 months of life. About 1.5 per 1000 live births among Europeans (Dandy & Edwards 2003) will persist unless treated.

DDH is a serious condition and needs to be identified as soon after birth as possible, certainly by the routine 6-week developmental check-up. Diagnostic neglect or improper treatment leads to painful arthritis from an early age. For this reason, examination of both hips should be a routine part of every newborn's first physical examination.

Causes of DDH include:

- genetically determined joint laxity (the incidence is higher if a relative is affected)
- hormonal laxity – it is possible that relaxin may be secreted by the fetal uterus in response to estrogen and progesterone reaching the fetal circulation. This could explain the greater incidence in females, and the low incidence among premature babies born before hormones reach their peak
- genetically determined dysplasia of the hip, which does predispose to dislocation
- breech malposition – the incidence is slightly higher when the infant is delivered breech than with normal delivery.

DDH is more common among children with torticollis, foot abnormalities and in certain ethnic groups.

Unless specifically looked for, the condition may not be noticed until the child begins to walk (which may be delayed), and there may be a limp, though the condition is painless.

Girls are affected 6–8 times more than boys (Adams & Hamblen 2001, Apley & Solomon 1993, Dandy & Edwards 2003).

The pathology of DDH involves the bony nucleus of the femoral head appearing late, its development is retarded, and it is dislocated superiorly and laterally from the acetabulum (Fig. 14.1). The femoral head must lie in correct relationship

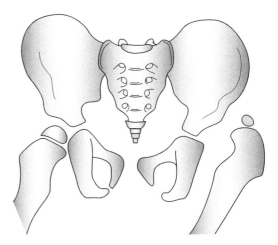

Figure 14.1 • The dislocated hip. Note the shallow dysplastic acetabulum, the hypoplastic femoral head with its lateral and superiorly displaced position.

with the acetabulum for each to develop and grow in a normal manner. In most cases the femoral neck is anteverted beyond the normal infant range of 12–25°. The ossification centre for the roof of the acetabulum is late in developing and the angle of the acetabular roof is shallow and steeper than the normal side. The joint capsule is gradually elongated as the femoral head is displaced upwards.

Diagnosis can almost always be determined in the first few days of life by clinical examination (Fig. 14.2), which includes:

- shortening of one limb
- asymmetry of the fat folds on the medial thigh
- widening of the perineum, especially in bilateral cases (one-third are bilateral)
- prominence of the trochanter on the involved side on palpation
- positive Allis or Galeazzi sign
- telescoping (piston movement) of the thigh
- Ortolani test positive:
  - The baby's thighs are held with the thumbs medially and the fingers on the greater trochanters; the hips are flexed to 90° and gently abducted. Normally there is smooth abduction to almost 90°. In CHD the movement is usually impeded, but if pressure is applied to the greater trochanter there is a soft 'clunk' as the dislocation reduces, and then the hip abducts fully
- Barlow test positive:
  - The examiner's thumb is placed in the groin and, by grasping the upper thigh, an attempt is made to lever the femoral head out of the acetabulum during adduction. If the femoral head is in the reduced position, but can be made to slip out of the socket and then back in again (with the Ortolani maneuver), the hip is unstable and should be examined by ultrasound.
- X-ray examination (not appropriate before 6 months):
  - the ossification center of the femoral head is late in appearing and development is retarded
  - the ossification center of the femoral head is displaced superiorly and laterally
  - the acetabular roof has an increased upward slope
- arthrography may be useful
- ultrasound scanning in the newborn determines the position of the femoral head, when X-rays tend to be inconclusive.

In older children (over 4 months) an important clinical sign is the restriction of abduction when the hip is flexed

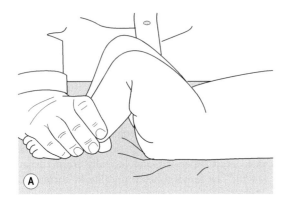
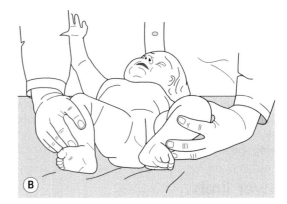
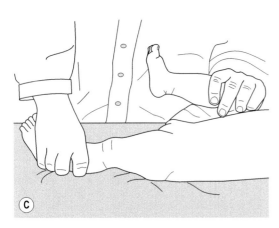
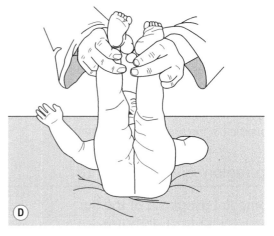

Figure 14.2 • Examination of the child with developmental dysplasia of the hip (DDH): (A) the Allis sign, in which one knee is lower than the other when the knees are flexed to 90° will be positive; (B) decreased abduction on the involved side; (C) loss of knee flexion which is normally characteristic of the neonate on the involved side as the opposite hip is flexed; and (D) a short leg on the involved side with asymmetrical fat folds in the medial thigh area.

(Chappel's or Hart's sign) which may be noticed by the mother as she puts on the child's diaper (nappy). In still older children, delay in walking, abnormality of gait, and an increase of the lumbar lordosis should raise suspicion.

In terms of prognosis, the earlier in life the dislocation is reduced, the better the chance for development of a normal hip. Treatment begun in the first week of life is very simple, and can nearly always ensure normal development of the hip.

In patients where treatment is begun after the first year, only about 50–66% can expect to remain permanently free from trouble, with problems including gradual redislocation and secondary arthritis in middle adult life. All children found to have DDH should be referred to a pediatric orthopedist. Treatment depends on the age at which DDH is detected.

Chiropractic co-management is always appropriate in such cases as the biomechanical dysfunction caused by the hip pathology will create spinal and pelvic subluxation. Significant modification of technique is necessary in order to avoid any pressure at all being applied to the affected hip. Techniques such as Logan Basic, Toftness, SOT, Thompson terminal point and Activator are safe and effective ways of managing children with DDH.

Transient synovitis (TS) of the hip (transient arthritis, observation hip)

Transient synovitis (TS) is the most common cause of limping in childhood (Hay et al 1997). TS is due to mild inflammation of the synovial membrane of the hip, resulting in synovial effusion within the joint capsule, initiated by minor trauma, such as a twisting sprain. TS is a short-lived affliction of childhood (3–10 year olds), affecting boys twice as often as girls, causing groin and anterior thigh pain (sometimes reaching the knee), muscle spasm about the hip, a limp during walking where the child decreases the time of weight-bearing on the involved hip, and limitation of hip internal rotation (best detected by the 'roll test') and abduction. Symptoms last 1–2 weeks and the child may have more than one episode.

X-ray examination will usually be normal, or may demonstrate evidence of joint capsule distension. TS is important because it resembles clinically the earliest signs of Perthes' (LCP) disease, or infection, before the characteristic X-ray changes are visible. Joint aspiration reveals sterile fluid.

The prognosis is good with a full recovery expected within 3–6 weeks, including a return to normal range of motion of all hip movements.

The treatment of TS is simple. Daily adjusting, bed rest, reassurance, and analgesic medication until the pain has settled and full hip movements have been restored are appropriate. A diagnosis of TS is only made after the hip has recovered but never while the symptoms and signs are present. While the symptoms and signs are present, a diagnosis of infective arthritis or Legge–Calvé–Perthes' disease (LCP) should be kept firmly in mind, and acted upon appropriately should further symptoms and signs appear, especially fever. Full recovery within a few weeks justifies the retrospective diagnosis of TS.

Occasionally a patient believed to have TS of the hip will eventually show radiographic changes in the femoral capital epiphysis characteristic of LCP. In these cases it is believed that distension of the hip joint capsule by fluid produces pressure, which cuts off the circulation to the femoral capital epiphysis. In cases of TS it is therefore advisable to perform follow-up X-ray assessment if there is persistent pain and/or limp.

Chiropractic management should consist of gentle hip joint mobilization, correction of the subluxation complex, usually found at the sacral segments, sacroiliac joint, lumbosacral junction, or upper cervical complex. Resolution usually occurs in a matter of a few days (Hay et al 1997.) Chiropractic care should never be commenced until the X-ray and laboratory examination is completed.

Perthes' disease

Perthes' disease has been variably referred to as Legg–Calvé–Perthes' disease, LCP, coxa plana and osteochondritis. It is an osteochondritis of the femoral head affecting children (5–10 years old), resulting in temporary softening of the femoral head, resulting in pain and deformity, and is one of the important causes of painful limping in childhood. The main importance is that it may lead to the development of osteoarthritis of the hip in later life.

LCP is thought to be due to a disturbance of the blood supply to the femoral head. Up to the age of 4 years, (1) metaphyseal vessels that penetrate the growth disc, (2) lateral epiphyseal vessels running in the retinacula, and (3) scanty vessels in the ligamentum teres supply the femoral head. The metaphyseal blood supply declines, until by age 4 it has virtually disappeared. By the age of 7 years the vessels in the ligamentum teres have developed. Therefore between the ages of 4 and 7 years the femoral head depends for its blood supply and venous drainage almost entirely on the lateral epiphyseal vessels, whose position within the retinacula makes them susceptible to stretching and pressure from effusion. Such pressure may be insufficient to block off the arterial flow, but it could easily cause venous stasis resulting in a rise in intraosseous pressure and consequent ischemia, leading to osteonecrosis of the femoral head. This then sets up a sequence of events, which will last 2–3 years.

LCP is more common in boys. Epidemiological studies have shown that there is a higher incidence in children of low birthweight who are not quite 'up to par' physically and among underprivileged communities. Affected children have retarded growth of the trunk and limbs, with notably small feet (Apley & Solomon 1993). LCP usually affects only one hip but can be bilateral. There is frequently a great deal of pain and muscle spasm about the hip secondary to an associated synovitis, and pain may be felt in the anterior thigh to the suprapatellar region.

Physical examination will generally show moderate limitation of all hip movements compared to the unaffected side. Usually the first motion lost is rotation, and is easily assessed by rolling the thigh internally and externally, which causes pain and muscle spasm if movement is forced. General health is usually unaffected.

On X-ray examination, LCP has a series of distinct radiological stages:

- X-ray changes are usually present at the time advice is sought, with the crescent sign (Fig. 14.3) and widening of the joint space (Waldenström's sign) being early signs.

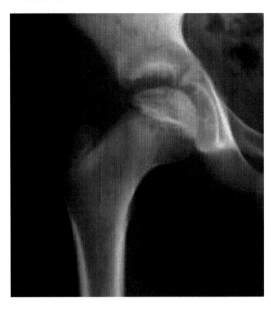

Figure 14.3 · The crescent sign, seen here, is the earliest radiological sign of LCP disease and is often seen in conjunction with slight widening of the joint space on the affected side.

- Ischemia and bone death. The bony nucleus appears to have shrunk within the surrounding bed of cartilage.
  The cartilaginous part of the femoral head, being nourished by synovial fluid, remains viable and becomes thicker than normal.
- New bone is laid down on the dead trabeculae ('creeping substitution'; on X-ray this gives a fragmented appearance) – dead bone is dense, and the neighboring hypervascularized bone is osteoporotic. During this phase structural rigidity is lost, and deformation of the epiphysis (larger and flatter) may occur from pressure across the joint.

- Distortion and remodeling. Both the acetabulum and femoral head ('mushrooming') are deformed (Fig. 14.4), causing the limb on that side to be shorter though the discrepancy is not great. Eventually the texture of the bone returns to normal.

Radioisotope scanning is also used when investigating a case of LCP which shows failure of the uptake of the isotope in the region of the bony nucleus. Since this 'void' is seen at an early stage, it may be important in early diagnosis.

In order to reach a definitive diagnosis, LCP has to be distinguished from infection, which it may resemble clinically. This is done mainly by clinical examination and X-ray. In LCP the child's general health is unaffected and the erythrocyte sedimentation rate (ESR) and blood counts are normal.

The prognosis in LCP is age-specific. The earlier in life the child is affected, the better the prognosis (under 6 years the prognosis is excellent). Permanent deformity usually results in secondary arthritis later in life (usually 40+). Prognosis is better if only part of the epiphysis is affected, as is often the case.

Treatment protocols often produce disappointing outcomes. The old method of treatment of preventing weight-bearing on the softened femoral head by prolonged recumbency (often for 2 years or more) has been abandoned, because results were not commensurate with the disruption to the child's life. Devices to prevent weight-bearing have also fallen into disfavor, because they were seldom effective and they embarrassed the child psychologically. In favorable cases where the whole head has not been affected, the only treatment is rest for a few weeks until the pain subsides. Some consider that it is best to hospitalize the child for a short time (until the spasm subsides), with the limb in traction to ensure complete bed rest. They are subsequently monitored with periodic X-ray review.

While it is essential for all cases of Perthes' disease to be actively managed by an orthopedic surgeon (Weinstein 1997), cooperatively managed care is to be strongly encouraged.

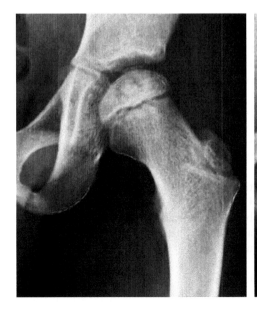
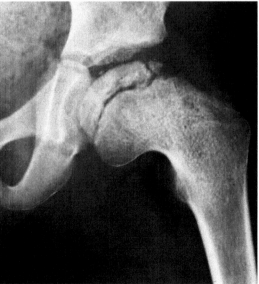

Figure 14.4 · Mushroom deformity of the femoral head is seen in the advanced stage of LCP disease. (Reproduced from Adams & Hamblen 2001.)

Given the effect of the chiropractic adjustment on the circulatory system (Gatterman 1995, Homewood 1977, Strang 1984), the chiropractor has a key role to play in management by correcting the lumbar and pelvic subluxation complex, affording the patient optimal vascular conditions to enhance the revascularization stage, and equal loading of the hip joints to enhance the remodeling stage and beyond by maximizing bone mineral density accrual (Bailey et al 1997). The obvious precaution should be taken of avoiding all adjustive procedures that place any stress on the proximal femur, such as Gonstead push–pull moves, diversified thigh stabilization procedures (thigh-ilio-deltoid, etc.) and extension techniques. Nutritional supplementation designed to optimize blood flow and assist bone and connective tissue healing is also useful.

Slipped upper femoral epiphysis (SUFE)

Slipped upper femoral epiphysis (SUFE) occurs more commonly in boys in the 10–16-year age group (girls usually 11–14, boys usually 14–16). The junction between the capital epiphysis and the neck of the femur loosens, and with the downward pressure of weight-bearing and the upward pull of muscles on the femur, the epiphysis is displaced, down and backwards. The cause is unknown, but an underlying endocrine disorder is suspected as two types of body build are seen: children who are above the 90th percentile for height and the obese child. In almost half of the cases, both hips are affected (one after the other).

The clinical features of SUFE include a gradual onset of pain in the groin region, and stiffness and limp in a 10–16-year-old. This is easily misdiagnosed as a sprain and often, unfortunately, disregarded. The limp may become a gluteal lurch (because of coxa vara) and the child may become aware that the leg is 'turning out' (because of femoral retroversion). A telltale sign is that the external rotation increases as the hip is flexed.

Sometimes the pain may be felt mainly in the knee, and SUFE should be suspected in any 10–16-year-old with aching about the knee, but no knee abnormality on examination. Forcing hip movements in the restricted range usually exacerbates the pain. A valuable diagnostic sign is when the hip is flexed, the thigh externally rotates (Fig. 14.5).

SUFE is not readily apparent on A-P X-ray because the slip is usually posterior. Therefore a frog-leg or lateral film is more appropriate and readily shows the slip (Fig. 14.6). Even cases involving slips of only minor degrees can be identified by drawing a line along the middle of the femur, with a second line drawn from the anterior to the posterior base of the epiphysis. The intersection of these two lines will normally form a right angle. If this angle is <87°, the epiphysis is deemed to have slipped posteriorly.

This condition may be discovered before actual slipping of the epiphysis occurs in the so-called 'pre-slipped' phase, characterized by an abnormally widened and irregular growth plate ('wide and woolly'), associated with some rarefaction in the metaphysis of the femur, but no actual displacement.

The diagnosis of SUFE should be suspected in every patient 10–20 years aged who complains of pain in the hip, thigh or knee (Fig. 14.7). The condition is often missed because of pain felt predominantly in the knee. Therefore, if physical and

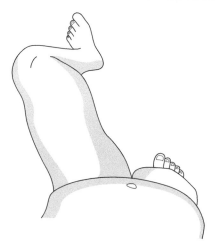

Figure 14.5 ● In SUFE, when the hip is flexed, the thigh externally rotates, as shown. (Reproduced with permission from Renshaw 1986.)

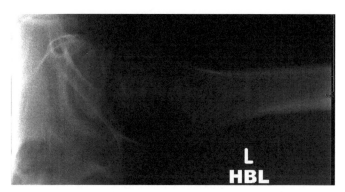

Figure 14.6 ● Frog-leg view demonstrating slippage of the upper femoral epiphysis. (Reproduced from Adams & Hamblen 2001.)

X-ray examination of the knee is negative, the hips should be X-rayed as well.

Clinical complications arising from SUFE include:

- avascular necrosis of the femoral head
- cartilage necrosis
- slipping of the opposite side which occurs in at least 20% of cases
- coxa vara
- femoral retroversion, because the head slips backwards, which results in an external rotation of the lower limb
- shortening of the femur by 1–2 cm
- later osteoarthritis (especially if severe displacement is allowed to remain uncorrected).

The typical medical management plan seeks to:

- preserve epiphyseal blood supply
- prevent further displacement of the physis
- correct any deformity.

To prevent further displacement, weight-bearing should be prohibited as soon as the diagnosis is made. Medical treatment depends on the degree of displacement. If the displacement is slight the position may be accepted, and to prevent further displacement, threaded wires or screws are inserted. When

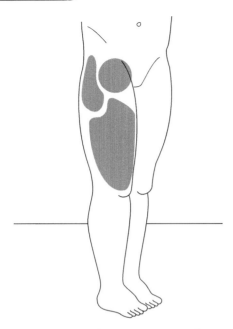

Figure 14.7 • Typical referred pain locations in children with hip disease. (Reproduced with permission from Renshaw 1986.)

Table 14.2 Tumors which may affect the knee area in children, adolescents and young adults

Tumor	Affected age group
Unicameral (or solitary) bone cyst	2–20
Aneurysmal bone cyst	5–25
Non-ossifying fibroma	8–20
Chondroblastoma	10–25
Osteosarcoma	10–25
Ewing's sarcoma	10–25
Chondromyxoid fibroma	10–30
Enchondroma	10–30

displacement is severe medical opinion differs, with some advocating manipulation of the femoral epiphysis to a better position (with the risk of avascular necrosis of the femoral head) and then securing it in place with threaded wires or screws. Others believe that the risk of avascular necrosis is too high (Apley & Solomon 1993, Dandy & Edwards 2003) and will not attempt to manipulate the head to a better position, but screw the epiphysis in its position to prevent any further dislocation and then perform an anterior wedge osteotomy below the trochanters (1–2 years after securing the epiphysis) to correct the position of the femoral head in the acetabulum.

The knee region

Owing to the elasticity of their connective tissue structures, it is very rare to see acute ligamentous injuries in children. For this reason, injuries involving damage to the menisci, lateral collateral ligaments, coronary and cruciate ligaments are deemed to be outside the scope of this text.

If a young person presents with knee pain which does not have an obvious cause, is worse at night (non-mechanical pain) and/or is increasing, an X-ray examination of the knees should be obtained because of the number of tumors that can affect this age group (Table 14.2). If nothing is found at the knee, then an X-ray examination of the hips should be obtained as hip conditions such as transient synovitis, Perthes' disease (5–10 years) and SUFE (10–20 years) can present as mainly knee and/or anterior thigh pain.

Benign genu varum of toddlers

This very common but seldom serious condition alarms many parents. A mild degree of outward bowing of the knees is so common in children 1–3 years old that it is considered

to be a normal stage of development which usually corrects itself spontaneously by the age of 3 years (Fig. 14.8) and does not require treatment unless it persists into later childhood. Before simply reassuring parents that it is normal, however, it is important to exclude serious disease. Under the age of 5 years this could be vitamin C or D deficiency, Blount's disease (Fig. 14.9) or growth disorders (epiphyseal injuries, epiphyseal dysplasia, rickets).

Monitoring for improvement or worsening over time can be determined by bringing the child's ankles together and measuring the distance between the medial epicondyles at the knee.

Benign genu valgum of childhood

This deformity can also alarm parents, but is so common in children 3–5 years old as to be considered a normal stage of development (Fig. 14.10), which in the absence of underlying disease usually corrects itself spontaneously by age 6 (soon after the child starts primary school) to reach the adult 5–8°.

Before reassuring parents of its normality, it is important to exclude serious disease.

Monitoring for improvement or worsening over time can be determined by goniometric measurement of the tibiofemoral angle, or by bringing the child's knees together and measuring

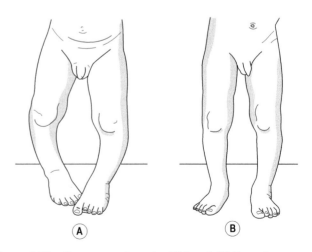

Figure 14.8 • Genu varum in early childhood. (A) Normal physiological genu varum in a toddler; (B) normally developed straight legs at 3 years of age.

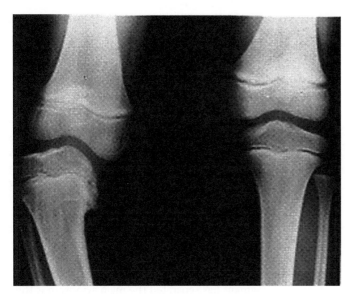

Figure 14.9 • Blount's disease in a child presenting with genu varum. (Reproduced with permission from Renshaw 1986.)

the distance between the medial malleoli at the ankles. It is acceptable to have 10 cm (4 inches) between the ankles at the age of 4 when the deformity is greatest.

If the condition persists after the age of 10, then a simple surgical treatment to retard the growth of the bone on one side of the tibia is employed. The procedure entails the use of metal staples to bridge the epiphysis (epiphysiodesis); these are removed after correction. Following cessation of epiphyseal growth, correction requires an osteotomy.

The vast majority of children brought to chiropractors because of either varum or valgum 'deformity' fall within the ranges of normal physiological development. While it is appropriate to carefully examine the spine and lower extremities in these children, care should be exercised to ensure that unnecessary levels of care are not given to correct a 'problem' that will resolve as a part of the natural development of the child.

Not all cases, however, are physiological. Persistence outside the normal developmental age range or the presence of other symptoms suggestive of disease warrant careful diagnostic evaluation. Lumbopelvic and lower extremity subluxation may contribute to persistence of either valgus or varus deformity, particularly when the deformity is of asymmetrical magnitude, as do a number of important pathologies with which the chiropractor should be familiar (Box 14.1).

Osgood–Schlatter's disease

Osgood–Schlatter's disease (OSD) is a traction apophysitis from the pull of the patella tendon on the developing tibial tubercle (Fig. 14.11), seen in 10–14-year-olds, more often a very active boy (Adams & Hamblen 2001). While it is a self-limiting condition, the name sounds so serious that often parents need to be reassured that their child will survive.

The typical presentation in OSD is a painful limp with the patient able to accurately localize the pain to the tibial tubercle, which appears swollen and sometimes reddened. Pain can be aggravated by palpation, kneeling on the area, active use of the quadriceps (running, stair climbing, bicycle riding), or strongly contracting the quadriceps against resistance with the knee held straight. The patient usually reports that the pain increases with physical activity and reduces after rest. The diagnosis is a clinical one and is easily made by age, activity, location of pain and aggravating factors.

In most cases treatment is not required, other than to advise against certain activities such as sports, kneeling, running, climbing and cycling. Ice may also be recommended.

If local pain and tenderness are severe, the limb may be immobilized for 6–8 weeks in a plaster cylinder extending from the groin to ankles. Extreme tenderness may respond to local hydrocortisone injection. As the condition resolves, the patient may be left with enlargement of the tibial tubercle, but apart from the appearance it causes no problems.

Despite the fact that OSD is a clinical and not a radiological diagnosis, it is always wise to perform an X-ray examination in

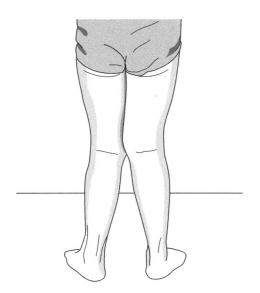

Figure 14.10 • Genu valgum at 4 years of age.

Box 14.1

Pathological causes of genu varum and genu valgum deformity in children

Genu varum

Blount's disease
Early walking
Obesity
Gait disturbance

Genu valgum

Paralytic conditions
Rheumatic diseases
Rickets
Trauma
Endocrine disease
Infection

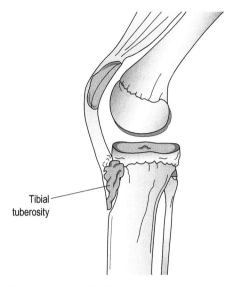

Figure 14.11 ● Osgood–Schlatter's disease is a traction apophysitis from the pull of the patella tendon on the developing tibial tubercle, often resulting in irregularity and fragmentation of the tibial tuberosity. (Reproduced with permission from Renshaw 1986.)

Tibial tuberosity

order to rule out the possibility of a tumor or avulsion of the tibial tubercle being the cause of the child's pain.

Collective clinical experience suggests that the pain over the tuberosity will respond symptomatically more quickly with chiropractic treatment, with many patients able to continue participating in sport without pain following care. Chiropractic management is dependent upon the demonstration of the anterior tibial subluxation complex, which is a triad of pain on palpation over the tibial tubercle, decreased drawer sign in the A-P direction when compared to the unaffected side, and weakness of the tibialis anterior muscle and variably also weakness of the quadriceps and popliteus muscles.

The tibial subluxation in these cases is best adjusted using a drop mechanism with a single firm thrust and hold procedure. Further to this, it may also be appropriate to use the knee shuttle technique with thigh extended off the table using a gentle rotatory motion so as to stretch any adhesions in the knee compartment, and advise the patient to engage in physical activity up to pain tolerance level. In the more severe cases, it may be necessary to immobilize the knee and relieve it from weight-bearing for a short time until the pain level decreases. Analgesic pain management strategies are seldom ever required.

Sinding–Larsen–Johansson's disease

Sinding–Larsen–Johansson's disease (SLJ) is a traction apophysitis similar to OSD. It occurs in young active patients in the same age group (10–14). Patients having both OSD and SLJ at the same time are not unusual. SLJ is due to traction of the patella tendon on the lower pole of the patella, causing point tenderness at the inferior pole of the patella, which is aggravated by activities such as running, jumping (basketball) and ascending stairs. SLJ is a clinical diagnosis and the condition usually responds to rest, ice, stretching of the hamstrings,

and strengthening of the quadriceps. Rarely is immobilization of the knee required.

Osteochondritis dissecans

Osteochondritis dissecans (OD) can occur in children, adolescents and young adults (8–20 years), and the knee is the most commonly affected joint (also affects the capitulum of the humerus and the dome of the talus). The subchondral bone becomes avascular and, with the articular cartilage that covers it, may slowly separate (2–3 months) from the surrounding bone to form a loose body in the knee joint, leaving a shallow cavity in the articular surface which is ultimately filled in with fibrocartilage (Fig. 14.12).

Initially, before separation of the fragment, the patient (usually a male) complains of intermittent aching and or discomfort in the knee after exercise (mechanical joint pain), a feeling of insecurity and intermittent swelling.

Once the fragment has separated the main symptom is then recurrent sudden locking, pain, and the knee giving way or collapsing. Both knees should be carefully examined as the condition is bilateral in 1 case in 4. Movements are not usually impaired, there may be effusion, and the vastus medialis may demonstrate atrophy (measure the thigh circumference 5 cm above the superior pole of the patella). With the knee flexed to 90°, tenderness may be elicited by deep palpation over the lateral aspect of the medial femoral condyle (just medial to the inferior pole of the patella). Wilson's sign may be positive. This is performed by flexing the patient's knee to 90°; the tibia is then internally rotated, then as the knee is taken into extension the patient reports experiencing pain. The pain is relieved by inducing external rotation of the tibia. An X-ray examination of both knees should be obtained, which usually shows

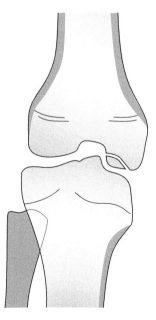

Figure 14.12 ● Osteochondritis dissecans is an osteochondritis that results in the formation of a loose body in the medial compartment of the knee joint, leaving a shallow cavity in the articular surface which is ultimately filled in with fibrocartilage.

the defect. The most productive projection for visualizing the defect is the intercondylar or tunnel view.

Medical investigations can include radionuclide scans which show increased activity around the lesion, MRI scans which consistently show the lesion, and arthroscopy which clearly shows the defect in both the later stages and in the early stages when the defect is concealed beneath the articular cartilage that looks normal. Prodding of the area may demonstrate softening.

In the early stages of the disease when the cartilage is intact, treatment is limited to supporting the knee and curtailing strenuous activities for 6–12 months, as in some cases, especially in the small and young, the lesion can heal spontaneously. When the lesion is 'ripe' (when a clear line of demarcation has formed between the fragment and the surrounding normal bone), surgical options can include removal of the fragment with the cavity filling with fibrocartilage, or pinning the fragment in place.

Patella dislocation/recurrent patella dislocation

Patella dislocation is most common in preadolescent and adolescent girls. The displacement is always lateral and often both knees are affected. The causes of lateral instability of the patella are shown in Box 14.2.

The initial dislocation does not usually involve a violent action, but some activity where the knees are flexed (often dancing), during which severe pain is felt in front of the knee, and the patient is unable to straighten it. The girl may fall to the ground.

Often the dislocation is recognized and immediately reduced by the patient or an onlooker. The knee is swollen, and the patella is seen and felt on the lateral side of the lateral femoral condyle. After reduction there is blood-stained effusion and tenderness over the medial part of the quadriceps expansion, which is usually strained or torn, in turn resulting in laxity of medial to lateral movement.

Some patients only suffer one or two episodes of dislocation and are not bothered again, but many patients suffer multiple dislocations at an increasing rate so that they are seriously handicapped. The repeated dislocation damages the contiguous surfaces of the patella and femoral condyle which increases the flattening of the condyle and facilitates further dislocations. Multiple dislocation events predispose the joint to later degenerative joint disease (DJD).

Box 14.2

Causes of lateral instability of the patella

- General ligamentous laxity (double jointedness/genu recurvatum)
- Underdevelopment of the lateral femoral condyle with a shallow intercondylar groove
- Smaller patella
- An abnormally high position of the patella (patella alta)
- Genu valgum, which causes the line of pull of the quadriceps to be further lateral
- muscle defect

During the 'apprehension test' the knee is slightly flexed and the patella is pushed laterally. When the patient feels the patella is going to dislocate laterally she will contract the quadriceps and have an apprehensive look on her face.

Chiropractic management includes exercises to strengthen the quadriceps muscle (especially vastus medialis), stretching of the iliotibial band, and mobilization of the knee joint, which is thought to facilitate the action of the vastus medialis muscle. If there is a pronated foot (which increases the tibiofemoral valgus angle and the Q angles) then an orthotic device may be appropriate to help prevent recurrences. As the patient grows older, the extensor mechanism often becomes more stable. If the patient is severely disabled by recurring dislocations and she has stopped growing, surgery is an advisable course of action.

Patella tracking dysfunction

Patella tracking dysfunction (PTD), previously referred to as chondromalacia patellae, is common among active adolescent (10–15-year-old) girls, and constitutes a large percentage of chronic, non-traumatic and post-traumatic knee problems. The term 'chondromalacia patellae' means softening of the cartilage of the patella. Because the articular cartilage is not a pain-sensitive structure, the term chondromalacia does not adequately describe the clinically significant features of the pathological process, nor does it take into account etiological considerations. In fact, surgical studies have suggested for many years now that the surface chondromalacia is a relatively normal characteristic of most adult patellae, and probably has little relationship in cause or effect to symptomatic knee problems (Abernathy et al 1978, Goodfellow et al 1976, Meachim & Emery 1974, Outerbridge 1961, Shoji 1974, Storigord 1975).

Biomechanically, the direction of pull of the quadriceps tends to be in line with the femur, whereas the pull of the patella ligament is in line with the long axis of the tibia. The angle formed between these lines of pull is the Q angle. The lateral vector component causes a tendency for the patella to be pulled laterally during contraction of the quadriceps. The anatomic factors which stabilize the patella to prevent lateral movement are shown in Box 14.3.

As the knee approaches full extension the patella moves superiorly out of the deep part of the patellar groove, and the patellofemoral compressive force decreases. In this position dynamic stabilizing factors then play an essential role. The most important dynamic factor is contraction of the vastus medialis obliquus muscle (VMO), which prevents excessive lateral movement of the patella during knee extension.

Chronic PTD is a condition in which the patella tends to be pulled too far laterally each time the knee is extended under load. During normal knee function the small odd medial facet of the patella only makes contact (compressive force) during the extremes of knee flexion, a position that they seldom assume. Thus, during normal use, the odd medial facet is non-articulating and does not receive much compressive force. Because of this the subchondral bone is less dense, softer, and weaker than the rest of the undersurface of the patella.

Box 14.3

The anatomic factors which stabilize the patella to prevent lateral movement

- The prominence of the lateral femoral condyle anteriorly
- The depth of the patella groove
- When the knee is flexed, the pull from the patella ligament and tendon results in a patellofemoral compression force that holds the patella firmly against the patella groove
- Proper position of the patella

If during knee extension the patella is pulled too far laterally, the patella will follow the contour of the patellar groove of the femur, causing the patella to undergo some rotation (tilting) in the transverse plane, bringing the odd medial facet into a contacting position. With such contact, the relatively weak subchondral bone of the odd medial facet may be unable to withstand the loads imposed on it. This results in an increased rate of trabecular microfracturing, which may incite a low-grade, painful inflammatory response.

Excessive lateral patella movement during repeated extension may cause abnormal tensile stresses to the medial retinaculum of the knee. This could also be a source of low-grade inflammation and pain. The symptoms which are characteristic of chronic PTD are shown in Box 14.4.

In terms of treatment, 60–80% of knees treated conservatively respond favorably to non-operative treatment. Success depends on the cooperation and compliance of an informed patient. Failures are often due to inadequate advice by the practitioner regarding restriction of activities and/or inappropriate VMO strengthening (Fig. 14.13). A typical conservative treatment protocol is outlined in Box 14.5.

Surgical treatment should be avoided, for although a variety of procedures have been devised the results are almost universally disappointing (Adams & Hamblen 2001). Surgical procedures have included scraping of the soft cartilage from the articular surface, division of the lateral retinaculum, repositioning the patella ligament insertion distally and medially, and patellectomy.

Chiropractic management of chondromalacia is multifactorial. Firstly, an attempt should be made to correct any contributing anomalies such as pronation (referral to a podiatrist), fixed flexion deformity of the hip (chiropractic correction of iliopsoas spasm), etc. Secondly, subluxation complex affecting the knee or ankle should be corrected and maintained, as should any spinal subluxation complex. Subluxation of the lower lumbar spine and pelvis is frequently associated with lower limb disorders and should be actively managed. Thirdly, exercise designed to strengthen the knee extensor and hamstring muscle groups should be prescribed (Figs 14.13 and 14.14). Fourthly, it may also be useful to apply cross-friction techniques to the genu articularis muscles to alleviate any tension they may cause in the tracking process of the patella during knee motion. Finally, mobilization of the patella may be performed, beginning with very passive movement and, as pain permits, the degree of distraction should be increased until the

Box 14.4

Symptoms characteristic of chronic patella tracking dysfunction

- Gradual onset of pain (there may be a recent increase in activities, or an injury or a period of disuse)
- Deep pain is felt in a generalized area over the medial aspect of the knee, and prepatellar region
- Pain is aggravated by activities involving patellofemoral compression, such as:
  - descending stairs
  - sitting with the knee bent for long periods of time
  - squatting
- Crepitus, easily felt if you palpate the knee while the patient does a deep knee bend from a standing position

Signs might include:

- Patella malalignment (glide component, tilt component, rotation component, anteroposterior position) (Hertling & Kessler 1996)
- A predisposing factor (femoral anteversion, external tibial torsion, increased foot pronation, genu recurvatum which may be associated with patella alta, generalized joint laxity, leg length discrepancies)
- Visible VMO atrophy
- Weakness of VMO
- Tightness of the lateral retinaculum
- Tightness of the iliotibial band
- Tight gastrocnemius and/or hamstrings may place increased demand on the quadriceps muscle during knee extension
- Weakness of hip abductors and external rotators has been associated with PTD
- Discomfort if the patella is passively moved laterally, if the medial retinaculum is irritated
- Patellofemoral grinding test is usually positive (*Note*: this test can be positive in asymptomatic patients)
- Tenderness to deep palpation of the back side of the medial patella
- Tenderness to palpation of the adductor tubercle, where the medial retinaculum attaches

PTD, patella tracking dysfunction; VMO, vastus medialis obliquus.

---

mobilization can be performed pain-free with the knee held in slight flexion.

The ankle and foot region

Sever's disease

Sever's disease is a traction apophysitis on the posterior calcaneus from the pull of the Achilles tendon, and, as with OSD and SLJ, occurs in active (jumping) children, usually boys about 10–14 years of age (Adams & Hamblen 2001, Apley & Solomon 1993, Dandy & Edwards 2003). Typically the child complains of pain behind the heel, slight swelling over the posterior aspect of the heel, which is tender to palpation, and may have a slight limp. The X-ray examination is usually

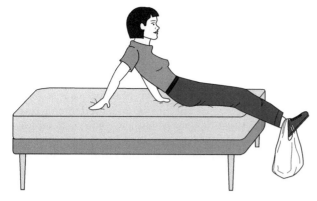

Figure 14.13 • Exercise for strengthening the quadriceps muscle group in patients with PTD. Place a 1–2 kg weight in a plastic supermarket or similar bag, place it over the foot as shown, lean back and slowly lift the foot until the knee is in full extension. Hold it there for 10 seconds, then slowly lower it again. The exercise is most effective if performed two to three times per day within pain tolerance.

Box 14.5

A typical conservative treatment protocol for PTD

- Decrease activities involving high and/or prolonged patellofemoral compressive loads (walking down stairs, bent knee sitting, etc.)
- VMO strengthening exercises
- If the lateral retinaculum appears tight it should be stretched (heat, ultrasound, stretch)
- If foot pronation is present consider referral to a podiatrist
- Stretching of the iliotibial band
- Manipulation of the knee joint medial to lateral to stretch tight lateral knee structures – which is believed to facilitate VMO training
- Tight hamstrings have long been recognized as a cause of various extensor mechanism disorders of the knee. It is therefore appropriate to stretch tight hamstrings
- Ice and/or anti-inflammatory medication

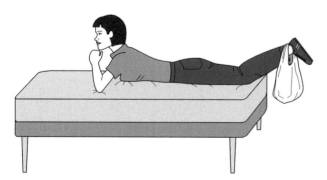

Figure 14.14 • Exercise for strengthening the hamstring muscle group in patients with PTD. Place a 1–2 kg weight in a plastic supermarket or similar bag, place it over the foot as shown and slowly lift the foot until the knee is flexed to approximately 30°. Hold it there for 10 seconds, then slowly lower it again. The exercise is most effective if performed two to three times per day within pain tolerance.

normal. Treatment usually consists of restricting activities, ice, raising the heel half an inch or, if pain is particularly troublesome, a below-the-knee walking plaster will give relief.

Köhler's disease

Köhler's disease is an osteochondritis of the developing nucleus of the navicular causing softening and deformity of the navicular in 3–5-year-olds (kindergarten–preschool children). Typically the child complains of pain in the inner (midtarsal) part of the foot, limping (may walk on the outer side of the foot), tenderness over the navicular, and sometimes there is pain on forced movement.

The X-ray examination shows the bone to be squashed and more dense than normal, and it may have a fragmented appearance. Over the 2–3-year span of the disease, the normal texture of the bone is restored, but the shape is compressed.

Treatment is often not necessary, but the pain may be reduced by strapping and restricting activity for a few weeks, or it may be necessary to rest the foot in a walking plaster.

Freiberg's disease

Freiberg's disease is an avascular necrosis causing pain in a metatarsal head (usually the second) which is aggravated by standing or walking and relieved by rest, in an adolescent (more commonly girls) during their growth spurt (13–18 years) (Adams & Hamblen 2001, Saidoff & McDonough 2002). The metatarsal head may become deformed under pressure of weight-bearing.

On examination the affected metatarsal head may be enlarged and tender. The joint is irritable (painful on movement) and X-rays show the head to be fragmented/granular, wider, and to have lost its dome shape to become more square. After about 2 years the texture of the bone returns to normal, but the squaring of the articular surface remains (which predisposes to later osteoarthritis of the joint).

In terms of treatment, if the disease is detected at an early stage before deformity of the joint surface has occurred, the patient should cease all sports activity and the area should be immobilized in a walking plaster in the hope that it will resolve with minimal deformity. Surgery is an option in the hope of preventing permanent distortion of the joint surface. Through a window cut in the dorsal surface of the metatarsal neck the necrotic bone of the head is curetted out and replaced by cancellous chip bone grafts, packed firmly enough to restore the normal dome-shaped contour of the articular surface. The foot is then placed in plaster for 6 weeks.

Intoeing/pigeon toeing

Intoeing (pigeon toeing) causes concern for many parents, but it is a normal part of development of the lower limbs (Fig. 14.15). When it is persistent, there are possible causes in the hip, tibia, and/or forefoot.

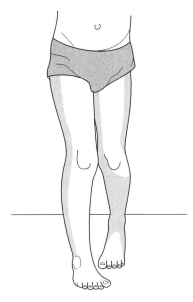

Figure 14.15 • Intoeing in a preschool-age child.

Femoral anteversion

The neck of the femur is directed more anteriorly, so that the only comfortable way for the child to keep the femoral head in the acetabulum without stretching the capsule is to rotate the femur internally, causing the knees and toes to point inwards (these children often find it more comfortable to sit with their legs in the 'W' position).

On examination it is appropriate to observe the position of the patellae. The whole leg will be internally rotated so that both the foot and the patella point medially. Secondly, with the child sitting, rotate the femur internally and externally by swinging the tibia medially and laterally. Normally these movements are equal but with femoral anteversion the foot will swing further out (i.e. internal thigh rotation is increased), and the foot will not swing as far inwards (i.e. external thigh rotation is decreased). Referral is advised if this persists beyond the age of 8 years.

Internal tibial torsion

The natural internal tibial torsion that is seen in newborn babies can persist up to age 4 years. The examination is performed by having the child sit on the examination table with the knees flexed at 90°. The examiner then places a finger on both the internal and external malleoli. By about age 4 this should reveal approximately 15° of external tibial torsion (relative to the edge of the table). Referral is advised if internal tribial torsion persists beyond the age of 4 years.

Metatarsus adductus/forefoot varus

On observation of the sole of the foot, a line along the long axis of the calcaneus should pass between the 2nd and 3rd toe space. In metatarsus adductus the forefoot adducts (i.e. the calcaneal line passes lateral to the 2nd–3rd toe space). If the deformity can be manually corrected beyond the neutral position, it can most likely be corrected by stretching of the foot during the first few weeks of life (which the parents can do).

A non-mobile foot (the forefoot cannot be adducted beyond the neutral position) should be referred, as it may indicate tarsal coalition. Referral is advised if this persists beyond the age of 2 years.

Out-toeing

Out-toeing (Fig. 14.16) has four principal causes: 'external rotation contracture of the hip in infancy, femoral retroversion, external tibial torsion' (Renshaw 1986), and subluxation of the lumbar spine, pelvis, hip and knee.

External rotation contracture is the result of tightness in the external rotators, probably arising from the baby's intrauterine position. It is seen on examination as very little internal rotation and excessive external rotation. In addition to adjusting the attendant chiropractic subluxation patterns, parents should be shown how to stretch the affected muscle group.

The upper limb

The shoulder region

Fracture of the clavicle

Fracture of the clavicle occurs in all pediatric age groups (e.g. due to a fall on the shoulder or a fall on an outstretched hand (FOOSH) injury), and the clavicle is the most commonly fractured bone at birth. Diagnosis is relatively simple. The child presents with a history of a difficult birth or trauma and loss of the normal contour of the affected clavicle (a painful lump over its middle one-third).

There is no active management for a fractured clavicle in a newborn apart from careful handling of the affected shoulder by the parents and other caregivers. As soon as the initial sharp pain begins to subside (usually 1–2 weeks), active shoulder exercises should begin to restore full mobility. In children the fracture will be solid after only 2–3 weeks. The callus at the fracture site in children can also be alarming to parents,

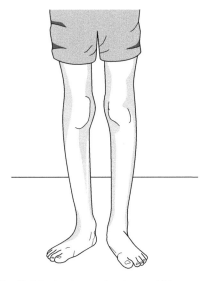

Figure 14.16 • Out-toeing in a school-age child.

as the clavicle may have looked normal immediately after the injury. In time the callus diminishes as the bone remodels.

After 6 weeks, or when union of the bone can be guaranteed, the acromioclavicular and sternoclavicular joints should be checked for functional integrity. There may also be chiropractic subluxations in the cervical spine and the first rib to deal with.

Sprengel's deformity

The Sprengel's deformity is the most frequent congenital deformity of the shoulder girdle, and represents a failure of the scapula to descend (the scapula is part of the C5–C6 sclerotome and myotome). It usually affects one scapula, which is small, hypomobile, associated with poorly developed muscles and an omovertebral band or bone which connects the scapula to the lower cervical spinous processes. Shoulder movements, especially abduction, may be restricted. Sprengel's deformity is known to be associated with spinal (Klippel–Feil) and renal anomalies.

Surgical treatment is not often recommended as it seldom improves function. It may, however, improve the appearance (and should be done before the age of 5–6 years), but can cause considerable scarring (Adams & Hamblen 2001, Renshaw 1986, Salter 1999). Full spine radiography is an essential investigation prior to chiropractic care. Adjustive thrusts have to be avoided in those motion segments affected by the omovertebral band or bone.

The elbow region

Pulled elbow

Pulled elbow is otherwise known as painful pronation or nursemaid's elbow. This is one of the more common pain syndromes encountered by chiropractors, with the diagnosis easily made on the basis of the characteristic history, posture, and physical examination findings.

Between the ages of 2 and 4 years (but reported up to 6 years) children are prone to subluxation of the cartilaginous radial head out of the annular ligament (Adams & Hamblen 2001, Illingworth 1982). The child presents with pain, crying and fretting, and refuses to use the arm. He or she will invariably hold the injured arm in pronation with the extended elbow hanging limply at the side. The child is very unwilling to be examined or even touched. The parent or caregiver, fearing that something is broken, will report a traumatic incident in which the child's pronated elbow was suddenly pulled by the forearm or wrist (as in catching a falling child, or pulling a child up stairs, for example) (Bretland 1994, Salter 1999). Post-mortem studies demonstrate that in young children a sudden pull on the extended pronated elbow produces a tear in the distal attachment of the annular ligament, and when the pull is released part of the annular ligament slips into the radiohumeral joint, the source of the pain being the pinched annular ligament. Post-mortem studies also indicate that, with the elbow flexed, sudden supination of the forearm frees the incarcerated part of the ligament which then resumes its normal position (Salter 1999).

The child is going to be reluctant to allow the chiropractor to examine the elbow and may become overanxious to the point of hysteria when an attempt is made to do so. Examination technique should be extremely gentle and performed slowly with constant reassurance given to the child that you will not hurt them. Characteristically there will be tenderness over the anteromedial aspect of the radial head, markedly decreased and painful supination of the forearm which is actively resisted, and lack of voluntary movement of the arm generally.

There is no useful evidence of injury on X-ray examination (Renshaw 1986). The radiographer may unwittingly 'treat' the condition by encouraging the child to 'be a brave little boy or girl' and position the elbow in supination for the anteroposterior X-ray view, causing the radial head to relocate.

The child with pulled elbow can be readily and successfully managed by the chiropractor without resort to assistance from either radiology or medical specialists. A number of methods of reduction which are usually easy and painless, and have most children using the elbow again within minutes, have been variously described by Bretland (1994), Renshaw (1986), Tachdjian (1972) and Salter (1999). The basic essentials are as follows:

- The practitioner's thumb is placed in the antecubital space. The other hand takes the wrist and firmly supinates the forearm, and gently flexes the arm acutely against the fulcrum of the thumb in the 'crotch' of the elbow. A slight 'click' may be felt, the pain is relieved, and normal use restored. No aftercare is required.
- Longitudinal pressure of the radius against the humerus with the elbow flexed. The forearm can be alternately pronated and supinated, and the radial head will pop back into position with dramatic relief of pain.

The mechanism of injury commonly causes joint-related problems reflexively at the acromioclavicular, sternoclavicular and first costovertebral joints as well as the lower cervical and/or upper thoracic motion segments, and on occasion in the wrist. All these areas need to be examined and corrections made as necessary. A failure of the symptoms associated with pulled elbow to resolve rapidly and permanently raises the possibility of an unrecognized injury, which should be assessed, and referred to an orthopedist if no cause can be found.

The wrist and hand region

Infantile trigger thumb

This condition is usually seen before the age of 2 years and can be mistaken for a dislocated thumb, or a congenital anomaly. Its presentation is similar to that of trigger finger in adults. Characteristically, the child is unable to straighten the thumb, which is locked in flexion. It is sometimes possible for the examiner to extend the thumb passively. A palpable nodule will be present at the base of the thumb, at the position of the mouth of the flexor tendon sheath (at the head of the first metacarpal bone).

Active treatment for this condition is not necessary. Spontaneous recovery often occurs after a few months. In the event it does not, injection of the tendon sheath with hydrocortisone is appropriate followed by open release of the tendon sheath if the condition has not resolved by age 4 years.

The cervical spine

Congenital infantile (muscular) torticollis

In pediatrics, congenital muscular torticollis, or 'wry neck' as it is sometimes referred to, is most frequently a benign cosmetic problem which may result in facial asymmetry (Lloyd-Roberts & Fixsen 1990) and plagiocephaly. The condition is a result of tightness in one sternocleidomastoid (SCM) muscle which is sometimes associated with a palpable non-tender 'tumor' or mass in the belly of the muscle at about the level of the angle of the mandible. This 'tumor' was shown by Sanerkin & Edwards (1966) to contain hemorrhage, fragmentation, muscle necrosis, and disruption of the endomysial sheaths which is known to lead to fibrosis. This description of the histopathology of the 'tumor' lends credence to an etiology of intrauterine malposition causing localized ischemia, or injury during birth interfering with the blood supply to the SCM (it is more common following difficult delivery, breech presentations and in infants of primaparas) (Lloyd-Roberts & Fixsen 1990).

Typically the presentation involves an infant whose head is tilted toward the involved side and rotated toward the shoulder on the side opposite the torticollis. The 'tumor' may regress or disappear in 3–6 months, but if it does not regress the affected muscle becomes shortened and replaced by fibrous tissue, with associated contractures in the soft tissues of the neck. If the deformity persists untreated, compensatory curvature of the cervical and thoracic spine with elevation of the shoulder on the affected side may occur.

Congenital muscular torticollis is most amenable to correction using a combination of chiropractic adjusting and home-based exercise. There are, however, some known causes of torticollis which would make such an approach to treatment catastrophic (Box 14.6) (Bussieres et al 1994, Toto 1993) and these should be ruled out before any treatment of a physical kind is implemented. It is essential to perform a full neurological examination in addition to a radiological assessment of the cervical spine in children presenting with congenital muscular torticollis (Shafrir & Kaufman 1992).

Once a pathological cause has been ruled out, it is appropriate to implement a home exercise program and chiropractic care. To assist with the correction of the problem, following application of a warm moist towel, parents are taught how to apply gentle stretching exercises (to increase the distance between the origin and insertion of the SCM muscle) several times a day. This is accomplished by gently bending the neck laterally, away from the side of the involved SCM, and then slowly providing maximum rotation of the head and face toward the side of the torticollis. This position should be held for 5 seconds, released, and then repeated 5–10 times at each exercise session. An exercise session should ideally be performed each time the baby is changed, if practicable (Renshaw 1986).

While some children with congenital muscular torticollis will not respond to chiropractic care and exercise, it is both safe and appropriate to continue care for at least the first 2 years of life regardless of facial asymmetry, since successful surgical outcome is not age-dependent and a good result may be expected in children right up to puberty (Lloyd-Roberts &

Box 14.6

Pathological causes of congenital muscular torticollis

- Neoplasms of the spinal column, spinal cord and soft tissues of the neck
- Infection of the spinal column, spinal cord and soft tissues of the neck
- Fracture of the skull, neck or clavicle
- Instability and dislocation of the upper cervical spine
- Congenital malformations of the cervical spine
- Oculomotor lesion(s) – cranial nerves III, IV and/or VI

Fixsen 1990, Renshaw 1986). Surgery is a last resort treatment approach and is usually performed at 3–4 years of age. It is essential that surgery should be followed by regular chiropractic care and the stretching exercises described above if the best possible results are to be obtained.

The thoracic spine

Scoliosis

Scoliosis is a lateral curvature of the spine, but is actually a triplanar deformity with lateral, anteroposterior and rotational components. Scoliosis describes the physical deformity, but is not a diagnosis per se. There are several types of scoliosis and these are detailed in Table 14.3.

Adolescent idiopathic scoliosis (AIS) is the most common type of structural scoliosis, more common in girls (females predominate with curves over 30°) who are significantly taller than matched controls (they begin their growth spurt earlier, but adult heights show no difference), with the onset usually between 10 and 12 years at the time of the adolescent growth spurt. The adolescent growth spurt spans a period of approximately 3½ years, with the greatest growth occurring during the first 1½ years. Of AIS patients requiring surgery, 85% are female. In the early stages the child does not normally have pain, despite the appearance of the deformity. The older child may complain of back fatigue and pain secondary to long-standing musculoskeletal imbalance.

Normally the thoracic curve is convex to the right (rib hump will be on the right), and the lumbar spine curves to the left. By thrusting the ribs backward on the convex side, this rotation increases the severity of the deformity. Progression is not inevitable. Most curves under 20° resolve spontaneously or remain unchanged. General predictors of progression are a female patient of young age with a severe curve.

Physical examination should determine whether there are any associated findings such as bony anomalies, neurological conditions, patches of hair along the midline and/or café-au-lait spots. The standing patient should be observed from both the posterior and the anterior for evidence of scoliotic deformity such as asymmetry of the waist, breasts, shoulder or hip height, winging of the scapulae or head tilt, and also from the side for an increase in the thoracic kyphosis and/or lumbar lordosis.

Table 14.3 Clinical characteristics of the types and subtypes of scoliosis in children and adolescents

Age-related common orthopedic syndromes in pediatrics

Non-structural scoliosis (changes with changes in posture)
- Postural scoliosis (secondary to a non-spinal condition – poor posture, short leg, hip contracture, muscle spasm)
- Sciatic scoliosis (seen with painful spinal conditions)

Structural scoliosis (does not change with changes in posture)
- Osteopathic scoliosis (seen with congenital bone anomalies, fracture, bone softening disease)
- Neuropathic and myopathic scoliosis (poliomyelitis, cerebral palsy, Friedrich's ataxia, neurofibromatosis, muscular dystrophy)
- Idiopathic scoliosis
  - 0–3 years, infantile idiopathic scoliosis (rare, 95% resolve spontaneously)
  - 4–9 years, juvenile idiopathic scoliosis (rare, similar to adolescent idiopathic scoliosis but with a poorer prognosis)
  - >10 years, adolescent (AIS – this section of Chapter 14 relates to this form of scoliosis)

Box 14.7

Five signs of scoliosis on physical examination
- Shoulder unleveling
- One prominent scapula
- Visual or palpable lateral curve
- Adam's position – persistence of the curve and rib humping
- Adam's position – unequal distance of the fingers from the floor

---

When the patient is sitting, if the curve disappears, then it is most likely due to a short leg. Because of the concealing effect of clothing, a scoliosis may reach considerable proportions before being noticed and it may initially be poorly fitting clothing that draws parents' attention to their child's back.

It is appropriate to perform an Adam's test and observe for the right rib hump on the convex side. The forward bending makes the curve and rib hump more obvious (as distinct from postural or mobile scoliosis). Five signs of scoliosis seen on physical examination are shown in Box 14.7.

X-ray examination is absolutely essential in all patients meeting the physical examination criteria for scoliosis. A full-spine (14′ × 36′) posterior to anterior view (taken standing) for signs of any bony anomalies, location of the curve, and pelvic unleveling is the appropriate examination. At least three measurements should then be determined: (1) the angle of the curve (Cobb method is most reliable); (2) assessment of vertebral body rotation (Nash–Moe method); and (3) determination of skeletal maturity using the Risser score (iliac crest apophysis).

Skeletal maturity is estimated by observing the extent of the ossification of the iliac apophysis (Risser's score) which progresses from lateral to medial around the iliac crest and fuses to the ilium at the same time as fusion of the vertebral ring apophyses, after which time further progression is minimal. A numerical value is assigned to Risser's score according to how extensive the iliac apophysis ossification is. The upper pelvic rim is divided into four equal parts and the criteria used to determine the numerical value for Risser's score are shown in Box 14.8.

By way of clinical interpretation, in a child who presents with a scoliosis, a Risser score of 0 means there is a 36% chance of progression, a score of 2 means there is an 11% chance of progression, and a score of 5 indicates there is little chance of progression (Yochum & Rowe 1996).

Other radiographic assessment can consist of studies to determine the degree of kyphosis using the Cobb method on the lateral X-ray (T1–T12), and studies to determine the degree of flexibility of the curve. X-ray examination is often repeated as often as every 3–4 months to determine if progression is occurring. It has been suggested the X-ray be taken P-A in order to take advantage of any decrease in radiation exposure to developing breast tissue that this position may offer (Souza 2005). Repeat X-rays are advised to be taken at the same time of day because diurnal variation has been shown to change the Cobb angle by as much as 5° (Beauchamp et al 1993).

Progression is not inevitable. Most curves under 20° resolve spontaneously or remain unchanged. Scoliosis is also far less likely to be progressive in male patients. Normally, if a curve does start to deteriorate, then it will usually continue to do so during the remainder of the growth period, and often slightly after that. The most important indicator of a good prognosis (little chance of progression) is closure of the vertebral growth plates (Risser score of 5).

The management, co-management or referral for surgery of a case by a chiropractor is dependent on the findings of the assessment mentioned above. The following parameters may be helpful:

Curves less than 20°

In the young child the chiropractor can institute treatment to correct biomechanical faults in the spine and lower limb, but the patient needs to be periodically reassessed to determine whether the curve is improving, remaining static or progressing. If it becomes apparent that the curve is deteriorating, the parents should be advised and the need for medical referral discussed. If the patient has reached skeletal maturity, further progression is unlikely.

Many chiropractors have claimed success in the treatment of scoliosis, but it is unclear what type of scoliosis they were dealing with. Other than a few isolated case reports, there is

Box 14.8

Criteria for applying a numerical value to Risser's score

1. Appearance of the apophysis in the outer 25% of the upper pelvic rim
2. Appearance of the apophysis in the outer 50% of the upper pelvic rim
3. Appearance of the apophysis in the outer 75% of the upper pelvic rim
4. Appearance of the apophysis in all four quarters of the upper pelvic rim
5. Apophysis is fused to the ilium

a dearth of research evidence to indicate that chiropractic care has any effect on the natural history of AIS. There is also no such evidence available for the medical practice of spinal bracing; however, anecdotal evidence suggests it may be effective in the 30–40° range.

One theory for the development and progression of idiopathic scoliosis which fits in well with the various chiropractic theories is that when abnormal sensory information from the spine is processed at the central nervous system level it is misinterpreted as normal leading to inappropriate output information regarding body orientation in space (Herman et al 1985).

Curves between 20° and 40°

A dilemma often exists for chiropractors faced with a patient with a progressive curve where the parents are seeking an alternative to bracing and surgery. The practitioner should explain to the patient and parents the consequences of allowing the curve to progress and weigh this against the possible advantages of bracing or surgery. It should be understood, however, that these curves (20–40°) are still within the conservative (chiropractic and medical) management range.

If the patient has not reached skeletal maturity and the curve is less than 30°, conservative chiropractic treatment can be offered. However, if progression is noted, the patient should be referred for bracing (this is the range in which bracing is believed by many to be most effective). Patients do not wear the brace for 24 hours (current prescription is more commonly for 16–18 hours a day), so even when a patient has been prescribed a brace, the patient can still be given chiropractic care. Girls who are braced at or before the time of menarche have the best results.

Braces are used during the period while waiting until the child is old enough for operation (surgery is usually deferred until early adolescence in order to minimize loss of height that may result from fusion of a significant length of the growing spine), and may diminish the severity of the curve sufficiently to make subsequent surgery less extensive and formidable. It needs to be appreciated that this is a very contentious point as opinion certainly differs about the effectiveness of bracing, as it has never been subjected to prospective controlled trials and may merely mask the natural history of variable rates of progression of the curves, meaning the 'successes' may have been in those cases that would not have progressed anyway (Adams & Hamblen 2001, Dandy & Edwards 2003).

Co-management with medical specialists is recommended when curves enter this equivocal range (20–40°) where clinical decisions become more difficult. The aims of chiropractic care include the following (Souza 2005):

- maintaining spinal intersegmental flexibility (a more flexible spine may be less likely to have scoliosis develop)
- manipulation of the cervical spine may influence righting mechanisms in an effort to balance the spine (Nansel et al 1993)
- removal of segmental dysfunction may eliminate sources of aberrant sensory input and consequent output problems such as pain and accompanying muscle spasm

- proprioceptive input would then be normalized, providing an appropriate database for higher cortical decisions of body positioning
- leveling of the pelvis.

If the patient is approaching skeletal maturity and the deformity is acceptable (<30°) and well balanced, medical treatment is unnecessary unless sequential X-rays show definite progression. If the patient has reached skeletal maturity, progression is not likely, and so chiropractic treatment is directed to correction of biomechanical faults.

Curves greater than 40°

The patient has now reached a stage where bracing may be tried; if that does not work surgery is the recommended treatment. As well as the appearance and chronic pain, severe scoliosis can have disastrous cardiopulmonary and neurological consequences and is associated with higher rates of psychosocial adjustment problems, unemployment, delayed marriage, or no marriage at all (Bunch & Patwardham 1989).

Scheuermann's disease

Scheuermann's disease (SD), otherwise known as adolescent kyphosis, is a growth disorder and is the most common cause of 'round back' deformity in teenagers (Fig. 14.17). The etiology is unknown but leads to the vertebral body becoming slightly wedge shaped, which results in an exaggeration of the normal thoracic kyphosis. Possibly half of the teenagers with SD have spinal pain, which commonly lasts 1–2 years. The patient is often brought to the practitioner because the parents have noticed that in an otherwise fit teenager there is 'poor posture' or 'round shoulders' and by this time they are often tired of the parent's nagging to 'stand up straight and stop slouching'.

The reported incidence varies greatly (from 0.4% to 8.3%) depending on whether the criteria for diagnosis are based on X-ray or clinical findings (Jahn 1978). Some authors say it is more common in boys (Adams & Hamblen 2001, Dandy & Edwards 2003), others say it is twice as common in girls (Apley & Solomon 1993) or occurs equally (Jahn 1978). SD is easily diagnosed by history, clinical appearance and X-ray examination.

The physical examination reveals a smooth, increased thoracic kyphosis below which is a compensatory increase in the lumbar lordosis. Percussion over the affected spinous processes may produce tenderness; palpation usually reveals paraspinal muscle spasm; and an associated scoliosis is found in 30–40% of the cases. The thoracic deformity cannot be corrected by changes in posture (as opposed to a postural kyphosis). The parents should be told that the child cannot help standing with rounded shoulders and that continually nagging their child to 'stand up straight' is unhelpful and frustrating. Movements are normal, but tight hamstrings often limit straight leg raising, and the pectoral muscle group is often found to be tight.

On the lateral X-ray, the endplates of the mid to lower thoracic vertebrae (usually T6–T10) appear irregular or fragmented, the changes being more marked anteriorly, and one or more vertebral bodies may become wedge shaped. Later in life

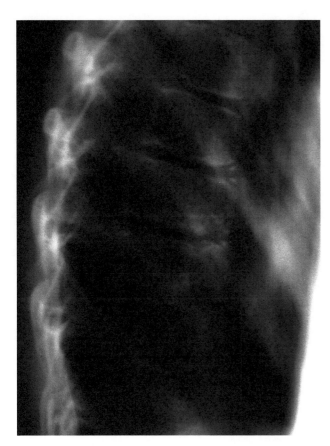

Figure 14.17 • Scheuermann's disease in an adolescent male. Note the irregular, fragmented endplates and the wedge-shaped vertebral bodies. (Reproduced from Adams & Hamblen 2001.)

the SD patient may develop degenerative changes secondary to the vertebral deformation. This is not an uncommon cause of adult thoracic pain where the origin is Scheuermann's disease during adolescence.

Assuming that sufficient growth time remains, chiropractic care based on empirical data seems to be clinically sound in its aim of preventing progression of the deformity of the vertebral bodies.

The lumbar spine

The chiropractic subluxation syndrome

In the lumbar spine and pelvis, the chiropractic subluxation occurs most commonly at the L5/S1 junction and at the sacro-iliac joints. The expected distribution of pain from the lumbo-pelvic subluxation complex is shown on an anatomical basis in Table 14.4. While there are many similarities between the adult and child, the most striking difference is the paucity of pain seen in children below the knee arising from the lumbar disc syndrome. The chiropractic subluxation syndrome is a diagnosis which is made by exclusion. A pain syndrome in the lumbar spine, pelvis or lower limb of a child should never be attributed to a mechanical cause alone until a careful search for pathology has been undertaken.

Pediatric low back pain

Recognition of pediatric low back pain (PLBP) as a serious health problem is increasing as studies are emerging showing it to be much more common than once believed. For decades, low back pain was thought to be uncommon among children and adolescents, and when present it was considered a serious pathological condition. This belief was largely based on hospital and clinic-based studies looking at presentation of PLBP to tertiary care practitioners such as pediatric orthopedists. More recent community and school-based studies have shown a much higher prevalence of this condition than previously suspected (Balague et al 1988, 1993, 1995; Burton et al 1996; Ebrall 1994b; Fairbank et al 1984; Kujala et al 1992, 1996, 1997; Leboeuf-Yde & Kyvik 1998; Mireau et al 1984; Newcomer et al 1997; Olsen et al 1992; Salimen et al 1992, 1995; Troussier et al 1994; Turner et al 1989), and that most cases of PLBP do not present to health professionals for treatment.

Taimela et al (1997), in a study of 1171 children aged 7–16 years, reported a LBP prevalence of 1% in 7-year-olds, 6% in 10-year-olds, and 18% in 14- and 16-year-olds, which was chronic or recurrent in 33% of females and 26% of males. A UK study of 216 students (Burton et al 1996) reported a prevalence of 11.6% in 11-year-olds, and 50.4% in 15-year-olds. Lebeouf-Yde & Kyvik 1998 (4884 12–17-year-olds), Ebrall 1994b (610 12–19-year-olds), Newcomer et al 1997 (96 10–19-year-olds) and Balague et al 1995 (615 12–17-year-olds) all reported a prevalence of over 50%.

Initial low back pain episodes most often occur at 12–14 years of age (Fairbank et al 1984, Newcomer & Sinaki 1996) with a 16-fold increase in prevalence by 16–20 years of age (Burton et al 1996). One study reported that almost 15% of children experience frequent or continual back pain (Troussier et al 1994). Olsen et al (1992) reported that one-third of children with back pain experienced restricted activity as a result of pain, demonstrating that this had a significant impact on these children.

Different levels of physical activity have been found to influence PLBP: children involved in competitive sports (Balague et al 1988; Burton et al 1996; Kujala et al 1996, 1997; Newcomer & Sinaki 1996; Troussier et al 1994) and children who are sedentary (Salimen et al 1995) have both been found to be at increased risk of developing PLBP, while moderate activity appears to have a protective effect (Newcomer & Sinaki 1996). However, other studies have not corroborated these results: Taimela et al (1997) reported no significant relationship to activity level; and studies by Balague et al (1993) and Fairbank et al (1984) found no relationship to sport.

Anthropometric factors such as increased height (in males) (Salimen et al 1992) and increased trunk length (Fairbank et al 1984) have been related to PLBP. Decreased spinal function including decreased lumbar range of motion (Salimen et al 1992), decreased strength of the supporting abdominal musculature (Kujala et al 1996), and sacroiliac joint dysfunction (Mireau et al 1984) have also been suggested as risk factors for PLBP. Other factors which appear related to PLBP occurrence are previous back injury (Troussier et al 1994), presence of increased degenerative disc disease (Salimen et al 1995), psychological factors (Balague et al 1995), smoking, and

Table 14.4 Common pain locations and patterns of weak muscles associated with various anatomical levels in the chiropractic subluxation syndrome

Subluxation location	Expected distribution of pain
Thoracolumbar junction	Subluxation at the thoracolumbar junction is often associated with suboccipital headache, flank pain similar to that seen with renal pathology and local pain at the site of subluxation similar to that seen with Scheuermann's disease
Midlumbar spine	Recurrent abdominal pain which is vague and migratory, in which growth factors are normal and there are no other signs of intra-abdominal pathology
Lumbosacral junction	Pain is usually seen locally at the L5/S1 area with radiation into the posterior acetabular area and into the upper half of the lateral or posterolateral thigh. Referred pain to the sacrococcygeal junction is common
PI innominate	Pain experienced in the involved sacroiliac joint with an aching quality with radiation into the hamstring group. Pain in the medial knee is also common
AS innominate	Groin pain, especially when associated with the 'In' innominate listing. Can also cause pain in the testes and aching in the gluteus maximus
In innominate	Frequently associated with the AS innominate listing, in which case it causes groin and sometimes testicular pain
Ex innominate	Pain in the gluteus medius/minimus muscles. Sometimes associated with the piriformis syndrome
Sacrum	Suboccipital headache, midthoracic pain, thoracolumbar pain, urinary incontinence and occasionally radiations into the posterolateral thigh on the side of rotary subluxation
Pubic symphysis	Medial thigh pain in the region of the hip adductors and gracilis muscles. Suprapubic pain and muscular tenderness at the costal insertions of the rectus abdominis muscles. Associated with dysfunction of the diaphragm on the side of pubic ramus superiority. Middle one-third groin pain is also a common occurrence
Coccyx	Pain is typically at the sacrococcygeal junction with the patient reporting a sense of inadequate rectal emptying on defecation and a feeling of constant pressure in the rectum, particularly after prolonged sitting

increased time spent watching television (Balague et al 1988, Troussier et al 1994). Reports on the influence of gender on PLBP risk have been inconclusive; two studies demonstrated an increased incidence for females (Troussier et al 1994), although these results have not been supported by other studies (Olsen et al 1992).

Medical clinic-based studies have estimated that 50% of PLBP cases are mechanical (often called non-specific or idiopathic in the literature) (Abril Martin et al 1997) with the remainder due to a specific or serious cause. Because the data for this study come from medical clinics, and many cases of PLBP fail to present to health professionals, the percentage of cases of mechanical PLBP is likely to be higher. This is supported by the suggested risk factors discussed above. In fact, the distribution of etiologies in PLBP has been suggested to be similar to that of adult low back pain (Combs & Caskey 1997).

Assessment of PLBP consists of a thorough history (children are often poor historians), complete physical examination, further diagnostic investigations including X-rays, bone scans and/or laboratory examination if indicated, and appropriate follow-up.

Warning signs and symptoms detected on history are spinal pain in a child under 4, pain duration of more than 4 weeks with increasing severity, associated constitutional features (weight loss, malaise, fever), neurological deficits (gait alterations, weakness, sensory loss, sphincter disturbances) and non-mechanical pain. Because children are often unable to

clearly describe the location and character of their complaint, and have a poor concept of time, it is helpful to determine the temporal relationship relative to events such as birthdays or holidays (King 1984). Because the child is often a poor historian it is important to question the child's parent or guardian about any observed changes. Inquiring about specific tasks such as climbing stairs or endurance is also helpful in investigation of the presence of possible neurological changes.

The physical examination is similar to the adult examination:

- observation for cutaneous lesions such as café-au-lait spots, dermal cysts or hairy patches, which may suggest a spinal anomaly or tumor
- postural examination, to assess for deformities such as scoliosis or kyphosis
- range of motion
- orthopedic tests
- gait analysis
- careful neurological examination of motor, sensory and reflex assessment
- temperature if the child is distressed, has a fever and/or pain on weight-bearing.

Differential diagnoses that should be considered in PLBP can be separated into two major categories: non-mechanical and mechanical. Non-mechanical causes of PLBP can be vascular, infectious, inflammatory, neoplastic, nutritional, degenerative, idiopathic, congenital, arthritide, traumatic, toxic, endocrine and metabolic, for which medical referral is indicated. Mechanical etiologies of PLBP are believed to be the most common, and are diagnosed after other causes have been considered and excluded. Mechanical etiologies include joint (capsuloligamentous sprain) and muscle/tendon dysfunction syndromes (strains, spasm, trigger points) due to postural (adolescent) kyphosis bony anomalies (spondylolisthesis), trauma and overuse syndromes. Chiropractors are ideally placed to treat mechanical syndromes, as they have a mechanical approach to management. If relief is forthcoming, the chiropractic treatment can be used retrospectively as a confirmatory diagnostic test for mechanical low back pain.

Failure to respond to mechanical (chiropractic) management after three treatment visits should prompt the clinician to reassess their examination and working hypothesis, and consider further investigation and possible medical referral. Children only rarely respond to stress with physical complaints that have no evidence of organic pathology. Therefore, PLBP should not be attributed to hysteria or malingering, and a diagnosis of psychological PLBP should be made only by exclusion (King 1984), and then only after consultation with an appropriate professional. Studies have shown that delayed diagnosis in PLBP is very common. One tertiary care facility reported that for serious causes of PLBP (such as metastasis, arthritides, etc.) 66% of correct diagnoses were delayed more than 1–3 months, while 16% were delayed more than 6 months (Turner et al 1989).

Recommended conservative medical treatment of PLBP has included: decreased activity, physical therapy modalities, heel lifts, injection, mobilization, and NSAIDs, with very little evidence of success.

A review of the literature investigating manipulative treatment of mechanical LBP in adults reveals numerous randomized controlled trials (Anderson et al 1992, Shekelle et al 1992) and several major evidence-based reviews (Bigos et al 1994, Haldeman et al 1993, Henderson et al 1994, Manga et al 1993, Rosen et al 1994, Shekelle et al 1991, Waddell et al 1996). These studies provide evidence that spinal manipulation is an efficacious form of therapy for uncomplicated LBP in terms of pain relief, improved activity and patient satisfaction.

Burton (1996) reported that there are similarities between childhood and adult LBP symptoms and suggested that management should follow the current clinical guidelines for adults. Studies have reported that 11–16% (Friis 1987, Spigelblatt et al 1994) of children utilize alternative or complementary therapies, including chiropractic. Kassak (1994) reported that in South Dakota approximately 17% of chiropractic patients were pediatric; another study reported that the most common presentation (39%) in this group was mechanical low back pain (Ebrall 1994a). A recent Canadian study reported similar results, with the majority of chiropractors reporting treating pediatric patients mainly for musculoskeletal complaints (Verhoef & Papadopoulos 1999). There is abundant anecdotal evidence to support chiropractic treatment of PLBP, but literature assessing and documenting this form of management is sparse.

Although there is a lack of evidence, the similarity of PLBP to adult low back pain, as well as anecdotal evidence, suggests that manipulation is an appropriate treatment; chiropractors need to prioritize research in the area of PLBP to better elucidate the role that chiropractic manipulation can play in the management of this condition.

The short-term prognosis for children with LBP appears to be very good. One longitudinal study reported that children often forgot about previous episodes of back pain. From this the authors hypothesized that this may indicate that PLBP may be just a trivial experience of life and of no significance (Burton et al 1996). However, other studies have suggested a less positive long-term prognosis, reporting that childhood back pain may lead to or predispose an individual to adult LBP. This hypothesis is based on several observations. The late childhood prevalence of LBP approaches the adult prevalence level (Balague et al 1988, 1995; Burton et al 1996; Ebrall 1994b; Leboeuf-Yde & Kyvik 1998; Mireau et al 1984; Olsen et al 1992). Salimen et al (1995) demonstrated that degenerative disc disease in childhood is a predictor for future back pain. In addition, a 25-year prospective cohort study found the occurrence of PLBP, along with a family history of back pain, to be highly correlated with adult back pain (Harreby et al 1995). There are, however, no studies that demonstrate that treatment of pediatric low back pain has any impact on future occurrences of adult low back pain. Chiropractic is in a good position to research this area further.

References

Abernathy, P.J., Townsend, P.R., Rose, R.M., et al., 1978. Is chondromalacia patellae a separate entity? J. Bone Joint Surg. 60B, 205–210.

Abril Martin, J.C., Martos Rodriguez, L.A., Queiruga Dios, J.A., et al., 1997. [Back pain in children.] Ann. Esp. Pediatr. 46, 133–137.

Adams, J.C., Hamblen, D.L., 2001. Outline of Orthopaedics. thirteenth ed. Churchill Livingstone, Edinburgh, p. 156, 178–184, 195–197, 305–315, 343, 359–360, 373, 405, 418–419.

Anderson, R., Meeker, W.C., Wirick, B.E., et al., 1992. A meta-analysis of clinical trials of

spinal manipulation. J. Manipulative Physiol. Ther. 15, 181–194.

Apley, A.G., Solomon, L., 1993. Apley's System of Orthopaedics and Fractures, seventh ed. Butterworth Heinemann, Oxford, pp. 68–71, 360–361, 387–397, 400–409, 493.

Bailey, D.A., Faulkner, R.A., Kimber, K., et al., 1997. Altered loading patterns and femoral bone mineral density in children with unilateral Legg–Calvé–Perthes disease. Med. Sci. Sports Exerc. 29 (11), 1395–1399.

Balague, F., Dutoit, G., Waldburger, M., 1988. Low back pain in schoolchildren. Scand. J. Rehabil. Med. 20, 175–179.

Balague, F., Damidot, P., Nordin, M., et al., 1993. Cross-sectional study of the isokinetic muscle trunk strength among school children. Spine 9, 1199–1205.

Balague, F., Skovron, M., Nordin, M., et al., 1995. Low back pain in schoolchildren – a study of familial and psychological factors. Spine 20, 1265–1270.

Beauchamp, M., Labelle, H., Grimard, G., et al., 1993. Diurnal variation of Cobb angle measurement in adolescent idiopathic scoliosis. Spine 18, 1581–1583.

Betz, R.R., 1990. Late sequelae of septic arthritis of the hip in infancy and childhood. J. Pediatr. Orthop. 10, 365.

Bigos, S., Bowyer, O., Braen, G., et al., 1994. Acute Low-Back Problems in Adults. Clinical Practice Guideline No. 14, AHCPR Publication No. 95-0642. Agency for Health Care Policy and Research Public Health Service, US Department of Health and Human Services, Rockville, MD.

Bretland, P.M., 1994. Pulled elbow in childhood. Br. J. Radiol. 67 (804), 1176–1185.

Bunch, W.H., Patwardham, A.G., 1989. Scoliosis: Making Clinical Decisions. Mosby, St Louis.

Burton, A.K., 1996. Low back pain in children and adolescents: to treat or not? Bull. Hosp. Joint Dis. 55, 127–129.

Burton, A.K., Clarke, R.D., McClune, T.D., et al., 1996. The natural history of low back pain in adolescents. Spine 21, 2323–2328.

Bussieres, A., Cassidy, J.D., Dzus, A., 1994. Spinal cord astrocytoma presenting as torticollis and scoliosis. J. Manipulative Physiol. Ther. 17 (2), 113–118.

Combs, J.A., Caskey, P.M., 1997. Back pain in children and adolescents: a retrospective review of 648 patients. South Med. J. 90, 789–792.

Dandy, D.J., Edwards, D.J., 2003. Essential Orthopaedics and Trauma, fourth ed. Churchill Livingstone, Edinburgh, p. 240, 318, 338–340, 345–346, 410, 434.

Ebrall, P.S., 1994a. A description of 320 chiropractic consultations of Australian adolescents. Chiropr. J. Aust. 24, 4–8.

Ebrall, P.S., 1994b. The epidemiology of male adolescent low back pain in a north suburban population of Melbourne, Australia. J. Manipulative Physiol. Ther. 17, 447–453.

Fairbank, J.C.T., Punsent, P.B., Van Poortvleit, J.A., et al., 1984. Influence of anthropometric factors and joint laxity in the incidence of adolescent back pain. Spine 9, 461–464.

Friis, B., 1987. Alternative treatment of children – why and how often? An interview investigation in a paediatric department. Ugeskr. Laeger 149, 806–808.

Fysh, P., 1998. Orthopedics. In: Anrig, C., Plaugher, G. (Eds), Pediatric Chiropractic. Williams & Wilkins, Baltimore.

Gatterman, M.I., 1995. Foundations of Chiropractic: Subluxation. Mosby, St Louis.

Goodfellow, J., Hungerford, D.S., Zindel, M., 1976. Patellofemoral joint mechanics and pathology, Part 1: functional anatomy of the patellofemoral joint. J. Bone Joint Surg. 58B, 287–290.

Haldeman, S., Chapman-Smith, D., Peterson, D.M., 1993. Guidelines for Chiropractic Quality Assurance and Practice Parameters. Proceedings of the Mercy Center Consensus Conference. Aspen Publishers, Gaithsburg, MD.

Harreby, M., Neergaard, K., Hesselsoe, G., 1995. Are radiologic changes in the thoracic and lumbar spine of adolescents risk factors for low back pain in adults? A 25-year prospective cohort study of 640 school children. Spine 20, 2298–2302.

Hay, W.W., Groothius, J.R., Hayward, A.R., et al., (Eds) 1997. Current Pediatric Diagnosis and Treatment, thirteenth ed. Appleton and Lange, Stamford, CT.

Henderson, D.J., Chapman-Smith, D.A., Mior, S., et al., 1994. Clinical guidelines for chiropractic practice in Canada. J. Can. Chiropr. Assoc. 38 (Suppl. 1), 1–203.

Herman, R.M., Mixon, J., Fisher, A., et al., 1985. Idiopathic scoliosis and the central nervous system: a motor control problem. Spine 10, 1–14.

Hertling, D., Kessler, R.M., 1996. Management of Common Musculoskeletal Disorders: Physical Therapy Principles and Methods, third ed. Lippincott, Philadelphia.

Homewood, A.E., 1977. The Neurodynamics of the Vertebral Subluxation. Valkyrie Press, St Petersburg, Florida.

Illingworth, R.S., 1982. Common Symptoms of Disease in Children, seventh ed. Blackwell Scientific, Oxford.

Jahn, W.T., 1978. Conservative management of Scheuermann's juvenile kyphosis. J. Manipulative Physiol. Ther. 1 (4), 228–245.

Kassak, K.M., 1994. The practice of chiropractic in South Dakota: a survey of chiropractors. J. Manipulative Physiol. Ther. 17, 523–529.

King, H.A., 1984. Back pain in children. Pediatr. Clin. North Am. 31, 1083–1095.

Kujala, U.M., Salimen, J.J., Taimela, S., et al., 1992. Subject characteristics and low back pain in young athletes and nonathletes. Med. Sci. Sports Exerc. 24, 6–32.

Kujala, U.M., Taimela, S., Erkintalo, M., et al., 1996. Low-back pain in adolescent athletes. Med. Sci. Sports Exerc. 28, 165–170.

Kujala, U.M., Taimela, S., Oksanen, A., et al., 1997. Lumbar mobility and low back pain during adolescence: a longitudinal three-year follow-up study in athletes and controls. Am. J. Sports Med. 25, 363–368.

Leboeuf-Yde, C., Kyvik, K., 1998. At what age does low back pain become a common problem? A study of 29,424 individuals aged 12–41 years. Spine 23, 228–234.

Lloyd-Roberts, G.C., Fixsen, J., 1990. Orthopaedics in Infancy and Childhood, second ed. Butterworth-Heinemann, London.

Manga, P., Angus, D., Papadopoulos, C., et al., 1993. The Effectiveness and Cost Effectiveness of Chiropractic Management of Low-Back Pain. University of Ottawa, Ottawa.

Meachim, G., Emery, I.H., 1974. Quantitative aspects of patellofemoral cartilage fibrillation in Liverpool necropsies. Ann. Rheum. Dis. 3, 39–47.

Mireau, D.R., Cassidy, J.D., Hamin, T., et al., 1984. Sacroiliac joint dysfunction and low back pain in school aged children. J. Manipulative Physiol. Ther. 7, 81–84.

Nansel, D.D., Waldorf, T., Cooperstein, R., 1993. Effect of cervical spinal adjustments on lumbar paraspinal muscle tone: evidence for facilitation of intersegmental tonic neck reflexes. J. Manipulative Physiol. Ther. 16, 91–95.

Newcomer, K., Sinaki, M., 1996. Low back pain and its relationship to back strength and physical activity in children. Acta. Paediatr. 85, 1433–1439.

Newcomer, K., Sinaki, M., Wollan, P.C., 1997. Physical activity and four-year development of back strength in children. Am. J. Phys. Med. Rehabil. 76, 52–58.

Olsen, T.L., Anderson, R.L., Dearwater, S.R., et al., 1992. The epidemiology of low back pain in an adolescent population. Am. J. Public Health 82, 606–608.

Outerbridge, R.E.E., 1961. The aetiology of chondromalacia patellae. J. Bone Joint Surg. 43B, 752–757.

Renshaw, T.S., 1986. Pediatric Orthopedics. WB Saunders, Philadelphia.

Risser, J.C., 1964. Scoliosis: past and present. J. Bone Joint Surg. Am. 46, 167–199.

Rosen, M., Breen, A., Hamann, W., et al., 1994. Report of a Clinical Standards Advisory Group Committee on Back Pain. HMSO, London.

Saidoff, D.C., McDonough, A.L., 2002. Critical Pathways in Therapeutic Intervention: Extremities and Spine. Mosby, St Louis.

Salimen, J.J., Maki, P., Oksanen, A., et al., 1992. Spinal mobility and trunk muscle strength in 15-year-old schoolchildren with and without low-back pain. Spine 17, 405–411.

Salimen, J.J., Erkintalo, M., Laine, M., et al., 1995. Low back pain in the young – a prospective three-year follow-up study of subjects with and without low back pain. Spine 20, 2101–2108.

Salter, R.B., 1999. Textbook of Disorders and Injuries of the Musculoskeletal System, third ed. Williams & Wilkins, Baltimore, pp. 161–162, 520–521.

Sanerkin, N.G., Edwards, P., 1966. Birth injury to the sternomastoid muscle. J. Bone Joint Surg. 48B, 441.

Shafrir, Y., Kaufman, B.A., 1992. Quadriplegia after chiropractic manipulation in an infant with congenital torticollis caused by a spinal cord astrocytoma. J. Pediatr. 120 (2/1), 266–269.

Shekelle, P.G., Adams, A.H., Chassin, M.R., et al., 1991. The Appropriateness of Spinal Manipulation for Low-Back Pain: Indications and Ratings by a Multidisciplinary Expert Panel. Monograph No. R-4025/2 - CCR/FCER. RAND, Santa Monica, CA.

Shekelle, P.C., Adams, A., Chassin, M.R., et al., 1992. Spinal manipulation for low back pain. Ann. Intern. Med. 117, 590–598.

Shoji, H., 1974. Chondromalacia patellae: histological and biochemical aspects. N. Y. State J. Med. 74, 507–510.

Souza, T.A., 2005. Differential Diagnosis and Management for the Chiropractor: Protocols and Algorithms. Jones and Bartlett, Boston, pp. 105–125.

Spigelblatt, L., Laine-Ammara, C., Pless, B., et al., 1994. The use of alternative medicine by children. Pediatrics 94, 811–814.

Storigord, J., 1975. Chondromalacia of the patella: physical signs in relation to operative findings. Acta. Orthop. Scand. 46, 685–694.

Strang, V.V., 1984. Essential Principles of Chiropractic. Palmer College of Chiropractic, Davenport, Iowa.

Tachdjian, M.O., 1972. Pediatric Orthopedics. WB Saunders, Philadelphia.

Taimela, S., Kujala, U.M., Salimen, J.J., et al., 1997. The prevalence of low back pain among children and adolescents – a nationwide, cohort-based questionnaire survey in Finland. Spine 22, 1132–1136.

Toto, B.J., 1993. Chiropractic correction of congenital muscular torticollis. J. Manipulative Physiol. Ther. 16 (8), 556–559.

Troussier, B., Davoine, P., deGaudemaris, R., et al., 1994. Back pain in school children: a study among 1178 pupils. Scand. J. Rehabil. Med. 26, 143–146.

Turner, P.C., Green, J.G., Galasko, C.S.B., 1989. Back pain in childhood. Spine 14, 812–814.

Verhoef, M.J., Papadopoulos, C., 1999. Chiropractors' involvement in the treatment of patients under the age of 18. J. Can. Chiropr. Assoc. 43, 50–57.

Waddell, G., Feder, G., McIntosh, A., et al., 1996. Low-Back Pain Evidence Review. Royal College of General Practitioners, London.

Weinstein, S.L., 1997. Natural history and treatment outcomes of childhood hip disorders. Clin. Orthop. Relat. Res. November (344), 227–242.

Yochum, T.R., Rowe, L.J., 1996. Scoliosis. In: Essentials of Skeletal Radiology, second ed. Williams & Wilkins, Baltimore.

Autism

15

Kylie M. Gray   Avril V. Brereton   Bruce J. Tonge

Autism was first described in 1943 by Leo Kanner. His vivid, detailed account described 11 children suffering from an 'inborn autistic disturbance of affective contact' (Kanner 1943). This lifelong condition has since been referred to as autism, early infantile autism, Kanner's autism, childhood schizophrenia and childhood autism. The official term for this condition as described by the Diagnostic and Statistical Manual of Mental Disorders (DSM-IV) (American Psychiatric Association (APA) 2000) is *autistic disorder*.

Kanner (1943) observed eight boys and three girls and described the main features of this syndrome as being an inability to relate in an ordinary way to other people, a failure to use language for the purpose of communication, an anxiously obsessive desire for the maintenance of sameness, limited spontaneous activity, a fascination for objects (handled with fine motor skill) and good cognitive potential. Onset was at birth or before 30 months, all children were physically normal, and all were from what Kanner described as highly intelligent families, although we now know that autism can occur in any child, from any family.

Diagnosis

The diagnosis of autism is based on the presence of an internationally agreed set of defined developmental and behavioral characteristics. It is not possible to diagnose autism through the use of medical tests, such as blood tests, or any other physiological feature. The most commonly used criteria for the diagnosis of autism in Australia are those outlined in the Diagnostic and Statistical Manual of Mental Disorders, fourth edition text revision (DSM-IV-TR) (APA 2000). This manual classifies autistic disorder (the term used by the DSM-IV for autism) as one of the pervasive developmental disorders. According to the DSM-IV, a diagnosis of autistic disorder requires specific criteria to be met in three areas: (1) impairment in social interaction, (2) impairments in communication, and (3) repetitive and stereotyped patterns of

behavior, interests and activities. Delays or abnormalities in functioning must be present before 3 years of age in one or more of these areas in order for the diagnosis to be made. The DSM-IV diagnostic criteria are conceptually identical to the other most commonly used set of criteria: the International Classification of Disorders, tenth revision (ICD-10), compiled by the World Health Organization (WHO 1992).

Other pervasive developmental disorders include Asperger's disorder and pervasive developmental disorder not otherwise specified (PDD-NOS). Asperger's disorder differs from autism and high functioning autism (autism with no cognitive impairment) in that there is no general delay in the onset of language, and no significant delay of cognitive development or adaptive behavioral skills (APA 2000). PDD-NOS is diagnosed when there are impairments in reciprocal social interaction and communication, and/or when stereotyped behaviors or interests are present, but not the degree that meets full criteria for autistic disorder. Collectively, autistic disorder, Asperger's disorder and PDD-NOS are now often referred to as *autism spectrum disorders*.

Features/characteristics of the disorder

Children with autism present with delayed and disordered development affecting three main areas: social interaction, communication and play, behavior and interests.

Intellectual disability

Approximately 70–80% of children with autism have an intellectual disability, the majority in the moderate to severe range (APA 2000, Fombonne 2005b, Wing & Gould 1979). Most children with autism have a scattered profile of ability in which they are relatively better at visual motor tasks compared with verbal and social comprehension tasks. For example, a young child with autism might be easily able to work a computer by observing someone, yet be unable to respond to a simple question. A minority of children with autism demonstrate an extraordinary specific skill, for example in drawing, memory or music, but are often unable to make effective social use of this splinter skill. When considering whether a child meets any given criterion for autism, it is important to take into account the child's intellectual level and evaluate the symptomatology of autism independently of the intellectual disability.

Social interaction

Children with autism share a fundamental deficit in reciprocal social interaction and are impaired in their ability to develop social relationships (Rutter & Schopler 1987). They lack the skills necessary to make friends and many are not disturbed by this, preferring to be on their own. Children with autism are unable to understand the feelings of others and lack empathy. They are unable to modify their behavior according to the requirements of a given social situation or context, or appreciate that this is required. Their behavior is therefore often considered inappropriate, for example a child who on seeing his mother crying climbed onto her lap and instead of offering her some comfort wanted to know 'Where is the water coming from?'. Children with autism show little or no interest in sharing pleasure with others. This is evident in their lack of pointing out or showing things of interest to parents (Baron-Cohen et al 1992, Gray & Tonge 2001). Most children with autism fail to use eye-to-eye gaze and do not seek out the company of other people. There is a lack of pretend and creative play, and a general failure to use toys and other objects for their intended purpose.

Communication

The abnormalities and delays exhibited by children with autism encompass all aspects and modalities of communication (Rutter & Schopler 1987). The fundamental deficit has been described as a failure in the capacity to use language as a means of social communication (Rutter & Schopler 1987). It has been estimated that 50% of children with autism do not develop the ability to speak (Prizant 1996, Schreibman 1994). This lack of verbal ability is distinctive in that no attempt is made to compensate for the lack of spoken language through the use of mime or gesture.

Children with autism who are verbal demonstrate specific deficits such as an inability to interpret tone of voice, facial expression and body language (Rapin 1991). As a result, they often misunderstand the intended meaning of statements and conversations. They also have difficulties in aspects of participating in a conversation, such as an inability to take turns, maintain eye contact with the person they are speaking to, and adhere to a topic of conversation (Rapin 1991).

Verbal children with autism may also demonstrate echolalia and pronoun reversal. Echolalia is the repeating of words or phrases that the child has heard or that he himself has spoken. Echolalia can be either delayed, repeating something heard or said earlier, or immediate, repeating something just heard or said. Pronoun reversal is the incorrect use of pronouns, such as substituting *you* for *I*. For example, a young child with

autism may approach a parent and say, 'You want a drink of water?' meaning 'I want a drink of water.' The child is demonstrating use of a delayed echolalic phrase together with an inability to use the pronoun.

Repetitive and stereotyped patterns of behavior, interests and activities

This category of behaviors consists of rigid adherence to rituals and routines, unusual interests and preoccupations, and motor or verbal stereotypes. Children with autism may become very distressed in response to even minor changes in their routine or environment. For example, driving a different way to the supermarket or a slight change in the arrangement of the furniture in the living room may provoke distress or tantrum. Unusual activities and preoccupations can include, for example, enjoying spending hours playing with water, shaking a piece of string, flicking a light switch repetitively, repeatedly doing the same puzzle, studying numbers and letters or the telephone book. Some children with autism have a particular narrow interest, which they study in great detail, such as dinosaurs, street directories or bus timetables. They will study their particular topic of interest to the point where they know everything there is to know about the subject and constantly talk to people in great detail about it, oblivious to the lack of interest of those with whom they are speaking. Children with autism may become abnormally attached to an unusual object or to part of an object, such as the lid of a blue felt pen, which has to be taken everywhere. An obsessive preoccupation with one type of toy, for example Thomas the Tank Engine, or idiosyncratic play with toys, such as lining them up or staring intently as the wheels spin around, are commonly seen. Attempts to change routines or disrupt repetitive activities and rituals frequently result in high levels of distress or severe tantrums.

Motor stereotypies may include flapping of the hands, twirling objects, flicking of the fingers, rocking, head banging or spinning the body. These actions are repeated over and over again. Verbal stereotypes may include non-verbal noises such as humming, or repetitively singing a particular song, telling a joke or asking a particular question over and over again.

Common behavioral and emotional problems

In addition to autism symptomatology, there are a number of behavioral and emotional problems that are common in children with autism. These may include, but are not limited to, overactivity, disruptive behavior, temper tantrums, aggressive behavior, self-injurious behavior (e.g. biting of self, head banging), fears and phobias, sleep disturbance, bedwetting or soiling (Rutter 1985). Behavioral problems occur at a high rate in children with autism, significantly higher than in children with an intellectual disability and higher than typically developing children (Brereton et al 2006, Herring et al 2006, Lecavalier 2006, Tonge & Einfeld 2003). High rates of behavioral and emotional problems have been shown to persist into adulthood (Tonge & Einfeld 2003). Such problem behaviors add considerably to the burden of the care and management of children and young people with autism.

It is of relevance to chiropractors that children with autism may have a reduced sensitivity and reaction to pain. A number of other sensory disturbances may also occur. These include intolerance of certain sounds, bright light and touch. Sensitivity to smell, taste, and differences in food texture may seriously limit a child's diet.

Assessment

A diagnosis of autism should be made through specialist diagnostic team assessment. An autism assessment should include pediatric medical consultation, communication–speech assessment, cognitive, audiological, sensori-integrative and psychosocial assessments, behavioral observations, child psychiatric consultation, and multidisciplinary case discussion. Assessment must include a detailed interview with the parents or carers of the child and observation of the child. Semistructured interviews are available to assist the clinician in the interview with the parents. One such interview, the Autism Diagnostic Interview-Revised (ADI-R) (Lord et al 1994, Rutter et al 2003b), produces an algorithm which is linked to ICD-10 (WHO 1992) and DSM-IV (APA 2000) diagnostic criteria. The interview takes approximately 90 minutes to administer and requires training in its use. A standardized observational measure is also available – the Autism Diagnostic Observation Schedule (ADOS) (Lord et al 1989, 2000, 2001).

A number of checklists and questionnaires have been developed to assist with screening and measurement of severity of symptoms. None of these instruments is able to make a diagnosis of autism; however, they can provide useful information to aid the clinician in assessment. They include the Modified Checklist for Autism (M-CHAT) (Robins et al 2001), the Social Responsiveness Scale (SRS) (Constantino et al 2003), the Social Communication Questionnaire (SCQ) (Corsello et al 2007, Rutter et al 2003a) and the Childhood Autism Rating Scale (CARS) (Schopler et al 1980), which requires a trained clinician to administer. Another instrument, the Developmental Behaviour Checklist (DBC) (Einfeld & Tonge 1995, 2002), is completed by parents or caregivers and surveys the broad range of emotional and behavioral problems that occur in young people with intellectual disability. The DBC can also be used to screen children for autism and describe the nature and severity of their symptoms (Brereton et al 2002, Gray & Tonge 2005, Gray et al 2008, Steinhausen & Metzke 2004).

Diagnoses of autism should always be made using current diagnostic criteria, as outlined in the DSM (APA 2000) and ICD (WHO 1992). A diagnosis should not be made on the basis of any single measure or assessment, but by incorporating all sources of information and assessment results.

Prevalence

Varying figures have been reported on the prevalence of autism worldwide, with the question having been raised of whether the true prevalence of autism is increasing.

Reported prevalence figures can be impacted by methodologies across studies (Fombonne 2005b, Wazana et al 2007), whether or not children without intellectual disability were included in the sample, whether only autism is measured or other pervasive developmental disorders (Asperger's disorder and PDD-NOS) are also included, and by increased public awareness. One of the most important issues is the use of different diagnostic and case inclusion criteria across studies.

Some recent prevalence studies report autism prevalence rates of 38.9 per 10 000 in a birth cohort of children (Baird et al 2006), 18.9 per 10 000 in preschool children (Chakrabarti & Fombonne 2005), and 20.5 per 10 000 (Gillberg et al 2006). Recent studies including autism, Asperger's disorder and PDD-NOS in case ascertainment provide prevalence rates of 116.1 per 10 000 (Baird et al 2006), 67 per 10 000 (Centers for Disease Control 2007), 53.3 per 10 000 (Gillberg et al 2006), and 62.5 per 10 000 in an Australian study (MacDermott et al 2007). In a review of epidemiological studies, Fombonne (2005a, 2005b) concluded that currently the best available estimate of the prevalence of pervasive developmental disorders is 60 per 10 000. It is well established that autism occurs more frequently in males than females, with a male to female ratio of 4.3:1.0 (Fombonne 2005b).

Associated medical conditions

Children and adolescents can present with the same range of medical conditions as typically developing children, with studies reporting rates of medical conditions ranging from 5% to 55% (Filipek 2005). As the degree of intellectual disability increases, the rate of associated medical conditions also increases (Lauritsen et al 2002, Ritvo et al 1990). These can include genetic conditions such fragile X syndrome, Down syndrome and other chromosomal and genetic abnormalities, tuberous sclerosis, cerebral palsy, congenital rubella embryopathy, deafness, sleep disturbances, inborn errors of metabolism and mitochondrial disorders (Lauritsen et al 2002). Approximately one-third of those with autism develop epilepsy (Minshew et al 2005), with a larger proportion developing epileptiform abnormalities (Kawasaki et al 1997). There is also a significantly increased risk of associated psychiatric conditions such as tic disorders, anxiety and depression. These may emerge during adolescence.

Etiology

The cause of autism is currently unknown. Early theories attributed the development of the condition to the parents', in particular the mother's, style of unresponsive, cold, detached parenting (Bettelheim 1967, Kanner 1973). Research and experience have proven this theory of causation to be false (Schopler 1971) and autism is now recognized as a disorder of neurobiological dysfunction (Anderson & Hoshino 1997, Filipek 2005, Minshew et al 1997) of unknown origin.

A link between autism, gastrointestinal disease and the measles–mumps–rubella immunization was proposed in 1998 (Wakefield et al 1999). Further research has not supported the claim of a causal link between autism and the MMR vaccine (Chen et al 2004, DeStefano & Thompson 2004, Fombonne & Chakrabarti 2001, Smeeth et al 2004, Taylor et al 1999) and a retraction was made by the authors (Murch et al 2004). Mercury and thimerosal poisoning from vaccines has also been posited as a cause of autism; however, research evidence does not support this claim (Andrews et al 2004, Fombonne 2008, Madsen et al, 2003, Ng et al 2007, Parker et al 2004, Stehr-Green et al 2003).

Genetics plays a prominent role in autism (Rutter et al 1997). Although the specifics of this role remain unknown, it is unlikely that autism is a single gene disorder (Bolton & Rutter 1990) and the evidence suggests that a small number of interacting genes are likely to be responsible for the condition (Bailey et al 1996, Rutter et al 1997). It has also been argued that the different features of autism may be caused by different genes (Happe et al 2006).

Treatment

There is no cure available for autism. Treatment must be a collaborative approach between the family and the professionals involved in the child's care. No single treatment modality will be appropriate for all children and all families (Howlin 1998). Treatment planning will include a range of services and approaches which may include speech and language therapy, early intensive intervention, special education, parent training, behavior therapy, pharmacotherapy and occupational therapy. Treatment and support service needs will also change as the child develops and moves into adolescence and adulthood. It is necessary to consider individually the needs and characteristics of each child and family, and adapt treatment accordingly. It is also necessary for any treatment program to include education for parents about the diagnosed condition. Along with general information about the condition, parents will want to know what this means for their child, for their family, and for their child's future. It is also the responsibility of the clinician to assist parents in understanding the range of treatment options, including which have established efficacy.

Although there is an abundance of literature reporting on intervention and treatment programs for autism, much of it suffers from inadequate study design or a lack of systematic evaluation. The list of therapeutic strategies for autism that have appeared in the literature is vast. Aversive therapy, behavior therapy, dance therapy, developmental therapy, fenfluramine treatment, electroconvulsive shock therapy, Goldfine treatment, holding therapy, interactive therapy, megavitamin therapy, mainstreaming, patterning therapy, psychical therapy, speech therapy, pony therapy, play therapy, music therapy and sensory integration have all been described (Schopler 1989).

Some of these interventions and treatments have begun to be systematically evaluated. However, a substantial proportion of proposed treatments have not been adequately or systematically evaluated, and they are often expensive and time consuming, have no supporting evidence, and frequently promise impossible cures (Howlin 1997, Werry 1996). These include auditory integration training, the option method, scotopic sensitivity training, holding therapy, facilitated communication, pet therapies, the Doman–Delacto method, daily life therapy, sensory integration therapy, cranial osteopathy, vitamin treatments, facilitated communication, and gluten- and casein-free diets to name just a few (Howlin 1997, Metz et al 2005). Other recent treatment 'fads' include chelation therapy and secretin. In terms of chelation therapy, there is no evidence of the efficacy of chelation as a treatment for autism, and serious concerns have been raised regarding safety (Sinha et al 2006), particularly in light of the death of a child undergoing chelation therapy. Secretin (a gastrointestinal hormone) was also proposed as a treatment for autism via a television program suggesting it as a possible cure for autism (Aman & Armstrong 2000). However, research has now clearly demonstrated that that secretin does not have a role in the treatment of autism (Owley et al 2001, Sandler & Bodfish 2000, Sandler et al 1999, Volkmar 1999).

Alternative and complementary therapies

A small number of studies have investigated the use of complementary and alternative medicines in the treatment of children with autism. Complementary and alternative therapies are numerous, and include meditation, prayer, creative therapies (for example art, music and dance), herbs, vitamins, minerals, foods, osteopathic manipulation, chiropractic, massage and reiki. While evaluating the efficacy of these alternative treatments, two studies have demonstrated that more than half of parents surveyed reported using at least one of these alternative treatments (Hanson et al 2007, Wong & Smith 2006). The majority of alternative therapies used were modified diets and vitamin and/or mineral supplements (Wong & Smith 2006).

There is no evidence at this point of the efficacy of chiropractic in the treatment of autism. A few cases studies, not published in peer-reviewed journals, have claimed that successful outcomes were achieved through the use of chiropractic with children with autism (Gleberzon 2006). Case reports and anecdotal reports do not provide evidence for the efficacy of a treatment; randomized clinical trials are needed to investigate the effects of any treatment. It has been noted that primary management of the treatment of a child with autism by a chiropractor is neither in keeping with knowledge of current best practice nor in the best interests of the child (Ferrance 2003, Gleberzon 2006). It is essential that professionals working with the families of children with autism are knowledgeable about the demonstrated efficacy, or lack thereof, of treatments that are available. It is important for professionals to be able to explain these issues to families and provide them with informed advice about their treatment options.

Early intervention

Early diagnosis of autism is important. It enables crucial treatment and intervention for both the child and the family to commence at an early age. Although the full effects of early intervention are not yet established (Baron-Cohen et al 1996) and research studies comparing programs are lacking (Corsello 2005), early intervention results in better child outcomes, particularly when it starts before the age of 4 years (Harris & Weiss 1998, Rogers 1996, Sheinkopf & Siegel 1998). Training parents to implement early intervention programs has also demonstrated gains in communicative behavior, knowledge of autism, parent communication style, parent–child interaction, and a reduction in parent stress and mental health problems (McConachie & Diggle 2005, Tonge et al 2006). Early intervention contributes to the prevention of the development of maladaptive behaviors, and may influence a family's ability to cope and deal with their child's disorder. Difficult behavior can escalate if left untreated and may become entrenched and beyond the control of parents, making intervention extremely difficult or unsuccessful, and negatively impact social, educational and community opportunities (Horner et al 2002, Howlin & Yates 1989). Early language intervention at the prelinguistic and early language stages of development can also have a significant positive impact (Lord & McGee 2001). Research is also now showing the improvements that can be made when intervening early to teach joint attention, symbolic play and imitation skills (Drew et al 2002; Kasari et al 2001, 2006).

Behavioral interventions

Behavioral interventions are the most frequently used treatment methods for the social, communication, adaptive and behavioral difficulties faced by children with autism (Bregman et al 2005). These approaches utilize behavioral techniques and principles to teach new skills and promote desirable behavior. There is a large amount of published research, although incomplete, on the efficacy of behavioral interventions for children with autism. The sample sizes of the majority of the studies are small, limited in length of treatment follow-up, and published reports of treatment failures are rare, possibly reflecting an unfortunate reluctance on the part of researchers to report such results or journal editors to publish them (Horner et al 2002).

Behavioral methods have proved to be useful in enhancing social behavior, communication skills and self-help skills, in reducing anxiety and undesirable behaviors such as obsessional activities, self-injury and aggression, and in reducing parent stress (Bregman & Gerdtz 1997; Koegel et al 1992a, 1992b; Lord 1995; Luiselli et al 2000; Moes et al 1992). Today the emphasis of behavioral teaching methods is on teaching replacement skills rather than simply removing the undesirable behavior. Care is taken to analyze the function or purpose that the behavior serves in order to develop more adaptable and appropriate behavior. Most problem behaviors are not random and meaningless but rather are communications from children who have limited and impaired ability to communicate their thoughts, feelings and needs. For example, in differing contexts, rocking and squealing may indicate a call for attention, distress from a painful ear, being overwhelmed with social anxiety in a busy classroom, or frustration at not understanding or being understood.

A useful methodological framework for intervention is that of parent training, emphasizing the key role that parents can play in their child's therapy. It has been recommended that parental involvement in treatments is an essential element of successful programs (Powers 1992, Simeonsson et al 1987). An advantage of this method is that the skills taught to parents can be varied to accommodate the needs of the child and deal with child-specific problems and reduce parent stress (Anastopoulos et al 1993, Graziano & Diament 1992, Johnson et al 2007, McConachie & Diggle 2005, Research Units on Pediatric Psychopharmacology Autism Network 2007). There is empirical evidence that a structured small group education and skills training program intervention for parents with young children with autism leads to persistent improvement in parental mental health, family functioning, and adaptive behavior in their children with autism (Brereton & Tonge 2005, Tonge et al 2006).

Teaching and special education

Special education programs for children with autism are individually designed by teachers using a problem-solving approach to address specific needs. These programs aim to provide predictable, consistent and highly organized teaching situations in the classroom. Studies indicate that approaches which provide a structured and predictable environment are most effective in promoting improved social and communication skills (Bartak & Rutter 1973, McClannahan & Krantz 1999, Olley 1999, Schopler 1987, Schreibman et al 2000). The response to treatment is related to the severity of intellectual and language impairment (Schopler 1987); however, most children make some gains in learning when behavioral methods and special education approaches are put in place. The move to integrate children with autism into as normal a learning situation as possible is generally appropriate. Placement in mainstream or special education schools is dependent upon the child's intellectual level. Integration is a desirable principle; however, some children with autism have difficulty coping without close supervision on a long-term basis. Without adequate special resources and teaching, children with autism are at risk of remaining isolated and unoccupied, unable to integrate themselves into class and peer activities, or to benefit from the educational environment. Early intervention programs employ both behavioral and special education techniques and are carried out in special group settings as well as in the home. Professional teaching support is vital for those family members and carers who are working on treatment programs at home, as they are generally intensive and demanding.

Pharmacotherapy

There are no drugs that specifically treat autism. Despite high rates of clinical use of psychopharmacotherapy in children with autism (Aman et al 2000, Martin et al 1999, Witwer & Lecavalier 2005), there is a paucity of clinical trials in this population. However, there are ranges of psychoactive drugs that have been shown to modify symptoms or treat associated psychiatric disorders. Drug therapy should only be used as part of a broader management plan. The purpose of the drug therapy and possible side-effects must be fully explained to the parents in order to ensure compliance. Neuroleptic drugs such as haloperidol have been shown to reduce aggressive disturbed behavior and arousal (Locascio et al 1991). Antidepressants such as selective serotonin reuptake inhibitors (SSRIs; e.g. fluoxetine) and tricylic antidepressants (e.g. imipramine and clomipramine) may reduce anxiety and obsessional and overactive behavior. Drugs that block the action of opiate receptors in the brain, such as naltrexone, may reduce self-injurious agitated behavior (Campbell et al 1990). Risperidone, a newer 'atypical' neuroleptic, has been shown to be effective in the treatment of severe behavioral problems such as aggression, severe tantrums and self-injurious behavior (Research Units on Pediatric Psychopharmacology (RUPP) Autism Network 2005a, 2005b). These neuroleptic drugs can be associated with significant side-effects such as dystonic reactions (e.g. tremor, muscular rigidity and motor restlessness) and weight gain with ultimate risk of metabolic problems such as diabetes. These side-effects are less likely on low dosages, which are usually sufficient for a therapeutic effect, with careful attention to diet and exercise. Although generally efficacious, the use of stimulant medication to treat any coexisting symptoms of pronounced inattention and hyperactivity can have a limited response or adverse effects in children with intellectual disability and children with autism (Aman et al 2003, Research Units on Pediatric Psychopharmacology (RUPP) Autism Network 2005a), but may be of use in a minority of children with clear-cut additional symptoms of attention deficit and hyperactivity (Tonge 2002).

Effects on the family

Parents of children with autism face a number of specific stressors (Marcus et al 2005). Parents may not understand their child's problems because the professional has not provided an accurate and informative description of the child's diagnosis. Parents may be confused and upset by changes in the pattern of autistic symptoms that occur at different developmental stages, for example the emergence of more obsessional symptoms in a teenager with autism. Not knowing whether the child with autism cannot or will not respond is a source of upset and frustration for parents. Many children with autism are physically attractive with none of the physical abnormalities often associated with disability, which may make it more difficult for parents and others to accept that the child has a severe developmental disorder with associated difficult behavior (Marcus et al 1997). Parents also face the stress of making a number of difficult decisions regarding management, such as time-consuming and expensive therapies which promise miracle cures, use of behavior-modifying drugs, and mainstream versus special schooling.

Having a child with autism has a significant impact upon parents, particularly in terms of stress (Bristol & Schopler 1983, Dunn et al 2001, Sanders & Morgan 1997), mental health (DeMyer 1979, Olsson & Hwang 2001, Yirmiya & Shaked 2005) and family functioning (Choutka 1999,

Johnson & Hastings 2002). Higher levels of psychosocial distress are present in families of children with autism than those of typically developing children (Fombonne et al 2001, Holroyd & McArthur 1976, Koegel et al 1992c) or children with other disabilities (Fombonne et al 2001, Sanders & Morgan 1997, Tonge & Einfeld 2003). Much of this psychosocial distress can be attributed to child behavior and emotional problems (Hastings 2004, Herring et al 2006, Lecavalier et al 2005).

It is important to convey to parents that these are normal grief reactions experienced by most parents of disabled children. The family as a whole also requires consideration. Parents may be consumed with caring for a demanding and difficult child and have little time for themselves or other children in the family. The siblings of a child with autism have their own needs and often benefit from psychological assistance and support that addresses the issues they face.

Outcome

Autism is a lifelong disorder and most individuals require care and support throughout their lives. Longitudinal studies have provided information on the long-term outcome of children diagnosed with autism. It has been established that slightly less than 10% are able to lead independent lives in adulthood (Gillberg 1991, Wing 1989), with the majority remaining highly dependent on their families or support services (Howlin et al 2004). Around 50% of children with autism remain without useful communicative speech (Lord & Rutter 1994). Studies have found that in the majority of cases social, behavioral and communication deficits and impairments persist through to adolescence and adulthood (Ballaban-Gil et al 1996, Gillberg 1998, Gillberg & Steffenburg 1987, Larsen & Mouridsen 1997, Rutter 1970, Rutter et al 1967, von Knorring & Hagglof 1993, Werry 1996), with a poor to very poor outcome in at least 60% of samples. Such outcomes have also been reported in studies of children with high functioning autism (Szatmari et al 1989). High levels of psychopathology, which persist into adulthood, have also been reported in children and adolescents with autism (Tonge & Einfeld 2003).

However, outcome in autism is variable, as demonstrated in case studies of children with positive outcomes (Schwartz et al 1998). Normal to good social adjustment was found in 14% of cases (9 out of 63) (Rutter et al 1967), improvement in 43.2% of children between 10 and 15 years of age (Kobayashi et al 1992), while Gillberg & Steffenburg (1987) reported fair to good outcomes in 17% of cases. A review of the outcome literature has concluded that a good outcome is seen in approximately 5–15% of cases, while a poor to very poor outcome in terms of social adjustment is seen in 60–75% of cases followed through to adolescence or early adulthood (Nordin & Gillberg 1998).

It has consistently been shown that IQ and language development are the most reliable predictors of outcome (Gillberg & Steffenburg 1987, Kobayashi et al 1992, Nordin & Gillberg 1998, Rutter et al 1967), specifically higher IQ and the development of communicative speech by the age of 5–6 years. However, the type and degree of support provided beyond school and into adulthood plays a crucial role in outcomes (Howlin 2005).

Conclusion

Parents of a young child with developmental and/or behavioral difficulties are likely to seek help from a range of professionals and services, including chiropractors. Early diagnosis and identification of autism facilitates access to early intervention and promotes the best possible outcome. Therefore, any professional who comes into contact with children who have developmental delays or unusual behavior should refer on to a pediatrician for further decision on whether referral to a specialist assessment team is indicated. Autism is a lifelong condition but symptoms change and modify with development, education, behavioral management and other appropriate treatments. Children with autism may also suffer from a number of other associated medical conditions such as epilepsy, tic disorders and mental health problems. Specific pharmacological and psychological treatments are indicated for these conditions. It is important that the diagnosis of autism does not overshadow the assessment of other conditions for which treatment may be available.

References

Aman, M.G., Armstrong, S.A., 2000. Regarding secretin for treating autistic disorder. J. Autism Dev. Disord. 30 (1), 71–72.

Aman, M.G., Collier-Crespin, A., Lindsay, R.L., 2000. Pharmacotherapy of disorders in mental retardation. Eur. Child Adolesc. Psychiatry 9, 98–107.

Aman, M.G., Buican, B., Arnold, L.E., 2003. Methylphenidate treatment in children with borderline IQ and mental retardation: analysis of three aggregated studies. J. Child Adolesc. Psychopharmacol. 13, 29–40.

American Psychiatric Association, 2000. Diagnostic and Statistical Manual of Mental Disorders – Text Revision, fourth ed. American Psychiatric Association, Washington, DC.

Anastopoulos, A.D., Shelton, T.L., DuPaul, G.J., et al., 1993. Parent training for attention-deficit hyperactivity disorder: its impact on parent functioning. J. Abnorm. Child Psychol. 21 (5), 581–596.

Anderson, G.M., Hoshino, Y., 1997. Neurochemical studies of autism. In: Cohen, D.J., Volkmar, F.R. (Eds), Handbook of Autism and Pervasive Developmental Disorders, second ed. John Wiley and Sons, New York, pp. 325–343.

Andrews, N., Miller, E., Grant, A., et al., 2004. Thimerosal exposure in infants and developmental disorders: a retrospective cohort study in the United Kingdom does not support a causal association. Pediatrics 114 (3), 584–591.

Bailey, A., Phillips, W., Rutter, M., 1996. Autism: towards an integration of clinical, genetic, neuropsychological, and neurobiological perspectives. J. Child Psychol. Psychiatry 37 (1), 89–126.

Baird, G., Simonoff, E., Pickles, A., et al., 2006. Prevalence of disorders of the autism spectrum in a population cohort of children in South Thames: the Special Needs and Autism Project (SNAP). Lancet 368 (9531), 210–215.

Ballaban-Gil, K., Rapin, I., Tuchman, R., et al., 1996. Longitudinal examination of the behavioural, language, and social changes in a population of adolescents and young adults with autistic disorder. Pediatr. Neurol. 15 (3), 217–223.

Baron-Cohen, S., Allen, J., Gillberg, C., 1992. Can autism be detected at 18 months? The needle, the haystack, and the CHAT. Br. J. Psychiatry 161, 839–843.

Baron-Cohen, S., Cox, A., Baird, G., et al., 1996. Psychological markers in the detection of autism in infancy in a large population. Br. J. Psychiatry 168 (2), 158–163.

Bartak, L., Rutter, M., 1973. Special educational treatment of autistic children: a comparative study: I. Design of study and characteristics of units. J. Child Psychol. Psychiatry 14 (3), 161–179.

Bettelheim, B., 1967. The Empty Fortress. The Free Press, New York.

Bolton, P., Rutter, M., 1990. Genetic influences in autism. Int. Rev. Psychiatry 2 (1), 67–80.

Bregman, J., Gerdtz, J., 1997. Behavioral interventions. In: Cohen, D.J., Volkmar, F.R. (Eds), Handbook of Autism and Pervasive Developmental Disorders, second ed. John Wiley and Sons, New York, pp. 606–630.

Bregman, J.D., Zager, D., Gerdtz, J., 2005. Behavioral interventions. In: Volkmar, F.R., Paul, A., Klin, A. et al. (Eds), Handbook of Autism and Pervasive Developmental Disorders, vol. 2. John Wiley and Sons, Hoboken, NJ, pp. 897–924.

Brereton, A.V., Tonge, B.J., 2005. Pre-schoolers with Autism: An Education and Skills Training Programme for Parents. Jessica Kingsley Publishers, London.

Brereton, A.V., Tonge, B.J., Mackinnon, A.J., et al., 2002. Screening young people for autism with the Developmental Behaviour Checklist. J. Am. Acad. Child Adolesc. Psychiatry 41 (11), 1369–1375.

Brereton, A.V., Tonge, B.J., Einfeld, S.L., 2006. Psychopathology in children and adolescents with autism compared to young people with intellectual disability. J Autism Dev. Disord. 36, 863–870.

Bristol, M.M., Schopler, E., 1983. Stress and coping in families of autistic adolescents. In: Schopler, G., Mesibov, G. (Eds), Autism in Adolescents and Adults. Plenum Press, New York, pp. 251–278.

Campbell, M., Anderson, L.Y., Small, A.M., et al., 1990. Naltrexone in autistic children: a double blind and placebo controlled study. Psychopharmacol. Bull. 26, 130–135.

Centers for Disease Control, 2007. Prevalence of autism spectrum disorders – Autism and Developmental Disabilities Monitoring Network, 2007. 14 sites, United States, 2002. Surveillance Summaries, February 9, 2007. Morb. Mortal. Wkly. Rep. 56 (SS-1), 12–28.

Chakrabarti, S., Fombonne, E., 2005. Pervasive developmental disorders in preschool children: confirmation of high prevalence. Am. J. Psychiatry 162 (6), 1133–1141.

Chen, W., Landau, S., Sham, P., et al., 2004. No evidence for links between autism, MMR and measles virus. Psychol. Med. 34 (3), 543–553.

Choutka, C.M., 1999. Experiencing the reality of service delivery: one parent's perspective. Journal of the Association for Persons with Severe Handicaps 24 (3), 213–217.

Constantino, J.N., Davis, S.A., Todd, R.D., et al., 2003. Validation of a brief quantitative measure of autistic traits: comparison of the social responsiveness scale with the autism diagnostic interview-revised. J. Autism Dev. Disord. 33 (4), 427–433.

Corsello, C., 2005. Early intervention in autism. Infants and Young Children 18 (2), 74–85.

Corsello, C., Hus, V., Pickles, A., et al., 2007. Between a ROC and a hard place: decision making and making decisions about using the SCQ. J. Child Psychol. Psychiatry 48 (9), 932–940.

DeMyer, M.K., 1979. Effect of early symptoms on the family. In: DeMyer, M.K. (Ed.), Parents and Children in Autism. VH Winston, Washington, DC, pp. 149–172.

DeStefano, F., Thompson, W.W., 2004. MMR vaccine and autism: an update of the scientific evidence. Expert Rev. Vaccines 3 (1), 19–22.

Drew, A., Baird, G., Baron-Cohen, S., et al., 2002. A pilot randomised control trial of a parent training intervention for pre-school children with autism: preliminary findings and methodological challenges. Eur. Child Adolesc. Psychiatry 11 (6), 266–272.

Dunn, M.E., Burbine, T., Bowers, C.A., et al., 2001. Moderators of stress in parents of children with autism. Community Ment. Health J. 37 (1), 39–52.

Einfeld, S.L., Tonge, B.J., 1995. The developmental behaviour checklist: the development and validation of an instrument to assess behavioural and emotional disturbance in children and adolescents with mental retardation. J. Autism Dev. Disord. 25 (2), 81–104.

Einfeld, S.L., Tonge, B.J., 2002. Manual for the Developmental Behaviour Checklist: Primary Carer Version (DBC-P) and Teacher Version (DBC-T), second ed. Monash University Centre for Developmental Psychiatry and Psychology, Clayton, Melbourne.

Ferrance, R.J., 2003. Autism – another topic often lacking facts when discussed within the chiropractic profession. J. Can. Chiropr. Assoc. 47 (1), 4–7.

Filipek, P., 2005. Medical aspects of autism. In: Volkmar, F.R., Paul, R., Klin, A. et al., (Eds), Handbook of Autism and Pervasive Developmental Disorders, vol. 1. John Wiley and Sons, Hoboken, NJ, pp. 534–578.

Fombonne, E., 2005a. The changing epidemiology of autism. J. Appl. Res. Intellect. Disabil. 18, 281–294.

Fombonne, E., 2005b. Epidemiological studies of pervasive developmental disorders. In: Volkmar, F.R., Paul, R., Klin, A. et al. (Eds), Handbook of Autism and Pervasive Developmental Disorders, vol. 1. John Wiley and Sons, Hoboken, NJ, pp. 42–69.

Fombonne, E., 2008. Thimerosal disappears but autism remains. Arch. Gen. Psychiatry 65 (1), 15–16.

Fombonne, E., Chakrabarti, S., 2001. No evidence for a new variant of measles-mumps-rubella-induced autism. Pediatrics 108 (4), E58.

Fombonne, E., Simmons, H., Ford, T., et al., 2001. Prevalence of pervasive developmental disorders in the British nationwide survey of child mental health. J. Am. Acad. Child Adolesc. Psychiatry 40 (7), 820–827.

Gillberg, C., 1991. Outcome in autism and autistic-like conditions. J. Am. Acad. Child Adolesc. Psychiatry 30 (3), 375–382.

Gillberg, C., 1998. The long-term course of autistic disorders: update on follow-up studies. Acta. Psychiatr. Scand. 97, 99–108.

Gillberg, C., Steffenburg, S., 1987. Outcome and prognostic factors in infantile autism and similar conditions: a population-based study of 46 cases followed through puberty. J. Autism Dev. Disord. 17 (2), 273–287.

Gillberg, C., Cederlund, M., Lamberg, K., et al., 2006. Brief report: 'The autism epidemic': the registered prevalence of autism in a Swedish urban area. J. Autism Dev. Disord. 36, 429–435.

Gleberzon, B.J., 2006. Chiropractic and the management of children with autism. Clin. Chiropr. 9, 176–181.

Gray, K.M., Tonge, B.J., 2001. Are there early features of autism in infants and preschool children? J. Paediatr. Child Health 37 (3), 221–226.

Gray, K.M., Tonge, B.J., 2005. Screening for autism in infants and preschool children with developmental delay. Aust. N. Z. J. Psychiatry 39 (5), 378–386.

Gray, K.M., Tonge, B.J., Sweeney, D.J., et al., 2008. Screening for autism in young children with developmental delay: an evaluation of the developmental behaviour checklist – early screen (DBC-ES). J. Autism Dev. Disord. 38 (6), 1003–1010.

Graziano, A.M., Diament, D.M., 1992. Parent behavioral training: an examination of the paradigm. Behav. Modif. 16 (1), 3–38.

Hanson, E., Kalish, L.A., Bunce, E., et al., 2007. Use of complementary and alternative medicine among children diagnosed with autism spectrum disorder. J. Autism Dev. Disord. 37, 628–636.

Happe, F., Ronald, A., Plomin, R., 2006. Time to give up on a single explanation for autism. Nat. Neurosci. 9 (10), 1218–1220.

Harris, S.L., Weiss, M.J., 1998. Right From the Start: Behavioral Intervention for Young Children with Autism. Woodbine House, Bethesda, MD.

Hastings, R., 2004. Child behaviour problems and partner mental health as correlates of stress in mothers and fathers of children with autism. J. Intellect. Disabil. Res. 47 (4–5), 231–237.

Herring, S., Gray, K., Taffe, J., et al., 2006. Behaviour and emotional problems in toddlers with pervasive developmental disorders and developmental delay: associations with parental mental health and family functioning. J. Intellect. Disabil. Res. 50 (12), 874–882.

Holroyd, J., McArthur, D., 1976. Mental retardation and stress on the parents: a contrast between Down's syndrome and childhood autism. Am. J. Ment. Defic. 80 (4), 431–436.

Horner, R.H., Carr, E.G., Strain, P.S., et al., 2002. Problem behavior interventions for young children with autism: a research synthesis. J. Autism Dev. Disord. 32 (5), 423–446.

Howlin, P., 1997. Prognosis in autism: do specialist treatments affect long-term outcome? Eur. Child Adolesc. Psychiatry 6 (2), 55–72.

Howlin, P., 1998. Practitioner review: psychological and educational treatments for autism. J. Child Psychol. Psychiatry 39 (3), 307–322.

Howlin, P., 2005. Outcomes in autism spectrum disorders. In: Volkmar, F.R., Paul, R., Klin, A., et al. (Eds), Handbook of Autism and Pervasive Developmental Disorders, vol. 1. John Wiley and Sons, Hoboken, NJ, pp. 201–220.

Howlin, P., Yates, P., 1989. Treating autistic children at home: a London based programme. In: Gillberg, C. (Ed.), Diagnosis and Treatment of Autism. Plenum Press, New York, pp. 307–322.

Howlin, P., Goode, S., Hutton, J., et al., 2004. Adult outcome for children with autism. J. Child Psychol. Psychiatry 45 (2), 212–229.

Johnson, C.R., Handen, B.L., Butter, E., et al., 2007. Development of a parent training program for children with pervasive developmental disorders. Behav. Intervent. 22, 201–221.

Johnson, E., Hastings, R.P., 2002. Facilitating factors and barriers to the implementation of intensive home-based behavioural intervention for young children with autism. Child Care Health Dev. 28 (2), 123–129.

Kanner, L., 1943. Autistic disturbances of affective contact. Nerv. Child 2, 217–250.

Kanner, L., 1973. To what extent is early infantile autism determined by constitutional inadequacies? In: Kanner, L. (Ed.), Childhood Psychosis: Initial Studies and New

Insights. H Winston, Washington, DC, pp. 69–75.

Kasari, C., Freeman, S., Paparella, T., 2001. Early intervention in autism: joint attention and symbolic play. Int. Rev. Res. Ment. Retard. 23 (23), 207–237.

Kasari, C., Freeman, S., Paparella, T., 2006. Joint attention and symbolic play in children with autism: a randomized controlled intervention study. J. Child Psychol. Psychiatry 47 (6), 611–620.

Kawasaki, Y., Yokota, K., Shinomiya, M., et al., 1997. Brief report: electroencephalographic paroxysmal activities in the frontal area emerged in middle childhood and during adolescence in a follow-up study of autism. J. Autism Dev. Disord. 27, 605–620.

Kobayashi, R., Murata, T., Yoshinaga, K., 1992. A follow-up study of 201 children with autism in Kyushu and Yamaguchi areas, Japan. J. Autism Dev. Disord. 22 (3), 395–411.

Koegel, L.K., Koegel, R.L., Hurley, C., et al., 1992a. Improving social skills and disruptive behavior in children with autism through self-management. J. Appl. Behav. Anal. 25, 341–353.

Koegel, L.K., Koegel, R.L., Surratt, A., 1992b. Language intervention and disruptive behavior in preschool children with autism. J. Autism Dev. Disord. 22, 141–153.

Koegel, R.L., Schriebman, L., Loos, L.M., et al., 1992c. Consistent stress profiles in mothers of children with autism. J. Autism Dev. Disord. 22 (2), 205–216.

Larsen, F.W., Mouridsen, S.E., 1997. The outcome in children with childhood autism and Asperger syndrome originally diagnosed as psychotic: a 30 year follow-up study of subjects hospitalized as children. Eur. Child Adolesc. Psychiatry 6 (4), 181–190.

Lauritsen, M.B., Mors, O., Mortensen, P.B., et al., 2002. Medical disorders among inpatients with autism in Denmark according to ICD-8: a nationwide register-based study. J. Autism Dev. Disord. 32 (2), 115–119.

Lecavalier, L., 2006. Behavioral and emotional problems in young people with pervasive developmental disorders: relative prevalence, effects of subject characteristics, and empirical classification. J. Autism Dev. Disord. 36, 1101–1114.

Lecavalier, L., Leone, S., Wiltz, J., 2005. The impact of behaviour problems on caregiver stress in young people with autism spectrum disorders. J. Intellect. Disabil. Res. 50 (3), 172–183.

Locascio, J.J., Malone, R.P., Small, A.M., et al., 1991. Factors related to haloperidol response and dyskinesias in autistic children. Psychopharmacol. Bull. 27, 483–499.

Lord, C., 1995. Facilitating social inclusion: examples from peer intervention programs. In: Schopler, E., Mesibov, G.B. (Eds), Learning and Cognition in Autism: Current Issues in Autism. Plenum Press, New York, pp. 221–240.

Lord, C., McGee, J., 2001. Social development. In: Lord, C., McGee, J. (Eds), Educating Children with Autism. National Academy of Sciences, Washington, DC, pp. 66–81.

Lord, C., Rutter, M., 1994. Autism and pervasive developmental disorders. In: Rutter M., Taylor E., Hersov B. (Eds), Child and Adolescent Psychiatry: Modern Approaches, third ed. Blackwell, Oxford, pp. 569–591.

Lord, C., Rutter, M.L., Goode, S., et al., 1989. Autism Diagnostic Observation Schedule: a standardized observation of communicative and social behavior. J. Autism Dev. Disord. 19 (2), 185–212.

Lord, C., Rutter, M., LeCouteur, A., 1994. Autism Diagnostic Interview-Revised: a revised version of a diagnostic interview for caregivers of individuals with possible pervasive developmental disorders. J. Autism Dev. Disord. 24 (5), 659–685.

Lord, C., Risi, S., Lambrecht, L., et al., 2000. The Autism Diagnostic Observation Schedule-Generic: a standard measure of social and communication deficits associated with the spectrum of autism. J. Autism Dev. Disord. 30 (3), 205–223.

Lord, C., Rutter, M., DiLavore, P., et al., 2001. Autism Diagnostic Observation Schedule (ADOS) Manual. Western Psychological Services, Los Angeles, CA.

Luiselli, J.K., Cannon, B.O.M., Ellis, J.T., et al., 2000. Home-based behavioral interventions for young children with autism/pervasive developmental disorder: a preliminary evaluation of outcome in relation to child age and intensity of service delivery. Autism 4 (4), 426–438.

McClannahan, L.E., Krantz, P.J., 1999. Activity Schedules for Children with Autism: Teaching Independent Behavior. Woodbine House, Bethesda, MD, p. 117.

McConachie, H., Diggle, T., 2005. Parent implemented early intervention for young children with autism spectrum disorder: a systematic review. J. Eval. Clin. Pract. 13, 129.

MacDermott, S., Williams, K., Ridley, G., et al., 2007. The Prevalence of Autism in Australia: Can it be Established from Existing Data? Australian Advisory Board on Autism Spectrum Disorders, Forestville, New South Wales.

Madsen, K.M., Lauritsen, M.B., Pedersen, C.B., et al., 2003. Thimerosal and the occurrence of autism: negative ecological evidence from Danish population-based data. Pediatrics 112 (3/1), 604–606.

Marcus, L., Kunce, L., Schopler, E., 1997. Working with families. In: Cohen, D.J., Volkmar, F.R. (Eds), Handbook of Autism and Pervasive Developmental Disorders, second ed. John Wiley and Sons, New York, pp. 631–649.

Marcus, L.M., Kunce, L.J., Schopler, E., 2005. Working with families. In: Volkmar, F.R., Paul, R., Klin, A. et al. (Eds), Handbook of Autism and Pervasive Developmental Disorders, third ed, vol. 2. John Wiley and Sons, Hoboken, NJ, pp. 1055–1086.

Martin, A., Scahill, L., Klin, A., et al., 1999. Higher-functioning pervasive developmental disorders: rates and patterns of psychotropic drug use. J. Am. Acad. Child Adolesc. Psychiatry 38 (7), 923–931.

Metz, B., Mulick, J.A., Butter, E.M., 2005. Autism: a late twentieth century fad magnet.

In: Jacobson, J.W., Foxx, R.M., Mulick, J.A. (Eds), Controversial Therapies for Developmental Disabilities: Fad, Fashion and Science in Professional Practice. Lawrence Erlbaum Associates, Mahwah, NJ, pp. 237–263.

Minshew, N.J., Sweeney, J.A., Bauman, M.L., 1997. Neurological aspects of autism. In: Cohen, D.J., Volkmar, F.R. (Eds), Handbook of Autism and Pervasive Developmental Disorders, second ed. John Wiley and Sons, New York, pp. 344–369.

Minshew, N.J., Sweeney, J.A., Bauman, M.L., et al., 2005. Neurologic aspects of autism. In: Volkmar, F.R., Paul, R., Klin, A., et al. (Eds), Hanbook of Autism and Pervasive Developmental Disorders, vol. 1. John Wiley and Sons, Hoboken, NJ, pp. 473–514.

Moes, D., Koegel, R.L., Schreibman, L., et al., 1992. Stress profiles for mothers and fathers of children with autism. Psychol. Rep. 71 (3/2), 1272–1274.

Murch, S.H., Anthony, A., Casson, D.H., et al., 2004. Retraction of an interpretation. Lancet 363 (9411), 750.

Ng, D., Chan, C., Soo, M., et al., 2007. Low-level chronic mercury exposure in children and adolescents: meta-analysis. Pediatr. Int. 49 (1), 80–87.

Nordin, V., Gillberg, C., 1998. The long-term course of autistic disorders: update on follow-up studies. Acta. Psychiatr. Scand. 97 (2), 99–108.

Olley, J.G., 1999. Curriculum for students with autism. School Psychol. Rev. 28 (4), 595–607.

Olsson, M.B., Hwang, C.P., 2001. Depression in mothers and fathers of children with intellectual disability. J. Intellect. Disabil. Res. 45 (6), 535–543.

Owley, T., McMahon, W., Cook, E.H., et al., 2001. Multisite, double-blind, placebo-controlled trial of porcine secretin in autism. J. Am. Acad. Child Adolesc. Psychiatry 40 (11), 1293–1299.

Parker, S.K., Schwartz, B., Todd, J., et al., 2004. Thimerosal-containing vaccines and autistic spectrum disorder: a critical review of published original data. Pediatrics 114 (3), 793–804.

Powers, M.D., 1992. Early intervention for children with autism. In: Berkell, D.E. (Ed.), Autism: Identification, Education, and Treatment. Lawrence Erlbaum, Hillside, NJ, pp. 225–252.

Prizant, B.M., 1996. Brief report: communication, language, social, and emotional development. J. Autism Dev. Disord. 26 (2), 173–178.

Rapin, I., 1991. Autistic children: diagnosis and clinical features. Pediatrics 87 (5/2), 751–760.

Research Units on Pediatric Psychopharmacology (RUPP) Autism Network, 2005a. Randomized, controlled, crossover trial of methylphenidate in pervasive developmental disorders with hyperactivity. Arch. Gen. Psychiatry 62, 1266–1274.

Research Units on Pediatric Psychopharmacology (RUPP) Autism Network, 2005b. Risperidone treatment of autistic disorder: longer-term benefits and blinded

discontinuation after 6 months. Am. J. Psychiatry 162 (7), 1361–1369.

Research Units on Pediatric Psychopharmacology (RUPP) Autism Network, 2007. Parent training for children with pervasive developmental disorders: a multi-site feasibility trial. Behavioral Interventions 22, 179–199.

Ritvo, E.R., Mason-Brothers, A., Freeman, B.J., et al., 1990. The UCLA–University of Utah epidemiologic survey of autism: the etiologic role of rare diseases. Am. J. Psychiatry 147 (12), 1614–1621.

Robins, D.L., Fein, D., Barton, M.L., et al., 2001. The Modified Checklist for Autism in Toddlers: an initial study investigating the early detection of autism and pervasive developmental disorders. J. Autism Dev. Disord. 31, (2), 131–144.

Rogers, S.J., 1996. Early intervention in autism. J. Autism Dev. Disord. 26 (2), 243–246.

Rutter, M., 1970. Autistic children: infancy to adulthood. Semin. Psychiatry 2 (4), 435–450.

Rutter, M., 1985. The treatment of autistic children. J. Child Psychol. Psychiatry 26 (2), 193–214.

Rutter, M., Schopler, E., 1987. Autism and pervasive developmental disorders: concepts and diagnostic issues. J. Autism Dev. Disord. 17 (2), 159–186.

Rutter, M., Greenfeld, D., Lockyer, L., 1967. A five to fifteen year follow-up study of infantile psychosis. II. Social and behavioural outcome. Br. J. Psychiatry 113 (504), 1183–1199.

Rutter, M., Bailey, A., Simonoff, E., et al., 1997. Genetic influences and autism. In: Cohen, D.J., Volkmar, F.R. (Eds), Handbook of Autism and Pervasive Developmental Disorders, second ed. John Wiley and Sons, New York, pp. 370–387.

Rutter, M., Bailey, A., Lord, C., 2003a. Social Communication Questionnaire (SCQ). Western Psychological Services, Los Angeles, CA.

Rutter, M., LeCouteur, A., Lord, C., 2003b. Autism Diagnostic Interview-Revised. Western Psychological Services, Los Angeles, CA.

Sanders, J.L., Morgan, S.B., 1997. Family stress and adjustment as perceived by parents of children with autism or Down-syndrome: implications for intervention. Child Fam. Behav. Ther. 19 (4), 15–32.

Sandler, A.D., Bodfish, J.W., 2000. Placebo effects in autism: lessons from secretin. J. Dev. Behav. Pediatr. 21 (5), 347–350.

Sandler, A.D., Sutton, K.A., DeWeese, J., et al., 1999. Lack of benefit of a single dose of synthetic human secretin in the treatment of autism and pervasive developmental disorder. N. Engl. J. Med. 341 (24), 1801–1806.

Schopler, E., 1971. Parents of psychotic children as scapegoats. J. Contemp. Psychother. 4 (1), 17–22.

Schopler, E., 1987. Specific and nonspecific factors in the effectiveness of a treatment system. Am. Psychol. 42 (4), 376–383.

Schopler, E., 1989. Principles for directing both educational treatment and research. In: Gillberg, C. (Ed.), Diagnosis and

Treatment of Autism. Plenum Press, New York, pp. 167–183.

Schopler, E., Reichler, R.J., DeVellis, R.F., et al., 1980. Toward objective classification of childhood autism: Childhood Autism Rating Scale (CARS). J. Autism Dev. Disord. 10 (1), 91–103.

Schreibman, L., 1994. Autism. In: Craighead, W.E., Craighead, W.E., Kazdin, A.E., et al. (Eds), Cognitive and Behavioral Interventions: An Empirical Approach to Mental Health Problems. Allyn & Bacon, Boston, MA, pp. 335–358.

Schreibman, L., Whalen, C., Stahmer, A.C., 2000. The use of video priming to reduce disruptive transition behavior in children with autism. J. Posit. Behav. Intervent. 2 (1), 3–11.

Schwartz, I.S., Sandall, S.R., Garfinkle, A.N., et al., 1998. Outcomes for children with autism: three case studies. Top. Early Child. Spec. Educ. 18 (3), 132–143.

Sheinkopf, S.J., Siegel, B., 1998. Home-based behavioral treatment of young children with autism. J. Autism Dev. Disord. 28 (1), 15–23.

Simeonsson, R.J., Olley, J.G., Rosenthal, S.L., 1987. Early intervention for children with autism. In: Guralnick, M.J., Bennett, F.C. (Eds), The Effectiveness of Early Intervention for At-Risk and Handicapped Children. Academic Press, Orlando, FL, pp. 275–296.

Sinha, Y., Silove, N., Williams, K., 2006. Chelation therapy and autism. Br. Med. J. 333 (7571), 756.

Smeeth, L., Cook, C., Fombonne, E., et al., 2004. MMR vaccination and pervasive developmental disorders: a case-control study. Lancet 364 (9438), 963–969.

Stehr-Green, P., Tull, P., Stellfeld, M., et al., 2003. Autism and thimerosal-containing vaccines: lack of consistent evidence for an association. Am. J. Prev. Med. 25 (2), 101–106.

Steinhausen, H.C., Metzke, C.W., 2004. Differentiating the behavioural profile in autism and mental retardation and testing of a screener. Eur. Child Adolesc. Psychiatry 13 (4), 214–220.

Szatmari, P., Bartolucci, G., Bremner, R., et al., 1989. A follow-up study of high-functioning autistic children. J. Autism Dev. Disord. 19 (2), 213–225.

Taylor, B., Miller, E., Farrington, C.P., et al., 1999. Autism and measles, mumps, and rubella vaccine: no epidemiological evidence for a causal association. Lancet 353 (9169), 2026–2029.

Tonge, B.J., 2002. Autism, autistic spectrum and the need for better definition. Med. J. Aust. 176 (9), 412–413.

Tonge, B.J., Einfeld, S.L., 2003. Psychopathology and intellectual disability: the Australian child to adult longitudinal study. In: Glidden, L.M. (Ed.), International Review of Research in Mental Retardation, vol. 26. Academic Press, San Diego, CA, pp. 61–91.

Tonge, B., Brereton, A.V., Kiomall, M., et al., 2006. Effects on parental mental health of an education and skills training program for parents of young children with autism: a randomized controlled trial. J. Am. Acad. Child Adolesc. Psychiatry 45 (5), 561–569.

Volkmar, F., 1999. Lessons from secretin. N. Engl. J. Med. 341 (24), 1842.

von Knorring, A.L., Hagglof, B., 1993. Autism in northern Sweden: a population based follow-up study: psychopathology. Eur. Child Adolesc. Psychiatry 2 (2), 91–97.

Wakefield, A.J., Murch, S.H., Anthony, A., et al., 1999. Ileal-lymphoid-nodular hyperplasia, non-specific colitis, and pervasive developmental disorder in children. Lancet 351 (9103), 637–641.

Wazana, A., Bresnahan, M., Kline, J., 2007. The autism epidemic: fact or fiction? J. Am. Acad. Child Adolesc. Psychiatry 46 (6), 721–730.

Werry, J.S., 1996. Pervasive Developmental, Psychotic, and Allied Disorders. In: Hechtman, L.T. (Ed.), Do they Grow Out of it? Long-term Outcomes of Childhood Disorders. American Psychiatric Press, Washington, DC, pp. 195–223.

Wing, L., 1989. Autistic adults. In: Gillberg, C. (Ed.), Diagnosis and Treatment of Autism. Plenum Press, New York, pp. 419–432.

Wing, L., Gould, J., 1979. Severe impairments of social interaction and associated abnormalities in children: epidemiology and classification. J. Autism Dev. Disord. 9 (1), 11–29.

Witwer, A., Lecavalier, L., 2005. Treatment rates and patterns in young people with autism spectrum disorders. J. Child Adolesc. Psychopharmacol. 15 (4), 671–681.

Wong, H.H.L., Smith, R.G., 2006. Patterns of complementary and alternative medical therapy use in children diagnosed with autism spectrum disorders. J. Autism Dev. Disord. 36, 901–909.

World Health Organization, 1992. ICD-10. Classification of Mental and Behavioural Disorders: Clinical Description and Diagnostic Guidelines. World Health Organization, Geneva.

Yirmiya, N., Shaked, M., 2005. Psychiatric disorders in parents of children with autism: a meta-analysis. J. Child Psychol. Psychiatry 46 (1), 69–83.

Accidental and intentional injury in children

16

Neil J. Davies

It is probably reasonable to make the assumption that the great majority of chiropractors regularly treat pediatric patients in the course of their professional life. In fact, as time goes by the percentage of chiropractic practice represented by the pediatric population group is escalating, particularly in the past two decades, as parents seek solutions to their children's health problems outside the mainstream western or allopathic medical models (Lee et al 2000, Petetti et al 2001).

As the chiropractic profession matures it becomes more and more of an imperative to be watchful and vigilant in helping parents, schools and the general community to protect children from harm, both intentional and accidental. The purpose of this chapter is to offer time-honored guidelines and basic information to empower the family chiropractor to do just that.

Intentional injury

Child abuse, or intentional injury as it is now referred to, is a major public health issue. It is also a criminal activity that the chiropractor is uniquely placed to identify and act upon in a social, legal (depending upon jurisdiction) and professionally responsible way. It has been estimated that some 100 000 children each year who have been the subject of abuse or neglect attend chiropractic clinics in the USA alone (Nash 1990). Child abuse in its various forms is not a phenomenon unique to the developed, western world (Chen et al 2006) but a growing worldwide problem which transcends all classes – national, gender, socioeconomic, religious and cultural. Given the exponential increase in the numbers of children attending chiropractic clinics over the past 20 years or so, it is not surprising that the chiropractic literature has begun to take seriously the challenge of alerting practitioners to the problem identifying the abused and at-risk child (Davies 1992, Ebrall & Davies 2000, Gier 1987, Mootz & Hansen 1999, Nash 1990, Stierwaldt 1976, Wyatt 2005).

While most child abuse happens in the home, increasing numbers of child abuse cases are occurring within organizations such as churches, schools, child care businesses and residential schools. Abusive behavior takes a variety of forms and is associated with poverty, family stress and family isolation. It includes domestic violence, sexual abuse/assault, neglect and emotional abuse (Christoffel 1994, Fontana 1989). Children suffer more from victimization than any other population group. Victimization has been categorized into three broad groups: *the pandemic*, such as sibling assault, which it is probably reasonable to assume will at some point affect most children (Christoffel 1994); *the acute*, including physical abuse which affects a smaller but still significant number; and *the extraordinary*, including homicide, which affects only a small number of children (Finkelhor & Dziuba-Leatherman 1994). Statistically, throughout 2005 there were 3.3 million referrals of incidents of child abuse to relevant authorities in the USA involving some 6 million children. Tragically, there were 1460 deaths (US Department of Health and Human Services 2005). In all, it has been estimated that 1% of all American children have been the subject of abuse (Gordon & Palusci 1991). The statistics are not dissimilar in the other developed countries such as Australia where, in 2004, there were nearly 200 000 reports made to relevant authorities (Kovacs & Richardson 2004).

This problem is not getting better with time. To determine the extent of non-fatal infant maltreatment in the USA, the Center of Disease Control and Prevention (CDCP) and the Federal Administration for Children and Families (ACF) analyzed data collected in fiscal year 2006 (the most recent data available) from the National Child Abuse and Neglect Data System (NCANDS). The findings in this report indicate that, in the fiscal year 2006, 23.2 children per 1000 population aged <1 year experienced substantiated non-fatal maltreatment in the USA. Among these infants, neglect was the maltreatment category most commonly cited, experienced by 68.5% of victims. Among infant victims aged <1 year who experienced

16

© 2010, Elsevier Ltd, Inc, BV
DOI: 10.1016/B978-0-7020-3129-8.00016-5

substantiated maltreatment, 32.7% were aged ≤ 1 week and 30.6% were aged <4 days. Neglect also was the maltreatment category most often cited among children aged ≤ 1 week (Centers for Disease Control 2008).

The clinical evidence of child abuse which confronts the chiropractor in private practice varies widely from being minimal, difficult to quantify, and often ambiguous at the lower end of the severity scale to being very obvious at the higher end. When one considers the current prevalence of child abuse, it is obvious that knowledge of the relevant fundamental principles of diagnosis is essential for every chiropractor. Alertness to the possibility of abuse may save a life or prevent ongoing trauma due to physical, sexual or psychological trauma, and neglect.

Definitions of abuse

In a broad, general sense, child abuse can be defined as any intentional act, an omission or commission that endangers or impairs a child's physical or emotional health and development (Davies 1992). In the USA, federal legislation provides a foundation for all states by identifying a minimum set of acts or behaviors that define child abuse and neglect. The Federal Child Abuse Prevention and Treatment Act (CAPTA) (42 U.S.C.A. §5106g), as amended by the Keeping Children and Families Safe Act of 2003, defines child abuse and neglect as, at minimum:

Any recent act or failure to act on the part of a parent or caregiver which results in death, serious physical or emotional harm, sexual abuse or exploitation; or

An act or failure to act which presents an imminent risk of serious harm.

The above definition of child abuse and neglect refers specifically to parents and other caregivers. A 'child' under this definition generally means a person who is under the age of 18 or who is not an emancipated minor.

While CAPTA provides definitions for sexual abuse and the special cases related to withholding or failing to provide medically indicated treatment, it does not provide specific definitions for other types of maltreatment such as physical abuse, neglect or emotional abuse. While US federal legislation sets minimum standards, each state is responsible for providing its own definition of maltreatment within civil and criminal contexts (Wikipedia 2008). The reader is directed to the Child Welfare Information Gateway website located at http://www.childwelfare.gov/can/defining/ for specific definitions of each of the categories of child abuse as they are dictated by the laws of each state.

Recognition of abuse

The child who has suffered abuse may present with either physical or behavioral indicators, non-specific indicators, or at times a combination of all three, depending upon what form the abuse has taken.

Physical abuse

Physical indicators

Typically, the child who has suffered physical trauma that is intentional may have bruises at different stages of healing. These bruises frequently have characteristic shapes reflective of the instrument used in inflicting the bruise such as a stick or electric cord, etc. Fractures, particularly to the face, skull and spine, are common in such cases and are usually accompanied by an explanation from the parent, caregiver or child that is incongruent with the nature of the injury. Pattern-shaped burns are also sometimes seen, again, the shape being reflective of the instrument used to inflict the wound (e.g. iron, rope, cigarette, etc.) (Department of Human Services 2008, Ebrall & Davies 2000).

Behavioral indicators

The behavior of the child who has been physically abused sometimes provides vital clues to the diagnosis. The injured child will often say straight out that someone has hurt them, or they (or their caregiver) offer an explanation for their injury which is incongruent with the nature of the injury. They may display antisocial behavior such as extreme aggression or being withdrawn, they may appear to be afraid of their caregivers or the chiropractor, or sometimes display a complete lack of emotion in a situation that would normally be at least a little intimidating to a small child. Finally, expressing a fear of going home or leaving the clinic at the end of a consultation is indicative of the child feeling insecure about their safety (Department of Human Services 2008, Ebrall & Davies 2000).

Emotional/psychological abuse

Physical indicators

The emotionally abused child seldom exhibits any physical evidence of having been abused, rendering the physical examination of little worth in making the diagnosis. The only exception to this is Ewart's sign which is sustained retraction and thinning of the upper lip (Ewart 1980).

Behavioral indicators

Behaviorally, the emotionally abused child appears to exhibit low self-esteem and often experiences the sudden onset of pathophysiological stress-related conditions such as asthma (Frost 2004, Weist et al 2000), constipation (Hobbs et al 1999) and secondary enuresis (Gowers 2005). A range of other behaviors may also be seen. These include depression, anxiety, developmental delay, poor social skills, persistent habit disorders (rocking back and forth, nail-biting, etc.), sudden change in temperament, being withdrawn and tearful, self-harm, sleep disorders, and declining or poor academic achievement (Department of Human Services 2008, Ebrall & Davies 2000).

Sexual abuse

Physical indicators

The diagnosis of Sexual abuse is not often diagnosed by demonstrating physical signs. The sexually abused child may, however, present with a range of physical indicators, all of which need to be approached in a highly sensitive and respectful, if not oblique, manner. Typically, the sort of physical signs which may be seen are genital irritation or infection, inadequately explained anogenital trauma, persistent vaginal discharge, pregnancy in the very young adolescent, difficulty walking and recurrent urinary tract infection (Ebrall & Davies 2000).

Behavioral indicators

Behaviorally, the sexually abused child may tell the chiropractor that sexual abuse has occurred; they may complain of headache or abdominal pain, experience difficulty with their schoolwork, display sexual behavior or demonstrate knowledge of sexual practice which is not age appropriate, experience difficulty in sleeping, and have difficulty relating to adults and peers (Department of Human Services 2008). Depression and suicidal tendencies are also associated with sexual abuse (Chen et al 2006). Developmental regression such as the onset of secondary enuresis may accompany sexual abuse (Gowers 2005) as well as sleep disturbances and 'night terrors'. Finally, antisocial behavior such as drug addiction and alcoholism may occur (Oates 1986), as may sexual promiscuity and prostitution (South Australian Department of Community Welfare Child Protection Unit 1990).

Non-specific indicators

A range of non-specific behaviors may result from sexual abuse. These include a sudden change in behavior or temperament, sleep disorders, complaints of headache or abdominal pain, school difficulties, difficulties relating to peers or adults, self-harm behaviors, persistent habit disorders, excessive and inappropriate demands for privacy, and a reluctance to go home from school or other places where the child feels safe (Ebrall & Davies 2000).

Neglect

As a category of abuse, neglect is an insidious, chronic problem that may end up proving to be fatal (Ebrall & Davies 2000, Margolin 1990). Helfer (1990) has described neglect in the following way:

1. Abandonment/desertion. The child is left destitute or without adequate support.

2. Medical neglect. The lack of adequate medical or dental treatment. There is no direct reference to mental health conditions.

3. Environmental neglect. Unhygienic and unsafe living conditions.

4. Failure to supply adequate clothing to protect the child from the elements.

5. Failure to ensure safety. The placing of a child in a situation in which there is no or insufficient adult supervision to protect the child from real and significant risk and harm.

6. Failure to provide adequate food/fluid. Lack of foods or fluids to sustain normal functioning.

7. Failure to thrive (inorganic). Failure to thrive is presented as a likely harmful outcome of neglect, whereas the other subtypes are presented primarily as parental or caregiver omissions. Failure to thrive is directly associated in this type with failure to provide food/fluid partly or entirely as a result of underlying interactive concerns, which contribute to the failure to thrive syndrome.

Physical indicators

The diagnosis of neglect is arrived at after due consideration has been given to a wide range of physical indicators such as constant hunger, failure to thrive, malnutrition, lack of subcutaneous tissue, poor hygiene, inappropriate dress for the climatic conditions, a lack of adult supervision, unattended medical needs, abandonment and poor dietary habits.

Behavioral indicators

Behavioral indicators of neglect include stealing food, extending days at school, constant fatigue and listlessness, alcohol and drug abuse, claims of there being no adult supervision, aggressive or otherwise inappropriate behavior, isolation from peer group and chronic school absenteeism. Depression and suicidal tendencies are also associated with sexual abuse (Chen et al 2006, Ebrall & Davies 2000).

Initiating intervention when abuse has occurred

In the event the chiropractor has taken a case history, performed a physical examination, and on balance believes the physical, behavioral and non-specific evidence suggests that abuse of the child has taken place, the law requires that a report be initiated. All 50 states in the USA require mandatory reporting, making it a breach of the law not to report suspected cases of abuse. It is critical that all chiropractors make themselves aware of the contact details of the appropriate authority relative to the jurisdiction in which they practice and have it on record in case it becomes necessary to make a report of suspected abusive behavior. It should also be remembered that the chiropractor is not responsible for the diagnosis of abuse, but only that the physical, behavioral and non-specific evidence is suggestive of abuse. In most jurisdictions there will generally be three possible ways a report can be initiated. The first is to a local child protection unit which are usually staffed by social workers with specialty training in abusive family situations. This is the appropriate referral if the child you are concerned about is not, in your opinion, in immediate physical danger or in need of urgent medical care. The second is the emergency department of the hospital, and the child who should be referred there is the one in need of immediate medical care. Thirdly, and finally, there is the police. The police should only be called in the first instance in cases where, in your opinion, the child is in immediate physical danger or will be if allowed to go home.

The role of the chiropractor does not stop at the point where a report has been initiated. Ongoing care and emotional support for the family during the likely stressful sequelae to a report of abuse is crucial to their recovery as a family unit in addition to assisting them to access whatever family, social or psychological services that may be needed.

The role of the chiropractor in preventive strategies

Like many other problems dealt with by the chiropractor, prevention is usually the best possible way to deal with a problem. The chiropractor, like other health care professionals, has an opportunity to impact the problem of child abuse and neglect by being proactive in participating in or initiating preventive strategies at both the community and family levels.

At the community level

Community level strategies are preventive, designed to impact families before abusive behavior occurs. These strategies include public education programs, parent education classes and family support programs. The chiropractor is strongly placed to offer classes on such subjects as feeding techniques for babies and toddlers, strategies for settling babies to sleep, as well as general health and wellness classes. The idea of these classes is to educate parents, make them aware of the help chiropractic can offer them and reduce the total stress a child necessarily brings to the home.

At the community level, the chiropractor can also be very helpful in pointing parents and caregivers towards community-based help programs directed towards stress management, family support and the development of parenting skills. Making patients aware of community-based services and personnel to contact at times when help is needed is also a valuable public health service that chiropractors can render to families of young children. It is also appropriate for chiropractors to act in an advocacy role on behalf of patients needing to access such services.

At the family level

This is more specific in that it entails identifying families which are under stress and who may need assistance from community-based services. In this situation it is appropriate from a public health perspective to intervene on behalf of that particular family and assist them in accessing the necessary services. A very useful strategy at the family level is to visit new parents in their homes soon after they return from hospital with their new baby to make sure they are coping with the stress of having a newborn in their home.

The role of the chiropractor in keeping children safe from accidental harm

A safe environment for children to grow up in extends beyond just being safe from intentional injury and neglect. There are many products available today which are aimed at the child market, and not all of these are in the best interests and safety of the child or their developmental well-being. While a summary of every available product on the market that falls into this category is outside the scope of this chapter, a description of two will suffice to demonstrate the responsibility a chiropractor has, in a public health sense, to educate and warn the consuming public. The chiropractic biomechanical understanding of body structure and function and its effect on development places the chiropractor in a unique position to assess such products on an individual basis from the perspective of their potential biological impact.

Trampolines

The recreational use of trampolines has increased dramatically during the past 10 years. There has been a striking parallel increase in the number of children presenting to fracture clinics with injuries associated with trampoline use in that same time period (Bhangal et al 2006, Hurson et al 2007, Nysted & Drogset 2006). To a large extent, the serious injuries that happen to children while trampolining do so when they have no adult supervision. In one study conducted in Ireland, of the children presenting to a public hospital orthopedic clinic over a 6-month period with injuries sustained while trampolining, 60% were unsupervised by an adult at the time (McDermott et al 2006). A study conducted in the USA demonstrated that there is no significant difference between the rate or type of injuries occurring with the so-called mini-trampolines as opposed to full-sized trampolines (Shields et al 2005).

Injuries related to trampolining are typically orthopedic in nature, involving the cervical spine and upper limb. However, more serious neurological injuries do occur, such as quadriplegia (Torq 1987, Torq & Das 1984), and conditions involving the vasculature are also seen to be on the rise. While strokes, thrombi and embolus formation in children related to sports injuries are rare, the incidence associated with trampoline use is increasing. Minor trauma to the vulnerable extracranial vertebral arteries as they travel superficially through the dorsum of the neck can begin a cascade of events that may result in arterial dissection, thrombus formation, and embolization with cerebral infarction (Wechsler et al 2001). Other vascular complications of trampoline injuries have also been recorded in the scientific literature and should be noted by chiropractors caring for children with such injuries (Kwolek et al 1998).

Some physicians and physiotherapists charged with caring for children with cystic fibrosis (CF) claim that cardiopulmonary performance, sputum production and general well-being are all enhanced by the judicious and supervised use of trampolining. However, a study conducted at the National Center for Cystic Fibrosis, Edmond and Lily Safra Children's

Hospital, Chaim Sheba Medical Center in Tel-Hashomer, Israel, in which the authors conducted an exhaustive search of the scientific literature on trampolining as a therapeutic modality for cystic fibrosis patients, concluded that the presumed benefits of trampoline use for CF patients are not proven and, furthermore, the suggested benefits could be acquired using other types of exercise. The authors further concluded that, weighing the known risks of trampolines against the potential benefits that are not unique to this particular exercise modality, the use of trampolines for CF should not be recommended (Barak et al 2005). The rate of increase in trampoline-related injury to children is becoming a serious public health issue (Shankar et al 2006) and has resulted in various calls in the scientific literature, ranging from those who favor a complete ban on sales of trampolines (Furnival et al 1999, Torq & Das 1984) to those who recommend that strict guidelines for the recreational use of trampolines be put in place, and further recommend that no child should be on a trampoline, either with another child or unsupervised by an adult (Bhangal et al 2006, McDermott et al 2006, Nysted & Drogset 2006, Purcell & Philpott 2007).

In 1999 the American Academy of Pediatrics (AAP) recommended that trampolines should never be used in the home environment, in routine physical education classes, or in outdoor playgrounds (American Academy of Pediatrics 1999). In 2006 this policy was reaffirmed based on the evolving data of recorded injuries from trampolining accidents, 30% of which were fractures, many resulting in hospitalization and surgery (American Academy of Pediatrics 2006).

Given the increasing frequency of serious injury to children using trampolines in a home environment and the less severe injuries, some of which are being seen by chiropractors, that are not being reported in the scientific literature, it seems that on balance the most appropriate advice for chiropractors to offer parents is that they should not buy a trampoline for home use. This advice would be in keeping with the official policy of the American Academy of Pediatrics and would be the most resonant with the opinions expressed in the scientific literature. Chiropractors can also play an important public health role by educating parents about the dangers of trampolines, thereby empowering them to make informed choices about the toys they buy their children.

Baby walkers

A baby walker is a device that allows a baby who has yet to develop the ability to walk unaided to be held in the upright position while bearing some weight through the legs. The child is then able to 'walk' around in the device. Some basic neurodevelopmental physiology should be considered here. Probably the most important thing to consider is the effect on motoric development by placing a child in the walking posture when their neurodevelopment is at the crawling stage. While there may be some convenience benefits to the parents/caregivers, the baby's gross motor development is far better served by being placed prone and allowed to roll and crawl around the floor (Davis et al 1998, Majnemer & Barr 2005, Salls et al 2002). The relationship between the prone position and

subsequent neurodevelopment has long been well understood and, now that prone sleeping has been causally linked to sudden infant death syndrome (Gunn et al 2000), placing baby in the prone position during waking hours has become far more critical.

Aside from their negative effect on neurodevelopment there is the important issue of potential injury, particularly from falling down stairs. The American Academy of Pediatrics has estimated that during 1999 there were 8800 children under 15 months of age treated in emergency departments across the USA for baby walker-related injuries (American Academy of Pediatrics 2001). In an attempt to reduce the number of such injuries, manufacturers have developed a braking mechanism, designed to stop the walker if one or more wheels drop off the riding surface. These braking systems, however, have been demonstrated to be ineffective and may offer parents a false sense of security (Ridenour 1997).

The American Academy of Pediatrics policy position on baby walkers is clear in that they recommend that baby walkers be banned from sale. Along with the pediatrician and family general practitioner, the chiropractor is in a powerful position to encourage parents to avoid purchasing baby walkers, and should take every opportunity to do so both during consultations and in a broader sense by providing information to the wider public about the dangers of walkers and advising the use of stationary activity centers instead. However, despite the best advice, there will be parents who insist upon buying a baby walker and in this event they should be advised to make certain the one they buy meets the revised voluntary performance standards.

Sleep posture and sudden infant death syndrome

In 1992 the American Academy of Pediatrics, following analysis of the growing evidence database suggesting that the prone sleeping posture in babies was a major factor contributing to the incidence of sudden infant death syndrome (SIDS), adopted a policy position recommending all babies sleep in any non-prone position (i.e. side-lying or supine) with the exception of those at risk of aspiration of vomitus from gastroesophageal reflux and other conditions. In 2000, on the basis of new evidence, the AAP advised that the supine position was the preferred position as it offered the greatest level of protection from SIDS, although side-posture sleeping, while not as good as supine sleeping, was still better than prone sleeping (Kattwinkel et al 2005).

In addition to the sleep posture, other factors that have been shown to be causative in SIDS are exposure to an environment where the parents smoke and bed sharing where the mother is a smoker (Gunn et al 2000, Kattwinkel et al 2005, Mitchell et al 1997). On the positive side, there is compelling evidence that pacifiers offered at sleep time reduce the risk of SIDS, even though the actual mechanism is not understood (Arnestad et al 1997, Carpenter et al 2004, Fleming et al 1999, Hauck et al 2003, L'Hoir et al 1999, McGarvey et al 2003, Tappin et al 2002). Breastfeeding has also been shown to be protective in some studies (Home et al 2004, Kattwinkel et al 1992, L'Hoir et al 1998, Mitchell et al 1993). While somewhat controversial, the research of Dr Jim Sprott (2004) in New Zealand is demanding of attention. Sprott has shown that, when wrapped in a specially prepared polyethylene cover, mattresses are prevented from giving off certain poisonous gases, which he claims cause cot death.

Chiropractors can make a significant contribution to the effort to reduce SIDS by advising parents, both during consultation and via health promotion initiatives to the broader community, on the following strategies which are largely consistent with those recommended by the American Academy of Pediatrics (Wennegren et al 1997):

1. Sleep infants on their back unless there is the danger of aspiration of vomitus.

2. Use a firm sleep surface and keep soft materials and objects out of the cot.

3. Do not smoke during pregnancy or inside the house after the birth of the child.

4. Keep the child in the maternal bedroom but separate from the parental bed, especially when the mother is a smoker.

5. Offer the baby a pacifier at nap time.

6. Avoid overheating the child with blankets, etc.

7. Avoid commercial home monitor devices which are marketed on the premise they reduce the risk of SIDS. They simply do not work.

8. Always fully wrap mattresses in a specially prepared polyethylene cover which is available commercially (www.eves-bestcom/babesafe-mattress-covers.htm).

Safety: a proactive approach

There is a huge number of child-safe products available to parents today, some very useful while others may be more of a gimmick than a genuinely valuable product. It is beyond the scope of this chapter to list and illustrate an exhaustive range of child-safe products, but the family chiropractor would do well to encourage parents to visit their local child-safe store to see what is available, or visit one of the plethora of websites selling these products on line. In an attempt to be proactive in the field of child safety protection, it should be considered well within the practice scope of the family chiropractor to be familiar with the range of useful safety products and to make parents and caregivers aware of what they can do to protect their child from accidental injury in the home, while traveling in the car, and around the garage and garden.

A final word

In terms of discharging public responsibility for health promotion and disease prevention, all that is really required is a little personal availability of the chiropractor to participate in public health education initiatives, and the investment of time and resources in providing written information to parents to empower them to make better choices for their children. Investing in the future health and well-being of the children who will one day constitute the adult population in the communities in which we live is a professionally responsible choice.

References

American Academy of Pediatrics, 1999. Committee on Injury and Poison Prevention and Committee on Sports Medicine and Fitness. Trampolines at home, school, and recreational centers. Pediatrics 103 (5/1), 1053–1056.

American Academy of Pediatrics, 2001. Committee on Injury and Poison Prevention. Injuries associated with infant walkers. Pediatrics 108 (3), 790–792.

American Academy of Pediatrics, 2006. Committee on Injury and Poison Prevention and Committee on Sports Medicine and Fitness. Trampolines at home, school, and recreational centers. Pediatrics 117 (5), 1846–1847.

Arnestad, M., Andersen, M., Rognum, T., 1997. Is the use of dummy or carry-cot of importance for sudden infant death? Eur. J. Pediatr. 156, 968–970.

Barak, A., Wexler, I.D., Efrati, O., et al., 2005. Trampoline use as physiotherapy for cystic fibrosis patients. Pediatr. Pulmonol. 39 (1), 70–73.

Bhangal, K.K., Neen, D., Dodds, R., 2006. Incidence of trampoline related pediatric fractures in a large district pediatric hospital in the United Kingdom: lessons to be learnt. Inj. Prev. 12 (2), 133–134.

Carpenter, R.G., Irgens, I.M., Blair, P.S., et al., 2004. Sudden unexplained infant death in 20 regions in Europe: case control study. Lancet 363, 185–191.

Center of Disease Control and Prevention, 2008. Nonfatal maltreatment of infants, United States, October 2005–September 2006. MMWR Morb. Mortal. Wkly. Rep. 57 (13), 336–339.

Chen, J., Dunne, M.P., Han, P., 2006. Child sexual abuse in Henan province, China: associations with sadness, suicidality, and risk behaviours amongst adolescent girls. Int. J. Adolesc. Med. Health 38 (5), 544–549.

Christoffel, K.K., 1994. Intentional injuries: homicide and violence. In: Pless, I.B. (Ed.), The epidemiology of childhood disorders. Oxford University Press, New York, pp. 392–411.

Davies, N.J., 1992. Recognizing the abused and at-risk child. Chiropr. J. Aust. 22 (1), 2–4.

Davis, B.E., Moon, R.Y., Sachs, H.C., et al., 1998. Effects of sleep position on infant motor development. Pediatrics 102 (5), 1135–1140.

Department of Human Services, State Government of Victoria, Australia, 2008. Child Protection 2008. Available at: http://www.office-for-children.vic.gov. au/child_protection/library/publications/ protection/what (accessed March 30, 2008).

Ebrall, P.S., Davies, N.J., 2000. Non-accidental injury and child maltreatment. In: Davies, N.J. (Ed.), Chiropractic pediatrics, a clinical handbook. Churchill Livingstone, Edinburgh.

Ewart, M., 1980. Physical indicators of emotional abuse in children [Letter]. Br. Med. J. 280 (6210), 334.

Finkelhor, D., Dziuba-Leatherman, J., 1994. Victimization of children. Am. Psychol. 49 (3), 173–183.

Fleming, P.J., Blair, P.S., Pollard, K., et al., 1999. Pacifier use and sudden infant death syndrome: results from the CESDI/SUDI case control study. Arch. Dis. Child. 81, 112–116.

Fontana, V., 1989. Child abuse: the physicians responsibility. N. Y. State J. Med. 89 (3), 152–155.

Frost, N., 2004. Child welfare: major themes in health and social welfare. Taylor and Francis, Abingdon.

Furnival, R.A., Street, K.A., Schunk, J.E., 1999. Too many pediatric trampoline injuries. Pediatrics 103 (5), e57.

Gier, J.L., 1987. Recognizing and treating the abuse victim. J. Am. Chiropr. Assoc. (April), 39–41.

Gordon, M., Palusci, V., 1991. Physician training in the recognition and reporting of child abuse, maltreatment and neglect. N. Y. State J. Med. 91 (1), 1–2.

Gowers, S.G. (Ed.), 2005. Seminars in child and adolescent psychiatry, second ed. Royal College of Psychiatrists, London.

Gunn, A.J., Gunn, T.R., Mitchell, E.A., 2000. Is changing the sleep environment enough? Current recommendations for SIDS. Sleep Med. Rev. 4 (5), 453–469.

Hauck, F.R., Herman, S.M., Donovan, M., et al., 2003. Sleep environment and the risk of sudden infant death syndrome in an urban population: the Chicago Infant Mortality Study. Pediatrics 11, 1207–1214.

Helfer, R.E., 1990. The neglect of our children. Pediatr. Clin. North Am. 37, 933–942.

Hobbs, C.J., Hawks, H.G., Wynn, J.M., 1999. Child abuse and neglect: a clinician's handbook. Churchill Livingstone, Edinburgh.

Home, R.S., Parslow, P.M., Ferens, D., et al., 2004. Comparison of evoked arousability in breast and formula fed infants. Arch. Dis. Child. 89, 22–25.

Hurson, C., Browne, K., Callender, O., et al., 2007. Pediatric trampoline injuries. J. Pediatr. Orthop. 27 (7), 729–732.

Kattwinkel, J., Brooks, J., Myerberg, D., 1992. American Academy of Pediatrics taskforce on infant positioning and sudden infant death syndrome. Pediatrics 89, 1120–1126.

Kattwinkel, J., Hauck, F.R., Keenan, M.E., et al., 2005. American Academy of Pediatrics. The changing concept of sudden infant death syndrome: diagnostic coding shifts, controversies regarding the sleep environment and new variables to consider in reducing risk. Pediatrics 116 (5), 1245–1255.

Kovacs, K., Richardson, N., 2004. Child abuse statistics. National Child Protection Clearinghouse. Australian Institute of Family Studies, Canberra.

Kwolek, C.J., Sundaram, S., Schwarcz, T.H., et al., 1998. Popliteal artery thrombosis associated with trampoline injuries and anterior knee dislocations in children. Am. Surg. 64 (12), 1183–1187.

Lee, A.C., Li, D.H., Kemper, K.J., 2000. Chiropractic care for children. Arch. Pediatr. Adolesc. Med. 154 (4), 401–407.

L'Hoir, M.P., Engleberts, A.C., van Well, G.T.J., et al., 1998. Case control study of current validity of previously described risk factors for SIDS in the Netherlands. Arch. Dis. Child. 79, 386–393.

L'Hoir, M.P., Engleberts, A.C., van Well, G.T.J., et al., 1999. Dummy use, thumb sucking, mouth breathing and cot death. Eur. J. Pediatr. 158, 896–901.

McDermott, C., Quinlan, J.F., Kelly, I.P., 2006. Trampoline injuries in children. J. Bone Joint Surg. Br. 88 (6), 796–798.

McGarvey, R.G., McDonnell, M., Chong, A., et al., 2003. Factors relating to the infant's last sleep environment in sudden infant death syndrome in the Republic of Ireland. Arch. Dis. Child. 88, 1058–1064.

Majnemer, A., Barr, R.G., 2005. Influence of supine sleep positioning on early motor milestone acquisition. Dev. Med. Child. Neurol. 47 (6), 370–376.

Margolin, L., 1990. Fatal child neglect. Child Welfare 69 (4), 309–319.

Mitchell, E.A., Taylor, B.J., Ford, R.P., et al., 1993. Dummies and the sudden infant death syndrome. Arch. Dis. Child. 68, 501–504.

Mitchell, E.A., Tuohy, P.G., Brunt, J.M., et al., 1997. Risk factors for sudden infant death syndrome following the prevention campaign in New Zealand: a prospective study. Pediatrics 100, 835–840.

Mootz, R., Hansen, D., 1999. Advances in Chiropractic. Mosby, St Louis.

Nash, E.M., 1990. Child abuse; recognizing and reporting. ICA Review of Chiropractic (March–April), 19–23.

Nysted, M., Drogset, J.O., 2006. Trampoline injuries. Br. J. Sports Med. 40 (12), 984–1977.

Oates, K., 1986. Sexual abuse of children. Aust. Fam. Physician 15, 786.

Petetti, R., Singh, S., Hornyak, D., et al., 2001. Complementary and alternative medicine use in children. Pediatr. Emerg. Care 17 (3), 165–169.

Purcell, L., Philpott, J., 2007. Trampolines at home and playgrounds: a joint statement with the Canadian Pediatric Society. Clin. J. Sport Med. 17 (5), 389–392.

Ridenour, M.V., 1997. How effective are brakes on infant walkers? Percept. Mot. Skills 84 (3/1), 1051–1057.

Salls, J.S., Silverman, L.N., Gatty, C.M., 2002. The relationship of infant sleep and play positioning to motor milestone achievement. Am. J. Occup. Ther. 56 (5), 577–580.

Shankar, A., Williams, K., Ryan, M., 2006. Trampoline-related injury in children. Pediatr. Emerg. Care 22 (9), 644–646.

Shields, B.J., Fernandez, S.A., Smith, G.A., 2005. Comparison of mini-trampoline- and full sized trampoline-related injuries in the United States, 1990–2002. Pediatrics 116 (1), 96–103.

South Australian Department of Community Welfare Child Protection Unit, 1990. Preventing and reporting child abuse. SADCW, Adelaide.

Sprott, T.J., 2004. Cot death – cause and prevention: experiences in New Zealand 1995–2004. J. Nutr. Environ. Med. 14 (3), 221–232.

Stierwaldt, D.D., 1976. Child abuse and the chiropractor. Digest of Chiropractic Economics (July–August), 138.

Tappin, D., Brooke, H., Ecob, R., et al., 2002. Used infant mattresses and sudden infant death syndrome in Scotland: case control study. Br. Med. J. 325 (7371), 1007.

Torq, J.S., 1987. Trampoline-induced quadriplegia. Clin. Sports Med. 6 (1), 73–85.

Torq, J.S., Das, M., 1984. Trampoline-related quadriplegia: review of the literature and reflections on the American Academy of Pediatrics' position statement. Pediatrics 74 (5), 804–812.

US Department of Health and Human Services, Administration on Children, Youth and Families, 2007, Child Maltreatment 2005. US Government Printing Office Washington, DC.

Wechsler, B., Kim, H., Hunter, J., 2001. Trampolines, children and strokes. Am. J. Phys. Med. Rehabil. 80 (8), 608–613.

Weist, K.B., Buisr, A.S., Sullivan, D., 2000. Asthma's impact on society, the social and economic burden. Lung biology. In: Health and Disease, vol. 138. Taylor and Francis/CRC Press, Chicago.

Wennegren, G., Alm, B., Oyen, N., et al., 1997. The decline in the incidence of SIDS in Scandinavia and its relation to risk intervention campaigns. Nordic epidemiological SIDS study. Acta Pediatr. 86, 963–968.

Wikipedia contributors, 2008. Child abuse. Wikipedia, The Free Encyclopedia. March 4, 2008, 23:11 UTC. Available at:http:// en.wikipedia.org/w/index.php? title=Child_abuse&oldid=195910710 (accessed March 5, 2008).

Wyatt, H., 2005. Handbook of Clinical Chiropractic Care. Jones and Bartlett, Sudbury.

Cancer in children

Neil J. Davies

Pediatric cancer represents only a small proportion of childhood illness. Cancer, however, remains the second most common cause of death behind trauma in children aged 1–14 years (Australian Bureau of Statistics 2004). A working knowledge of the common clinical presentations of pediatric malignancies and an understanding of the principles of diagnosis and management are important for all care practitioners who are involved in the care of children.

The approximate incidence of pediatric cancers is 10–12 cases per 100 000 children (Weir et al 2003). Adult cancers typically arise in epithelial tissues (skin, bowel, lung). In contrast, childhood cancers arise from mesodermal tissue (blood, connective tissue, bone). Children with cancer often remain asymptomatic until the disease has reached the advanced stage. The low incidence of childhood cancer combined with its propensity to present late in the course of the disease means that a high index of suspicion of common symptoms of pediatric malignancy should be maintained by all practitioners in order to facilitate an early and accurate diagnosis.

Remarkable progress has been made in both the diagnosis and management of pediatric malignancies. Many hospitals around the world are involved in cooperative group studies and most patients are enrolled on study protocols that aim to improve the treatment of childhood cancers. Overall patient mortality has decreased by 50% (Weir et al 2003). Patients with childhood cancer should always be treated in a major hospital with experience in pediatric oncology. Some tumors, unfortunately, continue to have a poor prognosis. Disseminated neuroblastoma in children older than 1 year, for example, continues to have an 80% mortality.

Treatment of childhood cancers can take many months to years. The population of children who are either currently being treated, or have been successfully treated for cancer is significant. Most health practitioners will encounter at least one patient or a relative of a patient with childhood cancer. Cancer treatment carries a certain morbidity and some of these patients may experience long-term side-effects of therapy. A basic knowledge of and ongoing vigilance for these potential side-effects is necessary to best manage these patients. All practitioners have a role to play in supporting both the child and the child's family in dealing with the unique emotional challenges that comes with the diagnosis of cancer. Unfortunately, a number of children will not respond favorably and will die from either their underlying malignancy or complications arising from their treatment. Supporting a patient and the family through the grieving process can be both a difficult and a personally rewarding experience, with scope for input from all practitioners involved in the child's care.

Acute leukemia

Acute leukemia is the most common childhood cancer. Once an incurable disease, leukemia can now be cured in up to 60–70% of cases. The incidence of acute leukemia is 4 per 100 000 children under the age of 15 years (Waters & Smith 1998).

Acute lymphoblastic leukemia

Acute lymphoblastic leukemia (ALL) is the most common form of childhood leukemia. ALL is more common in boys than girls and has a peak incidence in the 2–6-year-old age group (Waters & Smith 1998). The etiology of ALL remains unknown; however, certain genetic and inherited conditions confer a susceptibility to the development of ALL. Fanconi's anemia, Bloom syndrome, and the immunodeficiency states, ataxia telangiectasia, Wiskott–Aldrich and severe combined immunodeficiency syndromes also have an increased incidence of ALL (Pui at al 2008).

Clinical presentation

The uncontrolled proliferation of leukemic white cells in bone marrow significantly compromises the number of normal marrow cells and hence peripheral blood constituents. Symptoms,

© 2010, Elsevier Ltd, Inc, BV
DOI: 10.1016/B978-0-7020-3129-8.00017-7

therefore, are related to a reduction in red and white blood cells and platelets as well as the infiltration of leukemic cells outside the bone marrow. The most common symptoms are pallor, fever and easy bruising, with background symptoms of malaise, irritability and vague abdominal pains. Pallor is insidious in onset and children may not be seen until the anemia has become moderately severe, presenting with symptoms of cardiac failure (cardiovascular decompensation). Children are vulnerable to infections and may present with fever. Fever may also be due to the release of cytokines from the leukemic cells. Easy bruising can often be missed or rationalized as the child being clumsy.

Twenty-five percent of patients will present with apparent musculoskeletal symptoms (Gonçalves et al 2005, Pui et al 2008). Bone pain and joint pain of the bony pelvis, lower back and femur, or a refusal to walk in the younger child are common presentations. These vague symptoms may be mistaken for various musculoskeletal conditions or gross motor developmental delay. In children presenting with musculoskeletal symptoms it is a reasonable approach to exclude the diagnosis of leukemia before starting any form of therapy.

Examination usually reveals a pale, irritable child with various signs of extramedullary infiltration including hepatosplenomegaly, lymphadenopathy and, occasionally, skin infiltrates. Petechiae and bruising are often present. Testicular infiltration may present with a unilaterally enlarged testis, and other rare findings include renal enlargement, papilledema and nerve palsies.

Classification

ALL represents a heterogeneous group of cancers and a number of systems have been developed to classify the different types (Ries et al 1994, Pui & Crist 1994, Pui et al 2008). Cellular morphology, cell surface markers and cytogenic abnormalities have helped to classify different subgroups of ALL. It is known that most cases of ALL stem from an abnormal proliferation of B cell-committed progenitors.

The prognosis of each case of leukemia can be predicted according to its subgroup and features of the clinical presentation (i.e. age of the patient and peripheral total white cell count). Certain cytogenic abnormalities also help identify groups of children who may have a worse prognosis. Translocations between chromosomes 9 and 22 t(9:22) and chromosomes 4 and 11 t(4:11) are common translocations seen in ALL, and children with these chromosomal abnormalities are at risk of a worse prognosis (Pui & Crist 1994).

Investigations

The full blood count usually reveals varying degrees of anemia, thrombocytopenia and granulocytopenia. Absolute white cell counts are normal in approximately 50% of cases (Waters & Smith 1998). Leukemic cells (immature malignant white cells or blast cells) are often seen in the peripheral blood film. These leukemic cells are functionally impotent. Diagnosis is confirmed with a bone marrow examination showing infiltration of the normal cellular matrix with blast cells. In children, the usual practice is to take a sample of the bone marrow

from the posterior iliac crest under sedation or general anesthesia. Normal bone marrow aspirates show less than 5% of immature blast cells but patients with ALL will show a minimum of 25% blast cells present.

Other investigations may show multiorgan impairment. Liver function tests may be abnormal, renal function may be impaired, and calcium may be elevated. A chest X-ray may show signs of mediastinal lymphadenopathy or, rarely, leukemic lung infiltrates.

Examination of the cerebrospinal fluid (CSF), for evidence of leukemic blasts, is essential and will require a lumbar puncture at diagnosis. The cerebrospinal fluid is a known reservoir for leukemic cells and will require specific treatment if leukemic cells are detected in the CSF.

Treatment

Successful treatment for leukemia involves using specific antileukemic chemotherapy and supportive care. At diagnosis, infections are treated with intravenous antibiotics, and blood products are supplied to correct anemia and thrombocytopenia. Monitoring the nutritional status of the child is important and additional nutritional support may be required. Although the cure for ALL approaches 70–80% of all patients treated, research is still being performed to improve specific antileukemic therapy. Multinuclear studies involving hospitals and universities around the world aim to further increase the cure rate of ALL. These protocols use combination chemotherapy with the therapy divided into distinct phases of remission induction, consolidation and maintenance treatment. Remission induction usually lasts 4–5 weeks. A repeat bone marrow aspirate is then performed to confirm remission (normal cellular bone marrow) and 95% of children will be in remission after standard induction therapy.

Consolidation therapy aims to deliver multiple chemotherapeutic agents within a relatively short period to treat any residual leukemic cells and prevent the development of resistance of the leukemic cells to the chemotherapy. The consolidation phase includes therapy directed at preventing relapse of leukemic cells in the central nervous system. CNS prevention traditionally involved cranial irradiation, but this has been associated with significant side-effects. The advent of intrathecal chemotherapy has successfully reduced the incidence of CNS relapse from 60% in the early 1970s to less than 10% with current regimens. Most protocols involve a period of maintenance chemotherapy lasting 18 months to 3 years. Children usually have only monthly outpatient visits during this time and are able to return to their usual activities, including school.

Relapse of acute lymphoblastic leukemia

Twenty percent of children with ALL will experience a relapse of their leukemia. Relapse is usually detected during routine follow-up, but may not present with symptoms similar to those at first diagnosis. Relapse is most common in the first year after the cessation of maintenance chemotherapy. It is rare to relapse 4 years from the cessation of therapy. Treatment of relapsed ALL remains difficult. Allogeneic (genetically different but belonging to the same species) bone marrow transplantation offers the best prognosis for these patients. Up to 50% of patients with relapsed ALL can be cured with a suitably matched bone marrow transplant (Uderzo et al 2000).

Acute myeloid leukemia

Acute myeloid leukemia (AML), or acute non-lymphoid leukemia (ANLL), is only one-fifth as common as ALL. AML does not have a peak age of incidence and is equally as common in infants as in adolescents. AML results from proliferation of malignant myeloid cells and can be classified according to morphological and cytochemical staining patterns. The French–American–British (FAB) classification of AML recognizes seven subgroups (M0–M7). Each group has unique clinical and prognostic significance (Ebb & Weinstein 1997, Golub et al 1997, Kaspers & Zwaan 2007).

Clinical presentation

Like ALL, AML presents with symptoms related to bone marrow and extramedullary infiltration by leukemic cells. Gingival hyperplasia and skin infiltration are more common than in ALL.

Investigations

A full blood count will show varying degrees of pancytopenia with blasts seen in the peripheral blood smear. Other organ systems may be impaired by leukemic infiltrates. Renal function may also be impaired by leukemic infiltrates as well as by the precipitation of the by-products of rapidly dying leukemic cells. CNS infiltration has a higher prevalence than in ALL and will require specific therapy. A bone marrow aspirate will confirm the diagnosis by showing replacement of normal marrow cells with blast cells.

Treatment and prognosis

Successful therapy for AML will require intensive combination chemotherapy. Most protocols result in prolonged periods of bone marrow suppression as a side-effect of the intensive regimens, and bone marrow transplantation has become the standard of care for patients with AML. A transplantation involving harvesting the bone marrow of the patient prior to intensive 'myeloablative' chemotherapy and 'transplanting' the patient's own marrow after it has had some form of treatment to purge it of any residual leukemic cells is known as an autograft transplantation (Gorin 1998). Alternatively, an allogeneic transplant may be used if there is a suitably HLA-matched donor. Patients tend to spend prolonged periods of time in hospital as they are particularly vulnerable to infections and often require nutritional and blood product support. Most patients experience remission with current regimens but many patients relapse within 2 years. The prognosis of AML is not as good as that of ALL. Approximately 50% of patients with AML will experience long-term cure. Features of the clinical presentation and the initial white cell count, the subgroup of AML and the presence of certain cytogenic abnormalities all influence the prognosis (Kaspers & Zwaan 2007).

Tumors of the central nervous system (CNS)

Brain tumors represent almost one-fifth of all cases of childhood cancer and are the most common solid tumor in children (Ries et al 1994, Weir et al 2003).

Clinical presentation

CNS tumors generally present either as a result of raised intracranial pressure or by direct infiltration of brain structures and cranial nerves. Early morning headaches associated with vomiting are the classic symptoms of raised intracranial pressure. The headache is typically relieved by vomiting. The combination of bradycardia and hypertension, known as Cushing's response, is also a sign of raised intracranial pressure. Drowsiness is a late sign of raised intracranial pressure and should alert the physician to impending disaster. Papilledema is a sure sign of raised intracranial pressure. The normal optic disc, which is usually cupped, will become filled in at the onset of raised intracranial pressure. As the pressure increases, the optic nerve margins will become blurred and the disc becomes frankly swollen. In an infant, raised intracranial pressure may also be accompanied by a swollen and tense fontanel. Direct infiltration of CNS structures can produce symptoms and signs that may aid in the localization of the tumor. Truncal ataxia results from a central cerebellar tumor, whereas a peripheral cerebellar tumor is more likely to cause an intention tremor. Resultant cranial nerve palsies may also localize the tumor. A sixth nerve palsy can present as a result of direct infiltration or as a false localizing sign of increased intracranial pressure. A persistent head tilt may represent a palsy of one of the nerves to the muscles of the eye rather than a musculoskeletal disorder, and all patients presenting with 'wry neck' should have detailed neurological examination and referral for appropriate CNS imaging.

Endocrine disorders may occur when tumors infiltrate the pituitary gland. Diabetes insipidus, in particular, presenting as increased thirst, polyuria and growth failure, can herald the presence of a brain tumor.

Pathology

The cell of origin of the tumor has important management and prognostic considerations. Astrocytomas are tumors arising from the astrocyte glial cell and can be found in the supra- and infratentorial regions. Low-grade astrocytomas are the most common childhood CNS tumor and are usually found in the posterior fossa. High-grade astrocytomas are less common, the most anaplastic of which is glioblastoma multiforme, which has a poor prognosis.

Medulloblastoma is a common malignant childhood CNS tumor arising from undifferentiated neuroepithelial cells in the cerebellum close to the fourth ventricle. Histologically similar cells can be found outside the cerebellum and it has been proposed that these tumors be called primitive neuroectodermal tumors (PNET). These tumors have the propensity to disseminate along from the meninges and spinal cord. Ependymomas arise from the ependymal cells, usually from around the fourth ventricle. These represent only 10% of all

CNS tumors. Local invasion, presenting as cranial nerve involvement, is characteristic of an ependymoma. Brainstem gliomas arise from the glial cells in the pons and medulla. Because of their close proximity to many of the cranial nerve nuclei, brainstem gliomas usually present as cranial nerve palsies. These tumors are not amenable to surgery and have a particularly poor prognosis. Other rare tumors include optic nerve gliomas, craniopharyngiomas and pineal tumors, which may present with visual disturbance and hypothalamic–pituitary dysfunction.

Investigations

Children presenting with symptoms and signs suggestive of a brain tumor need urgent referral to a center experienced in treating childhood CNS tumors. Detailed imaging is the most important investigation and magnetic resonance imaging (MRI) is the preferred modality. MRI will show the position of the tumor and provides the neurosurgeon with important information regarding surgical options. Suspected raised intracranial pressure will be confirmed by the presence of hydrocephalus. Biopsy of the brain tumor is necessary to determine appropriate treatment and prognosis. Depending on the histological type of tumor, other staging procedures may be required, including nuclear bone scan and bone marrow biopsies to exclude metastases.

Treatment

Children with newly diagnosed brain tumors should be referred to a tertiary care center and each child should be enrolled on a multicenter group study to be treated according to study protocol. A multimodal approach to the treatment of brain tumors is usually necessary to achieve the best outcome (Kalfia & Grill 2005, Kun 1997). Low-grade astrocytomas, in favorable sites, may be treated with surgery alone, whereas high-grade gliomas will need initial surgery, intensive chemotherapy and radiotherapy. Brainstem gliomas are treated with radiotherapy alone but the prognosis remains very poor.

It is important to consider the potential complications of therapy when planning treatment of CNS tumors in childhood. The developing brain and spinal cord are susceptible to the side-effects of all modes of treatment. Radiotherapy in particular can affect intellectual development and cause endocrine deficiencies resulting in delayed growth and sexual development. Radiotherapy also has the potential to cause secondary tumors, most commonly meningiomas. Attempts at curative surgery may leave patients with significant neurological side-effects including weakness of limbs, altered personality and predisposition to seizures. Many of the long-term side-effects of chemotherapy when used to treat very young children are not fully understood. Parents need to be fully informed of potential side-effects and be given adequate counseling when discussing treatment options.

Hodgkin's disease and non-Hodgkin's lymphoma

Hodgkin's disease and non-Hodgkin's lymphoma are related malignancies that collectively represent the third most common malignancy in children.

Hodgkin's disease

Hodgkin's disease is uncommon in children less than 5 years of age and has a unique bimodal age distribution with one peak between the ages of 15 and 34 years and another peak after the age of 50 years (Celkan & Yildiz 2008).

Clinical presentation

Hodgkin's disease is a malignancy that typically presents as a painless enlargement of a single lymph node or group of lymph nodes, most commonly affecting the supraclavicular and cervical lymph nodes. Rarely will the liver and spleen or other organs be involved. Patients may be asymptomatic or may experience systemic symptoms such as loss of weight, night sweats or unexplained fever ('B' symptoms). The presence of 'B symptoms' relates to the prognosis.

Investigations

The diagnosis of Hodgkin's disease requires biopsy of the enlarged lymph node and histological identification of multinucleated cells known as Reed–Sternberg cells. These cells are thought to arise from primitive lymphoid cells and are characteristically surrounded by inflammatory cells.

Classification and staging

Classification of Hodgkin's disease depends on the type and arrangement of the cells in the biopsied specimen. The disease is typically divided into four subgroups; the nodular sclerosing subgroup is the most common type in children. The anatomical staging of Hodgkin's disease is the most important determinant of prognosis and classifies patients into four groups.

Treatment

Hodgkin's disease can be successfully treated with radiotherapy and combination chemotherapy. Newer therapeutic protocols rely on chemotherapy alone because of the well-recognized complications of radiotherapy in children. Patients who experience disease relapse on chemotherapy alone can be successfully treated with more intensive chemotherapy and/or radiotherapy (Hodgson et al 2007, Oberlin 1996).

Non-Hodgkin's lymphoma

Non-Hodgkin's lymphoma (NHL) is a group of tumors of lymphoreticular cell origin. NHL affects boys more than girls with a peak incidence at 11 years (Glotzbecker et al 2006, Magrath 1997).

Clinical presentation

Unlike Hodgkin's disease, NHL rarely presents with isolated peripheral lymphadenopathy. Mediastinal lymph node enlargement occurs in up to 25% of cases and may be large enough to obstruct venous return from the head and neck causing symptoms of headache, facial swelling and engorged veins of the neck consistent with superior vena cava syndrome (Shad & Magrath 1997b). Additionally, abdominal disease, usually presenting as pain in the right lower quadrant and abdominal distension is a typical presentation of SNCC-type lymphoma (Burkitt's lymphoma) (Shad & Magrath 1997b).

Investigations

The diagnosis of NHL is confirmed with a tissue diagnosis. This can be obtained by direct biopsy of the primary tumor mass or from exudative fluid from around the mass (ascites resulting from abdominal NHL). Other investigations, including assessment of renal function, serum uric acid level and a chest X-ray to rule out mediastinal masses, are also important. Imaging with abdominal and chest computed tomography (CT), bone scans and biopsy of the bone marrow are all necessary for adequate staging of NHL. A laparotomy is rarely needed to accurately stage patients presenting with abdominal disease.

Classification

The tissue sample obtained at diagnosis is classified according to the predominate cell type found. Classification of NHL, however, remains confusing. Most cases of NHL occurring in children can be classified into three subgroups:

1. Lymphoblastic lymphoma is mostly T cell in origin.
2. Small non-cleaved cell type (SNCC; Burkitt's and non-Burkitt's lymphoma) is derived from immature B cells.
3. Large cell lymphoma, the third group of NHL, is less common in children.

The classification of the disease provides important treatment and prognostic information.

Treatment and prognosis

As for Hodgkin's disease, staging has particularly important prognostic significance. Patients presenting with stage 1 or stage 2 disease can expect a cure rate of 80–90%. Patients with more advanced disease can expect a cure rate of only 60–70% (Sandlund et al 1996, Shad & Magrath 1997a, Shukla & Trippett 2006). Intensive combination chemotherapy is necessary for cure.

Neuroblastoma

Neuroblastoma is predominantly a tumor of infancy that develops from the neural crest cells of the adrenal medulla or the paraspinal sympathetic ganglia. The true incidence of neuroblastoma is probably much greater than is currently thought, as many of the undiagnosed cases in very young infants undergo spontaneous regression (Brodeur & Castleberry 1997).

Clinical presentation

Most cases of neuroblastoma arise from the adrenal glands, presenting as a large abdominal mass, typically in children less than 4 years of age. The second most common site is the posterior mediastinum, presenting as an atypical chest mass. This may compress other organs and present with signs or airway obstruction including cough, stridor, and even superior vena cava obstruction. Tumors may also arise in utero and can prevent normal growth of vital structures, including the spinal cord, leading to paraplegia. Rare presentations, including hypertension, flushing, perspiration and intractable diarrhea resulting from the release of catecholamines from the tumor, should alert the practitioner to the possibility of occult neuroblastoma (Dreyer & Fernbach 1994).

Investigations

Appropriate imaging, usually by CT scan, is necessary accurately to define the abdominal or chest mass. A tissue diagnosis is also important and provides information regarding prognosis. The diagnostic work-up for neuroblastoma should also include measurement of urinary metabolites of catecholamines, which are excreted by the tumor in 90% of cases and can be used as a useful tumor marker during treatment.

Staging

Nearly 70% of new diagnoses will present with metastases. Metastasis is usually to bone, bone marrow, skin and the liver. Accurate staging requires a CT scan of the abdomen, bone marrow biopsy and nuclear bone scan (Castleberry 1997, Park et al 2008).

Treatment and prognosis

Because many of the patients present with advanced disease, successful treatment of neuroblastoma is difficult. Most treatment regimens remain experimental and involve intensive combination chemotherapy and radiotherapy. Allogeneic bone marrow transplants are a therapeutic option, allowing more intensive chemotherapy to be directed against resistant or recurrent tumors. Stage 4 disease, however, still has only a 20% cure rate despite the use of intensive regimens, and is the focus of significant ongoing research (Australian and New Zealand Children's Cancer Study Group 1993). Early-stage disease in young infants can be treated with surgery alone with an excellent prognosis.

Renal tumors

Wilms' tumor, or nephroblastoma, is a rare renal malignancy usually occurring in children under 5 years of age (Waters & Smith 1998). The incidence is 0.75 cases per 100 000 children. It is thought that Wilms' tumor develops in utero from embryological cells. In utero diagnosis, however, is rare, and Wilms' tumor is usually detected in infancy. Certain congenital conditions are associated with an increase in the incidence of Wilms' tumors: Beckwith syndrome (macroglossia, omphalocele, pancreatic and renal hyperplasia, postnatal gigantism); WAGR syndrome (Wilms' tumor, genitourinary abnormalities, and mental retardation); and hemihypertrophy (asymmetrical development of one half of the body) all have an increased incidence of Wilms' tumor.

Clinical presentation

The classic presentation of Wilms' tumor is that of a silent abdominal mass, often detected in routine physical examination. Occasionally, children will present with hematuria associated with minor abdominal trauma. Hypertension is a frequent finding on examination. Twenty percent will present with distant metastases at diagnosis, usually to the lung (Prowse et al 1998, Siegel & Chung 2008).

Investigations

Ultrasound, CT scan or MRI is used to confirm the presence of a mass arising from the kidney and should also exclude bilateral renal tumors, which occur in 5% of cases. Often the inferior vena cava will contain a tongue of tumor tissue that can extend into the right atrium and is usually asymptomatic. Tissue diagnosis is important for confirmation of diagnosis and to plan treatment.

Treatment and prognosis

Ideally the tumor is removed by nephrectomy, followed by chemotherapy and radiotherapy to target undetectable micro-metastases. In practice, however, a very large tumor mass is often present at diagnosis and precludes safe surgery. The larger the tumor, the more likely it is that tumor spillage will occur during surgery, resulting in local tumor spread. As a result, chemotherapy is often used preoperatively to rapidly shrink the tumor and facilitate surgical removal (D'Angio et al 1989, Wu et al 2005). Prognosis depends on the stage of disease, age of the patient, tumor size and histopathology. Overall, Wilms' tumor has a 90% cure rate.

Malignant bone tumors

Osteosarcoma

Osteosarcoma is a rare tumor that accounts for 60% of all childhood bone tumors (Mahoney 1994). The peak incidence occurs in teenagers and the tumor is more common in children who are taller than average. The cause of osteosarcoma is unknown but appears to be associated with the period of rapid growth of long bones.

Clinical presentation

The typical presentation is of pain and swelling in one of the long bones; the distal femur, proximal tibia and proximal humerus are the sites most commonly affected (Meyers & Gorlick 1997). Minor trauma may precipitate the presentation, but delay the true diagnosis. Children with osteosarcoma are often treated for suspected traumatic pain and swelling until the duration of symptoms prompts further investigation. The astute practitioner will be wary of symptoms and signs that do not correlate with the history of trauma. Examination will reveal a palpable mass in most cases. Some loss of movement is expected and the child may walk with a painful gait.

Investigations

An X-ray will show lytic or sclerotic bony lesions, often accompanied by a periosteal reaction. An MRI scan of the involved bone is then required to delineate the full extent of the tumor within the medullary cavity and surrounding joints, and will guide surgical treatment (Damron et al 2007, Himelstein & Doormans 1996). A biopsy of the tumor is required to confirm diagnosis. Accurate staging to detect metastatic disease is important and will include a nuclear bone scan and CT scan of the chest. Twenty percent of children will have metastatic disease at presentation (Damron et al 2007, Himelstein & Doormans 1996).

Treatment and prognosis

Successful treatment of osteosarcoma remains a challenge and includes intensive chemotherapy, surgery and radiotherapy. Prognosis depends greatly on the individual response to chemotherapy. Appropriate surgery to the primary tumor is also important and often involves limb amputation. Limb salvage operations are possible in some cases. Overall prognosis is 50–60% cure; however, patients presenting with metastatic disease have a poorer prognosis (Damron et al 2007, Link & Eilber 1997).

Ewing's sarcoma

Ewing's sarcoma, while commonly a tumor of bone, may also occur in the soft tissues (Ahmad et al 1999, Damron et al 2007). The exact cell of origin is unknown. Ewing's sarcoma is twice as common in males and, like osteosarcoma, is more likely to affect taller children.

Clinical presentation

Presentation is similar to that of osteosarcoma but any bone may be affected, including the vertebrae. Systemic symptoms such as loss of weight and unexplained fever are more common (Damron et al 2007, Grier 1997). Metastasis can occur anywhere in the body: lung, other bones and bone marrow are the usual sites of spread.

Investigations

Radiology of the affected area may show a sclerotic or lytic bony lesion with a significant soft tissue component. MRI will be required to fully evaluate the extent of the primary lesion. CT of the chest, bone marrow biopsy and a nuclear bone scan are all necessary for accurate staging.

Treatment and prognosis

Chemotherapy remains the mainstay of treatment. As with osteosarcoma, response to chemotherapy is the most important prognostic factor. Local control of the tumor is also important. Lesions that are not surgically resectable are treated with radiotherapy. The long-term prognosis for children with Ewing's sarcoma varies depending on the stage, and ranges from 60% to 80% complete cure.

Rhabdomyosarcoma

Rhabdomyosarcoma accounts for approximately 5% of childhood cancers. The tumor arises from mesenchymal cells that usually differentiate into fibrous connective tissue, cartilage, muscle and bone. As a result, this tumor may occur anywhere in the body (Pappo et al 1997, Rodeberg & Paidas 2006).

Clinical presentation

Rhabdomyosarcoma presents as a progressive soft tissue swelling. The head and neck are the most common sites of tumor origin. The genitourinary tract, including the bladder, vagina and uterus, are also common sites. Rarely, adolescents present with rhabdomyosarcoma of the extremities (Cabral & Tucker 1999, Rodeberg & Paidas 2006). The swelling is usually present for many weeks and presentation may be precipitated by a minor trauma. Systemic symptoms are not common.

The mass is usually firm to hard on palpation and may be tender. Deformity of the surrounding tissues with infiltration of the mass should alert the practitioner to the possibility of a malignancy. Pelvic masses may present as recurrent urinary tract infections secondary to inadequate emptying of the bladder, or alternatively as a limp.

Investigations

Adequate imaging is necessary to delineate the mass. Initial investigation with ultrasound should be supplemented with CT scan or MRI. A biopsy of the mass is also necessary for diagnosis.

Treatment and prognosis

All patients with rhabdomyosarcoma will receive multimodal therapy. Therapy for rhabdomyosarcoma is stratified according to risk. The preferred option is surgical removal of the tumor followed by adjuvant chemotherapy. The variety of tumor sites means that primary surgery should be tailored to each case. Many head and neck tumors will not be fully resectable because of their relative size and proximity to vital structures (Pappo et al 1997, Rodeberg & Paidas 2006). Although complete resection confers a better prognosis in rhabdomyosarcoma, careful consideration should be given to the cosmetic and functional outcome of all surgical procedures. Adjuvant chemotherapy, second-look surgery and radiotherapy are used where necessary.

Approximately 60% of children with rhabdomyosarcoma will be cured. Prognosis depends on tumor site, degree of spread and histopathology. Patients with metastatic disease at diagnosis (stage IV) have a poor prognosis with current therapy, and new approaches to treatment are needed to improve survival in this group.

Hepatoblastoma

Hepatoblastoma is a rare liver tumor of childhood that presents as an abdominal mass. Serum alphafetoprotein, an embryonal protein produced by tumor cells, is elevated, and is an excellent marker for response to treatment. Biopsy of the liver mass confirms the diagnosis. Chemotherapy to reduce the tumor size is given prior to definitive surgery. Successful treatment depends on complete resection of the tumor. Cure rates with combination chemotherapy and surgery approach 70% (Isaacs 2007, Raney 1997).

Retinoblastoma

Retinoblastoma is a rare aggressive tumor of the retina of young children. It commonly presents as leukoria (a white pupillary reflex) or the onset of strabismus (squint) resulting from loss of vision in the affected eye. Treatment should ideally involve not only curing the child of the malignancy but also preserving the sight of the eye. New multimodal therapy involves combination chemotherapy and various local control modalities including laser therapy surgery.

Langerhans cell histiocytosis

This disease has been previously called histiocytosis X (Letterer–Siwe disease, Hand–Schüller–Christian syndrome). Langerhans cell histiocytosis (LCH) is not a true malignancy, but probably a disorder of immune regulation involving the histiocyte. The most common presentation is bony lesions of the skull associated with pain and swelling. An X-ray will show a lytic lesion that can be cured with local therapy alone. Multiple lesions in other bones require systemic chemotherapy. Soft tissue lesions may involve the liver, lung, tissues around the head and neck, and the pituitary, the latter presenting as diabetes insipidus (Ladish & Jaffe 1997).

Principles of cancer treatment

There are two components to the treatment of a child with cancer. Cure is the ultimate goal of treatment. Supportive treatment, however, is also fundamental to the child's management. Curative treatment involves administering specific cancer treatment drugs, curative surgery and radiotherapy. Supportive care aims to help deal with many of the side-effects of the cancer treatments and the effects of the tumor.

Chemotherapy is the mainstay of treatment of childhood cancer. Chemotherapeutic agents are developed with a sound understanding of the cellular and molecular biology. Most anticancer agents target molecules or pathways essential to cellular replication. Two main principles guide the administration of chemotherapy. Firstly, chemotherapy is given in maximum tolerated doses on the premise that most tumor cells demonstrate a steep dose–response curve (i.e. a small increment in the dose given can significantly increase the cell kill of the tumor). Secondly, multiple chemotherapeutic agents will be given together to prevent the development of resistance of a cancer cell to a single anticancer agent. On the basis of these two principles, chemotherapy protocols have been developed for specific groups of tumors. Most children with cancer are treated according to a specific protocol, many of which are part of national and international clinical trials.

Supportive care aims to alleviate the side-effects of cancer treatment as well as the physical and metabolic effects of the tumor. Side-effects of chemotherapy can usually be predicted because of the non-selective nature of most chemotherapeutic agents. Chemotherapy targets growing and dividing cells, both malignant and non-malignant. The organs most commonly affected by chemotherapy are those that demonstrate a high rate of cell turnover. The bone marrow is the most common organ affected and bone marrow suppression is a common side-effect of treatment. Multiple blood transfusions and intravenous antibiotics are necessary to treat the side-effects of bone marrow suppression. Skin, hair and mucous membranes also are affected and will return to normal after chemotherapy has ceased. A number of chemotherapeutic agents will have specific unpredictable side-effects: for example, anthracyclines, a commonly used group of drugs, have significant cardiotoxicity.

Radiotherapy is often used in the treatment of childhood cancer. Modern techniques using sophisticated three-dimensional computer models are capable of treating tumor cells while sparing normal tissues. Surgery remains an important mode of assessment and treatment for many of the solid cancers of childhood. The combination of surgery with chemotherapy and radiotherapy now allows the cure of tumors that previously were only treatable with radical, deforming surgery. Such multimodal therapy has an excellent functional and cosmetic result.

As the cure rate of childhood cancer increases, the late effects of treatment with chemotherapy and surgery are becoming more important. At present, 1 in 900 people are survivors of childhood cancer. Effects on the various organs of the body will become more functionally important as the patient ages. Late effects on cognition, sexual development, normal growth and the risk of secondary malignancies are all important considerations when treating children with cancer.

The dying patient

Modern treatment of the pediatric patient with cancer results in cure in almost 70% of patients. When cure is not possible, care of the dying patient and the family can be a clinical and emotional challenge. Whether or not to inform the child of impending death is a difficult dilemma and the decision depends very much on the age of the patient and the cultural background of the family. Whatever decisions are made, children must be treated in an atmosphere of trust and honesty. Current palliative care techniques enable practitioners to reassure children and their families that the dying process can be free of pain and anxiety and that appropriate treatment facilities will be available for the patient. Most patients and their families will prefer to be at home and this often requires a practitioner known to the family to be involved in the care of the dying child. Strong communication lines need to be established between the treating pediatric oncologist and the family practitioner. A caring and thoughtful approach, together with time to spend with the patient and family, is necessary to support the family and the child through the dying and grieving process.

Acknowledgment

The author wishes to acknowledge the contribution of the first edition authors, Dr David Ashley and Dr Chris Barnes of the Royal Children's Hospital, Melbourne, Australia.

References

Ahmad, R., Mayol, B.R., Davis, M., et al., 1999. Extraskeletal Ewing's sarcoma. Cancer 85 (3), 725–731.

Australian and New Zealand Children's Cancer Study Group, 1993. Protocol for advances neuroblastoma, opening date 01/07/93. Royal Children's Hospital, Melbourne.

Australian Bureau of Statistics, 2004. Health of Children, 2004. Australian Bureau of Statistics, Canberra.

Brodeur, G.M., Castleberry, R.P., 1997. Neuroblastoma. In: Pizzo, P.A., Poplack, D.G. (Eds), Principles and Practices of Pediatric Oncology, third ed. Lippincott Raven, Philadelphia.

Cabral, D.A., Tucker, L.B., 1999. Malignancies in children who initially present with rheumatic complaints. J. Pediatr. 134, 53–57.

Castleberry, R.P., 1997. Biology and treatment of neuroblastoma. Pediatr. Clin. North Am. 44 (4), 919–937.

Celkan, T., Yildiz, I., 2008. Prognostic factors in children with Hodgkin disease. Pediatr. Blood Cancer 51 (5), 712.

Damron, T.A., Ward, W.G., Stewart, A., 2007. Osteosarcoma, chondrosarcoma and Ewing's sarcoma: National Cancer Data Base Report. Clin. Orthop. Relat. Res. 459, 40–47.

D'Angio, G.J., Breslow, N., Beckwith, J.B., et al., 1989. Treatment of Wilms' tumor: results of the Third National Wilms' Tumor Study. Cancer 64 (2), 349–360.

Dreyer, Z.E., Fernbach, D.J., 1994. Neuroblastoma. In: Oski, F.A., Deangelis, C.D., Feigen, B.D. et al. (Eds), Principles and Practice of Pediatrics, second ed. JB Lippincott, Philadelphia.

Ebb, D.H., Weinstein, H.J., 1997. Diagnosis and treatment of childhood acute myelogenous leukemia. Pediatr. Clin. North Am. 44 (4), 847–862.

Golub, T.R., Weinstein, H.J., Holcombe, E.G., 1997. Acute myelogenous leukemia. In: Pizzo, P.A., Poplack, D.G. (Eds), Principles and Practice of Pediatric Oncology, third ed. Lipincott Raven, Philadelphia.

Gonçalves, M., Terreri, M.T., Barbosa, C.M., et al., 2005. Diagnosis of malignancies in children with musculoskeletal complaints. Sao Paulo Med. J. 123 (1), 21–23.

Gorin, N.C., 1998. Autologous stem cell transplantation in acute myelocytic leukemia. Blood 92 (4), 1073–1090.

Glotzbecker, M.P., Kersun, L.S., Choi, J.K., et al., 2006. Primary non-Hodgkin's lymphoma of bone in children. J. Bone Joint Surg. Am. 88 (3), 583–594.

Grier, H.E., 1997. The Ewing family of tumors: Ewing's sarcoma and primitive neuroectodermal tumors. Pediatr. Clin. North Am. 44 (4), 991–1004.

Himelstein, B.P., Doormans, J.P., 1996. Malignant bone tumors of childhood. Pediatr. Clin. North Am. 43 (4), 967–984.

Hodgson, D.C., Hudson, M.M., Constine, L.S., 2007. Pediatric Hodgkin lymphoma: maximizing efficacy and minimizing toxicity. Semin. Radiat. Oncol. 17 (3), 230–242.

Isaacs Jr., H., 2007. Fetal and neonatal hepatic tumors. J. Pediatr. Surg. 42 (11), 1797–1803.

Kalfia, C., Grill, J., 2005. The therapy of infantile malignant brain tumors: current status? J. Neurooncol. 75 (3), 279–285.

Kaspers, G.J., Zwaan, C.M., 2007. Pediatric acute myeloid leukemia: towards high-quality cure of all patients. Haematologica 92 (11), 1519–1532.

Kun, L.E., 1997. Brain tumors: challenges and direction. Pediatr. Clin. North Am. 44 (4), 907–917.

Ladish, S., Jaffe, E.S., 1997. The histiocytoses. In: Pizzo, P.A., Poplack, D.G. (Eds), Principles and Practices of Pediatric Oncology, third ed. Lippincott Raven, Philadelphia.

Link, M.P., Eilber, F., 1997. Osteosarcoma. In: Pizzo, P.A., Poplack, D.G. (Eds), Principles and Practices of Pediatric Oncology, third ed. Lippincott Raven, Philadelphia.

Magrath, I.T., 1997. Non-Hodgkin's lymphomas: epidemiology and treatment. Ann. N. Y. Acad. Sci. 824, 91–106.

Mahoney, D.H., 1994. Malignant bone tumors in children. In: Oski, F.A., Deangelis, C.D., Feigen, B.D. et al. (Eds), Principles and Practice of Pediatrics, second ed. JB Lippincott, Philadelphia.

Meyers, P.A., Gorlick, R., 1997. Osteosarcoma. Pediatr. Clin. North Am. 44 (4), 973–989.

Oberlin, O., 1996. Present and future strategies of treatment in childhood Hodgkin's lymphomas. Ann. Oncol. 7 (Suppl. 4), 73–78.

Pappo, A.S., Shapiro, D.N., Crist, W.M., 1997. Rhabdomyosarcoma: biology and treatment. Pediatr. Clin. North Am. 44 (4), 953–972.

Park, J.R., Eggert, A., Caron, H., 2008. Neuroblastoma: biology, prognosis, and treatment. Pediatr. Clin. North Am. 55 (1), 97–120.

Prowse, O.A., Reddy, P.P., Barrieras, D., et al., 1998. Pediatric genitourinary tumors. Curr. Opin. Oncol. 10 (3), 253–260.

Pui, C.H., Crist, W.M., 1994. Biology and treatment of acute lymphoblastic leukaemia. J. Pediatr. 124 (4), 253–260.

Pui, C.H., Robinson, L.L., Look, A.T., 2008. Acute lymphoblastic leukaemia. Lancet 371 (9617), 1030–1043.

Raney, B., 1997. Hepatoblastoma in children: a review. J. Pediatr. Hematol. Oncol. 19 (5), 418–422.

Ries, L.A.G., et al., 1994. SEER Cancer Statistics Review, 1973–91: tables and graphs, NIH Publication No. 94: 2739. National Cancer Institute, Bethesda, MD.

Rodeberg, D., Paidas, C., 2006. Childhood rhabdomyosarcoma. Semin. Pediatr. Surg. 15 (1), 57–62.

Sandlund, J.T., Downing, J.R., Crist, W.M., 1996. Non–Hodgkin's lymphoma in childhood. N. Engl. J. Med. 334 (19), 1238–1248.

Shad, A., Magrath, I., 1997a. Non-Hodgkin's lymphoma. Pediatr. Clin. North Am. 44 (4), 863–890.

Shad, A., Magrath, I.T., 1997b. Malignant non-Hodgkin's lymphoma in children. In: Pizzo, P.A., Poplack, D.G. (Eds), Principles and Practices of Pediatric

Oncology, third ed. Lippincott Raven, Philadelphia.

Shukla, N.N., Trippett, T.M., 2006. Non-Hodgkin's lymphoma in children and adolescents. Curr. Oncol. Rep. 8 (5), 387–394.

Siegel, M.J., Chung, E.M., 2008. Wilms' tumor and other pediatric renal masses. Magn. Reson. Imaging Clin. N. Am. 16 (3), 479–497.

Uderzo, C., Dini, G., Locatelli, F., et al., 2000. Treatment of childhood acute lymphoblastic leukemia after the first relapse: curative strategies. Haematologica 85 (11 Suppl.), 47–53.

Waters, K., Smith, P., 1998. Cancers in childhood: molecular biology and clinical features. In: Robinson, M.J., Roberton, D.M. (Eds), Practical Paediatrics, fourth ed. Churchill Livingstone, Edinburgh.

Weir, H.K., Thun, M.J., Hankey, B.F., et al., 2003. Annual report to the nation on the status of cancer, 1975–2000, featuring the uses of surveillance data for cancer prevention and control. J. Natl. Cancer Inst. 95 (17), 1258–1261.

Wu, H.Y., Snyder 3rd, H.M., D'Angio, G.J., 2005. Wilms' tumor management. Curr. Opin. Urol. 15 (4), 273–276.

Allergy, metabolic and endocrine disease in children

18

Philip J. Parry   Neil J. Davies

Allergy

Allergy is a common complaint estimated to affect up to 33% of the American population (Rapp 1991). Given this prevalence, it is likely that many chiropractors will see patients with allergies and they therefore need to recognize the symptoms of allergy and have a clear understanding of the potential causes. In treating children with allergies, the chiropractor should also be aware of the various diagnostic tests and therapies that may be made available to the patient through the chiropractic clinic, in addition to those available through other health care professionals, so that optimal patient care is provided.

The physiological basis of allergy

Traditionally, allergy is viewed as an excessive physiological response to an often common environmental substance (allergen) which is mediated by the immune system (Sly 1996). Disorders such as some adverse food and drug reactions where there is no evidence of immunological involvement do not fit this definition, although they are often considered to be forms of allergy.

The most common immunologically mediated response to an allergen (antigen) is a type I hypersensitivity reaction (Sly 1996). This encompasses immediate-type reactions such as rhinitis, hay fever and asthma as well as anaphylactic allergic reactions. In type I hypersensitivity reactions, mucosal immunoglobulin E (IgE), which is normally involved in defense against parasites, is responsible for 'sensitization' of mast cells and basophils, and the subsequent release of histamine and other inflammatory mediators such as cytokines, heparin, arachidonic acid, bradykinin and platelet aggregation factor. These mediators result in dilatation and increased permeability of local vasculature, smooth muscle contraction, chemotaxis, thromboxane and prostaglandin production. Effects include the production of a 'flare and wheal' at the site of allergen exposure, edema, bronchoconstriction and mucus production.

Erythema, edema and airway hyperirritability occur later in atopic dermatitis, allergic rhinitis and asthma.

Genetic factors are also partly responsible for IgE-mediated allergic reactions, there being an association between human leukocyte antigen (HLA) histocompatibility types and IgE-mediated hypersensitivity reactions (Sly 1996). It is thought that such individuals are thus more susceptible to, or 'atopic' for, allergies compared to others owing to differences in their ability to regulate IgE antibody production, dispose of allergens or control mediators.

Type II (cytotoxic) hypersensitivity involves activation of the complement system and cell lysis due to IgG and IgM reactions on cell membranes. A good example of a type II hypersensitivity is reaction to blood transfusions, drug-induced and other immune-related hemolytic anemias.

In type III immunopathological or immune complex mechanism allergic reactions, there is formation of tissue-damaging antibody–antigen complexes involving IgG or IgM in extracellular spaces (e.g. glomerulonephritis).

Type IV cell-mediated or delayed hypersensitivity involves the interaction of antigen with specifically sensitized thymus-dependent T lymphocytes, macrophages and cytotoxic cells, as seen in contact allergy such as poison ivy and chemically induced contact dermatitis, as well as some drug reactions.

The role of the nervous system in allergy

Although little has been written on nervous system dysfunction in allergy, its importance cannot be ignored owing to findings such as the hyperreactivity of the skin in individuals with atopic dermatitis, which is thought to result from autonomic imbalance where androgenic responses in lymphocytes and granulocytes are decreased and there is a disturbance of fatty acid metabolism (Sly 1996).

It has also been suggested that changes to viscerosomatic and viscerovisceral reflexes may be involved in the mediation of allergic effects in adverse food reactions. In patients with

DOI: 10.1016/B978-0-7020-3129-8.00018-9

functional neurological imbalance one wonders what effects may be occasioned upon their susceptibility to allergic responses, either via direct nervous system compromise and/or its effect upon the 'allergenic barrel'.

The barrel effect and adaptation

Symptoms of allergy may not always occur on every exposure to an allergen. The 'barrel effect' is an attempt to explain this phenomenon as physiological adaptation.

The barrel effect assumes that each potentially allergic person has a barrel for allergens. Symptoms do not occur if the barrel is not full, whereas if it overflows then symptoms ensue. This barrel may be filled with one or more types of allergen and can be emptied by reducing allergen exposure or its capacity increased via allergy injection (desensitization) therapy or improved nutrition, thus reducing the potential for symptoms. Factors that may decrease barrel capacity, and hence allergy potential, include infection, stress or poor diet. However, it is not always possible to keep the barrel from filling in sensitive people or those exposed to highly allergenic environments.

Adaptation is based on the idea that, after exposure to an allergen, sensitive people develop alarm symptoms. After this, a stage of addiction/adaptation appears and the body adjusts to the allergen and symptoms are no longer noticed. The patient may feel well or even better after exposure to the offending substance, often requiring frequent exposure to maintain this feeling (i.e. the person develops an 'addiction'). Eventually the body becomes exhausted and is unable to cope with developing illness, with symptoms now appearing after each allergenic exposure. This explains why frequently eaten or craved foods are often the allergenic ones, the so-called 'fatal attraction' phenomenon.

Types of allergy

Allergies may be classed as typical or atypical. Typical or classical allergies are those with easily recognizable symptoms such as hay fever, atopic dermatitis, adverse food reactions, allergic coughing or asthma, urticaria–angioedema, anaphylaxis, adverse drug reactions and insect allergies. Atypical allergies are usually less easy to recognize than typical allergies because of their subtle and delayed symptoms (Rapp 1991).

A relatively common example of a typical allergy is an adverse reaction to food (Briggs & Lennard 1997, Rapp 1991, Sly 1996), which may involve either immunological or non-immunological reactions. Allergy to a particular food develops when intact antigenic macromolecules pass through the gut epithelium into the circulation. This can happen in the first few months of life if the gut lining is damaged, as happens with gastroenteritis or if there is impaired digestive enzyme efficiency. Normally the absorption of these molecules is also limited by mucosal IgA, which may be deficient in some children, particularly in the neonate, thus allowing the formation of greater levels of antibodies to foods such as cow's milk (Briggs & Lennard 1997, Odze et al 1995, Sly 1996). A type I

reaction can result in angioedema of the lips, mouth, glottis and uvula, generalized urticaria, vomiting, asthma, and occasionally anaphylaxis and death. Offending foods may include peanuts, certain nuts and seeds, fish, shellfish, eggs, buckwheat, soy, corn and cow's milk. Delayed hypersensitivity reactions to foods may result in less severe symptoms such as bad breath, flatus, cramps, constipation, diarrhea, nausea and vomiting. In some cases overt gastrointestinal pathology may result, such as Crohn's disease and ulcerative colitis with milk, wheat, chocolate, egg, sugar or corn, or enteropathy in infants fed whole milk (Briggs & Lennard 1997, Odze et al 1995, Rapp 1991, Sly 1996). Non-intestinal symptoms may also occur.

Another example of a typical allergy that may present to the chiropractor is that of allergic polyarthritis, an uncommon transient allergic reaction that can arise after a mild upper respiratory tract infection, drug or food allergen exposure. Symptoms include synovitis and urticarial rash (Miller & Miller 1979). This needs to be differentiated from other rheumatic disease.

Atypical allergies may result in a myriad of non-specific symptoms. The more common of these are shown in Box 18.1.

Other less common allergy-related reactions include attention-deficit disorder, allergic tension fatigue syndrome, aggression, learning difficulties, delinquency, depression, suicide, Tourette syndrome and hypoglycemia (Hull & Johnston 1987, Miller & Miller 1979, Rapp 1991). Another important association between allergy and illness in children is that of otitis media (Arroyave 2001, Nsouli et al 1994). The more

Box 18.1

Common non-specific symptoms seen in patients with atypical allergy

- Pruritus
- Irritability
- Rash around the mouth
- Redness at the tip of the nose, ears, cheeks or buttocks
- Wrinkles under the eyes
- Mouth ulcers
- Geographic tongue
- Constant talking
- Speech changes
- Cold hands and feet
- Aching legs
- Joint stiffness
- Enuresis and encopresis
- Sleep disturbance
- Fatigue
- Headaches
- Tics and seizures
- Excessive perspiration
- Excessive drooling
- Thirst
- Pallor
- Decreased alertness
- Unpleasant body or foot odor

common allergens are cow's milk, eggs, chocolate, wheat, soy, nuts, shellfish, sugar and cigarette smoke (Nsouli et al 1994, Schmidt 1990). Sesame is a less common allergen, but important in some Middle Eastern countries (Aaranov et al 2008).

Allergy in different age groups

Although a similar approach can be used for allergy in various age groups, there are often differences in presentation. It is thought that signs of allergy may even be evident in utero, where the fetus may become hyperactive, kick vigorously and/or hiccup frequently upon exposure to the allergen (Rapp 1991). The offending substance is often a food to which the mother is allergic or eats frequently, such as milk, cheese, etc. (Rapp 1991).

In the neonatal period, affected infants may respond to an allergen by vomiting or spitting up frequently, drooling excessively, becoming irritable, not sleeping well, seeking constant attention, screaming, throwing temper tantrums, banging the head and demanding frequent rocking. They may appear unhappy and present with dark circles under the eyes, nasal congestion, repeated ear infections, a bloated abdomen with flatus, colic-like symptoms, moist chest and throat sounds, coughing, unpleasant foot or body odor, bright red buttocks, atopic dermatitis, frequent genital touching and early walking.

In breastfed infants, potential allergens may pass to the infant via breastmilk with symptoms usually developing within 2–4 hours after a feed (Machida et al 1994, Odze et al 1995, Rapp 1991). Cow's milk is frequently the culprit owing to protein intolerance (Odze et al 1995, Rapp 1991).

Breastfeeding, although shown not to have any bearing on atopic disease, may have a role to play in the prevention of some allergic conditions such as non-atopic wheeze (Siltanen et al 2003). While breastfeeding has also been reported to have the effect of delaying the onset and dampening the severity of symptoms (Beaudry et al 1995, Odze et al 1995, Rapp 1991), it remains a controversial proposition given the outcomes of some recent studies suggesting otherwise (Nagel et al 2009, Sears et al 2002, Siltanen et al 2003).

During infancy, the introduction of solid food may also be a time when allergy develops. This is why it is important to gradually introduce one food at a time and introduce foods that are harder to digest and potentially more allergenic last, such as eggs, fish and nuts (Briggs & Lennard 1997, Davies 1997, Rapp 1991).

Toddlers may present with both classical and less obvious symptoms of allergy. Sometimes symptoms of allergies that were present in infancy change so that the allergy is thought to have disappeared. Classical nasal symptoms and recurrent ear infections may be common in allergic toddlers and they may also present with dark circles, bags and wrinkles under the eyes, red ear lobes and cheeks, restless or aching legs, recurrent chest and sinus infections, diarrhea, constipation, abdominal pains, nausea, vomiting and headache. These children may also dislike being cuddled or touched, whine a lot, have incredible tantrums (although tantrums in 2–3-year-olds are often a normal part of development), be clingy, depressed, tire easily, display aggression or hyperactivity, and have

difficulty going to sleep (Rapp 1991). By 2 years of age, seasonal hay fever or asthma may develop (Rapp 1991, Sly 1996).

Children can suffer from many different allergies, both classical and atypical. They may have suffered with these during infancy or as toddlers, but the allergy remained undiagnosed despite numerous visits to different specialists. During this stage, symptoms may include recurrent infections, aggression, intestinal complaints such as nausea, flatus and halitosis, dry skin and hives, red nose tip, ears and cheeks, urinary complaints such as enuresis and frequency, and muscle aches and 'growing pains' (Rapp 1991).

During adolescence there may be more behaviorally related problems such as depression, suicidal tendencies and poor school performance (Rapp 1991). Even though adolescents may have suffered with the allergy since infancy with hyperactivity, as they grow older they may become tired, irritable and depressed. Symptoms may also change after puberty. For example, in males asthma may subside whereas in females it may worsen (Rapp 1991). Females may also suffer with cold hands and feet, menstrual irregularities and weight gain because of possible effects upon the endocrine system (Rapp 1991).

Clinical evaluation of the allergic child

A great deal of information can be attained from the case history and physical examination of the allergic child within the chiropractic setting. The use of a diary, food elimination diet and laboratory tests may aid in the diagnosis.

History

It is important to inquire about the nature, frequency, timing, severity, location, aggravating and relieving factors, and progression of symptoms. A previous history of symptoms and other allergies is also important as is a family history of similar or other allergies.

Physical examination

Anthropometry is essential as any deviation from normal can be an indicator of an underlying disorder. Occasionally in children with severe asthma, for example, chronic corticosteroid treatment can result in decreased growth (Sly 1996). Observation may reveal signs common to allergy such as dark circles and wrinkles under the eyes, mouth breathing, rhinorrhea, a transverse crease across the nose from constant rubbing, or skin rashes suggestive of atopic dermatitis. Cardiovascular signs, including increased anterior–posterior diameter of the chest, may be evident in chronic cases of asthma, while acute cases may produce nasal flaring, supraclavicular and/or intercostal retractions, and an increased pulsus paradoxus. In hay fever the nasal mucosa may appear pale, blue or pink with a profuse watery discharge. The tonsils and adenoids may also appear enlarged. Upon auscultation of the lungs, there may be a wheeze with prolonged expiration in asthma or an increase in the transfer of moist sounds with upper airway involvement in cases of hay fever or some food allergies, particularly cow's milk allergy.

Table 18.1 Example of a diary for a child with suspected cow's milk allergy

Date	Time	Reaction	Foods eaten	Chemicals contacted
10/11	10 a.m.	Red eyes	Corn flakes and milk Orange juice	Soap Toothpaste
	1 p.m.	Runny nose Tantrum	Cheese burger Fries Milk shake (chocolate)	Car fumes Plastic cup
	4 p.m.	Runny nose	Chocolate frog	
	8 p.m.	Tantrum Red eyes	Sausages Mashed potato Tinned peaches Ice-cream	Shampoo Soap

Record-keeping

When there is an allergy but the cause is unknown, keeping detailed records of symptoms and any possible aggravating factors/exposures may be a good start to detecting the offending substance. Table 18.1 gives an example of such a diary.

In vitro tests

Eosinophilia can be established by a white cell count (WCC) from analysis of secretions recovered from the respiratory tract. Eosinophil counts are not used specifically for allergy and can increase with drug hypersensitivity, rheumatic disorders and various malignancies (Rapp 1991, Sly 1996). Immunological tests can determine the general serum level of IgE (Prist test) or the presence of specific IgE antibodies (radio-allergosorbent test; RAST). Parasitic infestation, immunodeficiency disorders, nephronic disorders, cystic fibrosis and rheumatoid arthritis may also affect these tests. While immunological tests are less sensitive than skin tests, they appear to correlate reasonably well with them (Sly 1996).

In vivo tests

Skin tests, where an extract of allergen is introduced into the skin either superficially into the dermis (scratch test) or injected deeper (prick test), may detect strong sensitivities to pollen, molds, pets, dust or foods, and can test up to 40 substances at once. A positive reaction is one that produces a flare and wheal reaction on the skin in around 15 minutes. They are not always clinically reliable and have, on occasion, produced clinical symptoms and signs including anaphylaxis (Rapp 1991, Sly 1996).

Provocation testing, which involves direct exposure of the mucous membranes or skin to the suspected allergen, may be used to find a correct allergy extract for treatment (neutralization). It may be suitable for those children in whom many foods produce allergy, those that live in very allergenic environments, or those who have had little success with other methods of treatment. These tests are supposedly more sensitive and accurate because they test for one allergen at a time; however, their use is controversial amongst allergists (Rapp 1991).

Oral provocation testing is the gold standard for the diagnosis of food allergy and can be used to diagnose IgE-mediated food allergy and food-induced atopic dermatitis (Rapp 1991, Sly 1996). Suspected foods are blindly ingested in gelatin capsules, following an elimination diet, and symptoms and signs such as wheezing, a macular rash, sneezing, nausea, vomiting or abdominal pain observed for. Tests are contraindicated if there is a history of anaphylaxis and need to be carried out in an appropriate clinic under strict medical supervision. Progressively weaker dilutions of the allergen may also be given until symptoms ease, which signifies the treatment dose (neutralization). Disadvantages of this testing lie in the fact that it is very time-consuming, costly, and a limited number of allergists are able to do it.

Food elimination diets offer another way in which to identify the source of an allergy. The simplest and fastest of these is the single food elimination diet which is suitable for chiropractic use. One suspected food is eliminated entirely from the diet over 4 days. The food is then reintroduced in abundance while the patient is observed for the appearance of symptoms and signs. Reactions normally occur within 15–60 minutes of eating the offending food (Rapp 1991). A decrease in any of symptoms present prior to the diet may also occur while the offending food is not eaten. Detailed records should be kept while on the diet. This diet is helpful for testing those foods normally eaten but should not be used for foods where there is a known severe reaction. It should also not be used during an infection (Rapp 1991).

Although the single food elimination diet is easy to utilize, it does not test the effect of eliminating a combination of foods, with the result that the child who is allergic to more than one food may show little change in symptoms during the dietary period. The multiple food elimination diet eliminates several suspected or common food sources of allergy at once over several days and then reintroduces them one at a time. Care has to be taken in case severe symptoms develop and a food diary must be kept.

The practical rotation diet, where foods of the same category are eaten at 4-day intervals, is even more time-consuming and complex, and basically tests all foods in the way that the single food elimination diet tests one food. It may also be used in the treatment of some food allergies. It takes about a month before changes are evident, and clear instructions to the child and parent are necessary. Again, this type of diet is best managed by an allergist.

Treatment of allergy

Management of the allergic child is generally multifactorial and may involve chiropractic care, preventive environmental measures, immunotherapy, pharmacological therapy and dietary measures, either singly or in combination along with naturopathic medicine. Prophylaxis is also important (for example, breastfeeding should be encouraged and nursing mothers advised to avoid highly allergenic foods and environments). For those children with an already established allergy where the allergen(s) have been identified, prevention alone may be enough to keep the child's 'barrel' from overflowing and hence ease symptoms (e.g. the maintenance of a dust-free environment in the case of dust mite allergy, or the total avoidance or rotation of food in food allergies). These measures should form part of the chiropractic management of the allergic child that should also concentrate on correcting neurological imbalance. If conservative chiropractic and preventive measures prove to be incapable of controlling allergic symptoms fully, immunotherapy and/or drug therapy may be utilized.

In immunotherapy or hyposensitization, an aqueous extract of the known allergen is injected intradermally several times a week, using increasing doses of extract until the patient reaches an optimal treatment dose which signifies blockage of IgE owing to increased IgG production. This usually takes 5–6 months and the benefits may persist for several years, although renewed treatments are sometimes required (Rapp 1991, Sly 1996). It is usually used for IgE-mediated reactions and when there is a good correlation between symptoms, exposure and positive skin tests. It is not often used for atopic dermatitis or food allergies (Sly 1996). This treatment requires considerable patient compliance, is costly, and has the capacity to induce anaphylaxis. Hence, it must be conducted at an appropriately equipped medical center.

In provocation/neutralization testing a similar approach to allergy extract treatment is followed; however, progressively weaker dilutions of extract are given to the patient during testing until the correct treatment dose is arrived at.

Sometimes, when all else fails, or when other treatments have not been offered as an option, drug therapy may be employed. The drugs used in allergy generally interrupt pathways of the antibody–antigen reaction that result in tissue damage. Some modulate the release of chemical mediators such as terfenadine (Carter 1997), an antihistamine; others affect smooth muscle tension via adrenergic bronchodilators, such as salbutamol (Carter 1997); while others prevent inflammatory cell migration to the site of reaction. Other adrenergic drugs, such as phenylephrine, may reduce congestion and edema through their vasoconstrictive effects (Carter 1997). However, these drugs are not without a variety of potential side-effects, including nausea, vomiting, headache, epigastric pain, cardiac stimulation, insomnia, irritability, tremors and hypokalemia (Carter 1997, Rapp 1991, Sly 1996). Nasal sprays may provide temporary relief from nasal congestion but their long-term use may result in rebound vasodilation (Carter 1997, Rapp 1991, Sly 1996). Alka-Seltzer may also be useful in reducing food allergy symptoms in emergency situations.

The most potent drugs used in allergy are topical or systemic corticosteroids which decrease local edema, mucus production and inflammation, or exhibit anti-inflammatory actions, suppress mediator release and decrease hypersensitivity responses (e.g. prednisolone, betamethasone, fludrocortisone). Potential side-effects from their long-term use include osteoporosis, hypertension, diabetes mellitus, Cushing's habitus, myopathy, gastritis, pancreatitis and suppression of linear

growth (Carter 1997, Sly 1996). Topical skin preparations may lead to skin atrophy and hirsutism of the affected area. Such effects must be taken into consideration in the chiropractic management of children on corticosteroid medication and symptoms may include the constant reactivation of the primary subluxation complex. One has also to consider non-pharmacological medication ingredients that may be allergenic, such as sugar, corn, dyes or flavorings, which are common in some medications used for children.

Another area that needs to be taken into consideration in the management of allergy is the overall nutritional status of the individual. Some allergic children may develop deficiencies, and deficiencies may also reduce a child's general health, making the child more susceptible to illness, including allergy. Having a naturopath co-manage allergy patients is therefore highly recommended.

Several of the above measures can easily be assimilated into the overall chiropractic management of the child with allergy (e.g. advice on prevention and prophylaxis of allergy, the use of the clinical history, examination, and single food elimination diet findings for the detection of an allergy, etc.). In more complex cases, however, it is advisable to include the advice and treatment of other health care professionals such as an allergist or general medical physician.

Managing the primary subluxation complex in the pediatric population is usually a very sequential and systematic process. In allergy-affected children, when the primary subluxation complex is shown to be recurrent, the allergy must be considered to be uncontrolled and steps must be taken to address the symptoms. This may include a detailed and aggressive search for allergenic triggers, and, in more complex resistant cases, the advice and treatment of other health care professionals such as an allergist or general medical physician should be sought.

Evidence for a bidirectional link between the nervous and immune systems has been constantly growing since a landmark study published in 1975 (Ader & Cohen 1993). While still poorly understood, communication between the nervous and immune systems appears to occur via chemical messengers. The immune system, in association with an activated hypothalamic–pituitary–adrenocortical axis (HPA) acts as a sensory system, signaling the brain in the presence of a threat from the external environment to trigger a classical stress response (Blalock & Smith 1985). It has been suggested that the role of HPA activation is to provide a negative-feedback mechanism provided by the immunosuppressive activity of the glucocorticoids. The inhibitory activity of the glucocorticoids limits inflammatory responses and prevents the immune system from over-reacting and causing autoimmunity (Besedovsky et al 1986, Munck & Guyre 1986).

On a functional level, the chiropractic subluxation is known to adversely affect cortical afferentation, a process referred to as dysafferentation, and is therefore likely to be a component in the overall etiology. Adequate correction of the various levels of cortical dysafferentation is therefore vital in the management of the 'allergenic barrel'.

Anecdotal evidence has repeatedly shown that the pediatric patient will often show some level of deviation from normal anthropometric development in one particular area, usually weight. After the first visit to the chiropractic office, the child's parents will often report that the child has considerably increased their intake of food. After adequate sustainable correction of cortical dysafferentation has taken place, parents often comment that their child appears healthier and less susceptible to upper respiratory and ear infections. This common response is thought to be due to the bidirectional link between the nervous and immune systems described earlier in this chapter. A return to normal patterns of growth and development is usually seen once the child's allergic condition is stabilized.

Endocrine and metabolic diseases

Although chiropractors are not often involved in the treatment of metabolic or endocrine disorders in children, it is important to be familiar with such disorders because of their profound negative effects. Some of these disorders may also produce symptoms suggestive of a musculoskeletal problem, from which they must be differentiated. It is also possible that the endocrine system and metabolic function in children may be affected by allergy (Rapp 1991).

Disorders of the pituitary gland

Disorders of the pituitary gland may have widespread effects owing to the influence of the pituitary on almost all other endocrine glands. The main conditions seen are hypopituitarism, hyperpituitarism, and antidiuretic hormone (ADH) deficiency or hypersecretion.

Hypopituitarism and hyperpituitarism

These are rare in childhood and are mainly associated with abnormal production of growth hormone (GH) (DiGeorge et al 1996, Hull & Johnston 1987). Hypopituitarism usually occurs as a consequence of a functional or idiopathic defect of the hypothalamus rather than developmental abnormalities or pituitary pathology. Hyperpituitarism may arise when there is decreased feedback from target organs, as in hypothyroidism (DiGeorge et al 1996).

Presentation of the child with hyper- or hypopituitarism
The most common sign in hypopituitarism is short stature due to GH deficiency. These children are often of normal height and weight at birth and in the first 1–2 years, but growth then slows. They also tend to appear younger than their chronological age and have delayed dentition (DiGeorge et al 1996, Hughes 1975). If the cause is traumatic, such as head trauma, then growth may slow down (Yamanaka et al 1993). This contrasts with hyperpituitarism where there are excessive levels of GH with resultant gigantism. If other hormones as well as GH are also affected then other endocrine manifestations can occur (e.g. those associated with diabetes insipidus or Cushing syndrome). Symptoms of increased intracranial pressure may be prominent in both hypopituitarism and hyperpituitarism if due to a tumor.

Laboratory findings
These will demonstrate abnormal levels of GH.

X-ray findings
In hyperpituitarism there may be an increase in the size of the paranasal sinuses, tufting of the phalanges, and an increase in the size of the sella turcica (DiGeorge et al 1996, Yamanaka et al 1993).

Differential diagnoses
The short stature of hypopituitarism needs to be differentiated from that due to genetic causes, constitutional growth delay, Turner syndrome, skeletal, nutritional or metabolic disorders. Tall stature due to excess GH needs to be differentiated from that due to genetic causes, hyperthyroidism, arachnodactyly, sexual precocity and Marfan syndrome (DiGeorge et al 1996, Hughes 1975).

Treatment
In functional cases of hypopituitarism, administration of GH may alleviate the growth problems; the younger the child, the better will be the prognosis. In cases of tumor, excision, irradiation and administration of deficient hormones may be utilized. Treatment of hyperpituitarism is difficult and controversial. If the cause is a tumor then external irradiation, radioactive implants or hypophysectomy may be carried out. Sometimes thyroid extract, hydrocortisone and sex hormones are administered. In some cases, correction of the causal condition resolves the hyperpituitarism.

Antidiuretic hormone (ADH) deficiency

ADH deficiency results in diabetes insipidus and can occur with lesions of the hypothalamus, hypothalamicohypophyseal tracts, or posterior lobe of the pituitary. Causes include tumors, head or operative trauma, genetic causes and, less commonly, histiocytosis, encephalitis, leukemia, sarcoidosis and tuberosclerosis (DiGeorge et al 1996, Hughes 1975).

Presentation of the child with ADH deficiency

The child with diabetes insipidus presents with polyuria and polydipsia. In the infant this polydipsia is evident as excessive crying alleviated by water rather than milk (Hughes 1975). Hyperthermia, rapid weight loss, collapse, vomiting, constipation, growth failure and dehydration are also common features (DiGeorge et al 1996, Hughes 1975). If a destructive lesion such as a tumor is present, then neurological signs may also be demonstrable.

Laboratory findings
In diabetes insipidus, an increase in daily urinary output will be seen. In cases where the ADH deficiency is severe, water deprivation leads to a rise in plasma osmolality while urine osmolality remains below that of the plasma. The urine osmolality is a measure of the concentration of the urine and is primarily determined by the level of antidiuretic hormone (ADH). The urine osmolality is determined by the number of particles in the solution. In contrast, the urine specific gravity, which is a measure of the weight of the solution compared to that of an equal volume of distilled water, is determined by both the number and size of particles in the solution. In most cases, the urine specific gravity varies in a relatively predictable way

with the osmolality, with the specific gravity rising by 0.001 for every 35–40 mosmol/kg increase in osmolality. Thus, a urine osmolality of 280 mosmol/kg (which is isosmotic to plasma) is usually associated with a specific gravity of 1.008 or 1.009. Although urine osmolality is a more accurate marker of urinary concentration, specific gravity can be used if an osmometer is not available and if there is no reason to suspect increased excretion of larger solutes. Furthermore, a very low specific gravity ($\leq$1.003) is indicative of a maximally dilute urine (osmolality $\leq$100 mosmol/kg), since there are no causes of falsely low specific gravity measurements.

X-ray findings
Skull X-rays are sometimes useful in revealing abnormalities associated with the cause. However, MRI is the radiological imaging investigation of choice.

Differential diagnoses
These include hypocalcemia or potassium deficiency, primary renal disease, decreased kidney response to ADH, adipsia due to impairment of the thirst center and, rarely, a psychogenic syndrome (DiGeorge et al 1996, Hughes 1975).

Treatment
Uncomplicated cases of diabetes insipidus may go for years without treatment, with the affected patient able to cope as long as they have enough water. Occasionally, it may be necessary to use desmopressin administered via an intranasal spray. This drug is effective, but costly.

Hypersecretion of ADH

This is more common that a deficiency of ADH and can develop as a result of disorders of the central nervous system, drugs and ADH-secreting tumors.

Presentation of the child with hypersecretion of ADH
This condition may be latent and asymptomatic. Manifestations arise because of hypotonic body fluids and water intoxication and include decreased appetite, nausea, vomiting, irritability, personality changes, and neurological abnormalities including seizures.

Laboratory findings
There is hypo-osmolality of serum, with urine of a greater osmolality, and often hypouricemia.

Treatment
Correction of the causal disorder and restriction of fluids and hypertonic solutions often leads to spontaneous remission.

Juvenile diabetes mellitus

Juvenile or type 1 diabetes mellitus is a relatively common disorder affecting about 186 300 people younger than 20 years of age in the USA, which represents 0.2% of all people in this age group (NDIC 2008). It is rare in infancy, with a mean age of onset of 8 years (Hull & Johnston 1987). Males and females are affected equally and it may be less common in children who were breastfed (Ball 1997, Hull & Johnston 1987). Type 1 diabetes accounts for 10–15% of all cases of diabetes mellitus (Merck Manual 1999). Unlike type 2 or adult-onset diabetes mellitus, its onset may be rapid, insulin levels may be lowered in the prediabetic phase, insulin replacement is necessary, variations in insulin response can occur with swings between hyper- and hypoglycemia (Ball 1997, Carter 1997, Hughes 1975), and blood glucose levels may be lowered by exercise. Irreversible pancreatic B-cell failure occurs with decreased levels of insulin production. The exact cause of this is unknown but genetic HLA and autoimmune factors play a role (DiGeorge et al 1996). Other possible causes are those that produce hyperglycemia such as Cushing syndrome, hyperpituitarism, hyperthyroidism, congenital pancreatic defects, exhaustion of islet tissue, infections and toxins (DiGeorge et al 1996). The metabolic state is greatly altered so that ketonemia and metabolic acidosis result with dehydration and altered kidney function.

Presentation of the child with diabetes mellitus
It is possible for pancreatic B-cell damage to occur years before clinical manifestations are evident. Clinical symptoms and signs may be rapid in onset and include polyuria which sometimes presents as enuresis, polydipsia, weight loss, anorexia, pyogenic skin infections, vaginal candidiasis and constipation. If ketoacidosis develops, then vomiting, dehydration, hyperventilation, with an acetone odor on the breath and abdominal pains may also present as well as lethargy, shock and coma.

Laboratory findings
Urinalysis shows acid retention, high specific gravity, glycosuria and ketonuria. Blood analysis demonstrates glycemia and ketonuria. If dehydration is present, then blood urea nitrogen is raised as well as serum phosphate levels and hemoglobin. There is also an increase in blood polymorphonuclear leukocytes. The most commonly used blood test is the fasting blood glucose test, which will demonstrate increased levels after fasting.

Differential diagnoses
The differentials when considering a diagnosis of juvenile diabetes mellitus include salicylism, lead intoxication, cerebral injury, infection or neoplasm, Cushing syndrome, galactosemia, hyperthyroidism and glycosuria; as well as renal glycosuria and other renal tubular defects (DiGeorge et al 1996, Hughes 1975).

Management
Once a diagnosis of juvenile diabetes mellitus is made, very active and aggressive clinical management needs to be implemented. In cases of ketoacidosis and circulatory collapse, emergency treatment with saline or plasma and insulin administration is necessary. Long-term management aims at a compromise between the child leading a full life and normal growth with the best possible control of the diabetes (Hull & Johnston 1987). Effective control helps to reduce the long-term risks. Management of diet with appropriate nutrition is essential. High-fiber carbohydrates, regular small meals and snacks are recommended (Ball 1997). A dietician may be helpful in this respect.

Physical exercise can improve psychological well-being by increasing self-esteem and enhancing quality of life, and therefore should be encouraged (Giannini et al 2006). Education focusing on safe and appropriate insulin administration, other control measures, and the condition itself is important and is generally carried out by the child's general medical practitioner. Most children require insulin injections twice a day with the dosage dependent upon the individual. Regular capillary blood glucose measurement is a useful form of monitoring.

Problems secondary to diabetes which may arise are hypoglycemia, refractory hyperglycemia in the early part of the day owing to waning insulin action from the previous evening's injection (dawn phenomenon), and psychological problems in both parents and the child (Hull & Johnston 1987). Long-term complications may arise within 20 years of onset of the disorder and include renal failure, myocardial infarction, diabetic eye disease, gangrene and peripheral neuropathies.

Hypoglycemia

Hypoglycemia is rare beyond the newborn period (Gruppuso & Schwartz 1989). However, it needs to be considered when non-febrile seizures occur, especially in the early morning or after fasting in the diabetic child (Hull & Johnston 1987). There are two main forms that are differentiated by the presence or absence of ketones. Causes include ketotic hypoglycemia, hepatic enzyme deficiencies, hepatotoxins, endocrine deficiencies, pancreatic or hepatic tumors, and pre-diabetes mellitus (DiGeorge et al 1996, Hughes 1975). Reducing the overall amount of refined carbohydrates may also be important in the treatment of idiopathic hypoglycemia (Saunders et al 1982), as well as known food allergies (Rapp 1991).

Presentation of the child with hypoglycemia
Children with hypoglycemia may appear irritable, nervous, tired, pale and confused. They may demonstrate behavioral problems such as tantrums and complain of headaches, paresthesias and muscle weakness (DiGeorge et al 1996, Hull & Johnston 1987, Rapp 1991). Food may be demanded urgently by these children who may subsequently improve upon eating. This needs to be differentiated from allergic causes. In severe untreated cases, tachycardia, shock and coma may follow (DiGeorge et al 1996, Hull & Johnston 1987). Young infants may also demonstrate flushing, sweating, cyanosis, limpness, twitching, apneic spells and abnormal neurological signs (DiGeorge et al 1996, Hughes 1975).

Laboratory findings and management
In severe cases, treatment may be necessary before any tests can be performed. Screening tests may include a 12-hour fasting blood glucose test, prolonged oral glucose tolerance test, urinalysis for glucose and reducing substances, serum thyroxine test, and fasting and postprandial insulin levels. In acute cases, glucose infusions are given followed by frequent feeding of carbohydrates and protein. Pathological causes need to be dealt with accordingly and idiopathic cases managed through dietary measures.

Disorders of the thyroid and parathyroid glands

Hypothyroidism

Hypothyroidism is one of the most common endocrine abnormalities of childhood affecting approximately 1 in every

4000 live births (DiGeorge et al 1996, Hull & Johnston 1987). It may be evident in the neonate (cretinism) or develop after a period of apparently normal thyroid functioning. Girls are twice as likely as boys to be affected (DiGeorge et al 1996). It may arise through congenital causes, often associated with embryonic developmental abnormalities, or be acquired, as is the case in autoimmunization disorders, surgery, irradiation, iodine deficiency, or ingestion of goitrogens.

Presentation of the child with hypothyroidism
Clinical manifestations of hypothyroidism depend upon the degree and duration of thyroid dysfunction. Diagnosis prior to 6 months of age is often difficult (Rapp 1991). There are numerous signs suggestive of this disorder, including an increased birth weight, prolonged physiological icterus, feeding and respiratory difficulties, coarse facies, excessive sleeping and decreased crying. Both physical and mental growth and development may be retarded and facial features of wide-set eyes, a large tongue and short, thick neck may be present. Muscles will be hypotonic, deep tendon reflexes 'hung up', and rheumatic symptoms (Keenan et al 1993) such as myalgia and arthralgia have been shown to occur. The thyroid gland may be enlarged or there may be an associated thyroglossal cyst.

Laboratory findings
Thyroxin (T4) and tri-iodothyronine (T3) levels will be decreased. If the condition is due to a primary thyroid defect, then plasma levels of thyroid-stimulating hormone (TSH) will be increased. Anemia may also be detected and in children over 2 years of age cholesterol levels can be increased. GH and thyroglobulin levels may be decreased.

X-ray findings
Approximately 60% of children with hypothyroidism will demonstrate a delay in bone age upon X-ray with epiphyseal dysgenesis (DiGeorge et al 1996). Deformities of the thoracic and lumbar vertebrae are sometimes evident and an increase in sella turcica size, widening of sutures and wormian bones (bone islands within sutures) in the skull.

Treatment
Early diagnosis and treatment are imperative owing to the possibility of permanent mental retardation. Therapy is aimed at restoring normal physical and mental development. Treatment includes medication, usually with synthetically prepared thyroxine. Evaluation of bone age gives an indication of response to treatment. It should be noted that 50% of infants with severe hypothyroidism will retain some degree of mental retardation (DiGeorge et al 1996). In cases where the onset is more gradual, there is a corresponding improvement in prognosis. For children in whom the onset is after the second year of life, there is usually no mental retardation provided adequate treatment has been implemented and continued (DiGeorge et al 1996, Hughes 1975).

Hyperthyroidism

In childhood, hyperthyroidism is less common than hypothyroidism. It is sometimes called Graves disease (Hughes 1975). Females are affected five times more often than males and it often arises just prior to puberty (Imrie et al 2001). Immune factors are partly responsible for its occurrence and hereditary factors may play a role in its development. Affected individuals produce an immunoglobulin that binds with the TSH receptor, stimulating it to produce excessive amounts of thyroid hormone, thus leading to hyperthyroidism.

Presentation of the child with hyperthyroidism

Symptoms of hyperthyroidism usually develop gradually over a 6–12 month period (DiGeorge et al 1996). The thyroid, thymus, spleen and lymph nodes enlarge, and the child may exhibit a voracious appetite, smooth flushed skin, excessive sweating, exophthalmos and emotional disturbances. There may also be muscular weakness or motor hyperactivity. Hyperthyroidism is sometimes associated with tall-for-age stature.

Laboratory findings

T3 and T4 levels are increased and TSH levels decreased.

Treatment

Correction of hyperthyroidism involves either a partial thyroidectomy or antithyroid medication. The child should also be given regular chiropractic care as excessive thyroid hormone has the potential to produce widespread changes in muscle tone and thereafter contribute to the subluxation complex.

Hyperparathyroidism

This is a rare condition. It may arise from primary causes such as a parathyroid adenoma in the older child and idiopathic hyperplasia in the infant, or secondary causes such as renal insufficiency, vitamin D insufficiency rickets, and malabsorption syndromes (DiGeorge et al 1996).

Presentation of the child with hyperparathyroidism

Affected children present with vomiting, nausea, weight loss, polydipsia and polyuria. Musculoskeletal manifestations may include back and extremity pain, gait disturbance, muscular weakness, bony deformities and fracture (DiGeorge et al 1996, Hughes 1975). In a parathyroid crisis, oliguria, azotemia, stupor and coma may occur, and with progression, mental retardation, convulsions and blindness can result (DiGeorge et al 1996, Hughes 1975).

Laboratory findings

Serum calcium and parathyroid hormone (PTH) levels will be increased.

X-ray findings

On X-ray, subperiosteal resorption of bone with loss of cortical definition in the phalanges of the hands, trabeculation of the skull and, later, bone cysts, fractures and deformities may be seen (DiGeorge et al 1996, Hughes 1975, Rowe & Yochum 1987). Approximately 10% of affected children will develop rickets (DiGeorge et al 1996).

Differential diagnoses

Hyperparathyroidism needs to be differentiated from idiopathic hyperglycemia and malignancies such as Wilms' tumor and non-Hodgkin's lymphoma (Hughes 1975). Other uncommon causes are vitamin D intoxication, prolonged immobilization and lithium use (Allergheiligen et al 1998).

Treatment

Surgical exploration is common, with removal of any tumor if found.

Hypoparathyroidism

Hypoparathyroidism may arise from removal or damage to the parathyroid glands during thyroid surgery or from aplasia. However, permanent hypoparathyroidism is rare in childhood, with a transient form being common in the neonate in the first 12–72 hours of life, especially in cases of prematurity, asphyxia at birth, and in infants of diabetic mothers (DiGeorge et al 1996, Hughes 1975, Hull & Johnston 1987). Infants of mothers with hypoparathyroidism may also develop a transient form of the disease (Hughes 1975).

Presentation of the child with hypoparathyroidism

Affected infants present with generalized or focal convulsions, laryngospasm and apneic episodes (Hull & Johnston 1987). With increasing age there may also be associated anemia, Addison's disease, thyroiditis, hypothyroidism, diabetes mellitus and hepatitis (DiGeorge et al 1996).

Laboratory findings

Serum calcium is low and phosphorus level high.

X-ray findings

Calcification of the basal ganglia is sometimes seen.

Differential diagnoses

Hypoparathyroidism needs to be differentiated from magnesium deficiency, poisoning with inorganic phosphate, acute leukemia, renal insufficiency, and pseudohypoparathyroidism that is hereditary (DiGeorge et al 1996, Hughes 1975).

Disorders of the adrenal glands

Disorders of the adrenal medulla are rare and usually less obvious than those of the adrenal cortex. Only cortex disorders will be considered in this chapter.

Adrenocortical insufficiency

Adrenocortical insufficiency occurs when cortisol and/or aldosterone production is deficient. It is uncommon in childhood and may present as either a primary or chronic form (Addison's disease) (Merck Manual 1999). Causes include congenital aplasia, hypoplasia or hyperplasia of the adrenals, hemorrhage due to trauma and fulminating infections. Addison's disease may arise idiopathically or be due to destruction of the adrenal gland by granuloma (e.g. tuberculosis, which has become increasingly common recently, especially in developing countries), tumor, amyloidosis or inflammatory necrosis (Merck Manual 1999). Lesions of the pituitary and hypothalamus can also affect adrenal function.

Presentation of the child with adrenocortical insufficiency

In the acute form, shock-like symptoms such as hypotension, a weak and rapid pulse, cyanosis, cold clammy skin and hyperpyrexia are seen. The child may also vomit and have diarrhea and rapid respiration, and fall into a coma. In the infant, it may be indistinguishable from more common conditions such as pulmonary infection, sepsis or intracranial hemorrhage (Hughes 1975). In Addison's disease, manifestations arise more gradually and include weakness, anorexia, weight loss, vomiting attacks, diarrhea, abdominal pain, episodes of hypoglycemia, salt cravings, low blood pressure and recurrent convulsions. Hyperpigmentation of exposed areas of skin and the umbilicus, axillae, nipples and joints may also develop.

Laboratory findings

Serum sodium, chloride and glucose may be lowered and potassium increased. There is a decrease in 24-hour measurement of urinary 17-hydroxycorticosteroids.

Treatment

Acute cases require immediate referral for intensive emergency treatment with the administration of cortisol, glucose and saline solution. In chronic cases, long-term replacement therapy with cortisol and sometimes salt-retaining drugs such as flurohydrocortisone is utilized. Referral for concurrent naturopathic care to support adrenal function is appropriate and regular chiropractic care is essential.

Adrenocortical hyperfunction

The predominant manifestations of adrenocortical hyperfunction depend upon whether androgenic hormones, cortisol, aldosterone or estrogens are produced in excess.

Adrenogenital syndrome

Adrenogenital syndrome arises when there is an increase in androgenic hormone production because of adrenal hyperplasia or tumor. Effects are variable and virilization occurs in newborn females owing to increased testosterone levels. If untreated, there is early growth of pubic and axillary hair, acne, deepening of the voice, and acceleration of linear growth. Defects are only occasionally evident at birth in males but excessive growth and precocious puberty develop at around 4–5 years of age. One-third of those affected also have manifestations of adrenal insufficiency, with anorexia, diarrhea, failure to thrive or weight loss, and eventually a salt-losing crisis (Hughes 1975).

Laboratory findings

Urinary steroids, serum sodium, chloride, potassium and renin levels are all assessed.

Treatment

Cortisone is administered to decrease androgen production and retard the process of virilization.

Cushing syndrome

Cushing syndrome arises as a result of excessive levels of cortisol. Although a rare condition in childhood, it is more commonly seen in young girls than in boys. Causes include adrenocortical tumors in infants, adrenal hyperplasia in older children, and ACTH-producing extra-adrenal tumors.

Presentation of the child with Cushing syndrome

Children usually present with centripetal obesity, hirsutism, and impaired growth with delayed puberty, hypertension, headache and emotional lability. They may also suffer with backache and muscular weakness and have skin that bruises easily with stretch marks.

Laboratory findings

There is often glycosuria, hyperglycemia and eosinophilia as well as abnormal diurnal rhythms of plasma cortisol levels and increased urinary corticosteroids.

X-ray findings

Osteoporosis and osteonecrosis of the vertebrae may be evident on X-ray and sometimes sella turcica enlargement (Carter 1997, Rowe & Yochum 1987).

Differential diagnoses

The main differential of Cushing syndrome is the benignly obese child. However, these children are usually tall, not short, in stature.

Treatment

Surgical exploration for tumors is carried out with excision and/or radiotherapy if necessary. Occasionally ACTH agonists are given. For the chiropractor, bone weakening vertebral changes must be taken into consideration when adjusting these children.

Hyperaldosteronism

Hyperaldosteronism is usually caused by a tumor and associated with adrenal hyperplasia. It results in hypersecretion of aldosterone with an inability to concentrate urine. Affected children suffer with polyuria, polydipsia and muscular weakness. Sometimes there are also paresthesias, periodic paralysis, tetany and edema (DiGeorge et al 1996, Hughes 1975).

Laboratory findings

Serum sodium, calcium, phosphorus and chlorides are usually increased, and urinary aldosterone secretion is also increased.

Metabolic disease

There are numerous metabolic diseases that may affect children. These include defects in amino acid, lipid and carbohydrate metabolism as well as disorders of mucopolysaccharide, purine and heme metabolism. Hypoglycemia may also be considered a metabolic disorder and there are several metabolic myopathies.

Clinically, the more severe of these disorders are usually evident in the neonate as non-specific manifestations which need to be differentiated from severe generalized infections (Rezvani & Rosenblatt 1996). Without treatment, some can be fatal. Milder forms of metabolic disease may not be recognized for several months or years after the neonatal period as early manifestations are often non-specific and attributable to prenatal insults (Rezvani & Rosenblatt 1996). Signs may vary depending upon the type of disorder and the age of onset. In general, suspicion of metabolic disease should be raised in a child with unexplained mental retardation, developmental delays, motor deficits or convulsions. Affected children may also suffer episodes of unexplained vomiting, acidosis, mental deterioration and coma, and have an unusual body odor, particularly during times of illness (e.g. urine that smells of maple syrup in maple syrup urine disease, or a mousy smell in phenylketonuria). Other manifestations include hepatomegaly and renal stones. Often there is a family history of metabolic disease. All cases where the suspicion index for metabolic disease is heightened should be referred in the first instance for further investigation prior to the administration of chiropractic care.

References

Aaronov, D., Tasher, D., Levine, A., et al., 2008. Natural history of food allergy in infants and children in Israel. Ann. Allergy Asthma Immunol. 101 (6), 637–640.

Ader, R., Cohen, N., 1993. Psychoneuroimmunology: conditioning and stress. Annu. Rev. Psychol. 44, 53–85.

Allerheiligen, D.A., Schoeber, J., Houston, R.E., et al., 1998. Hyperparathyroidism. Am. Fam. Physician 57 (8), 1795–1802.

Arroyave, C.M., 2001. Recurrent otitis media with effusion and food allergy in pediatric patients. Rev. Alerg. Mex. 48 (5), 141–144.

Ball, M., 1997. Diabetes. In: Walqvist, M.L. (Ed.), Food and Nutrition. Allen and Unwin, St Leonards.

Beaudry, M., Dufour, R., Marcoux, S., 1995. Relation between infant feeding and infections during the first six months of life. J. Pediatr. 126 (2), 191–197.

Besedovsky, H.O., del Rey, A., Sorkin, E., et al., 1986. Immunoregulatory feedback between interleukin-1 and glucocorticoid hormones. Science 233, 652–654.

Blalock, J.E., Smith, E.M., 1985. A complete regulatory loop between the immune and neuroendocrine systems. Fed. Proc. 44, 108–111.

Briggs, D.R., Lennard, L.B., 1997. Food sensitivities. In: Walqvist, M.L. (Ed.), Food and Nutrition. Allen and Unwin, St Leonards.

Carter, W., 1997. The Australian Home Guide to Medication. Redwood Editions, Dingley.

Davies, N.J., 1997. A Reader for Clinical Chiropractic Paediatrics. RMIT Press, Bundoora, p. 249.

DiGeorge, A.M., Parks, J.S., Garibaldi, L., et al., 1996. The endocrine system. In: Behrman, R., Kliegman, R., Arvin, A. (Eds), Nelson Textbook of Paediatrics, fifteenth ed. WB Saunders, Philadelphia.

Giannini, C., Mohn, A., Chiarelli, F., 2006. Physical exercise and diabetes during childhood. Acta Biomed. 77 (Suppl. 1), 18–25.

Gruppuso, P.A., Schwartz, R., 1989. Hypoglycemia in children. Pediatr. Rev. 11, 117–124.

Hughes, J.G., 1975. Synopsis of paediatrics, fourteenth ed. Mosby, St Louis.

Hull, D., Johnston, D.I., 1987. Essential Paediatrics, second ed. Churchill Livingstone, Edinburgh.

Imrie, H., Vaidya, B., Perros, P., et al., 2001. Evidence for a Graves' disease susceptibility locus at chromosome Xp11 in a United Kingdom population. J. Clin. Endocrinol. Metab. 86 (2), 626–630.

Keenan, G.F., Ostrov, B.E., Goldsmith, D.P., et al., 1993. Rheumatic symptoms associated with hypothyroidism in children. J. Pediatr. 123 (4), 586–588.

Machida, H.M., Catto-Smith, A.G., Gall, D.G., et al., 1994. Allergic colitis in infancy: clinical and pathological aspects. J. Pediatr. Gastroenterol. Nutr. 19 (1), 22–26.

Merck Manual, 1999. Merck Manual of Diagnosis and Therapy, seventeenth ed. Merck Research Laboratories, Rahway, NJ.

Miller, S., Miller, J., 1979. Food for Thought: A New Look at Food and Behaviour, Prentice-Hall, New Jersey.

Munck, A., Guyre, P., 1986. Glucocorticoid physiology, pharmacology and stress. Adv. Exp. Med. Biol. 196, 81–96.

Nagel, G., Büchele, G., Weinmayr, G., et al.; ISAAC Phase Two Study Group, 2009. Effect of breastfeeding on asthma, lung function and bronchial hyperreactivity in ISAAC phase II. Eur. Respir. J. 33 (5), 993–1002.

National Diabetes Information Clearinghouse (NDIC), 2008. Available at: http://diabetes. niddk.nih.gov/dm/pubs/statistics/ (accessed April 2009).

Nsouli, T.M., Nsouli, S.M., Linde, R.E., et al., 1994. Role of food allergy in serous otitis media. Ann. Allergy 73, 216–219.

Odze, R.D., Wershill, B.K., Leichter, A.M., et al., 1995. Allergic colitis in infants. J. Pediatr. 126 (2), 163–167.

Rapp, D., 1991. Is This Your Child? Discovering and Treating Unrecognised Allergies in Children and Adults. William Morrow, New York.

Rezvani, I., Rosenblatt, D.S., 1996. Metabolic diseases. In: Behrman, R., Kliegman, R., Arvin, A. (Eds), Nelson Textbook of Paediatrics, fifteenth ed. WB Saunders, Philadelphia.

Rowe, L.J., Yochum, T.R., 1987. Essentials of Skeletal Radiology. Williams and Wilkins, Baltimore.

Saunders, L.R., Hofeldt, F.D., Kirk, M.C., et al., 1982. Refined carbohydrate as a contributing factor in reactive hypoglycaemia. South Med. J. 75 (9), 1072–1075.

Schmidt, M.A., 1990. Healing Childhood Ear Infections. North Atlantic Books, Berkeley.

Sears, M.R., Greene, J.M., Willan, A.R., et al., 2002. Long-term relation between breastfeeding and development of atopy and asthma in children and young adults: a longitudinal study. Lancet 360 (9337), 901–907.

Siltanen, M., Kaiosaari, M., Poussa, T., et al., 2003. A dual long-term effect of breastfeeding on atopy in relation to heredity in children at 4 years of age. Allergy 58 (6), 524–530.

Sly, M.R., 1996. Allergic disorders. In: Behrman, R., Kliegman, R., Arvin, A. (Eds), Nelson Textbook of Paediatrics, fifteenth ed. WB Saunders, Philadelphia.

Yamanaka, C., Momoi, T., Fujisawa, I., et al., 1993. Acquired growth hormone deficiency due to pituitary stalk transaction after head trauma in childhood. Eur. J. Pediatr. 152 (2), 99–101.

Pediatric nutrition

19

Neil J. Davies

In the so-called developed or western world, we have progressively moved further and further away from sound principles of nutrition. Packaged, processed everything has replaced natural, whole foods eaten as close to raw as possible. A good example of this is the breakfast cereals that specifically target children. A *Choice Magazine* survey (2007) of breakfast cereals available in supermarkets, for example, revealed that 'around 70% of the kids' cereals have too little fiber to be worth recommending. Of the kids' ones that make the grade for fiber, only six aren't spoilt by being too salty or sugary.' Similar observations could be made for the plethora of take away and 'fast foods' that are increasingly forming a regular part of the staple diet of today's child and adolescent.

There remains a critical role for the chiropractor to play in the field of pediatric nutrition. The chiropractor often meets the child and family for the first time at a point of ill health, at which time an opportunity to address longstanding poor nutritional practices presents itself. Taking the opportunity to steer the child and wider family away from processed, packaged, over-salted and sugary foods back to sound nutritional principles is a health promotion, disease prevention strategy that falls comfortably within the chiropractic paradigm of wellness.

In order to take this opportunity, the chiropractor needs to be familiar with the general principles of nutritional practice and the fundamental strategies used to measure, assess and advise patients accordingly. To provide patients and their families with sound, reliable information that will impact their health in the longer term, a knowledge of the nutritional requirements of infants and children, best feeding practices for the various age levels in pediatrics, and techniques for collecting and assessing food intake information is needed. Familiarity with the more common disorders of metabolism and nutrition that may be encountered in chiropractic practice is also essential.

Nutritional requirements of infants and children

Infants grow rapidly during the first year of life, increasing their weight threefold and their length twofold in that time. The rate of growth slows beyond the end of the first year, but still imposes a significant and unique nutritional demand. The nutrient turnover rate and higher metabolic rate of children as compared to adults, when superimposed on the need to support these rates of growth, create high maintenance needs as the clinician considers the various factors of health promotion in the child and adolescent patient. Failure to provide consistently adequate nutrition to children is also likely to affect not only growth but also development, both somatic and organic.

Recommended (or reference) intakes of most nutrients have been established, and these appear to fulfill the unique nutritional needs of the infant and young child. These requirements are summarized for the 0–6-month-old infant, the 6–12-month-old infant, the 1–3-year-old child, and the 4–8-year-old child in Table 19.1 (Heird 2004).

Feeding the child in the first year of life

Breastfeeding or bottlefeeding?

Infant nursing is a time-honored practice in all cultures and ages in human history. Breastfeeding is an unequalled way of providing ideal food for the healthy growth and development of infants; it is also an integral part of the reproductive process with important implications for the health of mothers. Human breastmilk is widely accepted to be the optimal source of nutrition for the newborn infant as it contains all the proteins, lipids, carbohydrates, micronutrients and trace elements necessary for optimal growth, development and immune protection.

© 2010, Elsevier Ltd, Inc, BV
DOI: 10.1016/B978-0-7020-3129-8.00019-0

Table 19.1 Daily reference intake of nutrients for normal infants

Nutrient	Reference intake per day			
	0–6 Mo (6 kg)	7–12 Mo (9 kg)	1–3 Yr (13 kg)	4–8 Yr (22 kg)
Energy (kcal (kJ)/24 h*	550 (2310)	720 (3013)	1074 (4494)	–
Fat (g/24 h)	31 (AI)	30 (AI)	–	–
Linoleic acid (g/24 h)	4.4 (AI)	4.6 (AI)	7 (AI)	10 (AI)
α-Linoleic acid (g/24 h)	0.5 (AI)	0.5 (AI)	0.7 (AI)	0.9 (AI)
Carbohydrate (g/24 h)	60 (EAR)	95 (EAR)	130 (RDA)	130 (RDA)
Protein (g/24 h)*	9.3 (EAR)	11 (RDA)	–	21 (RDA)
Electrolytes and minerals:				
Calcium (mg/24 h)	210[†]	270[†]	500[†]	800[†]
Phosphorus (mg/24 h)	100[†]	275[†]	460*	500
Magnesium (mg/24 h)	30[†]	75[†]	80*	130*
Sodium (mg/24 h)*	120	200	225	300
Chloride (mg/24 h)*	180	300	350	500
Potassium (mg/24 h)*	500	700	1000 (1 yr)	1400
Iron (mg/24 h)	0.27[†]	11*	7*	10*
Zinc (mg/24 h)	2[†]	3*	3*	5*
Copper (μg/24 h)	200[†]	220*	340*	440*
Iodine (μg/24 h)	110[†]	130[†]	90*	90*
Selenium (μg/24 h)	15[†]	20[†]	20*	30*
Manganese (mg/24 h)	0.003[†]	0.6[†]	102[†]	1.5[†]
Fluoride (mg/24 h)	0.01[†]	0.5[†]	0.7[†]	1.0[†]
Chromium (μg/24 h)	0.2[†]	5.5[†]	11[†]	15[†]
Molybdenum (μg/24 h)	2[†]	3[†]	17	22
Vitamins:				
Vitamin A (μg/24 h)	400[†]	500[†]	300*	400*
Vitamin E (mg α-TE/24 h)	4[†]	6[†]	6*	7*
Vitamin K (μg/24 h)	2.0[†]	2.5[†]	30[†]	55[†]
Vitamin C (mg/24 h)	40[†]	50[†]	15*	25*
Thiamine (mg/24 h)	0.2[†]	0.3[†]	0.5*	0.6*
Riboflavin (mg/24 h)	0.3[†]	0.4[†]	0.5*	0.6*
Vitamin B_6 (μg/24 h)	0.1[†]	0.3[†]	0.5*	0.6*
Folate (μg)	65[†]	80[†]	150*	200*
Vitamin B_{12} (μg/24 h)	0.4[†]	0.5[†]	0.9*	1.2*

Continued

Nutrient	Reference intake per day			
	0–6 Mo (6 kg)	7–12 Mo (9 kg)	1–3 Yr (13 kg)	4–8 Yr (22 kg)
Biotin (μg/24 h)	5[†]	6[†]	8[†]	12[†]
Pantothenic acid (mg/24 h)	1.7[†]	1.8[†]	2[†]	3[†]
Choline (mg/24 h)	125[†]	150[†]	200[†]	250[†]

AI, adequate intake; RDA, recommended daily amount; EAR, estimated average requirement; α-TE, alpha-tocopherol.

*RDA.

[†]AI (e.g. for infants <1year of age, this is the mean intake of normal breastfed infants).

Heird WC 2004 Nutritional requirements during infancy. In: Bowman BA, Russell RM (eds) Present knowledge in nutrition, 8th edn. International Life Sciences Institute (ILSI) Press, Washington, DC, pp 416–425.

The importance of breastmilk and its superiority as a source of infant nutrition is highlighted in the recent overhaul of the World Health Organization growth charts that are now based on exclusively breastfed infants. As a global public health recommendation, infants should be exclusively breastfed for the first 6 months of life to achieve optimal growth, development and health (World Health Organization 2003). In Australia, the 2001 National Health Survey showed that 87% of infants aged between 0 and 3 years had at some stage obtained nutrition from breastmilk – a similar figure (86%) to that identified in the 1995 survey (Australian Bureau of Statistics 2003).

Breastfeeding should be initiated as soon after the birth of the child as possible, depending, of course, on the infant's ability to tolerate enteral nutrition. Putting the newborn baby to the breast immediately postpartum facilitates the delivery of the placenta since the sucking of the areola stimulates the release of the nanopeptide hormone oxytocin from the adeno-hypophysis of the pituitary gland, which in turn causes myometrial contractions of the uterine wall (Sherwood 2006).

Breastfeeding in the immediate postpartum period also fosters mother–infant bonding (Feldman et al 2007, Kennell & McGrath 2005), with oxytocin levels having been shown to be critical in the promotion of successful bonding (Debiec 2007). Breastfeeding in the first hours of life also plays a role in maintaining normal metabolism as the baby progresses from fetal to extrauterine life. Breastfeeding has demonstrated long-term benefits for the overall health of the infant, with a reduced risk of the development of serious disorders. For example, infants who have been breastfed for a period in excess of 6 months have been shown to be less likely to develop autistic disorder than their counterparts who were artificially fed infant formula without docosahexaenoic acid/arachidonic acid supplementation (Schultz et al 2006). Breastfeeding has also been shown to play a significant role in the prevention of conditions such as obesity, gastrointestinal diseases (Kristin et al 2007), childhood cancers including leukemia (Shu et al 1999), bedwetting (Barone et al 2006), and the later development of asthma and allergies (Fulhan et al 2003).

It is axiomatic, therefore, that mothers should be encouraged and supported in their efforts to commence nursing their newborn infants as soon after delivery as possible. In the words of one young mother, when asked why she breastfed:

I breastfeed because it is how human females were designed to nurture their young. I breastfeed because it allows me precious close time with my daughter. I breastfeed because it ensures my daughter is getting optimum nutrition, antibodies, and will have smaller chances of contracting major diseases. I breastfeed because it is convenient, portable, easy and because she can have access to it anytime she wants. If I wanted to go out without her I could express enough milk for her to drink. I breastfeed because it eases her discomforts, it nurtures her soul as well as her body, and it offers a warm, safe and peaceful place to be when she is sad or hurts herself.

(Day 2006)

Introducing solid food

Solid foods should ideally be introduced to the infant at 6 months. Prior to that, wholly breastfeeding is not only adequate, it is highly desirable as it provides all the necessary nutrients for growth and development and avoids the possibility of an allergic or hypersensitivity reaction to solid foods, especially where there is a positive family history for atopic disease. The infantile gut is not mature enough to handle food other than mother's milk in the first 4–6 months of life, making the addition of solid foods undesirable until then.

There is also a commonly held belief that if a baby is given solid food late in the day it will aid sleeping though the night as it will create a feeling of fullness in the baby's stomach. This is, of course, patently untrue as food passes from the stomach into the small intestine in a short period, especially when the food is essentially carbohydrate as would be the case in a baby. It is also important to note that the potential for choking is much higher in a baby taking solids in the first 6 months of life than after that time.

When confronted with the question from parents as to whether or not their baby is ready for solid foods, the chiropractor needs first to determine the following:

- Can the baby hold its head steady when sitting?
- Does the baby open the mouth when food is offered?
- Does the baby show interest in food when other family members are eating?
- Does the baby effortlessly swallow food that is placed on its tongue?

Having determined that a baby is ready to start solid foods, the next question will be what foods to offer first. The most easily digested food for a baby starting out on solids is iron-fortified rice cereal. This product is readily available at any supermarket or health food store and is best mixed with mother's milk until it has a consistency much like nectar. Small portions are placed on the middle of the baby's tongue using a teaspoon. It is not uncommon for babies to initially reject a new food, perhaps due to the different texture and/or taste. Persistence is sometimes required to get the baby to begin taking the new food. Once the nectar-consistency cereal is being taken comfortably, it should be made thicker, more like a paste. This prepares baby for the addition of other foods of a similar consistency.

Adding new foods

Once the baby is comfortable with and is obviously enjoying cereal, other foods should be introduced at a rate of about two each week. The best foods to add next are vegetables that have been steamed and then pureed, and the sweeter fruits, such as pears, mango, etc. Each time a new food is added, the baby should be monitored for any evidence of allergic or hypersensitivity reaction such as diarrhea, vomiting, or the appearance of a new skin rash. It is worth pointing out that fruit juices are not appropriate in the first year of life and are best left out of the child's diet at least until he or she can drink competently from a cup. Offering fruit juices in baby bottles creates an unacceptable risk of tooth decay.

By the age of 7–8 months, babies should be having two meals of vegetables and fruit per day (8 tablespoons total) as well as regular breastfeeds on demand. The solid food component can be increased as demand requires and this may be associated with a reduction in the number of breastfeeds. By the age of 12 months, most babies can eat small portions of the soft table foods those in the wider family are eating. Table 19.2 provides a good general guide to offer parents.

The soy milk controversy

Artificial feeding of infants using soy milk formulae is promoted to the general public and health care practitioners alike as having significant health-enhancing benefits, including the care of babies with cow's milk intolerance (CMI) and cow's milk allergy (CMA), both of which are widely, and inappropriately, referred to as 'lactose intolerance'. Research on the use of soy milk baby formulae as an alternative in babies with CMI and CMA began to appear in the scientific literature in the 1970s and accelerated exponentially in the 1980s, and from there onwards to the present day. There is now a plethora of reported research trials on the effect of soy milk artificial formulae on CMI and CMA in particular. Results vary widely, but one thing is clear: there is an unacceptably high cross-reactivity between cow's milk and soy milk, making the advertising claims suspicious at best. In addition, a review of the epidemiological literature has not shown there to be any substance to the assertion that soy products confer a degree of protection from certain forms of cancer (Peeters et al 2003) or the prevention of infantile colic, regurgitation, or prolonged crying (Agostoni et al 2006).

What does not appear to have been widely disseminated, however, is the possibility of harmful effects of soy products designed for consumption by infants. Soy milk contains extraordinarily high levels of bioactive phytoestrogens, up to

Table 19.2 Use of food pyramid guidelines	
Age	**May begin. . .**
At 6 months	Iron-fortified baby rice cereal
	Strained/pureed vegetables (sweet potato, pumpkin, peas, carrots)
	Sweet and semi-sweet fruits (mango, pear, paw paw, banana, avocado)
6–9 months	Mixtures of pureed vegetables (broccoli, zucchini, etc.)
	Sweet and semi-sweet fruits (apple, peach, melon, nectarines, apricots)
	Chunky, soft prepared baby foods (soft carrot sticks and other vegetables)
	Yogurt, custard
	Rusks and other hand-held foods
	Porridge
9–12 months	Soft, finely chopped foods, soft combination foods such as casseroles, pasta and cheese, rice dishes, firm cheeses, beans, lentils
12+ months	Potato
	Minced meat, poultry or fish
	General family foods
	Fiber foods such as bran, wheat germ, whole wheat cereals, etc.)
	Whole cow's milk

11 times higher than the levels demonstrated to exert a wide range of hormonal and non-hormonal effects in adults (Setchell et al 1997). While research aimed at determining the digestibility and absorption of bioactive phytoestrogens has concluded that the consumption of soy products in infancy should be regarded as being generally safe, the actual rate of uptake of genestein and daidzeine, which is so much higher than that seen in infants who are breastfed or artificially fed with cow's milk formulae, has raised concerns among researchers. Irvine et al (1998), for example, raise the issue that since neonates are generally more susceptible than adults to perturbations of the sex steroid milieu it would be highly desirable to study the effects of soy isoflavones on steroid-dependent developmental processes in human babies. This reluctance to endorse soy outright is also found among other investigators (Miniello et al 2003, Strom et al 2001).

In addition to the phytoestrogen issue, soy infant formula is manufactured, at least in part, from soy beans which have been sourced from growers using genetically modified (GM) engineering techniques. In 1999 Baby Milk Action, a UK-based group campaigning for safer infant feeding, surveyed the leading UK artificial baby milk companies to find out if they claimed their artificial baby milks (both soya-based and modified cow's milk) were GM free or not. This survey was conducted in response to numerous calls from worried parents. At that time Heinz Farley's, Cow & Gate and Milupa responded that they did not use GM-grown soy beans in their infant formula manufacture. Mead Johnson did not respond to the query and SMA admitted that they had used GM soya in 1997, but withdrew it due to consumer concern. In the author's own survey conducted in Australia, food scientists at all the manufacturers polled were unable to give an assurance there were no GM-sourced soy beans used in the manufacture of infant formula.

There has been much debate among the scientific fraternity now for years over the safety of GM products. Some scientists claim there is no problem while others claim it produces new toxins and may damage the immune system and potentially cause allergy and some forms of cancer. What is critical to understand in all this is the fact that adults have a widely varied diet while the formula-fed child receives only milk, meaning of course that whatever effect there is will be greatly amplified in the infant. The reality is that the effects of GM-grown foods on short- and long-term child development is simply unknown.

Given the present state of knowledge of the effects of soy on development, immune function, and later life, the unacceptable levels of aluminum and other toxic substances, and the apparent uncertainty within the scientific community, the most responsible reaction from the chiropractor confronted with the mother of a child in their first year of life is to advise that the use of soy baby formulae cannot be recommended.

Feeding the child in the second year of life

Once into their second year, children begin to adopt the eating practices of their wider family very quickly and begin to participate in family mealtimes. As a general guide,

children of this age should be having 500–700 ml of breast-milk, cereal milk, or whole cow's milk, in addition to 6–8 tablespoons of fruit and vegetables, four servings of cereal, bread or pasta, and two servings of a tablespoon each of meat, poultry or fish.

Feeding the older child

Guidelines for providing nutrition that leads to health promotion and disease prevention in growing, developing children have been well established and widely published for many years. There is a plethora of internet websites offering such advice with nearly as many versions of the good food pyramid for children available as well. In one sense, the advice to eat as wide a range of foods in as near to their natural state as possible is excellent, but to help practitioners and their patients to plan in a more detailed way, the use of the food pyramid for children (Fig. 19.1) and the information in Table 19.3 will be invaluable. Provision of this information to parents may help to enhance the chiropractic consultation and also place information in the hands of parents that will allow them to better protect their growing child's health and well-being.

To allow parents to better understand and utilize the detail found in the food pyramid, the generally accepted meaning of 'one serving' is as follows:

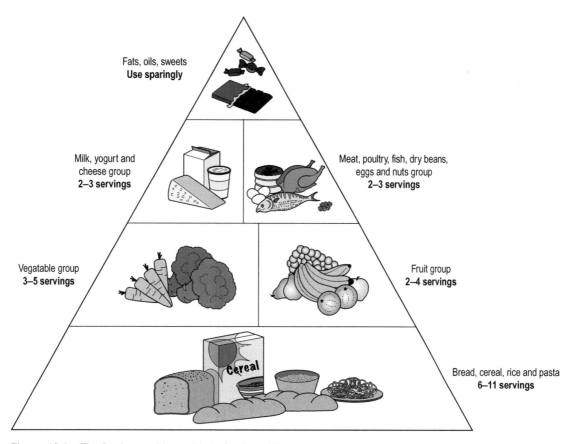

Figure 19.1 • The food pyramid: a guide to feeding children.

Table 19.3 General guideline for the introduction of solid foods in the first year of life

Food group	Serving size*	Servings/day
Grain	1 slice bread ½ cup rice (cooked) ½ cup pasta	6
Vegetables	½ cup raw or cooked 1 cup leafy	3
Fruit	¼ medium melon 1 whole fruit ¾ cup juice ½ cup canned ½ cup berries, grapes	2
Milk	1 cup milk, yogurt 2 oz cheese	2
Meat	2–3 oz cooked, lean ½ cup dried beans† 1 egg† 2 tbsp peanut butter	2
Fats/sweets		Limit

*These serving sizes are for 4–6-year-old children; serving sizes for 2–3-year-old children, except for milk, should be about two-thirds of those shown.
†These amounts are equal to 1 oz lean meat; two servings are equal to one meat serving.

Grain group

One serving is represented by 1 slice of bread, ½ cup of cooked rice or pasta, ½ cup of cooked cereal or 30 g of ready-to-eat cereal.

Vegetable group

One serving is represented by ½ cup of chopped or raw vegetables or 1 cup of raw green leafy vegetables.

Fruit group

One serving is represented by 1 piece of fruit or a melon wedge, ¾ cup of 100% fruit juice, ½ cup of canned fruit, or ¼ cup of dried fruit.

Milk group

One serving is represented by 1 cup of milk or yogurt or 60 g of cheese.

Meat group

One serving is represented by 60–80 g of cooked lean meat, poultry or fish, one egg, or ½ cup of cooked dry beans.

Collecting and assessing food intake information

Generally speaking, food intake assessment followed by very detailed dietary advice and monitoring is the professional domain of the dietitian or nutritionist. It is not the purpose of this section, or indeed this chapter, to suggest that this function be served by the family chiropractor. However, given the ready availability of reliable food nutrient information, it would seem reasonable for the family chiropractor to collect dietary information on appropriate patients in order to make an overall assessment of food categories it contains (i.e. total energy, protein, carbohydrate, total fat, calcium and iron), so that general dietary advice can be given which is specific to the presenting patient and within the guidelines of established nutritional requirements.

In Table 19.4, total food intake for a male child aged 5 years and 3 months is recorded and the nutrient breakdown calculated. This information is readily available using any of the multitude of on-line resources available today (Health Canada 2007) in addition to having the caregiver take the information directly from the nutritional information tables printed on packaging labels where this is available. The level to which the family chiropractor should go in assessing this information and advising the patient should reasonably be restricted to the percentiles of protein, carbohydrate and fat which make up the child's diet and the adequacy of the calcium and iron levels. This is by no means exhaustive, but does provide a well-balanced general look at the presenting patient's diet which will allow the family chiropractor to offer sound, evidenced-based advice.

From the information summary in Table 19.5, it is evident that this child's total energy intake at 5.3 MJ is inadequate (recommended level 7.6), the protein percentage is a little too high, the carbohydrate level is too high, and the total fat level is a little too low. In addition, the iron level is above that recommended and the calcium is extremely low.

Confronted with this information, the sort of advice the family chiropractor can offer to bring this diet more into line with internationally accepted standards could be as follows:

- Increase fat intake, preferably from vegetables, nuts, cold pressed oils, etc.
- Change protein source derivation from dependence upon highly refined foods such as white bread to wholemeal breads, dairy products, nuts, quality meat cuts, range-fed chicken, fish, etc.
- Increase the number of servings of fresh fruit and vegetables, which while still providing adequate carbohydrates will also provide essential vitamins, minerals and trace elements.
- Increase the number of foods per day which provide bioavailable calcium. This child needs adequate calcium for strong bone growth at this age and at present his levels are very low. It is urgent to address this issue in this case. The foods which should be recommended as containing the best sources of bioavailable calcium are as follows:
  - *Excellent sources*: spinach, turnip greens, mustard greens and collard greens.
  - *Very good sources*: blackstrap molasses, Swiss chard, yogurt, kale, mozzarella cheese, cow's milk and goat's milk. Basil, thyme, dill seed, cinnamon and peppermint leaves are also very good sources of calcium.
  - *Good sources*: romaine lettuce, celery, broccoli, sesame seeds, fennel, cabbage, summer squash, green beans,

Table 19.4 Three-day food intake record for a male child aged 5 years and 3 months

Day 1 Food	Energy kJ	Protein g/kJ (% total kJ)	Carbohydrate g/kJ (% total kJ)	Total fat g/kJ (% total kJ)	Calcium mg	Iron mg
Grape juice 110 ml	303	1.1/16.8	16.7/281.4	0.1/4.2	50.6	0.6
75 g white bread roll	780	6.8/113.4	36/604.8	1.5/58.8	64.5	2.1
1 dessert spoon chocolate paste	341	1.1/21	8.9/151.2	4.6/172.2	40	0.4
20 g wholemeal biscuit	370	1.3/21	10.9/184.8	4.5/172.2	9.8	1.5
2 brown slices of bread (50 g)	564	6/100.8	23.4/394.8	1.8/67.2	49.2	1.4
150 g tomato soup	270	2.3/37.8	11.3/189	1.5/58.8	52.5	1.4
50 g sausage	690	9/151.2	0.3/4.2	14.5/550.2	11.5	3.4
1 200 g pear	420	1/16.8	25/420	0	18	0.4
100 ml Fanta	220	0	14/235	0	1	0
100 ml Coke	175	0	11/184.4	0	11	0.2
1 chocolate cream cake	954	3.6/58.8	19.5/327.6	15.6/588	40.8	0.4
3 peppermint sweets	128	0	7.6/126	0	0	0
200 ml fruit drink	360	0	0	0.5/5	0	0.6
1 small portion chips (fried)	840	0	25/420	11/415.8	0	0
15 ml mayonnaise	310	0.2/4.2	4/67.2	6.5/247.8	1.6	0
50 g apple mousse	207	0.5/8.4	12.5/210	0	5	1.6
4 deep fried chicken nuggets	840	14.7/247.8	14.4/239.4	12/449.4	13	0.9
Total	7772	47.6/798 (10.3%)	240.5/4039.4 (51.9%)	74.1/2789.6 (35.9%)	368.5	14.9
Day 2 Food	**Energy kJ**	**Protein g/kJ (% total kJ)**	**Carbohydrate g/kJ (% total kJ)**	**Total fat g/kJ (% total kJ)**	**Calcium mg**	**Iron mg**
1 brown slice of bread	282	3/50.4	11.7/197.4	0.9/33.6	24.6	0.7
½ dessert spoon chocolate paste	170.5	0.55/10.5	4.45/75.6	2.3/86.1	20	0.4
50 ml grape juice	138	0.5/8.4	7.6/126	0.1/0	23	0.6
3 white rolls (150 g)	1560	13.6/226.8	72/1209.6	3/117.6	129	4.2
75 ml soya milk drink	123	1.9/33.6	1.9/33.6	1.5/58.8	11.3	0.1
40 g sasusage	552	7.2/121.8	0.2/4.2	11.6/436.8	9.2	2.72
1 dessert spoon raw beef paste	129	1.9/33.6	1.2/21	2.1/79.8	30	0.75
500 ml tinned tomato soup	900	7.5/126	37.5/630	5/189	175	1.4
6 small slices of French stick	520	4.5/75.6	24/403.2	1/37.8	43	1.4
1 dessertspoon herb butter	592	0.3/4.2	1.4/25.2	15.0/56.7	1	0
1 dessertspoon soya dessert	71	0.7/12.6	2.7/46.2	0.4/16,8	27.8	0.1
Total	5037.5	37.65/703.5 (13.9%)	164.65/2772 (55%)	42.9/1623.3 (32.3%)	493.9	12.37

Continued

Table 19.4 Three-day food intake record for a male child aged 5 years and 3 months—Continued

Day 3 Food	Energy kJ	Protein g/kJ (% total kJ)	Carbohydrate g/kJ (% total kJ)	Total fat g/kJ (% total kJ)	Calcium mg	Iron mg
1 50 g white roll	520	4.5/75.6	24/403.2	1/37.8	43	1.4
1 dessertspoon chocolate paste	341	1.1/21	8.9/151.2	4.6/172.2	40	0.4
20 ml grape juice	55	0.2/4.2	3.0/50.4	0	9.2	0.6
15 g Kit Kat	325	1.1/16.8	9.2/155.4	4.1/155.4	0	0 4
25 g wholemeal slice of bread	282	3/50.4	11.7/197.4	0.9/33.6	24.6	0.7
50 ml apple juice	89	0	5.3/88.2	0	17	0.9
200 ml lemon/lime drink	304	0.1/0	17.8/298.2	0.1/4.2	0	0.6
50 g egg noodles	250	2.5/42	37/199	0.2/8.4	16	2.6
120 g mixed vegetables	196	2.9/50.4	7.4/126	0.6/21	0	0.6
20 g prawn crackers	432	0.7/12.6	13.3/222.6	5.3/201.6	10.4	0.2
1 small banana	358	1.5/25.2	20/336	0	5	0.4
Total	3152	17.6/298.2 (9.4%)	157.6/2227.6 (70.6%)	16.8/634.2 (20.1%)	165.2	8.8

Table 19.5 Summary of nutrient content

Nutrient	Recommended value*	Measured value for this patient
Total energy MJ	7.6	5.3
Protein kJ	18–24	34
Carbohydrate kJ	130	187
Total fats kJ	90	45
Calcium mg	800	342
Iron mg	6–8	12

*The recommended values cited above are based on a total energy derivation ratio of protein 10%, carbohydrate 50% and total fats 40%.

garlic, tofu, Brussels sprouts, oranges, asparagus and crimini mushrooms. Oregano, rosemary, parsley, kombu and kelp are also good sources of calcium.

In summary, attention to the calcium and fat intake, the quality of the protein, and an improved intake of fruit and vegetables would radically improve this child's diet. Advice in addition to the above could also be given in the form of the *food guide pyramid* and, if more detailed counseling is required, a referral to a professional dietitian or nutritionist is appropriate.

References

Agostoni, C., Axelsson, I., Goulet, O., 2006. Soy protein infant formulae and follow-on formulae: a commentary by the ESPGHAN Committee on Nutrition. J. Pediatr. Gastroenterol. Nutr. 42 (4), 352–361.

Australian Bureau of Statistics, 2003. Breastfeeding in Australia. Publication 4810.0.55.001.Australian Bureau of Statistics, Canberra.

Barone, J.G., Ramasamy, R., Farkas, A., et al., 2006. Breastfeeding during infancy may protect against bed-wetting during childhood. Pediatrics 18 (1), 254–259.

Choice Magazine Online, 2007. Available at: www.choice.com.au/goArticle.aspx? id=104654 (accessed 29 August 2009).

Day, J. (Ed.) 2006. Breastfeeding...naturally. Australian Breastfeeding Association, East Malvern, Victoria.

Debiec, J., 2007. From affiliative behaviours to romantic feelings: a role of nanopeptides. FEBS Lett. 581 (14), 2580–2586.

Feldman, R., Weller, A., Zagoory-Sharon, O., et al., 2007. Evidence for a neuroendocrinological foundation of human affiliation: plasma oxytocin levels across pregnancy and the postpartum period predict mother–infant bonding. Psychol. Sci. 18 (11), 965–970.

Fulhan, J., Collier, S., Duggan, C., 2003. Update on pediatric nutrition: breastfeeding, infant nutrition and growth. Curr. Opin. Pediatr. 15, 323–332.

Health Canada, 2007. The Canadian Nutrient File. Available at: http://www.hc-sc.gc.ca/fn-an/nutrition/fiche-nutri-data/index-eng.php (accessed 29 August 2009).

Heird, W.C., 2004. Nutritional requirements. In: Behrman, R.E., Kliegman, R.M., Jenson, H.B. (Eds), Nelson Textbook of Pediatrics. seventeenth ed. Saunders, Philadelphia.

Irvine, C.H., Fitzpatrick, M.G., Alexander, S.L., 1998. Phytoestrogens in soy-based infant foods: concentrations, daily intake, and possible biological effects. Proc. Soc. Exp. Biol. Med. 217 (3), 247–253.

Kennell, J., McGrath, S., 2005. Starting the process of mother infant bonding. Acta Paediatr. 94 (6), 775–777.

Kristin, M.E., Berry, C.A., Cregan, M.D., 2007. The bioactive nature of human breastmilk. Breastfeed. Rev. 15 (3), 5–10.

Miniello, V.L., Moro, G.E., Tarantino, M., et al., 2003. Soy-based formulas and phyto-oestrogens: a safety profile. Acta Paediatr. Suppl. 91 (441), 93–100.

Peeters, P.H., Keinan-Boker, L., van der Schouw, Y.T., 2003. Phytoestrogens and breast cancer risk: review of the epidemiological evidence. Breast Cancer Res. Treat. 77 (2), 171–183.

Schultz, S.T., Klonoff-Cohen, H.S., Wingard, D.L., et al., 2006. Breastfeeding, infant formula supplementation, and autistic disorder: the results of a parent survey. Int. Breastfeed. J. 1, 16.

Setchell, K.D., Zimmer-Nechemias, L., Cai, J., et al., 1997. Exposure of infants to phyto-oestrogens from soy-based infant formula. Lancet 350 (9070), 23–27.

Sherwood, L., 2006. Fundamentals of Physiology, a Human Perspective. Thomson Brooks/Cole, Belmont, USA.

Shu, X.O., Linet, M.S., Steinbuch, M., et al., 1999. Breastfeeding and risk of acute childhood leukaemia. J. Natl. Cancer Inst. 91 (20), 1765–1772.

Strom, B.L., Schinnar, R., Zieglar, E.E., et al., 2001. Exposure to soy-based formula in infancy and endocrinological and reproductive outcomes in young adulthood. J. Am. Med. Assoc. 286 (10), 2402–2403.

World Health Organization, 2003. Global Strategy for Infant and Young Child Feeding. World Health Organization, Geneva.

Pain assessment and management in children

20

Neil J. Davies

Pain in the pediatric patient

Pain is a distressing situation for both the affected child and the parents. In a situation where correction of cerebral dysafferentation is unlikely to have an immediate pain-modulating effect, it becomes essential for the chiropractor to have a firm understanding of how to make an appropriate assessment and plan a management strategy. Failure on the part of the attending chiropractor to fully address the problem of a child's pain may well be perceived by the parents as a failure to adequately address and attempt to resolve their concerns for their child.

Despite the frequency of pediatric presentations where pain is a principal feature, and often the most traumatizing aspect of the child's condition, it still remains common for the immediate problem of pain to remain poorly addressed. Indeed, retrospective studies have demonstrated unequivocal evidence of underprescription of analgesics in clinical pain syndromes affecting neonates, infants and young children, to some degree based on the erroneous presumption that pain intensity cannot be accurately estimated in the very young, preverbal child (McGrath & Brigham 1992). It is interesting to note that while pain has been written about for many centuries, only in very recent times have the first standard, seminal textbooks on the subject of pain in the pediatric patient been published (McGrath 1990, McGrath & Unruh 1987, Ross & Ross 1988, Tyler & Krane 1990).

Pain is a sensation communicated to the brain from the periphery via highly specialized nerves termed 'nociceptors' and therefore the perception of pain by the brain is referred to as 'nociception'. Commonly (and incorrectly), the nerve endings of these specialized nerves are referred to as 'pain receptors'. Pain is not simply a sensory phenomenon passively transduced and conveyed by the peripheral and sensory nervous systems as once thought. Indeed, pain is a highly subjective human experience, modulated by a wide variety of behavioral, genetic, cultural, psychological and biological factors. At the physiological level, painful stimuli trigger biological processes that lead to amplification or inhibition of the pain signal. After tissue damage has occurred, peripheral nociceptors become sensitized to noxious stimuli due to the formation and accumulation of algogenic and inflammatory mediators in the periphery such as prostanoids, interleukins, bradykinin and histamine (Cepeda & Carr 2003). Peripheral sensitization and heightened afferent activity in pain fibers elicit functional, chemical and anatomical reorganization in neurons of the spinal cord that lead to long-term central potentiation, a form of pain memory (Dickenson et al 1997). The effect, therefore, of repeated stimulation of pain fibers is to produce a state of persistent spinal hypersensitivity characterized by progressively exaggerated and prolonged responses following each successive stimulus (Woolf & Thompson 1991). It has also been noted by various investigators that pain memory in neonates who had previously experienced the highest number of invasive procedures had the least behavioral response to a further painful procedure such as a heel stick. This lack of responsiveness has been ascribed to interrupted neurological development and may also reflect a degree of 'learned helplessness' (Berd & Masek 2003).

The biomedical model of pain assessment has historically focused on pain intensity and how to modulate it. Towards the end of the last century, however, behavioral scientists developed alternatives to the narrow, reductionist focus of the biomedical viewpoint with models of pain assessment and management which conceptualize and individualize the pain experience, highlighting motivational elements and their developmental origins in an attempt to fully address the social and cognitive nature of pain (Bush & Harkins 1991).

It is somewhat ironic, given the reductionist nature of the biomedical model and the avowed non-reductionist, holistic approach of chiropractic in general, that it remains the most useful model for the chiropractor confronted with a child in whom pain is a significant element of their condition. The reason for this apparent paradox is simple. The correction of cerebral dysafferentation generally has a powerful modulating

© 2010, Elsevier Ltd, Inc, BV
DOI: 10.1016/B978-0-7020-3129-8.00020-7

effect on the process of nociception, presumably through changing the amplifying effects that occur at the spinal cord. The effect of this pain-modulating influence of the chiropractic adjustment is by and large, to, reduce the pain experience of the child to the short term, thereby reducing most clinical decisions relating to pain management to a choice between pharmacological and home-based, non-pharmacological strategies which include active, intentional non-reinforcement of illness behavior. To this end, the biomedical model serves the chiropractor very well indeed, since children who have an ongoing need for pain management outside the protocol of the chiropractic adjustment will generally have clinical conditions which require medical management. They will therefore either self-select medical care, or they will be referred by the chiropractor.

A comprehensive, validated measure of pain is often necessary in order to establish an accurate clinical diagnosis. McGrath (1995) suggests that pain measurement in children is deceptively simple and may be accomplished by the addition of a few structured questions to the usual pain history and the use of a simple quantitative rating scale about sensory characteristics and critical situational factors which have the effect of modifying pain perception in a child.

Pain characteristics in pediatrics

Price (1985) has described how the perception of pain experienced by children is dependent upon complex, multidimensional neural interactions, where impulses generated by tissue damage are modified by ascending systems activated by innocuous stimuli such as touch and descending pain-suppressing systems activated by situational factors such as understanding, use of pain control strategies, etc. A child's pain is not merely an immediate and inevitable consequence of tissue damage. Due to the inherent plasticity of their nervous systems, children's nociceptive systems have the capacity to respond differently to the same degree of tissue damage. This plasticity is a unique feature of the pain system in children, even neonates. Diverse physical, environmental and psychological factors can affect nociceptive processing, so that, even though a child's pain is often initiated by tissue damage, the subsequent pain experienced depends on these factors in relation to the actual tissue damage (McGrath & Brigham 1992). A model depicting how the interaction of situational, behavioral and emotional factors bear on a child's pain experience is shown in Fig. 20.1.

Pain measurement in pediatrics

Neonates, infants and toddlers

In the chiropractic setting, an estimate of pain intensity in this age group is arrived at by the addition of a few basic pain-related questions added to the usual history (McGrath 1995), the observation of pain-related behavior (i.e. crying frequency, pitch and intensity, facial and verbal expression)

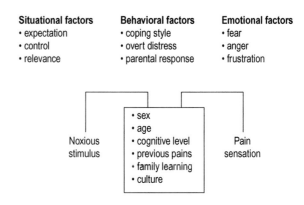

Figure 20.1 • A model depicting the interaction of situational, behavioral and emotional factors that bear on the total pain experience of a child. From McGrath & Brigham (1992) In: Turk DC, Melzack R (eds) 1992 Handbook of pain assessment. Guilford Press, London, p. 296. Reprinted by permission of Elsevier Science Publishing Co., Inc.

and measurement of autonomic functions such as heart rate, respiratory rate and blood pressure (Cooper & Keneally 1993).

The measurement of metabolic response to pain-related stress, such as catecholamines, cortisol, insulin and endorphin levels, have all been demonstrated to have inherent value in evaluating perceived pain levels (Bush & Harkins 1991, Cooper & Keneally 1993). While the chiropractic setting does not lend itself to the measurement of these biochemical markers, in individual cases it may become necessary to make an appropriate referral to a facility where this is possible.

Preschool and school-age children

For children aged from 4 years to approximately 7 years, a combination of pain drawings and the use of the Wong–Baker faces rating scale, when used against a background of consideration of the items shown in Fig. 20.1, offers the most valid method of assessing pain intensity. Pain drawings and the use of the faces rating scale are equally easy to administer, both within the chiropractic setting and in the home environment, thereby offering the chiropractor the opportunity to evaluate pain intensity in a longitudinal sense.

Pain drawings are administered using the Varni/Thompson Pediatric Pain Questionnaire: Form C (Child). The drawing blanks are shown in Fig. 20.2. The child to be assessed is shown the diagram and given the following instructions:

Pick the colors that mean *No hurt, A little hurt, More hurt* or *A lot of hurt* to you. Now, using those colors, color in the body to show how you feel. Where you have no hurt, use the *No hurt* color to color in the body. If a part of your body hurts, use the color that tells how much hurt you have to color in that part.

The faces used to assess pain in the Wong–Baker faces rating scale are shown in Fig. 20.3. The child to be assessed is shown the faces and instructed as follows:

Step 1: Explain to the child, in simple language, that each face is for a person who either feels no pain (hurt, or other adjective used by the child) or feels sad because they have some or a lot of pain.

No pain   Mild pain   Moderate pain   Severe pain
No hurt   A little hurt   More hurt   A lot of hurt

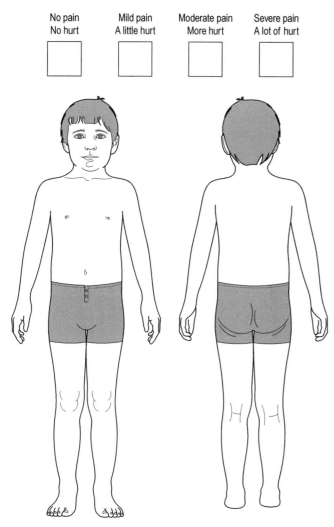

Figure 20.2 • Pain diagrams from the Varni/Thompson Pediatric Pain Questionnaire: Form C (Child) for use with preschool and school-age children. (Adapted from Walco & Varni 1991 with permission.)

Step 2: Point to each face in turn and explain to the child that this person feels:

0 Very happy because they have no pain at all
1 Hurts just a little bit
2 Hurts a little more
3 Hurts even more
4 Hurts a whole lot
5 Hurts as much as you can imagine, although you don't have to be crying to feel this bad.

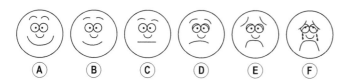

Figure 20.3 • The Wong–Baker faces rating scale (adapted from Whaley & Wong 1991 with permission).

In a clinical presentation in which pain is likely to be an ongoing concern and analgesia is necessary, the Wong–Baker faces scale may be administered at home by the child's parents as a means of deciding when to give the child medication. A record of each administration of the faces rating scale should be kept by the parents for entry into the patient's file at the next visit. It also acts as a valuable tool for evaluating the pain relief afforded the child by the chiropractic adjustment. The faces rating scale method of pain assessment focuses on the emotional distress aspect of pain and should not be interpreted as a direct measure of the pain the patient is experiencing. It should be noted that if a child identifies a number 4 face this does not necessarily imply that they are experiencing twice as much pain as if the number 2 face was chosen. Children do not necessarily record distress in direct proportion to their pain.

From the age of 7 years, a visual analog scale (VAS) may be employed in addition to pain drawings and the faces rating scale. The Varni/Thompson Pediatric Pain Questionnaire: Form C (Child) (Walco & Varni 1991; see Appendix 4) may be used for this purpose along with the Wong–Baker faces rating scale shown in Fig. 20.3.

Activator Methods Inc. has also produced an excellent VAS instrument which may be used for older children. It consists of a short steel ruler with a moveable marker attached to it. One side of the ruler is blank while the other side has a centimeter scale from 0 to 10. The chiropractor shows the blank side of the ruler to the child and explains that the 0 represents no pain whatsoever, while 10 is the worst pain they can imagine. The child is then asked to move the marker to the appropriate place on the scale that represents how they are presently feeling.

Another method in common use is a drawing of a numbered thermometer where the child is asked to place a mark at the number that they feel indicates the degree of pain.

In the case of chronic pain, it is most useful to ask the child's parents to keep a pain diary (Fig. 20.4). Faces from the faces rating scale or a brief description can be used each day to identify how the child has been feeling. It is also appropriate for parents to make a brief comment under the face for the day if they believe there are extenuating circumstances which may have exacerbated the child's condition. An example of a pain diary kept for a child who suffers from recurrent headache is shown in Fig. 20.5. From this pain diary, it can be readily ascertained on how many days of the month the child had headache, how intense each headache was, the effect of the upset tummy, when medication was required, and, by deductive reasoning, how effective the chiropractic adjustments were.

Common clinical problems in chiropractic practice which may require pain management

Pain in children that has a musculoskeletal origin is so responsive to the chiropractic adjustment that the use of pain control agents and methods is seldom required. The most common presentations to chiropractors which will necessitate active pain management are related to infection, head pain, teething

Headache history and pain information
(to be completed by parent)

Child's name ——————— Sex ——————— Age ———————

Date of birth ————————————————————————

Brothers/sisters (names and ages) ————————————————

Form completed by   Mother ————   Father ————   Other ————

Child's school ———————— Child's grade ————————

In general what is your child's attitude towards school? (please circle one)

Very negative   Negative   Neutral   Positive   Very positive

Overall, please indicate the level of your child's grades/academic performance.
(please circle one)

Nearly   Below   Average   Above   Superior
failing   average   average

Has your child's school teacher expressed any concerns regarding academic
performance, behaviour, or social relationships during the past year? (please specify)
————————————————————————————————
————————————————————————————————
————————————————————————————————

List your child's favourite three pastimes, hobbies, extracurricular activities.
————————————————————————————————
————————————————————————————————
————————————————————————————————

Number of school days missed in this year due to headaches ————————

Number of school days missed in last month ————————————

Number of doctor's visits in last month because of headaches ————————

Average frequency of headaches ————————————————

Average duration of headaches ————————————————

Parent: Married/seperated/divorced/remarried/widowed (please circle one)

Parents' principal ocupation during last 5 years:

Mother ——————————————————————————

Father ——————————————————————————

Parents' school level: ————— Mother ————— Father —————

Principal residence during last 5 years ————————————————

What causes your child's headaches? ————————————————
————————————————————————————————

Can he/she lessen the pain completely during a headache?
————————————————————————————————

What can you do to help your child when he/she has headaches?————————
————————————————————————————————

Is there any family history of regular headaches? (if so, please explain which family
member and what type of headaches) ————————————————
————————————————————————————————

Do any of your children or other family members have a chronic disease or illness (e.g.
diabetes, cancer, etc.)? ————————————————————
————————————————————————————————
————————————————————————————————

Do any of your children experience frequent problems with any type of pain (e.g.
stomach aches, back ache)? ————————————————————
————————————————————————————————
————————————————————————————————

Can you lessen the pain completely when you have a headache? ————————
————————————————————————————————
————————————————————————————————

Do any of these trigger your child's headache? (respond with A, always; S, sometimes;
N, never; D, dont know.)

Foods:
__ Chocolate
__ Wheat
__ Cheese
__ Sugar
__ Yeast
__ Eggs
__ Meat with nitrates
__ Other ——————

Weather:
__ Humidity, barometric pressure
__ Sudden or large temperature shift
__ Hot weather
__ Cold weather
__ Sun

Emotions:
__ Anger
__ Fear
__ Anxiety, worry
__ Other ——————

Social activities:
__ Party
__ Dance
__ Concert
__ Movie
__ Other ——————

School:
__ Class
__ Tests
__ Bus
__ Breaks
__ Other ——————

Other:
__ Physical activity
__ Fatigue
__ Mental concentration
__ Noise
__ Siblings

Figure 20.4 • Headache History and Pain Information form (reproduced with kind permission from McGrath 1993).

Sunday	Monday	Tuesday	Wednesday	Thursday	Friday	Saturday
1 ☺	2 ☺	3 ☺	4 ☹ Panadol	5 ☺	6 ☹	7 ☺
8 ☹	9 ☹ Adjustment	10 ☺	11 ☺	12 ☺	13 ☺	14 ☺
15 ☹	16 ☺	17 ☹	18 ☹	19 ☺	20 ☺	21 ☹
22 ☹ Upset tummy	23 ☹ Upset tummy	24 ☹ Adjustment	25 ☹ Panadol	26 ☹ Panadol	27 ☺ Adjustment	28 ☺
29 ☺	30 ☺	31 ☺				

Figure 20.5 • Pain diary for an 8-year-old child suffering from recurrent headache.

and joint pain. By far the most common of these clinical problems are otitis media, pharyngitis, mouth ulcers, urinary tract infection and headache. Joint-related problems in which inflammation is an issue which needs to be addressed (e.g. transient synovitis, sprain/strain injuries, etc.) may occasionally require short-term active pain management during the early stages of chiropractic care.

Otitis media

The majority of children who present with otitis media have pain. Otalgia is an understandable symptom of middle ear infection given the sensory innervation of the ear. There are many pain-sensitive structures in the ear which are irritated by inflammation associated with infection. Pain may result from the presence of toxic products, irritation, or stretching of the tympanic membrane, periosteum of the mastoid and the mucoperiosteum of the middle ear, which are all richly innervated structures.

In the medical model these children are routinely prescribed antibiotics despite a distinct lack of evidence confirming their clinical efficacy as an antibacterial agent in this condition. Recent studies have identified, however, that the reason children with ear infections who are given antibiotics report improvement more quickly than those who are not given antibiotics is because the antibiotics actually have an analgesic effect. Given that the same symptomatic outcome can be reliably produced using an analgesic agent such as acetaminophen (paracetamol), which is free of the immune-suppressing effect of antibiotics, and treatments which may be administered at home, it would seem unnecessary to prescribe them at all.

Children presenting with otitis media commonly have an upper cervical subluxation complex and almost invariably have disturbance of the reciprocal tension system. Adjusting the upper cervical complex has been shown to have a pain-reducing effect via the release of endorphins and substance P in addition to stimulating the immune system. Cranial correction is also a powerful tool in reducing pain from otitis media and facilitating middle ear drainage. In particular, the cranial procedure can be repeated two or three times per day if necessary during the peak severity period of the pain.

In addition to chiropractic care, the use of pediatric preparations of acetaminophen or ibuprofen, local treatments including the insertion of warm olive oil into the ear canal, the application of warm compresses, and blowing into the ear may be implemented. The patency of the tympanic membrane should be definitely established prior to advising parents to put oil in the child's ear (Schechter 1995).

Pharyngitis/tonsillitis

Acute pharyngitis and tonsillitis is a common pediatric presentation. Bacteria (usually streptococcus) and viruses are both capable of causing inflammation of the pharyngeal and lymphoid tissue. Once again, the medical model is the immediate prescription of antibiotics whose effects, as mentioned above, are analgesic rather than antibacterial. Since the presence of a streptococcal organism in pharyngitis has been reported in the literature to be as low as 10% in sample populations, the prescription of antibiotics in the first 72 hours would seem to be unnecessary.

The critical first step is the correction of cortical dysafferentation and the resultant neurological imbalance. Stimulation of local lymphoid tissue with zinc lozenges enhances the immune response, while gargling with a hypersaline solution offers a degree of pain relief. The use of local anesthetic agents such as sprays and lozenges should be avoided in young children as they may impair swallowing and increase the risk of aspiration. In particular, parents should be strongly advised against the use of aspirin gargles owing to the association of aspirin with Reye syndrome in prepubescent patients.

Some children who have pharyngitis or tonsillitis will have an intercurrent high-velocity cough. The effect of such coughing is to dry out the mucous membranes, which impairs healing, aggravates the already sore throat, and provides sufficient tracheobronchial irritation to initiate further coughing. It is therefore very useful in these circumstances to use steam inhalation in order to moisturize the mucous membranes. Direct methods of employing steam inhalation, usually with the head covered by a towel, should be avoided in preschool-age children in favor of steaming up a room such as the bathroom by running all the hot taps and simply keeping the child in the steam environment for 10–15 minutes. When direct steam inhalation methods are employed, care should be taken to cover the child's eyes with a towel to avoid irritation. In addition to using steam as required by the frequency of coughing throughout the day, a vaporizer should be kept running 24 hours per day in the child's room.

If, despite implementation of the above protocols, the child shows no sign of improvement within 72 hours, referral for antibiotic therapy is appropriate because of the high rate of development of secondary bacterial infection at this point in the natural history of both pharyngitis and tonsillitis (Schechter 1995).

Viral infections of the mouth

The oral cavity is richly innervated and therefore any viral infection such as herpes gingivostomatitis and mouth ulcers is extremely painful. For children with painful oral lesions, effective measures for pain control include drinking through a straw, using only filtered water, and avoiding excessively salty or acidic foods. In addition, it is helpful to apply a local anesthetic agent using a cotton-tipped applicator. This procedure can be repeated at home as required. Once again, it is not appropriate to use a spray in the mouth of young children as it can impair swallowing and increase the risk of aspiration.

Children with lesions involving herpes simplex infection may benefit from supplementation with lysine and B-group vitamins (Schechter 1995).

Urinary tract infections

Pain is commonly associated with both upper and lower urinary tract infection. Non-pharmacological pain control measures which can be suggested to parents by chiropractors include urinating in a warm bath, drinking lots of fluids, which has the effect of diluting the urine and thus reducing the burning on voiding, and drinking fluids such as cranberry juice which have the effect of altering urinary pH. These measures should always be attempted before the implementation of pharmacological measures to control pain because drugs such as phenazopyridine have been demonstrated to produce hemolytic anemia and hepatic toxicity if used for as long as a week.

From the chiropractic standpoint, the Logan Basic Technique tends to reduce pain from urinary tract infection,

particularly that caused by cystitis, in a significant proportion of children. While definitive studies into this phenomenon are lacking, it is thought at this stage to be possibly due to the adjustment causing a change in the urinary pH.

Headache

Headache is a common pediatric presentation but responds so well to chiropractic care that pain management is often not an issue. In cases where some form of pain management becomes necessary, pharmacological agents such as acetaminophen (paracetamol) may be used, albeit sparingly and then only when controlled by a pain diary, chiropractic headache log, visual analog scale, and, in the case of preschool-age children, the Wong–Baker faces scale.

In a child with headache, it is important at the first consultation to establish a care paradigm that is clearly understood and agreed to by both the child and the parents. Understanding the breadth and depth of the effect of the headaches on the child's life and identifying any triggering factor(s) will enhance management planning. Use of either the 'Headache History and Pain Information' form (McGrath 1993) (see Fig. 20.4) or the Varni/Thompson Pediatric Pain Questionnaire Form P (Parent) (Walco & Varni 1991; see Appendix 4) is also strongly suggested to assist with management planning.

The child should be counseled in relation to the cognitive and behavioral factors that may impact on the progress of the care program, and the parents should be instructed on how to assuage such emotions as fear and anxiety, etc. Blank diary forms with a sample copy, such as that shown in Fig. 20.5, should be given to the parents along with a number of chiropractic headache log forms and a copy of the faces scale. An example of a chiropractic headache log form is shown in Fig. 20.6.

Instructions to parents in the use of the pain diary should include the following:

1. Draw the face selected by the child from the face scale on the appropriate square.
2. Identify pain severity using the VAS and record it on days when headache is reported.
3. Make an appropriate remark, if necessary, on days when headache is reported.

In addition to providing the chiropractor with valuable clinical information, the keeping of a diary, headache log and visual analog record allows the parents to be actively involved in their child's care and affords the child comfort in knowing that the pain is not being ignored, but closely monitored with the option of either a return visit to the chiropractor or an analgesic to relieve the pain in the immediate short term. The child should be brought back for chiropractic evaluation when the headache is reported on three consecutive days or the severity of a headache is reported as higher than usual on the visual analog scale. Such measures assist greatly in negating the impact of cognitive, behavioral and emotional factors, and provide necessary reassurance for the child.

Children's Chiropractic Headache Pain Log *(fill in separate sheet after each headache)*

Patient's name: _____ Date of Birth: _____

My headache started at _____ a.m./p.m. on *(fill in day and date)* _____

My headache came on ☐ gradually and got stronger or ☐ suddenly

When my headache started I was *(fill in what you were doing at the time)* _____

_____

When the pain started I had been feeling *(describe your feelings)* _____

_____

To help me with the pain when my headache started I:

Describe what you did   Time   How much did it help?

                              Not at all   A little   Heaps   It killed the pain

                              Not at all   A little   Heaps   It killed the pain

My headache: ☐ suddenly stopped   ☐ slowly went away

After I get adjusted my headache: ☐ suddenly stops   ☐ slowly eases off

                       ☐ gets worse, then goes away

It has been _____ days/weeks/months *(circle one)* since my last adjustment

This is my _____ headache since my last adjustment

Since my last adjustment I have been feeling *(describe your feelings)* _____

_____

Please don't forget to fill in your headache diary and complete the pain diagrams.

Figure 20.6 • An example of a chiropractic pediatric headache log.

References

Berd, C.B., Masek, B., 2003. In: Melzack, R., Wall, P.D. (Eds), Handbook of Pain Management: A Clinical Companion to Wall and Melzack's Textbook of Pain. Churchill Livingstone, Edinburgh.

Bush, J.P., Harkins, S.W., 1991. Children in Pain: Clinical and Research Issues from a Developmental Perspective. Springer-Verlag, New York.

Cepeda, M.S., Carr, D.B., 2003. In: Approaches to Pain Management, an Essential Guide for Clinical Leaders. Joint Commission on Accreditation of Healthcare Organizations, Oakbrook Terrace, USA.

Cooper, M., Keneally, J., 1993. Pediatric pain and its treatment. Modern Medicine of Australia (Aug), 131–136.

Dickenson, A.H., Chapman, V., Green, G.M., 1997. The pharmacology of excitatory and inhibitory amino acid-mediated events in the transmission and modulation of pain in the spinal cord. Gen. Pharmacol. 28 (5), 633–638.

McGrath, P.A., 1990. Pain in Children: Nature, Assessment, and Treatment. Guilford Press, New York.

McGrath, P.A., 1993. Pain in Children: Nature, Assessment and Treatment. Guilford Press, New York.

McGrath, P.A., 1995. Pain in the pediatric patient: practical aspects of assessment. Pediatr. Ann. 24 (3), 126–133, 137–138.

McGrath, P.A., Brigham, M.C., 1992. The assessment of pain in children and adolescents. In: Turk, D.C., Melzak, R. (Eds), Handbook of Pain Assessment. Guilford Press, New York, pp. 195–314.

McGrath, P.J., Unruh, A.M., 1987. Pain in Children and Adolescents. Elsevier, New York.

Price, D.D., 1985. Psychological and Neural Mechanisms of Pain. Raven Press, New York.

Ross, R.M., Ross, S.A., 1988. Childhood Pain: Current Issues, Research, and Management. Urban & Schwarzenberg, Baltimore.

Schechter, N.L., 1995. Common pain problems in the general pediatric setting. Pediatr. Ann. 24 (3), 143–146.

Tyler, D.C., Krane, E.J., 1990. Pediatric Pain. Raven Press, New York.

Walco, G.A., Varni, J.W., 1991. Chronic and recurrent pain. In: Bush, J.P., Harkins, S.W. (Eds), Children in Pain. Clinical and Research Issues from a Developmental Perspective. Springer-Verlag, New York.

Whaley, L., Wong, D., 1991. Nursing Care of Infants and Children, fourth ed. Mosby Year Book, St Louis, p. 1148.

Woolf, C.J., Thompson, S.W., 1991. The induction and maintenance of central desensitization is dependent on N-methyl-D-aspartic acid receptor activation; implications for the treatment of post-injury pain hypersensitivity states. Pain 44 (3), 293–299.

The neuropathological basis of the subluxation

21

Ailsa van Poecke   Neil J. Davies

It has been common practice in chiropractic academia and clinical research to refer to the subluxation as the vertebral subluxation complex (VSC) (Gattermann 1995), a term that served the profession well in the latter part of last century but is now outdated, largely irrelevant and even misleading. The key element of the VSC model advanced by Lantz (1995) that is taught in chiropractic institutions around the world is unquestionably kinesiopathology, despite the fact that the model clearly calls for an equal focus on the neuropathological element. This unifocal approach has led to a serious deterioration of clinical standards among graduating chiropractors who begin their practice years identifying diminished joint function as the sole substance of the subluxation. As generations of chiropractors graduate and practice joint fixation manipulation, and call it chiropractic, the net result has been reduction of the art of chiropractic to the lowest possible common denominator with the neurological element of the subluxation largely ignored, or in some cases actively denied, despite the evolving body of knowledge to the contrary.

The subluxation complex, pictorially represented in Fig. 21.1, is based on precise, predictable patterns of neuropathology, kinesiopathology, and the compensation pattern. The term chosen to best describe these patterns of dysfunction, and used interchangeably with the subluxation or subluxation complex, is *dysafferentation*. Collective clinical experience has shown that there may be many layers of dysafferentation at the cerebral cortex, but they are not all obvious on first examination. Indeed, deeply dysafferentated patients may show changing patterns over many months as each one is identified and corrected by highly precise, anatomically specific adjustments. It is the ability to elicit these interacting patterns of biomechanical and neurological dysfunction which provides the chiropractor with the tools to make a highly precise diagnosis.

Allowing, in particular, the neuropathology to guide examination and diagnosis provides for the identification and correction of one layer of dysafferentation at a time and avoids the unnecessary and harmful prospect of adjusting many compensations, a compensation being defined as biomechanical dysfunction whose characteristics lack those required to confirm the diagnosis of dysafferentation. Additionally, these precise and predictable patterns allow for the testing and proving of subluxation correction before any care is implemented. An understanding of the neuropathology as it relates to the presence of the subluxation complex provides for an appreciation of the specific, yet complex, effects that the subluxation can exert on body function.

There are essentially four main neurological mechanisms. These are described in detail below.

Mechanism 1: the effect of dural tension

The major mechanical attachments of the dura are at the cranium, upper cervical spine and lumbaosacral junction. Dural attachments have been noted at the atlanto-occipital and atlantoaxial intervals. Dean & Mitchell (2002) have reported continuity between the nuchal ligament and the posterior spinal dura at these levels. Furthermore, the tendinous fibers of the rectus capitis posterior minor have been found to be continuous with the anterior spinal dura (Humphreys et al 2003,

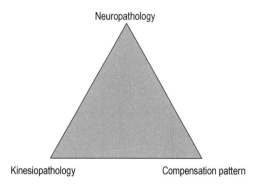

Figure 21.1 • The basic elements of the subluxation complex.

DOI: 10.1016/B978-0-7020-3129-8.00021-9

Nash et al 2005) and attachments have been identified between the ligamentum nuchae and the spinal dura (Humphreys et al 2003).

Dural attachments at the lumbosacral spine include Trolard's ligaments (anterior sacral–dural ligaments) and Hoffman's ligaments (Barbaix et al 1996, Wadhwani et al 2004) attaching the dura to the posterior longitudinal ligament (PLL) (Wiltse et al 1993). Additionally, a peridural membrane has been noted attaching to the pedicles anterior to the deep PLL (Loughenbury et al 2006).

Cerebrospinal fluid (CSF) flow is dependent upon, among other things, the appropriate function of the contractible meninges (Greitz 1993). Given the attachments of the dura to the musculoskeletal system it would seem reasonable that the presence of spinal kinesiopathology (i.e. aberrant biomechanics) could alter the anatomical lie of the dura. This in turn changes the dural tension and influences the contractible function of the meninges, contributing to a change in CSF flow dynamics, thereby changing the CSF pressure. Elevations in intracranial pressure in the critically ill patient have been associated with neurological dysfunction (Kofke & Stiefel 2007). Additionally, mild traumatic brain injury has been associated with (transient) deficits in motor and cognitive function (Sosnoff et al 2008). Given that the traumatic or seriously ill patient can experience obvious pathological changes in neurological function, it may be possible to suggest a gradation of neurological dysfunction resulting from subtle functional changes in the central nervous system such as those effected by cortical dysafferentation and the resulting distortion at the periphery.

The effects of subtle changes in intracranial pressure globally affect the central nervous system and its processing centers. The reticular formation is an excellent example of a key central nervous system structure and processing point (Snell 1992). It plays a pivotal role in the modulation of pain, the motor reactions associated with pain, postural and locomotor control, and the activity of the neck muscles during horizontal gaze (Leite-Almeida et al 2006, Reed et al 2008, Warren et al 2008). Change to the internal environment of the CNS may result in altered reticular formation function causing the inappropriate or ineffective processing of afferent neurological signals, which in turn reach the cerebral cortex as aberrant signals requiring processing into a meaningful efferent output that lies outside the normal sensory processing paradigm.

The cerebral cortex is also challenged by a change in CSF pressure and in so doing may fail adequately to synthesize the sensory information resulting in inappropriate efferent output. This process is known as dysafferentation (Knutson 1999, Seaman & Winterstein 1998) and represents the foundational neurological basis of the chiropractic subluxation.

Given the pivotal role which the reticular formation plays, a change in pain perception is also possible and its role in autonomic nervous function through the reticulospinal tract must not be disregarded. Additionally, the effect of a change in the internal environment of the CNS will also have an effect on other, if not all, CNS structures, including the cerebellum, limbic system and brainstem. Indeed, the exit point of the cranial nerves through the dura enveloping the brainstem will be directly affected by dural torsion providing a possible source of direct cranial nerve dysfunction.

Mechanism 2: noxious mechanoreceptor input from the dura

The major innervation of the dura is through slow-reacting type C fibers and fast-reacting type A fibers, principally at the cervicocranial junction (Snell 1992). The ventral dura is richly innervated by the sinuvertebral nerve plexus and from a number of perivascular nerve plexi (Fricke et al 2001, Groen et al 1988). Additionally, extensive networks of nerve fibers have been found in the dura and longitudinal ligaments (Kallakuri et al 1998), which has prompted the proposal that the dura may be a source of low back pain (Kallakuri et al 1998). Konnai et al (2000) also investigated the innervation of the lumbar dura and found that sensory fibers from the upper lumbar sympathetic ganglia directly innervate the lower lumbar dura mater. This suggests two possible pain pathways associated with the lumbar dura, namely the conventionally discussed noxious mechanoreceptor innervation and autonomic fibers from the upper lumbar sympathetic ganglia (Konnai et al 2000).

Discussion has also occurred regarding the innervation of the cervical and cranial dura and possible convergence of nociceptive fibers. It has been recognized that the PLL of the cervical spine and the cervical dura have differing innervations but that these include sympathetic fibers (Yamada et al 2001). It has also been noted that the supratentorial dura is innervated by small afferents originating from the trigeminal nerve (Bartsch & Goadsby 2003). Nociceptive fibers from the cranial dura and the upper cervical roots appear to converge on to the same second-order neurons at the trigeminocervical complex (Bartsch & Goadsby 2002, 2003). This may go some way to explaining some of the motor and nociceptive responses which occur as a result of dural stimulation, such as those seen in migraine patients (Bartsch & Goadsby 2003). This would also appear to demonstrate that the bombardment or sensory overload of the trigeminocervical nucleus results in aberrant or inappropriate output, similar to the process named above as dysafferentation.

As with any general ascending sensory information, the ascending tract for the transmission of nociceptive information from the spinal dura in the form of C or A type nociceptors is mainly via the spinothalamic tract. This tract communicates directly with the thalamus but also communicates with the reticular formation. The spinoreticular tract is also thought to be involved in nociception (Mense 2004).

Creating nociceptor stimulation by changing the contractibility of the meninges through kinesiopathology can provide for sensory overload from the dura into the central nervous system, whether via the spinothalamic tract or convergence at the trigeminocervical nucleus. The inability adequately to synthesize this information is referred to as dysafferentation.

Mechanism 3: noxious mechanoreceptor input from the facet joints

The facet joints are innervated by a variety of types of nerve ending. Principally, types I, II, III and IV have been recognized (McLain 1994, McLain & Pickar 1998, Snell 1992).

The lumbar and cervical facet joints are heavily innervated both with mechanoreceptors, sensitized during injury and inflammation, and a number of free nerve endings responsible for nociception (Cavanaugh et al 1996, 2006). Receptor types I–II have been recognized as mechanoreceptors and types III–IV as free nerve endings, also known as A delta and C fibers, which are particularly relevant to nociception.

Type I receptors are superficial, slow reacting, and very sensitive to movement. Their firing rate decreases with approximation of joint ends. They contribute a number of functions such as posture and joint tension, and have tonic effects on the lower motor neurons (LMNs) of the neck, limbs, jaw and eyes, and thus, given these functions, it is possible to postulate about the effects that resetting this aberrant input through chiropractic adjustment could have on postural conditions.

Type II receptors are low threshold and sense minor change in inner joint tension. They are rapidly adapting and dynamic. They function to monitor joint movement for reflex activity. Types III and IV are associated with pain perception and have an intimate physical relationship with types I and II.

The mechanoreceptor and nociceptor pathways which feed into the central nervous system are the spinothalamic and spinocerebellar tracts and the posterior columns. This contribution of sensory information is transmitted via a number of central nervous system structures including the cerebellum, reticular formation and thalamus to the cerebral cortex for processing into appropriate efferent output.

Aberrant kinesiopathology changes the orientation of the facet joint and its capsule and may expose the synovium to mechanical stress (Inami et al 2000). Aberrant facet position and the physiological irritation of the anatomical structures may result in the sensory overload discussed in the above mechanism and therefore contribute to dysafferentation.

Mechanism 4: aberrant sympathetic activity

Control of the blood supply to the cranium is achieved through the actions of the sympathetic nervous system. It is particularly influenced by the cephalic and cervical portions of the sympathetic nervous system (Coutsoukis 2007). The internal carotid nerve appears to be directly derived from the superior cervical ganglion and innervates the internal carotid artery as it travels superiorly to form the circle of Willis. The circle of Willis in turn is made up of both the internal carotid arteries and the vertebral arteries, the latter arising from the subclavian arteries. The vertebral arteries are innervated by the inferior cardiac nerve, arising from the inferior cervical ganglion (Coutsoukis 2007).

It is of importance to note that the sympathetic initiation of the flight or fight response tends to use the above-named innervation to redirect blood flow away from the central nervous system to supply the demands of the skeletal muscle. This minimal decrease in blood supply to the cerebrum may alter the internal environment of the CNS, providing more challenges to neurological homeostasis, and further affect the working of key CNS structures such as the reticular formation and cerebrum as previously mentioned.

Additionally, the direct connections of the sympathetic nervous system via the gray rami communicantes into the spinal nerves may provide for a source of sensory overload or afferent imbalance in the presence of the fight or flight response. The sympathetic fibers can also be stimulated through prolonged stress (Kadojic et al 1999) or excessive facet irritation (Suseki et al 1996). The presence of excessive sensory input or overload is of particular relevance at the sensitive upper cervical complex and sacral areas, which must also process afferent innervation from the richly innervated dura at these levels, and provides another possible mechanism of dysafferentation.

The fight or flight response from the sympathetic nervous system occurs as a reaction to stress in many different forms. The subluxation complex can certainly represent a form of chronic stress and it is in the presence of this prolonged stress that the process of dysafferentation will be exacerbated.

The adjustment

The chiropractic adjustment is a precise and highly specific intrusion into the nervous system. Delivering any adjustive thrust and, in particular, repeated adjustive thrusts to a segment or region of the spine or extremities must be assiduously avoided at all times if inappropriate neurological input is to be avoided. Repeated adjustive thrusts will put the patient at risk of developing an iatrogenic hypermobility syndrome at that level (Cox 1997).

The chiropractic adjustment can be seen as providing a sort of resetting mechanism to the nervous system. When applied in a highly skilful manner, the adjustment overrides the sensory gating mechanism and activates specific neurological pathways (Carrick 1997). Other studies have also discussed and investigated the effect of the chiropractic adjustment. An alteration of sensory processing by removing sub-threshold and chemical stimuli from paraspinal tissues (Pickar 2002) has been one mechanism suggested in addition to a possible change in reflex neural output to muscle and visceral organs. Furthermore, direct central corticospinal activation has also been noted (Dishman et al 2002, 2008). While recent studies such as these have attempted to define and clarify the neurological and biological mechanisms associated with the chiropractic adjustment, it remains an imperative that these mechanisms require further extensive investigation in order to be able to effectively explain the effects of the chiropractic adjustment to the wider scientific community.

The fundamental principle of the adjusting techniques described in Chapters 23–27 is the delivery of appropriate impulse directed to the higher cortical structures. Impulse is described in physics as the product of force and time and is expressed in the formula:

$$I = (F)(T)$$

In order to generate the maximum possible impulse in any adjustment in a way that is not blocked by sensory gating mechanisms, a prolonged light contact is held for approximately 10 seconds followed by a very high acceleration thrust of extremely short duration and shallow depth. The first aspect maximizes the time element and the latter the force element.

References

Barbaix, E., Girardin, M.D., Hoppner, J.P., et al., 1996. Anterior sacrodural attachments – Trolard's ligaments revisited. Man. Ther. 1 (2), 88–91.

Bartsch, T., Goadsby, P.J., 2002. Stimulation of the greater occipital nerve induces increased excitability of dural afferent output. Brain 125, 1496–1509.

Bartsch, T., Goadsby, P.J., 2003. Sensitization of cervical input and dural stimulation. Brain 126, 1801–1813.

Carrick, F.R., 1997. Changes in brain function after manipulation of the cervical spine. J. Manipulative Physiol. Ther. 20 (8), 529–545.

Cavanaugh, J.M., Ozatakay, A.C., Yamashita, H. T., et al., 1996. Lumbar facet pain: biomechanics, neuroanatomy and neurophysiology. J. Biomech. 29 (9), 1117–1129.

Cavanaugh, J.M., Lu, Y., Chen, C., et al., 2006. Pain generation in lumbar and cervical facet joints. J. Bone Joint Surg. Am. 88 (Suppl. 2), 63–67.

Coutsoukis, P., 2007. The Cephalic Portion of the Sympathetic System. Available at: http://www.theodora.com/anatomy/the_cephalic_portion_of_the_sympathetic_system.html (accessed 31 August 2009).

Cox, A., 1997. Proceedings of Gonstead Seminar of Chiropractic. Gonstead Clinical Studies Society (GCSS), Melbourne.

Dean, N.A., Mitchell, B.S., 2002. Anatomic relation between the nuchal ligament (ligamentum nuchae) and the spinal dura mater in the craniocervical region. Clin. Anat. 15 (3), 182–185.

Dishman, J.D., Ball, K.A., Burke, J., 2002. First Prize: Central motor excitability changes after spinal manipulation: a transcranial magnetic stimulation study. J. Manipulative Physiol. Ther. 25 (1), 1–9.

Dishman, J.D., Greco, D.S., Burke, J.R., 2008. Motor-evoked potentials recorded from lumbar erector spinae muscles: a study of corticospinal excitability changes associated with spinal manipulation. J. Manipulative Physiol. Ther. 31 (4), 258–270.

Fricke, B., Andres, K.H., Von Düring, M., 2001. Nerve fibers innervating the cranial and spinal meninges: morphology of nerve fiber terminals and their structural integration. Microsc. Res. Tech. 53, 96–105.

Gatterman, M.I. (Ed.), 1995. Foundations of Chiropractic: Subluxation. Mosby, St Louis.

Greitz, D., 1993. Cerebrospinal fluid circulation and associated intracranial dynamics: a radiologic investigation using MR imaging and radionuclide cisternography. Acta Radiol. Suppl. 386, 1–23.

Groen, G.J., Baljet, B., Drukker, J., 1988. The innervations of the spinal dura mater: anatomy and clinical implications. Acta Neurochir. (Wien) 92 (1–4), 39–46.

Humphreys, B.K., Kenin, S., Hubbard, B.B., et al., 2003. Investigation of connective tissue attachments to the cervical spinal dura mater. Clin. Anat. 16 (2), 152–159.

Inami, A., Kaneoka, K., Hayashi, K., et al., 2000. Types of synovial fold in the cervical facet joint. J. Orthop. Sci. 5, 475–480.

Kadojic, D., Demarin, V., Kadojic, M., et al., 1999. Influence of prolonged stress on cerebral hemodynamics. Coll. Antropol. 23 (2), 665–672.

Kallakuri, S., Cavanaugh, J.M., Blagoev, D.C., 1998. An immunohistochemical study of innervation of lumbar spinal dura and longitudinal ligaments. Spine 23 (4), 403–411.

Knutson, G.A., 1999. Dysafferentation: a novel term to describe the neuropathologic effects of joint complex dysfunction – a look at the likely mechanisms of symptom generation. J. Manipulative Physiol. Ther. 22 (1), 45–48.

Kofke, W.A., Stiefel, M., 2007. Monitoring and intraoperative management of elevated intracranial pressure and decompressive craniectomy. Anesthesiol. Clin. 25 (3), 579–603.

Konnai, Y., Honda, T., Sekiguchi, Y., et al., 2000. Sensory innervation of the lumbar dura mater passing through the sympathetic trunk in rats. Spine 25 (7), 776–782.

Lantz, C., 1995. The vertebral subluxation complex. In: Gatterman, M.I. (Ed.), Foundations of Chiropractic: Subluxation. Mosby, St Louis.

Leite-Almeida, H., Valle-Fernandez, A., Almeida, A., 2006. Brain projections from the medullary dorsal reticular nucleus: an anterograde and retrograde tracing study in the rat. Neuroscience 140 (2), 577–595.

Loughenbury, P.R., Wadhwani, S., Soames, R.W., 2006. The posterior longitudinal ligament and peridural (epidural) membrane. Clin. Anat. 19 (6), 487–492.

McLain, R.F., 1994. Mechanoreceptor endings in human cervical facet joints. Spine 19 (5), 495–501.

McLain, R.F., Pickar, J.G., 1998. Mechanoreceptor endings in human thoracic and lumbar facet joints. Spine 23 (2), 168–173.

Mense, S.S., 2004. Functional neuroanatomy for pain stimuli: reception, transmission and processing. Schmerz 18 (3), 225–237.

Nash, L., Nicholson, H., Lee, A.S., et al., 2005. Configuration of the connective tissue in the posterior atlanto-occipital interspace: a sheet plastination and confocal microscopy study. Spine 30 (12), 1359–1366.

Pickar, J.G., 2002. Neurophysiological effects of spinal manipulation. Spine J. 2 (5), 357–371.

Reed, W.R., Shum-Siu, A., Magnuson, D.S., 2008. Reticulospinal pathways in the ventrolateral funiculus with terminations in the cervical and lumbar enlargements of the adult rat spinal cord. Neuroscience 151 (2), 505–517.

Seaman, D.R., Winterstein, J.F., 1998. Dysafferentation: a novel term to describe the neuropathologic effects of joint complex dysfunction – a look at the likely mechanisms of symptom generation. J. Manipulative Physiol. Ther. 21 (4), 267–280.

Snell, R.S., 1992. Clinical Neuroanatomy for Medical Students, third ed. Little, Brown, Boston.

Sosnoff, J.J., Broglio, S.P., Ferrara, M.S., 2008. Cognitive and motor function are associated following mild traumatic brain injury. Exp. Brain Res. 187 (4), 563–571.

Suseki, K., Takahashi, K., Chiba, T., et al., 1996. CGRP-immunoreactive nerve fibres projecting to lumbar facet joints through paravertebral sympathetic trunk in rats. Neurosci. Lett. 221, 41–44.

Wadhwani, S., Loughenbury, P., Soames, R., 2004. The anterior dural (Hoffmann) ligaments. Spine 29 (6), 623–627.

Warren, S., Waitzmann, D.M., May, P.J., 2008. Anatomical evidence for interconnections between the central mesencephalic reticular formation andcervical spinal cord in the cat and macaque. Anat. Rec. 291 (2), 141–160.

Wiltse, L.L., Fonseca, A.S., Master, J., et al., 1993. Relationship of the dura, Hoffman's ligament, Batson's plexus, and a fibrovascular membrane lying on the posterior surface of the vertebral bodies and attaching to the deep layer of the posterior longitudinal ligament: an anatomical, radiologic, and clinical study. Spine 18 (8), 1030–1043.

Yamada, H., Honda, T., Yaginuma, H., et al., 2001. Comparison of sensory and sympathetic innervation of the dura mater and posterior longitudinal ligament in the cervical spine after removal of the stellate ganglion. J. Comp. Neurol. 434 (1), 86–100.

Measurement of the spinal subluxation in children

22

Neil J. Davies   Neil Cox

Kinesiopathology: a precise reflection of cerebral dysafferentation

Kinesiopathology as it relates to the measurement of the subluxation may reasonably be defined as abnormal biomechanical variance, the precise elements being dictated by the dysfunctional pattern of motor outflow arising from disturbed sensory integration principally at the cortical level, but at other levels within the brain as well. The neurological mechanisms involved in this phenomenon are described in Chapter 21.

Kinesiopathology may be represented by frank joint fixation, relative hypomobility, relative hypermobility, or aberrant motion within the normal physiological range, otherwise known as dyskinesia. At a gross level, dyskinesia is seen as a tic or the characteristic movement seen in Tourette syndrome, but when applied to joint movement it is taken to mean poorly coordinated, distorted, non-smooth movement within the normal physiological range of the joint being assessed.

In subluxation identification, kinesiopathology is defined as elements or vectors that are rotational in nature and occur about the three universal axes of motion described routinely in modern texts on biomechanics. These vectors apply equally to the joints of the spine and the extremities and offer the chiropractor a window of opportunity to be absolutely precise in the measurement of the biomechanical or somatic effects of the pattern of cortical dysafferentation affecting any given patient at any given point in time. These vectors are recorded as the traditional 'listing' for the sake of brevity and precision.

Use of listings in chiropractic practice

A listing provides the chiropractor with a simple and convenient way to describe, in detail, the directional vectors, usually three-dimensional, involved in the kinesiopathological states of fixation and hypomobility that may be involved as a manifestation of dysafferentation. Listings applied to each spinal motion segment or extremity joint provide the chiropractor with a mechanism for kinesiopathological vector resolution in order to facilitate precise, directionally accurate, adjusting.

Listings are also very useful for quick and accurate clinical record-keeping. In essence, they represent a description of the kinesiopathology of the affected joint at a given point in time as a reflection of one pattern of cortical dysafferentation. Frequently, as care is rendered to a chiropractic patient over time, a record of the listings on each consultation forms a pattern for that patient which may provide interpretive opportunity for the chiropractor and be made use of in future clinical decision-making. The listings used in this text are principally those formulated and taught by Dr Clarence Gonstead (Herbst 1968). There are, however, significant variations in the total system proposed in order to accommodate those biomechanical derangements not allowed for in the original or current Gonstead system. There are also some minor omissions from the traditional Gonstead system, which reflect new knowledge produced by biomechanical research in recent years.

Terminology

Listings use a single letter to identify each of the vectors represented by translation and or rotational movement about each of the three axes universally referred to as the x, y and z axes of rotation (Bergmann et al 1993, Gatterman 1990). The common origin of the three axes as they relate to the axial skeleton is a point midway between the cornua of the sacrum. The y-axis is described as the line occurring vertically through this origin, the x-axis being at 90° to this line parallel to the coronal plane, and the z-axis being at 90° to both the x and y axes in the sagittal plane, as shown in Fig. 22.1.

1

© 2010, Elsevier Ltd, Inc, BV
DOI: 10.1016/B978-0-7020-3129-8.00022-0

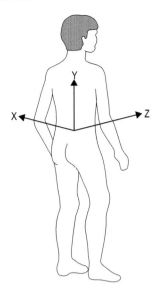

Figure 22.1 • Central coordinate system with the patient in anatomical position.

Table 22.1 Letters used in the compilation of listings to define vectors of kinesiopathology

Designated letter		Description of movement
P	Posterior	Describes extension movement about the x-axis
A	Anterior	Describes flexion movement about the x-axis
R	Right	Describes rotation about the y-axis
L	Left	Also describes rotation about the y-axis
S	Superior	Describes lateral flexion movement about the z-axis
I	Inferior	Also describes lateral flexion movement about the z-axis
Ex	External	Applies to iliac rotation on the sacrum about the y-axis
In	Internal	Also applies to iliac rotation on the sacrum about the y-axis

The letters used in the formulation of a listing describing kinesiopathology at the typical vertebral motion segment and what they signify are shown in Table 22.1. It should be noted that certain variations to this usage occur at the atypical spinal motion segments such as occiput/atlas, L5/sacrum, etc. Where this is the case, the precise usage will be identified.

It is an important clinical point to note that the cardinal rule of chiropractic adjusting for typical vertebral motion segments is that all adjustive thrusts should be made against the convexity of any scoliotic curve with the primary goal of reducing the intervertebral disc distortion designated by the letter 'S' or 'I' in the listing.

The cervical spinal motion segments

The atlanto-occipital articulation

The anatomical reference point for flexion/extension components of occipital listings has by convention been twofold according to the direction of movement. When the occiput moves into extension, the anterior rim of the foramen magnum moves anteriorly and superiorly. This movement about the x-axis is therefore designated by the listing 'AS' (Fig. 22.2)

Conversely, when the occiput moves into flexion, the posterior rim of the foramen magnum moves posteriorly and superiorly about the x-axis and is thus designated by the listing 'PS' (Fig. 22.3). The convex shape of the long axis of the occipital condyle is the reason why both listings contain the letter 'S', indicating that the nominated reference point has moved superiorly.

The anatomical reference point for lateral movement of the occiput is the condyle on the affected side which will always move superiorly owing to the convex shape of its transverse axis. This lateral and superior movement is designated by the listings 'RS' or 'LS', according to which side is affected.

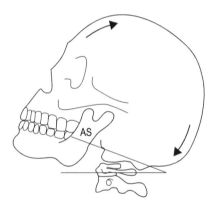

Figure 22.2 • AS component of the occipital listing. Notice how the anterior rim of the foramen magnum has moved anteriorly and superiorly about the x-axis.

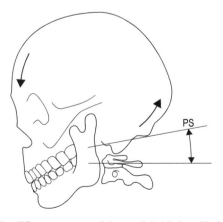

Figure 22.3 • PS component of the occipital listing. Notice how the posterior rim of the foramen magnum has moved posteriorly and superiorly about the x-axis.

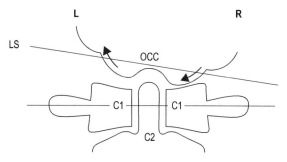

Figure 22.4 • LS component of the occipital listing. Notice how the left condyle has moved superiorly about the z-axis.

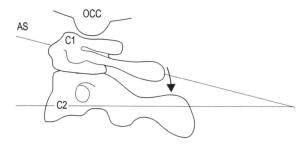

Figure 22.6 • The AS component of the atlas listing. Note the superiority of the anterior tubercle about the x-axis.

Table 22.2 Full complement of occipital listings	
AS occipital listings	**PS occipital listings**
AS (straight or bilateral)	PS (straight or bilateral)
AS-LS, AS-RS	PS-LS, PS-RS

For example, in Fig. 22.4, the left condyle has moved laterally and superiorly in accordance with the joint shape. The full complement of occipital listings is shown in Table 22.2.

The atlantoaxial articulation

Movement of the atlas on the axis is very complex and requires a four-letter listing to adequately describe all the usual vectors. The first letter is always 'A' which denotes the small anterior translation of the entire segment along the z-axis. This movement occurs concurrently with either flexion or extension.

The anatomical reference point used to describe flexion and extension of the atlas on the axis about the x-axis is the atlas anterior tubercle. In flexion, the anterior tubercle moves inferiorly and is denoted by the listing 'AI' (Fig. 22.5), while in extension the anterior tubercle moves superiorly and is denoted by the listing 'AS' (Fig. 22.6).

There is no lateral translation of the atlas on the axis along the x-axis. Rather, the atlas may become 'wedged' on one side owing to capsular swelling between the atlas inferior articular surface and the corresponding superior articular surface of axis (Herbst 1968, Plaugher 1993). When viewed from the

anterior, the atlas appears to have rotated about the z-axis with the side of superiority being denoted as the side of atlas 'laterality'. This is designated by the third letter of the atlas listing, the anatomical reference point being the tip of the transverse process on the side that has moved superiorly. For example, in Fig. 22.7, the atlas is lateral on the right.

The atlas also moves very significantly in rotation about the y-axis, the instantaneous axis of rotation being at the odontoid process. This movement accounts for 50% of all cervical rotation and is a simple rotary movement in the transverse plane about the instantaneous axis. The anatomical reference point is the transverse process on the side of 'laterality' which may move either anteriorly or posteriorly. Anterior rotation is denoted by the letter 'A' while posterior rotation is denoted by the letter 'P'. These letters represent the fourth component of the atlas listing.

The atlas may subluxate with greater or lesser degrees of rotation, and in some cases may have no rotation at all, although this is very much the exception rather than the rule. The full complement of atlas listings is shown in Table 22.3.

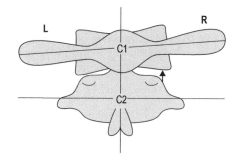

Figure 22.5 • The AI component of the atlas listing. Note the inferiority of the anterior tubercle about the x-axis.

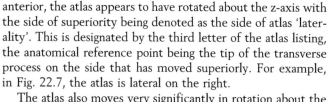

Figure 22.7 • Right atlas 'laterality' seen as rotation about the z-axis caused by swelling of the articular capsule.

Table 22.3 Full complement of atlas listings	
AS atlas listings	**AI atlas listings**
ASL, ASR	AIL, AIR
ASLA, ASRA	AILA, AIRA
ASLP, ASRP	AILP, AIRP

Axis/C3 and the lower cervical motion segments

The anatomical reference point for listing the axis and lower cervical spinal motion segments is the spinous process for rotation about the x-axis (extension) and rotation about the y-axis. Extension is denoted by the letter 'P' and is always the first letter used in the listings applicable to these segments. Posteriority, or extension about the x-axis, is the result of distortion of the annular fibers of the C2/C3 disc with anterior wedging of the intervertebral disc (Fig. 22.8). Spinous process movement to the right is denoted by the letter 'R' and to the left by the letter 'L'. These letters appear second in the listing.

The transverse process on the side to which the spinous process has rotated is used to list lateral flexion, by definition resulting in a wedging open of the intervertebral disc about the z-axis. The letters 'S' (Fig. 22.9) and 'I' (Fig. 22.10) are used

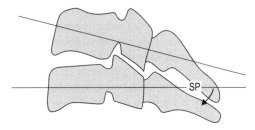

Figure 22.8 • The P component of the typical listing in the cervical spine. Note the distortion of the intervertebral disc anteriorly.

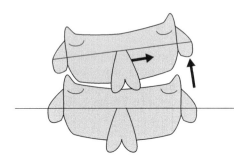

Figure 22.9 • The R and S components of the typical cervical listing. This configuration would be listed as PRS since the spinous process has deviated towards the side of the open wedge.

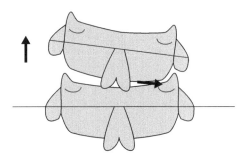

Figure 22.10 • The R and I components of the typical cervical listing. This configuration would be listed as PRI-La since the spinous process has deviated to the side opposite that of the open wedge. The reason why the -La is attached to the listing is to indicate the need to make the adjustive thrust on the left side of the spine in order to conform with the convention of adjusting into the scoliotic convexity created by the open wedge.

Table 22.4 Full complement of lower cervical listings	
Typical listings	**Atypical listings**
PLS, PRS	ESL, ESR
PLI-La, PRI-La	PI (straight posterior)

to reflect the distortion in the annular fibers of the lateral aspect of the disc (i.e. in the listing C2 PRS, the S means that the C2/3 disc is wedged open on the right side).

The listings in the cervical spine which have a '-La' component indicate that the spinous process is rotated to the side opposite the open wedge and therefore the adjustive thrust should be applied to the lamina on the side opposite that of the spinous rotation. This is, of course, in keeping with the convention of always applying the adjustive thrust against the convexity of the lateral spinal curve.

Atypical axis listings

The axis also has two atypical listings. The first is the entire segment lateral listing denoted as 'ESL' or 'ESR'. In this case, translation of the entire axis segment relative to C3 has occurred along the x-axis in addition to rotation about the z-axis, the superiority being on the side to which the segment has translated. There is also some degree of extension about the x-axis, although it is not denoted within the letters of the listing.

The second atypical listing is the PI axis, a listing that involves only rotation into extension about the x-axis.

The full complement of lower cervical listings is shown in Table 22.4.

The thoracic and lumbar spinal motion segments

The anatomical reference points used in the thoracic and lumbar spinal motion segments are identical to those used in the cervical spine and the listings are derived in exactly the same manner. It should be noted that the Gonstead system has not historically described the flexion subluxation in the thoracic spine owing to the anatomical inability of the segments to translate anteriorly along the z-axis. For the same reason, of course, thoracic segments are unable to translate posteriorly, which makes the use of 'P' in the thoracic listings something of a misnomer.

In order to resolve this anomaly, the use of the letters 'P' and 'A' in thoracic listings will be construed to mean rotation into extension about the x-axis and rotation into flexion about the x-axis respectively.

The listings in the thoracic spine which have a '-t' component indicate that the adjustive thrust should be applied to the contralateral transverse process; while in the lumbar spine, '-m' indicates that the thrust should be applied to the contralateral mamillary process, in keeping with the convention of always applying the adjustive thrust against the convexity of the lateral spinal curve.

Table 22.5 Full complement of thoracic and lumbar listings

Thoracic listings	Typical lumbar listings	Atypical lumbar listings (L5)
P (straight posterior)	P (straight posterior)	PLI, PRI
A (straight anterior)	PLS, PRS	PLS-M, PRS-M
PLS, PRS	PLI-M, PRI-M	
PLI-T, PRI-T		

Atypical listings at L5

The lumbosacral spinal motion segment, owing to several factors related to pelvic structure and function, presents a number of atypical configurations which have to be taken into account in order to respect the cardinal rule of adjusting – application of the thrust against the convexity of the lateral spinal curve. The atypical listings arise because of the relationship between the sacrum and its effects on the lumbar curve at the lumbosacral junction. It is possible at this level to have the closed wedge on the convex side of the lumbar scoliosis, in which case the contact for adjusting has to be taken on that side. When adjusting these atypical listings, the convexity of the lumbar scoliosis always takes precedence over the side of the open wedge.

The full complement of thoracic and lumbar listings is shown in Table 22.5.

The lumbosacral junction and pelvis

The sacroiliac joints and pubic symphysis

At the sacroiliac joint, listings of both the innominate and sacrum apply. The anatomical reference point for innominate listings is the PSIS (posterior superior iliac spine) and for sacrum listings either the ala or second sacral tubercle. The ala is used when the sacrum is rotated and the tubercle is used for midline flexion/extension subluxations.

Historically, the Gonstead system has only listed posterior rotations of the sacrum about the y-axis and lateral flexion about the z-axis. The posterior rotation of the sacrum is designated as 'P-R' or 'P-L', depending upon which sacral ala has rotated posteriorly. Should there be an inferior component, evidenced by rotation of the sacrum about the z-axis, then the listing is designated as 'PI-R' or 'PI-L'.

Recent investigations using CT scanning techniques and reported in the literature by Gatterman (1995), however, have clearly quantified anterior rotations of the sacrum about the y-axis. In addition, many chiropractic investigators have identified consistent and predictable physical signs that imply the existence of the anterior–inferior or 'AI' configuration of the sacrum (Coggins 1975, Kirk et al 1985, Logan & Murray 1950). In order to correct this anomaly, the AI sacral listing has been added.

As well as the rotational configurations of the sacrum, it is common to find extension of the sacral base in its relationship to the inferior end-plate of L5, distorting the intervertebral

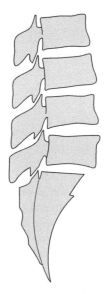

Figure 22.11 • Base posterior sacrum. Notice how the lumbosacral disc is distorted at its posterior aspect producing a parallel disc space and a reduced lumbar lordosis.

disc posteriorly and being listed as a base posterior sacrum or 'BP' (Fig. 22.11). Additionally, the sacrum occasionally moves into flexion about the x-axis, grossly distorting the intervertebral disc at its anterior margin. This is referred to as a base anterior sacrum, the listing being designated as 'BA' (Fig. 22.12).

Neither the base anterior nor the posterior listings have any rotational factors. There is also the possibility of the sacral segments being posterior in the midline or in rotation either singularly or in combination (i.e. S2 post or S2 P-R and S3 P-L).

The full complement of sacral listings is shown in Table 22.6.

The innominate is listed as having moved into extension (listed as 'PI') or flexion (listed as 'AS') about the x-axis as well as internal rotation (listed as 'In') or external rotation (listed as 'Ex') about the y-axis. Given the published data by

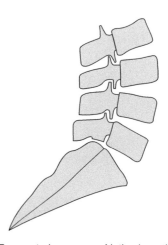

Figure 22.12 • Base anterior sacrum. Notice how the lumbosacral disc is distorted at its anterior aspect producing a large anterior wedging anteriorly and an increased lumbar lordosis.

Table 22.6 The full complement of sacral listings

Posterior sacrum	Anterior sacrum
BP (base posterior)	BA (base anterior)
P-L, P-R	LAIS, RAIS
PI-L, PI-R	
S2 P (2nd sacral segment posterior)	

Gatterman (1995) and Bergmann et al (1993), identifying the translational movement of the ilium on the sacrum in the oblique sagittal plane as an integral part of sacroiliac motion, it is reasonable to conclude that in all probability innominate listings will be compound (i.e. involving vector components of both flexion/extension and rotation) rather than simple.

The atypical innominate listings

These are all related to bilateral listings. They are nominated here as atypical owing to the relative infrequency with which they occur when compared to the unilateral compound listings described above. The full complement of typical and atypical innominate listings is shown in Table 22.7.

The pubic symphysis

The pubic symphysis has only minor capacity for movement as a shearing action about both the x and y axes. Considerably more movement is seen in the child than in the adult, although pregnancy is atypical due to the high circulating levels of the hormone relaxin. In the case of trauma where the symphysis is separated, the listing 'R-L' is used, implying that both the right and left pubic rami have moved laterally. When one of the pubic rami has moved superiorly, the listing 'RS' or 'LS' is applied, as the case may be. Conversely, when one of the pubic rami has moved inferiorly, the listing 'RI' or 'LI' is used. The full complement of pubic symphysis listings is shown in Table 22.8.

Table 22.7 Full complement of innominate listings

Typical listings	Atypical listings
PI, AS	In-Ex pelvis
In, Ex	Double PI, double AS
PIIn, PIEx, ASIn, ASEx	Double PIIn, PIEx
	Double ASIn, ASEx
	Double Ex, In

Table 22.8 Full complement of pubic symphysis listings

LLat-RLat (separation of the pubic synchondrosis)
LS, RS
LI, RI

Table 22.9 Full complement of coccygeal listings

Apex		
Anterior		**Posterior**
A-L, A-R		P-L, P-R
Base		
Anterior		**Posterior**
A-L, A-R		P-L, P-R
AI-L, AI-R		PI-L, PI-R

The sacrococcygeal articulation

While there is motion at the sacrococcygeal junction normally, a subluxation complex affecting the coccygeal apex is most often only evident after trauma, which may be sudden or prolonged. Listings of the coccygeal base, however, are more often related to dural tension subluxation. The coccyx moves in flexion/extension about the x-axis, rotation about the y-axis and, if ligament damage is present, rotation about the z-axis which is seen as lateral deviation of the coccygeal apex. The coccygeal apex and base may both be used as the anatomical reference point depending on the location of the subluxation. The listings used to describe movement of the coccygeal apex are 'A' for anteriority or flexion about the x-axis, with the addition of 'L' or 'R' to denote rotation of the base against the sacral apex about the z-axis. With respect to the coccygeal base, the 'A' listing also refers to anteriority but in this case now represents translation along the z-axis. The addition of 'L' or 'R' continues to denote rotation of the coccygeal base against the sacral apex, this time about the y-axis. Lateral deviation of the coccygeal apex is also identified by the open wedge it produces at the sacrococcygeal articulation.

The full complement of coccygeal listings is shown in Table 22.9.

Subluxation of the upper cervical complex

For the purpose of this discussion, the upper cervical complex is deemed to include the occiput/atlas, atlas/axis and axis/C3 motion segments. Examination of this area of the spine is the first step in the subluxation assessment of the patient. The upper cervical complex will exhibit motion loss in predictable patterns consistent with both local subluxation and compensation to subluxation in other areas. In addition, since it is the most freely mobile area of the spine, the upper cervical complex compensates most readily for subluxation elsewhere in the body. The examination findings here will therefore help to direct the remainder of the kinesiological assessment should the upper cervical spine fail to meet all the diagnostic criteria for subluxation (kinesiopathology, neuropathology and compensation pattern). The common denominator of movement loss in the upper cervical complex from which all the listings are finally derived is lateral flexion, not at any particular level, but generally. That is, if subluxation exists at any level in the upper cervical complex, a palpatory appreciation of restricted lateral flexion of the whole complex will be felt. Delineation of which level is affected is made possible by performing the other steps of the upper cervical kinesiological examination. In order to achieve an accurate, reproducible clinical assessment of the upper cervical complex, the patient must be placed in a position that is absolutely neutral in relation to the x, y and z axes, as shown in Fig. 22.13. For the infant and toddler seated in mother's lap, it will be necessary for the mother to provide support by firmly holding her child with one hand over the chest and the other over the upper back, as shown in Fig. 22.14.

Lateral flexion of the upper cervical complex

The first step in examination of the upper cervical complex is lateral flexion of the entire upper cervical spine. This is best appreciated by taking a contact over the articular pillars of axis and C3 with the thumb and index finger of the preferred palpating hand while the other hand is placed on the top of the head. Just as precise patient positioning is essential in order to achieve accurate and reproducible clinical assessment of the upper cervical complex, so too is the positioning of the examiner. It is important that the examiner approach the patient from the side with their z-axis aligned with the x-axis of the patient. The non-palpating hand must be placed on top of the head and not on the forehead in order to avoid creating unnecessary and unwanted extension of the cervical spine. Movement below C2/C3 is blocked and analysis of the movement to each side is then performed, as shown in Fig. 22.15.

This analysis will result in one of the following conclusions:

- unilaterally diminished movement to either the right or left
- bilaterally diminished movement of equal magnitude
- bilaterally diminished movement of asymmetrical magnitude (i.e. R>L or L>R).

In terms of clinical interpretation it is axiomatic that when a spinal motion segment is subluxated movement of the superior segment further into subluxation will occur while movement out of the subluxated position will be restricted. Therefore, unilaterally diminished movement implies ipsilateral upper cervical subluxation. This will be confirmed by demonstration of a predictable pattern of neurological deficit seen as Shimizu and pectoral hyperreflexia. Bilaterally diminished lateral flexion of either equal or asymmetrical magnitude may also imply a midline upper cervical subluxation (i.e. C2 PI, C0 double AS or double PS). In this case, the neurological assessment will show the Shimizu and pectoral reflexes to be bilaterally hyperreflexive. Loss of lateral flexion of the upper

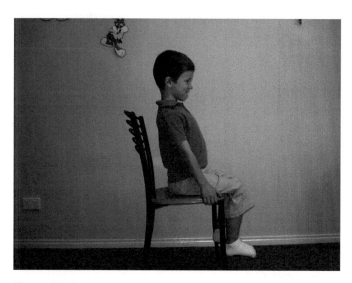

Figure 22.13 • Patient position for assessment of the upper cervical complex.

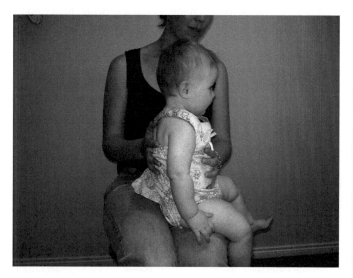

Figure 22.14 • The infant seated in a supported position on the mother's lap for the motion palpation examination of the upper cervical complex.

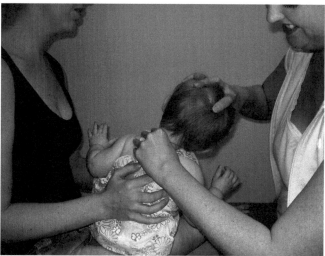

Figure 22.15 • Examination of lateral flexion of the upper cervical complex.

cervical complex will, however, only sometimes be associated with subluxation of the upper cervical spine. At other times such a loss may be a compensatory response to subluxation elsewhere in the body. When related to local subluxation, loss of lateral flexion at the upper cervical complex specifically identifies the z-axis elements of the subluxation (i.e. lateral occiput, lateral atlas or open wedge at C2/C3, the S or -La components of the listing used in the Gonstead system).

Once the lateral flexion component has been established, the remainder of the steps are utilized to identify both the motion segment level and the exact directional elements of the subluxation complex. Occiput/atlas is examined first, followed by axis/C3, and finally atlas/axis.

Assessment of long axis motion at the occipital condyle

Anatomically, the occipital condyles lie in a roughly horizontal plane converging at approximately 45° towards the anterior. This anatomical lie necessitates an examination protocol that maximizes motion of the occiput on the atlas across the z-axis, first in extension (Fig. 22.16), then in flexion (Fig. 22.17). While the examiner's non-palpating hand moves the patient's head into the appropriate quadrant, the thumb or index finger of the palpating hand palpates for the atlanto-occipital space to either open (flexion) or close (extension). Movement of the cervical spine below the atlas is blocked using the rest of the palpating hand.

In terms of clinical interpretation, movement along the long axis of the occipital condyle will be determined to be normal, excessive, or restricted. Excessive motion is a compensatory reaction to either an axis/C3 subluxation or a sacral subluxation, either midline or torsional. Conversely, axis/C3 motion in flexion will be excessive in the presence of an occipital subluxation. It can be seen, therefore, that the occiput/atlas and C2/C3 motion segments act in harmony in maintaining motion balance in the upper cervical spine. When a loss of motion occurs in flexion or extension at one level, the other level will

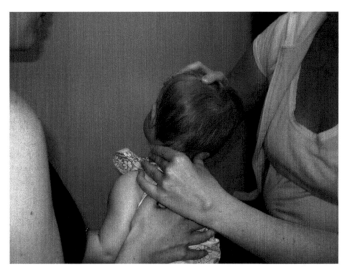

Figure 22.17 ● Examination of flexion of the left occipital condyle.

compensate by becoming hypermobile. When there is subluxation of the upper cervical complex, normal occipital motion is generally seen in association with the atlas/axis subluxation. Unilaterally restricted movement, when seen on the side of restricted lateral flexion, is indicative of ipsilateral occiput/atlas subluxation. Specifically, restricted flexion identifies the anterior occiput listing and restricted extension identifies the posterior occiput listing. The possible combinations of motion loss at occiput/atlas and their clinical interpretations are shown in Table 22.10.

Assessment of motion between axis and C3

The next step is to examine the axis/C3 motion segment in flexion as shown in Fig. 22.18. Normally, significant motion can be felt in this position. When the axis is subluxated, the combination of both occipital condyles being hypermobile along their long axis in both flexion and extension along with restricted flexion between C2 and C3 is diagnostic, provided the expected neuropathology has been identified. Once this

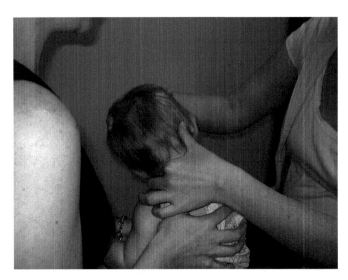

Figure 22.16 ● Examination of extension of the left occipital condyle.

Table 22.10 Possible combinations of motion loss at occiput/atlas and their clinical interpretations

Lateral flexion	Extension	Flexion	Listing
Right restriction	Right restriction	Normal	PS-RS
Left restriction	Left restriction	Normal	PS-LS
Right restriction	Normal	Left restriction	AS-RS
Left restriction	Normal	Right restriction	AS-LS
Bilateral restriction	Bilateral restriction	Normal	Double PS
Bilateral restriction	Normal	Bilateral restriction	Double AS

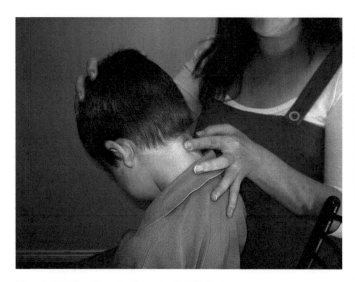

Figure 22.18 • Examination of axis/C3 flexion.

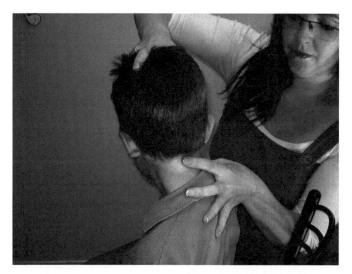

Figure 22.19 • Examination of axis/C3 in rotation. In this case restricted motion on right head rotation implies that the C2 spinous process is to the right.

Table 22.11 Possible combinations of motion loss at axis/C3 and their clinical interpretations

Lateral flexion	Flexion	Rotation	Listing
Right restriction	Restricted	R-L restricted	PRS
Left restriction	Restricted	L-R restricted	PLS
Right restriction	Restricted	L-R restricted	PLI-La
Left restriction	Restricted	R-L restricted	PRI-La
Bilateral restriction	Restricted	L-R/R-L restricted	PI

at both the occipital condyles and the C2/C3 motion segment, the only possible level at which the subluxation can be found is atlas/axis. It is well documented that 50% of cervical gross rotation occurs at this motion segment and this makes its identification as the subluxated level very simple. The arc of motion provided by the atlantoaxial articulation is mostly from 45–90° of head rotation and there will often be a quite obvious loss of this arc when the level of subluxation is at the atlas. Normal full range of motion is shown in Fig. 22.20. It is important to note that, in the case of the older child being examined in the seated position, the examiner has changed position and is now standing behind the patient so that their z-axis is aligned with the z-axis of the patient. This allows the doctor to place both hands symmetrically about the head, ensuring that the fingers are pointing inferiorly and able to lightly palpate the sternocleidomastoid (SCM) muscle, while looking down on the patient's head observing the extent of rotation by using the patient's nose as a guide. The doctor's position remains the same for the baby, the contact over the SCM in this case being the pisiform area with the fingers pointing cephalad.

A loss of gross rotation, as shown in Fig. 22.20, appreciated as the premature tightening of the SCM muscle at rotational end-range, implies that the atlas is rotated anteriorly on that side or, more rarely, posteriorly on the opposite side. A right

relationship has been demonstrated, and only then, should the motion segment be examined in rotation. The reference point for rotational loss is the spinous process, and it may, of course, be to the left or the right. It is deemed to be left when no motion can be detected between the C2 and C3 spinous processes on left head rotation and the same principle holds true with loss of motion on right head rotation (Fig. 22.19). The possible combinations of motion loss at axis/C3 and their clinical interpretations are shown in Table 22.11.

Assessment of motion between atlas and axis

The final step in the kinesiological examination of the upper cervical complex is gross cervical rotation. Given that there is a loss of lateral flexion to one side and normal movement

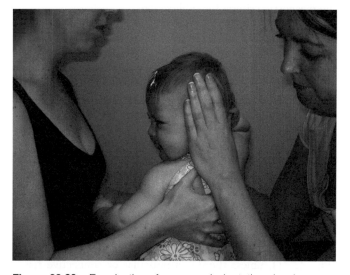

Figure 22.20 • Examination of gross cervical rotation showing restriction to the right side.

Table 22.12 Possible combinations of motion loss at atlas/axis and their clinical interpretations

Lateral flexion	Occiput/ atlas	Axis/C3	Gross rotation	Listing
Right restriction	Normal	Normal	Restricted to right	ASRA AIRA
Left restriction	Normal	Normal	Restricted to left	ASLA AILA
Right restriction	Normal	Normal	Restricted to left	ASRP AIRP
Left restriction	Normal	Normal	Restricted to right	ASLP AILP

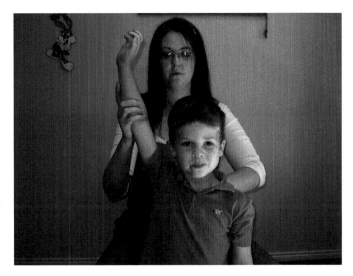

Figure 22.21 • Normal full range of glenohumeral abduction. Note the position of the hand.

anterior atlas, for example, would therefore be manifest as a combination of restricted lateral flexion and gross rotation on the right. The AS or AI component of the atlas listing also needs to be determined, either by X-ray examination or direct neurological measurement. The technique for neurological assessment is described later in this chapter. The possible combinations of motion loss at atlas/axis and the clinical interpretations are shown in Table 22.12.

In summary, there are four critical steps to examining motion at the upper cervical complex:

1. lateral flexion
2. condylar motion
3. axis/C3 flexion
4. gross cervical rotation.

Diligence in following these steps will allow for precise and reproducible identification of the vectors of kinesiopathology in the upper cervical complex. It should be remembered, however, that kinesiopathology is only one component of the subluxation complex and that these findings must be carefully correlated with the neurological, postural, and connective tissue findings, all of which are predictable, in order to meet the diagnostic criteria for subluxation.

While it is true that in the aging population the degree to which the upper cervical motion segments can move is affected by a multitude of pathological factors, such is rarely the case in the child and even the adolescent patient. The examiner can reasonably expect to see full and free ranges of motion in what are almost universally pristine joints. The outstanding contradiction to this is, of course, the child with aberrant developmental morphology, block vertebrae and platybasia being two good examples.

Role of the shoulder girdle in the upper cervical subluxation

Abduction of the humerus in the XY plane should normally be possible in a smooth, unbroken arc of movement to 180° (Fig. 22.21), unless there is a muscular or connective tissue pathology present. When performing this examination, the hand is held with the palm facing directly away from the body

in the x-axis and the arm is raised into full abduction at the glenohumeral joint. Care must be taken to keep the arm in the XY plane at all times throughout the procedure as rotation of the humerus during the test procedure will result in false-negative findings.

It is common for movement to stop between 90° and 135° when there is subluxation of the upper cervical complex, the shoulder itself, certain cranial complexes, the thoracic spine, the rib cage, or the pelvis and its appendages.

Neuropathology

When an upper cervical subluxation complex is present, the following neurological findings will be in evidence:

• hyperactive Shimizu reflex
• hyperactive pectoral reflex
• normal scapulohumeral reflex.

The Shimizu reflex, as it has been called here, is correctly termed the scapulohumeral reflex (Shimizu) (Shimizu et al 1993). However, owing to the existence of the entirely separate scapulohumeral reflex which is mediated via cervical nerves C5–C7, this reflex will be termed Shimizu's reflex or the Shimizu reflex for the purposes of this chapter. The Shimizu reflex response is elicited by 'tapping the tip of the spine of the scapula and acromion in a caudal direction'. The Shimizu reflex is classified as hyperactive only when an elevation of the scapula, an abduction of the humerus, or both have been clearly defined after striking these points with the reflex hammer (Shimizu et al 1993). The technique for examining this reflex is shown in Fig. 22.22. The reflex was discovered by Shimizu, a Japanese neurologist, and his colleagues when studying patients with disease causing neural compression at the brainstem, specifically between C1 and C3, and its presence is therefore deemed to indicate upper cervical cord pressure. Hyperactivity of the pectoral reflex has also been shown to be related to mechanical compression at the same level (Watson et al 1997). It is incumbent upon the

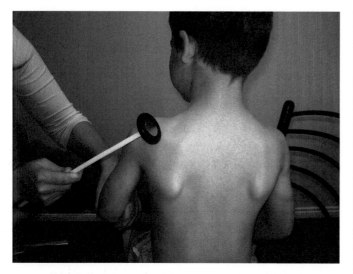

Figure 22.22 • Examination of the Shimizu reflex. It is important to ensure that the patient's head is in a neutral position when eliciting this reflex.

Table 22.13 Relationship of point-specific pain findings and upper cervical listings

Level	Description of location of pain points
Occiput	Pain over the nuchal lines on the side of subluxation. More reliable in the posterior listing than the anterior listing
Atlas	Pain over the styloid process of the side of laterality and over the posterior arch on the side of posterior rotation
Axis PRS and PRI-La	Pain over the right side of the axis spinous and the left lamina
Axis PLS and PLI-La	Pain over the left side of the axis spinous and the right lamina
Axis PI	Pain over the point of bifurcation of the axis spinous process in the segmental midline
Axis ESL or ESR	Pain over the lateral margin of the spinous process and the ipsilateral lamina on the involved side

chiropractor, therefore, to be certain that the presence of hyperactivity in the Shimizu and pectoral reflexes is due to mechanical forces related to the subluxation complex and not to any pathological process. Since the reflex center for the scapulohumeral reflex is in the lower cervical cord, it is spared in the presence of upper cervical subluxation. Weakness of both the sternocleidomastoid and upper trapezius muscles is also associated with upper cervical subluxation. The neurological deficits outlined above will be ipsilateral in cases of unilateral upper cervical subluxation and bilateral when the subluxation is in the midline.

Myopathology and connective tissue pathology

For each of the upper cervical listings there will be a reliably predictable pattern of bony and soft tissue point-specific pain findings, the pain being generated by stretch of the myotendinous attachment to bone or compression of muscular bundles. The pattern of painful points associated with upper cervical subluxation is identified in Table 22.13. In the older child a qualitative response is usually able to be reliably derived, while in the infant and toddler tenderness to palpation is generally seen as a primitive extensor response and sometimes crying. It is worth highlighting the fact that the only way to differentiate an entire segment right (ESR) listing of C2 from a PRS listing is to use the pain findings. The same is true for an entire segment left (ESL) and a PLS listing. The entire segment left or right listings tend to produce severe symptoms in the patient, who commonly experiences pain behind the eye on the affected side.

Postural examination

Each of the upper cervical listings causes the head to tilt away from the involved side, making the ear high on the affected side. That is, the mastoid process will be elevated on the side of restricted lateral flexion. The posteriorly rotated atlas subluxation (i.e. ASLP, ASRP, AILP and AIRP), however, is an exception to the rule as it makes the head tilt towards the side of subluxation (Herbst 1968).

The AS occiput listing causes the patient to 'crane the neck' forward, resulting in a compensatory hypolordosis of the cervical spine. While this pattern may indicate subluxation of the occiput, it is also commonly seen as compensation to subluxation of the lower cervical/upper thoracic motion segments and the rotated sacrum listings – either anterior or posterior. The PS occiput tends to cause a cervical hyperlordosis with the head maintained in a relatively normal position.

Infants tend to hold their head into rotation opposite the side of subluxation. Breastfed infants also tend to be irritable and feed poorly on the breast which requires them to lie with the subluxated side down. For example, a child with an AS-LS occiput will usually not nurse comfortably on the right breast because the child's left side is down when the mother is in the seated position. It is usually helpful to suggest to the mother that feeding may be less stressful for both herself and her baby if she feeds lying down.

In addition to the head tilt, there will be a physiological short leg arising from pelvic contracture measured in the supine position. The short leg will be ipsilateral to the side of occiput laterality and axis superiority (open wedge at the axis/C3 disc) but contralateral to the side of atlas rotation in atlas/axis subluxation. During examination of gross cervical rotation (step 4 of the kinesiological examination of the upper cervical spine), an attempt should be made to quantify the degree of rotation restriction in order to ascertain the major kinesiopathological vector in the atlas listing. When rotation is the major element, as it almost always is, the patient will demonstrate a contralateral short leg in the supine position, while minimal rotation loss will be associated with an ipsilateral short leg.

The information discussed up to this point represents the complete subluxation assessment of the upper cervical complex. It is worth highlighting, therefore, that the subluxation is a neurological entity and as such behaves predictably. In order to qualify as a subluxation, the appropriate kinesiopathology, neuropathology, and the expected compensation pattern must all be demonstrated. This includes the point-specific pain findings and the postural aberrations described above. When there is incongruity in the findings such that they do not all match the expected pattern exactly, the examiner must accept that the findings are compensatory and continue the search for the specific, primary subluxation.

Subluxation of the lumbopelvic region

The role of the upper cervical complex and shoulder girdle in the assessment of the lumbopelvic subluxation

As a global starting point, it is reasonable to assert that diminished total range of motion at the upper cervical complex in rotation about the z and y axes (lateral flexion and rotation) is universally seen in all dural tension subluxation complexes. Coupled with a diminished range of motion at the glenohumeral joints and a standard, orthodox neurological assessment of the Shimizu and pectoral reflexes, this phenomenon offers the chiropractor a great deal of clinical information about the specifics of the lumbosacral subluxation complex.

When the primary subluxation is in the lower lumbar spine or within the pelvic structures, there will be a predictable compensatory pattern of kinesiopathology and neuropathology at the upper cervical complex and the shoulder girdle. The patterns of movement loss which lead the chiropractor to the lumbopelvic area are as follows.

At the upper cervical complex:

- bilaterally diminished lateral flexion
- bilaterally diminished gross rotation.

At the glenohumeral joint:

- bilaterally diminished abduction in the XY plane.

It is worth noting that it is the rule rather than the exception that movement loss at both the upper cervical complex and the glenohumeral joint, while bilateral, will be asymmetrical in terms of magnitude.

The typical pattern of compensatory kinesiopathology is only half the equation, however, in determining that a primary pelvic subluxation exists. There will also be a definite, predictable pattern of neurological loss which will accord with the nature of the pelvic subluxation. When upper cervical lateral flexion and rotation are bilaterally diminished, the presence of the Shimizu reflex bilaterally with a normal pectoral and scapulohumeral reflex response is indicative of a midline pelvic subluxation (i.e. base anterior or base posterior sacrum). When the Shimizu reflex is absent in this same situation, this implies a torsional subluxation of the pelvis (anteriorly or posteriorly rotated sacrum, rotated sacral segment, etc.).

There is no value in examining the pelvis until after a thorough upper cervical assessment has been performed and the kinesiological and neurological compensation elements have been identified.

Assessment of pelvic motion

The pelvis may be considered to be made up of the lumbosacral junction, the sacroiliac joints and the pubic symphysis. The common denominator of movement loss in the pelvis from which all the listings are derived is flexion/extension at the L5/S1 junction. It is important to understand from the outset that in standard kinesiopathological patterns the loss of movement at the sacroiliac joints is opposite in direction to that which occurs at the L5/S1 junction.

L5 and the anterior sacral subluxation

The first step in the examination of the pelvis is L5/S1 flexion. This is best appreciated by palpating the space between the L5 spinous and the sacrum as the patient is slumped, as shown in Fig. 22.23. Just as in the examination of the upper cervical complex, precise patient and doctor positioning is essential in order to produce accurate and reliably reproducible clinical assessment outcomes. It is important that the patient does not have the ankles crossed and that they slump rather than bend forward. This slumping motion produces rotation about the x-axis at both the L5/S1 junction and sacroiliac joints. This x-axis rotation is produced in the baby by direct motion initiation at the L5/S1 level with the baby prone over the mother's lap (Fig. 22.24), and in the toddler the patient position is prone across the doctor's lap (Fig. 22.25).

Once it has been determined that flexion is impaired at L5/S1, the sacroiliac joints should be examined in extension. The technique for this examination in older children is in the sitting position (Fig. 22.26), and prone in infants and toddlers (Figs 22.27 and 22.28). This movement is best appreciated by

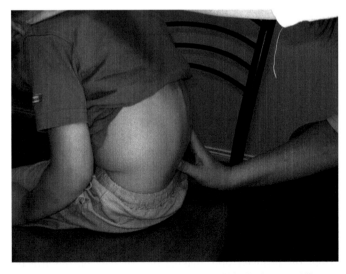

Figure 22.23 • Examination of the older child in flexion at L5/S1.

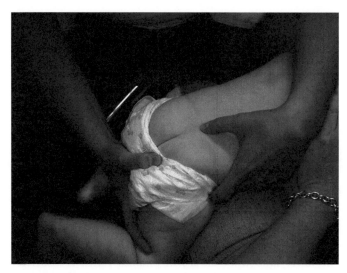

Figure 22.24 • Examination of the infant in flexion at L5/S1.

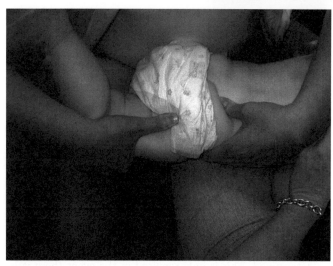

Figure 22.27 • Examination of the infant in extension at the sacroiliac joint.

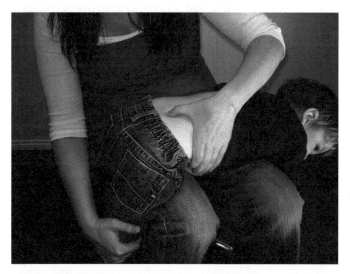

Figure 22.25 • Examination of the toddler in flexion at L5/S1.

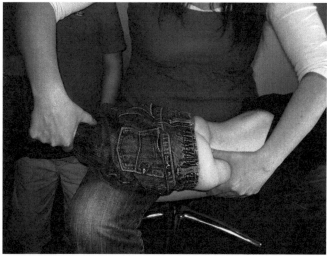

Figure 22.28 • Examination of the toddler in extension at the sacroiliac joint.

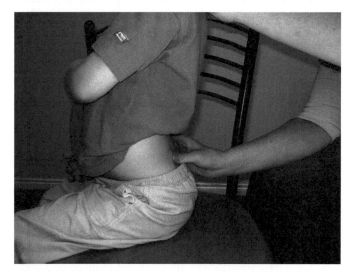

Figure 22.26 • Examination of the older child in extension at the sacroiliac joint.

placing the thumb horizontally across the sacroiliac joint and palpating the movement which occurs at physiological end-range as movement is initiated about the x-axis at the lumbo-sacral junction. Movement is maximally appreciated at the upper end of the sacroiliac joint when examining the patient in extension.

In terms of clinical interpretation, loss of motion in flexion at L5/S1 implies widening of the anterior aspect of the L5/S1 disc, a result of either an L5 subluxation or an anterior sacral subluxation. Both entities produce the same effect at the L5/S1 disc. Differentiation between the two will depend on the findings at the sacroiliac joints and the L4/L5 motion segment. When L5 is the site of primary subluxation, both sacroiliac joints will be normal in extension and L4/L5 will be hypermobile in flexion. When an anterior sacrum is the primary subluxation, there will be a loss of flexion at L5/S1 and diminished extension at one or both sacroiliac joints, depending on whether the sacral subluxation is midline or rotary, while flexion at L4/L5 will be normal.

Regardless of whether the subluxation is at L5 or sacrum, the Shimizu reflex will determine whether it is midline (bilateral), or torsional and therefore unilateral. Neurological loss in the lower limb will be consistent with the Shimizu indications and the kinesiopathology in the pelvis. A Shimizu reflex present bilaterally will be associated with bilateral neurological deficit in the lower limb while an absent Shimizu reflex is associated with a unilateral neurological loss in the lower limb.

Completing the three-dimensional L5 listing

Once it has been determined that L5 is the primary subluxation, the remainder of the three-dimensional vectors need to be determined. This is only required in the event there is no Shimizu reflex present as this is the key neurological indicator for torsional subluxation.

The first element to be determined is rotation about the y-axis. This is accomplished in the older child, who is seated, by rotating the trunk to the right and then to the left while palpating the L5/S1 interspace for movement of the spinous. The spinous will fail to move right to left on right trunk rotation when it is fixated towards the right side. The same holds true for movement on the left side of the body. In the infant and toddler, this rotational movement is generated in a similar way with the patient prone across the mother's lap or the doctor's lap respectively.

The second element to be determined is rotation about the z-axis. This is accomplished by depressing the shoulder as the L5/S1 interspinous space is palpated. When the L5/S1 disc is widened, motion about the z-axis to the affected side will be impaired. Again, this lateral flexion movement is initiated in the infant and toddler in the prone position.

These elements are now combined to put together the complete three-dimensional listing.

The S1 and posterior sacral subluxation

The second step in the examination of the pelvis is L5/S1 extension. This is best appreciated by palpating the space between the L5 spinous process and the sacrum as the patient arches their back, keeping the shoulders vertically above the pelvis as much as possible. In the infant and toddler, this motion is initiated with the child prone. This back-arching motion produces rotation about the x-axis.

Once it has been determined that extension is impaired at L5/S1, the sacroiliac joints should be examined in flexion. This movement is best appreciated by placing the thumb horizontally across the sacroiliac joint and palpating the movement which occurs at physiological end-range as the patient slumps, creating flexion at the lumbosacral junction. Movement is maximally appreciated at the lower end of the sacroiliac joint when examining the patient in flexion.

In terms of clinical interpretation, loss of motion in extension at L5/S1 implies widening of the posterior aspect of the L5/S1 disc, a result of either a posterior S1 segment subluxation or a base posterior sacral subluxation. Both entities produce the same effect at the L5/S1 disc. Differentiation between the two will depend upon the findings at the sacroiliac joints. When the S1 segment is the site of primary subluxation, the sacroiliac joints will exhibit normal flexion. When the subluxation complex involves the entire sacrum, there will be loss of extension at L5/S1 and loss of flexion at one or both sacroiliac joints depending on whether the subluxation is midline or torsional.

It is worth highlighting once again that regardless of whether the subluxation is at S1 or involves the entire sacrum, the Shimizu reflex will determine whether it is midline (bilateral), or torsional (unilateral). Neurological loss in the lower limb will be consistent with the Shimizu indications and the kinesiopathology in the pelvis. A Shimizu reflex present bilaterally will be associated with bilateral neurological deficit in the lower limb while an absent Shimizu reflex is associated with a unilateral neurological loss in the lower limb.

The posterior sacral segment subluxation

Sacral segment subluxation is identified by examining each intersegmental primordial disc, such as S2/S3, in extension. Posterior subluxation of a sacral segment widens the disc immediately above the affected segment and therefore prevents full extension at that primordial disc space. A loss of extension at S2/S3 would therefore indicate subluxation of the inferior segment, S3. This relationship is different to that in the movable spine where loss of flexion at a motion unit implies subluxation of the superior segment due to widening of the disc immediately below the subluxated vertebra. Sacral segments may subluxate posteriorly in the sacral midline (i.e. rotate about the x-axis) or rotate posteriorly on one side (i.e. about the y-axis). There can also be multiple segment subluxation with individual segments rotating posteriorly in opposite directions or towards the same side. In cases of multiple segment subluxation, the involved segments may or may not be adjacent. The neurological examination will clearly identify whether the sacral subluxation is midline or unilaterally rotated. Counter-rotated segments will appear, neurologically, as a midline subluxation. That is, there will be bilateral neurological deficits in the lower limb and the Shimizu reflex will be present, also bilaterally. Differentiation between midline sacral segment subluxation and counter-rotated segment subluxation is made possible by careful motion palpation, examination of point-specific pain findings, and the adjustive pre-test, which will be described later in this chapter.

The coccygeal subluxation

Unless the patient interview reveals a history of direct trauma leading to local pain, the coccyx, as a potential site of primary subluxation, is often overlooked. This is despite its potential to cause significant dural tension through the attachment of the filum terminale. The coccyx may subluxate at its base or apex. Coccygeal base subluxations are often not induced by trauma but are related to dural tension, while the anterior apex listings are much more likely to be caused by local trauma, which may be sudden or prolonged. Due to its relationship to the dura, subluxations of the coccyx are very often related to cranial subluxation, particularly the dropped sphenoid. Either the dropped sphenoid or the coccyx may represent the primary layer of subluxation and it is essential that when either listing has been identified and corrected the patient is thoroughly assessed for the presence of the other.

The coccygeal subluxation is evidenced by the usual loss of upper cervical and shoulder girdle motion accompanied by loss of extension at all sacral segmental levels with normal motion of the sacroiliac joints. Midline coccygeal subluxation will result in the presence of a Shimizu reflex bilaterally associated with bilateral neurological deficits in the lower limb, while in torsional subluxation the Shimizu reflex will be absent and the lower limb neurological deficit unilateral.

The innominate subluxation

The innominate must be considered to have met the criteria for subluxation only when there is normal flexion and extension at L5/S1. In order for there to be an innominate subluxation, firstly there would need to be a loss of movement at one or both sacroiliac joints in either flexion or extension. The affected joint would then be examined in internal and external rotation. Loss of internal rotation implies an externally rotated innominate, while loss of external rotation implies an internally rotated innominate.

Again, it is important to ensure that pure y-axis rotation of the patient's trunk is initiated and that any circumduction movement is avoided. Postural examination and point-specific pain findings, as described later in this chapter, will confirm the listing.

The pubic symphysis subluxation

Apart from subluxation of the three-joint complex which makes up the posterior elements of the pelvis, there is always the possibility of subluxation occurring at the pubic symphysis. Pubic symphysis subluxation should be suspected in the event there is the usual loss of upper cervical and shoulder girdle motion accompanied by either hypermobility at the L5/S1 junction and the sacroiliac joints, or motion losses inconsistent with any known subluxation pattern such as a loss of flexion at both the sacroiliac joints and the lumbosacral junction – a condition referred to as paradoxical kinesiopathology.

Pubic symphysis subluxation may take the form of a separation of the synchondrosis, torsion of the pubic rami with one side superior and the other inferior (a true midline subluxation), or unilateral superior or inferior movement of one pubic ramus. The same motion losses in the upper cervical complex and shoulder girdle that are associated with the posterior element subluxation complexes will apply equally to the pubic symphysis.

Rather than attempt to motion palpate this joint, confirmation of the listing is arrived at by the identification of point-specific pain findings and assessment of the psoas and rectus abdominis muscles. The psoas will be universally weak on the involved side and there will be pain over the origin of the rectus abdominis on the involved side – ipsilateral in unilateral subluxation and both sides with midline subluxation. Point-specific pain findings will also be evident at the pubic symphysis itself, over the anterior surface of the pubis in a synchondrosis separation, pubic tubercle when the ramus is superior, and inferior pubic arch when the ramus is inferior.

The pubic symphysis subluxation, while common in late pregnancy and postpartum females, is capable of causing severe symptom patterns, not necessarily related to local discomfort, in both men and women. It is often related to cranial dysfunction as a second layer of subluxation and, particularly midline pubic symphysis subluxation, may be easily mistaken for cranial kinesiopathology pattern no. 1 (see Chapter 27) if the examination is not done carefully enough – particularly with regard to the pectoral reflex.

The pelvis was previously described in this text as being made up of the lumbosacral junction, the sacroiliac joints and the pubic symphysis. It has already been shown that the sacral segments and the coccyx also make up part of the functional pelvis and it will be seen later that structures outside of this bony ring are related in subluxation pattern and effect to the pelvis, and will therefore also be associated with loss of both gross rotation and lateral flexion at the upper cervical complex. In such a case, where the upper cervical and shoulder girdle motion implies a pelvic subluxation, but examination of the pelvis posteriorly and anteriorly fails to identify a subluxation complex, the problem may be found at the xiphoid process, the diaphragm, or somewhere in the lower extremity. The rules of bilaterality and unilaterality associated with the pelvis apply equally to these areas.

Pelvic neuropathology

Apart from the pattern of neurological deficit seen as a present or absent Shimizu reflex, there will be a lost or diminished S1 reflex and weakness in the L4, L5 and S1 myotomes. When the Shimizu reflex is absent, one can expect unilateral loss of the reflexes and myotomes in the lower extremity and, conversely, when the Shimizu reflex is present bilaterally, one can expect to see bilateral loss of the reflexes and myotomes in the lower extremity.

In the subluxated condition, there will always be predictable consistency between the presence or absence of the Shimizu reflex and the bilateral or unilateral neurological deficits in the lower extremities, as the case may be. Inconsistency implies that the true primary subluxation has not been identified. The relationship between the level of subluxation and the expected neuropathology is shown in Table 22.14. In unilateral pelvic subluxation, the neurological deficit in the lower limb will be specific to the side of subluxation and it is worth highlighting, therefore, the muscles making up the hamstring group as a special case scenario. These muscles, in any combination of individual weakness, will be affected on the side of the open wedge in L5 subluxation, on the side of subluxation in posteriorly rotated sacral segments and when the ilium is affected. However, the hamstrings will be weak contralaterally when the sacrum is rotated unilaterally, either anteriorly or posteriorly.

Table 22.14 Neuropathology associated with pelvic subluxation complexes

Level	Muscles affected	Reflex changes
L5 PRS, PLI-m, PLS-m	Weak right hip flexion, right hamstring and right extensor hallucis longus (EHL)	Decreased right S1
L5 PLS, PRI-m, PRS-m	Weak left hip flexion, left hamstring and left EHL	Decreased left S1
L5P	Weak bilateral hip flexion, bilateral hamstring and bilateral EHL	Shimizu +ve bilaterally Decreased bilateral S1
RAIS, P-R sacrum	Weak right hip flexion, right psoas, left hamstring, restricted movement of right diaphragm	Decreased right S1
LAIS, P-L sacrum	Weak left hip flexion, left psoas, right hamstring, restricted movement of left diaphragm	Decreased left S1
BA, BP and counter-rotated sacrum	Weak bilateral hip flexion, bilateral psoas, bilateral hamstring, restricted movement of diaphragm bilaterally	Shimizu +ve bilaterally Decreased bilateral S1
PI, AS, In or Ex right ilium	Weak right hip flexion, right hamstring	Decreased right S1
PI, AS, In or Ex left ilium	Weak left hip flexion, left hamstring	Decreased left S1
Double PI, AS, In or Ex ilium	Weak bilateral hip flexion, bilateral hamstring	Shimizu +ve bilaterally Decreased bilateral S1
P-R sacral segment, P-R coccyx	Weak right hip flexion	Decreased right S1
P-L sacral segment, P-L Coccyx	Weak left hip flexion	Decreased left S1
Straight P or counter-rotated sacral segments, BP coccyx	Weak bilateral hip flexion	Shimizu +ve bilaterally Decreased bilateral S1
Right superior pubis, right inferior pubis	Weak right hip flexion, right psoas, decreased movement of right diaphragm	Decreased right S1
Left superior pubis, left inferior pubis	Weak left hip flexion, left psoas, decreased movement of left diaphragm	Decreased left S1
Pubic symphysis separation (R-Lat - L-Lat)	Weak bilateral hip flexion, bilateral psoas, decreased movement of diaphragm bilaterally	Shimizu +ve bilaterally Decreased bilateral S1

Myopathology and connective tissue pathology

For each of the pelvic listings there will be a reliably reproducible pattern of bony, muscular or connective tissue-related point-specific pain. These tender points, elicited by gentle and precisely accurate palpation, are extremely helpful to the chiropractor in quantifying the lower lumbar and pelvic subluxation. It should be noted, however, that false-positive and false-negative findings occur with a great enough frequency that these points should never be relied upon solely to make chiropractic clinical decisions. These tender points, like all the examination findings, should always be correlated to the other evidences of subluxation. The pattern of painful points associated with the pelvic subluxation complexes are identified in Table 22.15.

Postural examination

For each of the pelvic listings there will be a predictable pattern of postural distortion, both within the pelvis and more globally throughout the axial skeleton. These relationships, which are particularly useful in the lumbar spine and pelvis, are shown in Table 22.16.

In summary of the subluxation examination of the lower lumbar spine and pelvis, it is worth highlighting once more that the subluxation is a neurological entity and as such behaves predictably. In order to qualify as a subluxation, the appropriate kinesiopathology, neuropathology, and expected compensation pattern must all be demonstrated. This includes the point-specific pain findings and the postural distortions described above. When there is incongruity in the findings such that they do not all match the expected pattern exactly, the examiner must accept that the findings are compensatory and continue the search for the specific, primary subluxation.

Subluxation of the lower cervical spine

While there are no predictable patterns of kinesiopathology in the upper cervical complex that will lead the examiner directly to the lower cervical spine, there are various clues that may be detected in the examination steps so far described that will lead the chiropractor to this area. The first and most

Table 22.15 Pattern of painful points related to specific pelvic listings

Listing	Description of location of pain points
BP sacrum	S2 tubercle and the inferior tip of the L5 spinous
BA sacrum	Inferior tip of the L5 spinous and upper half of both sacroiliac joints
Posterior sacral rotation	Lower half of the affected sacroiliac joint and immediately lateral to the contralateral PSIS in the substance of the gluteus medius muscle
Anterior sacral rotation	Inferior tip of the L5 spinous and upper half of the right sacroiliac joint ipsilaterally
PI component of ilium	Upper half of the sacroiliac joint
AS component of ilium	Lower half of the sacroiliac joint
Ex component of ilium	Immediately lateral to the PSIS in the substance of the gluteus medius muscle
L5 rotation	Ipsilateral side of spinous and opposite mamillary process. There is no relationship to the lateral widening of the disc
Pubic symphysis	Over the anterior surface of the pubis in a synchondrosis separation, pubic tubercle when the ramus is superior, and inferior pubic arch when the ramus is inferior

Table 22.16 Relationship of postural findings and pelvic listings

Postural finding	Associated listing
Elevated iliac crest	PI innominate, anterior sacrum
Low iliac crest	AS innominate, posterior sacrum
Increased lumbar lordosis	PI innominate, anterior sacrum
Decreased lumbar lordosis	AS innominate, posterior sacrum, L5
Narrowed gluteal bulk	Ex innominate
Widened gluteal bulk	In innominate

reliable of these clues is that examination of the upper cervical complex and lumbopelvis will not reveal the site of primary subluxation. That is, while there may be compensatory kinesiopathology in these areas, the examination will not reveal the requisite combination of kinesiopathology, neuropathology and compensation pattern. The second indication is found in the quality of end-feel when assessing lateral flexion of the upper cervical complex. The loss of lateral flexion associated with local subluxation in the upper cervical complex or with subluxation in the pelvis is abrupt and firm, while the loss of lateral flexion associated with lower cervical lateral flexion is more spongy in end-feel. That is, it is muscular rather than articular. Given that the initial assessment of the patient

always begins with a kinesiological examination of the upper cervical complex and the shoulder girdle, followed by assessment of the Shimizu, pectoral and scapulohumeral reflexes, there will also be a predictable pattern of neurological deficit that will lead the chiropractor to the lower cervical spine (diminished or lost pectoral and scapulohumeral reflexes ipsilateral to the side of subluxation). An alternative indication of lower cervical subluxation may be persistent loss of upper cervical lateral flexion, of muscular type end-feel, even after correction of the primary dural tension subluxation.

All movements of the spinal motion segments in this area of the spine are coupled. As such, it follows that fixation/hypomobility must be demonstrated in all three body axes at any given level in order to be considered a possible site of subluxation.

Assessment of lower cervical spine motion

When a lower cervical spine subluxation exists, the lateral flexion motion will exhibit generalized loss on the side of the open wedge. Once the lower cervical spine has been identified as an area of possible subluxation, the first step is to examine the motion segments of the lower cervical spine in flexion (Fig. 22.29). Again, the precise positioning of both the doctor and the patient is vitally important when palpating the interspinous space as the lower cervical spine is examined. Loss of flexion occurs at the subluxated level accompanied by hypermobility at the level above. For example, when C6 is subluxated, flexion will be impaired at the C6/C7 level and the C5/C6 level will be hypermobile in flexion.

Once this relationship has been demonstrated, and only then, the affected motion segment should be examined in rotation (Fig. 22.30) and lateral flexion (Fig. 22.31). The reference point for rotational and lateral flexion loss is the spinous process. In rotation, the spinous process may be to the left or the right.

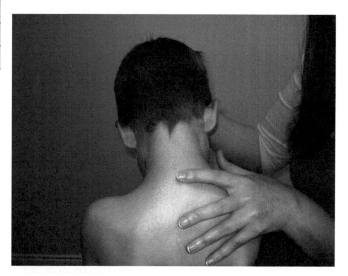

Figure 22.29 • Examination of the affected lower cervical spine motion segments in flexion.

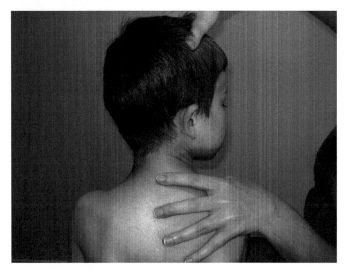

Figure 22.30 • Examination of the affected lower cervical spine motion segment in rotation.

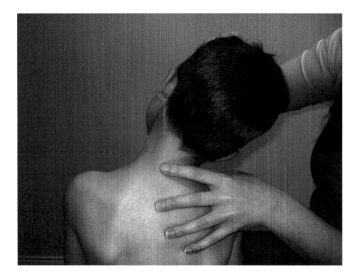

Figure 22.31 • Examination of the affected lower cervical spine motion segment in lateral flexion.

Table 22.17 Possible combinations of motion loss at the lower cervical spine and their clinical interpretations

Flexion	Rotation	Lateral flexion	Listing
Restricted	R-L restricted	Right restriction	PRS
Restricted	L-R restricted	Left restriction	PLS
Restricted	L-R restricted	Right restriction	PLI-La
Restricted	R-L restricted	Left restriction	PRI-La
Restricted	L-R/R-L restricted	Bilateral restriction	PI

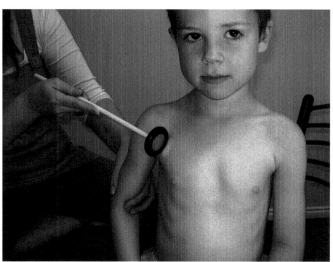

Figure 22.32 • Examination of the pectoral reflex.

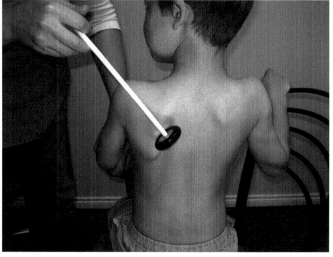

Figure 22.33 • Examination of the scapulohumeral reflex.

It is deemed to be right when no motion can be detected between the C6 and C7 spinous processes on right head rotation (Fig. 22.30), and of course the same principle holds true with loss of motion on left head rotation. In lateral flexion, the spinous process fails to move in rotation when lateral flexion is initiated, indicating an open wedge at the disc ipsilaterally. Table 22.17 shows the possible combinations of motion loss at the lower cervical spine and their clinical interpretations.

Neuropathology

When a lower cervical subluxation is present, reflexes, myotomes and sclerotomes may all show deficits related to the affected spinal level.

Reflexes

The pectoral reflex (Fig. 22.32) and scapulohumeral reflex (Fig. 22.33) are either both present or both absent when the lower cervical spine is the site of primary subluxation.

The nerves which are involved in both the pectoral (medial and lateral pectoral nerves) and scapulohumeral (long thoracic nerve) reflexes have a common root level at C5–T1 (Reuter 2005, Schwartzman 2006). It is therefore illogical to think that a lower cervical subluxation can affect one but not the other. In reality, loss of these reflexes due to lower cervical subluxation is a variable finding, being more consistent when the subluxated level involves the C5 nerve root and less consistent when C8 and T1 nerve roots are affected.

In order to obtain a valid and reliable assessment of the pectoral reflex, the technique of examination is critical. The goal is to strike the inferior aspect of the pectoral tendon with an upward motion of the reflex hammer, the head of which is oriented across the tendon as shown in Fig. 22.32. It is incorrect to strike the anterior aspect of the pectoralis tendon with the reflex hammer traveling in a horizontal arc. It is also important to avoid striking the anterior deltoid muscle belly. A normal pectoral reflex response involves observable contraction of the pectoral muscle (Schwartzman 2006). An obvious, rapid movement of the arm constitutes hyperreflexia. The importance of correct technique applies equally to assessment of the scapulohumeral reflex. This reflex is elicited by striking the lower medial scapula border, being careful to strike bone and not muscle (Reuter 2005). Again, the head of the reflex hammer should be oriented so that it strikes across the lower medial border of the scapula as shown in Fig. 22.33. A normal response is retraction of the scapula as the rhomboid muscle contracts.

While the pectoral and scapulohumeral reflexes may be diminished by subluxation anywhere from C5 to T1, there will also be level-specific reflex changes which will correlate with the findings from the kinesiological examination (Figs 22.34–22.36). The affected nerve root will always be at the level of the hypermobile disc as opposed to the level of fixation. For example, in the event there is a C6 subluxation, the C6 nerve root (brachioradialis), which emanates from the C5/C6 level, will be affected (Gatterman 1995).

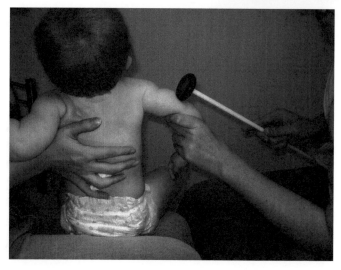

Figure 22.35 • C6 – brachioradialis reflex. Absent or diminished with C6 subluxation.

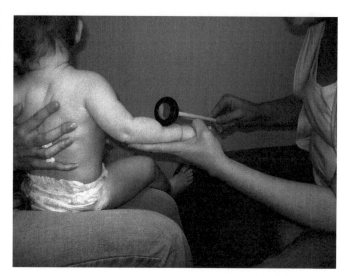

Figure 22.36 • C7 – triceps reflex. Absent or diminished with C7 subluxation.

Myotomes

The myotomes relative to the C5, C6 and C7 levels are readily assessable. The examiner tests the strength of the biceps (C5), brachioradialis (C6) and triceps (C7) in children old enough to cooperate with the examination procedure (Figs 22.37–22.39). As is the case for the reflex, it should be noted that a myotome weakness is related to the level of hypermobility.

Sclerotomes

While dermatomes and particularly myotomes are very spinal level specific at any given point in the body, sclerotomes demonstrate a lot of overlap in the bony tissue. In the upper limb, there are two areas of exception to this rule. The distal radial head is exclusively innervated by the C6 sclerotome and the proximal radial head is innervated exclusively by the

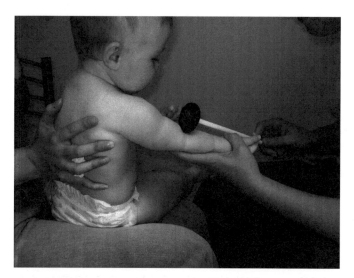

Figure 22.34 • C5 – biceps reflex. Absent or diminished with C5 subluxation.

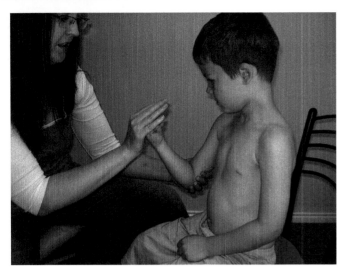

Figure 22.37 • C5 myotome, the biceps. The patient is asked to push their fist towards the ceiling.

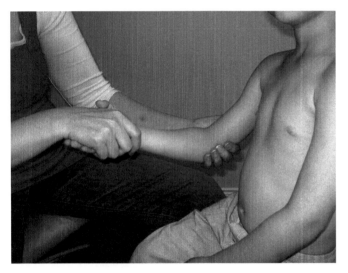

Figure 22.38 • C6 myotome, the brachioradialis.

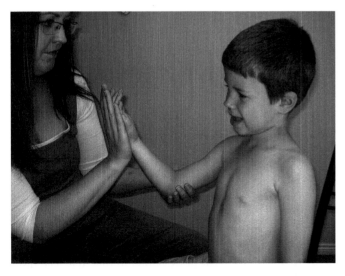

Figure 22.39 • C7 myotome, the triceps. Note how the patient's fingers are pointing upward with no flexion or extension of the wrist.

C7 sclerotome. These two areas offering the chiropractor a unique and valuable assessment opportunity. The clinical evaluation involves the application of sustained moderate pressure over the bony area innervated by the C6 sclerotome and then the C7 sclerotome. Sharp pain suggests subluxation at that level.

This clinical impression is reinforced if the pain can be significantly reduced by placing the head in such a position as to reduce the subluxation vectors which have been previously identified on examination. Conversely, pain can be produced or intensified in sclerotomes when the subluxation vectors are exacerbated by head position. This point introduces the concepts of exacerbation testing of the subluxation and adjustive pre-testing – major strengths of the Neuroimpulse Protocol method of treating children. These phenomena are discussed later in this chapter.

Myopathology and connective tissue pathology

For each of the lower cervical listings there will be a reliably reproducible pattern of bony and soft tissue point-specific pain. The patterns of painful points are identified in Table 22.18.

Postural examination

Forward head carriage is characteristic of lower cervical subluxation, it being axiomatic that the lower in the cervical spine (and even into the upper thoracic spine) the subluxation occurs, the more obvious the forward head carriage will be.

Subluxation of the thoracic and lumbar spine

The thoracic spine behaves in a similar way to the lower cervical spine when affected by subluxation. Loss of glenohumeral abduction is the most consistent and reliable indicator of thoracic subluxation; it occurs on the side of the open wedge with the degree of lost abduction correlating with the level of subluxation. This relationship is described later in this chapter. The loss of glenohumeral abduction must be viewed, however, within the context of upper cervical and lumbopelvic examination findings that do not meet the diagnostic criteria for subluxation in those areas. Alternatively, if a thoracic

Table 22.18 Relationship of point-specific pain findings and lower cervical listings

Listing	Description of location of pain points
PRS and PRI-La	Pain over the right side of the axis spinous and the left lamina
PLS and PLI-La	Pain over the left side of the axis spinous and the right lamina
Axis PI	Pain over the point of bifurcation of the axis spinous process in the segmental midline

subluxation does not present as the primary subluxation, but rather as a secondary layer, this may manifest as persistent loss of glenohumeral abduction against a background of normalized upper cervical function following correction of the primary dural tension subluxation.

Another reliable indicator of subluxation within the thoracic spine may be found in the clinical history. A complaint of pain at a specific, highly localized point within the thoracic spine is suggestive of local subluxation. This is in contrast to a complaint of more generalized pain, often burning in character and felt between the scapulae, usually either bilaterally or centrally. This presentation is characteristic of dural tension subluxation, making adjusting the thoracic spine at the level of pain counterproductive and technically wrong.

Subluxation of the upper lumbar spine will result in loss of lateral flexion and rotation bilaterally at the upper cervical complex; however, there will be no loss of glenohumeral abduction and, consequently, no Shimizu reflex. This is thought to be due to the lack of attachments of the trapezius muscle below T12. Examination of L5/S1 and the sacroiliac joints will be normal, as will examination of the front of the body. The psoas muscle is usually strong in upper lumbar presentations. At this point in the examination a subluxation of the upper lumbar spine must be considered along with the possibility of a muscle compartment syndrome or lower limb subluxation complex.

As was the case in the lower cervical area, all movements of the spinal motion segments in this area of the spine are coupled. As such, it follows that fixation/hypomobility must be demonstrated in all three body axes at any given level in order to be considered a possible site of subluxation.

Assessment of thoracic and upper lumbar spine motion

Once the initial examination of the patient has indicated that the primary subluxation complex may be located within the thoracic or upper lumbar spine, kinesiological assessment of these areas is appropriate. Motion assessment of the thoracic and upper lumbar spinal motion segments follows exactly the same protocols as those described for the lower cervical spine. In order to examine flexion at the upper four to six thoracic motion segments, the patient's head may be flexed forward using a similar technique to that used when assessing flexion of the lower cervical spinal motion segments. For levels lower than T4–T6, the patient will be required to slump in a similar fashion to when the lumbopelvis is being examined in flexion (Fig. 22.40), the goal being to create x-axis rotation at the level being examined.

Flexion is followed by rotation (Fig. 22.41), and then finally lateral flexion (Fig. 22.42), with similar principles of examination being applied to those movements. The interspinous space is the palpatory location, and the spinous process of the upper vertebra in the motion segment being examined is the reference point for clinical interpretation of the assessment findings. Restricted flexion is always associated with hypermobility in the motion segment above when that restricted flexion represents subluxation. It should be noted that thoracic vertebral

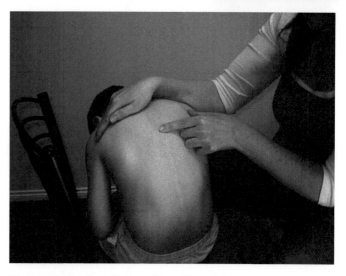

Figure 22.40 • Examination of the affected thoracic spine motion segments in flexion.

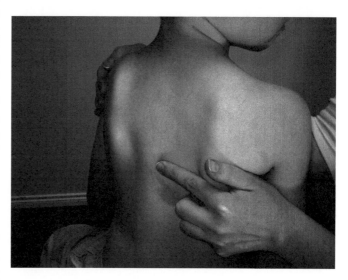

Figure 22.41 • Examination of the affected thoracic spine motion segment in rotation.

subluxation does not affect motion of the adjacent rib head in either flexion of extension. Table 22.19 sets out the range of possible outcomes of the motion assessment.

Neuropathology

When a thoracic or upper lumbar subluxation is present, pain will be elicited on gentle percussion with the reflex hammer over the spinous process of the subluxated vertebra. In a special case scenario, paraspinal skin rolling will produce severe pain on the side of the open wedge when the subluxation is at the thoracolumbar junction.

As mentioned in the introduction to this section, abduction of the arms at the glenohumeral joint will also be affected by thoracic subluxation, the degree to which the abduction is impaired being associated with the level of the subluxation, as described in Table 22.20.

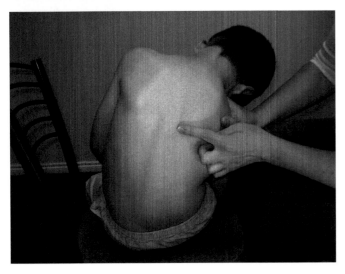

Figure 22.42 ● Examination of the affected thoracic spine motion segment in lateral flexion.

Table 22.19 Possible combinations of motion loss in the thoracic and upper lumbar spinal areas and their clinical interpretations

Flexion	Rotation	Lateral flexion	Listing
Restricted	R-L restricted	Right restriction	PRS
Restricted	L-R restricted	Left restriction	PLS
Restricted	L-R restricted	Right restriction	PLI-T (Thoracic) Or PRI-M (Lumbar)
Restricted	R-L restricted	Left restriction	PLI-T (Thoracic) Or PRI-M (Lumbar)
Restricted	L-R/R-L restricted	Bilateral restriction	PI

Table 22.20 Relationship between degree of reduction of abduction of the humerus and the thoracic subluxation

Degree of abduction reduction	Expected level of thoracic subluxation
90° of reduction	Upper one-third of the thoracic spine (T9–T12)
45–60° of reduction	Middle one-third of the thoracic spine (T5–T8)
10–15° of reduction	Lower one-third of the thoracic spine (T1–T4)

Sclerotomes

Embryologically, the ribs are formed by outcropping of the sclerotomal layer from the adjacent vertebrae. This makes specific rib angle tenderness to palpation a useful clinical tool in the subluxation assessment of the thoracic spinal motion segments. For example, rib 5 emanates from between the T5 and T6 vertebrae, and indeed articulates with both. Therefore, subluxation at the T6/7 level (with subsequent hypermobility at T5/6) will make the angle of the fifth rib painful to palpate on the side of the open wedge. This would mean that in a T6 PRS subluxation, the angle of the right fifth rib would be painful to palpation. As is the case in the lower cervical spine, exacerbation of the subluxation vectors worsens the sclerotomal pain and reduction of the vectors lessens it. In addition, when pain is present due to subluxation, gentle pressure applied to the affected vertebra in the direction of vector correction will lessen or obliterate it. In addition to glenohumeral abduction, sclerotomal pain offers the chiropractor a very reliable adjustive pre-test for the thoracic spine.

Myopathology and connective tissue pathology

For each of the thoracic and upper lumbar listings there will be a reliably reproducible pattern of bony and soft tissue point-specific pain findings. The patterns of painful points are identified in Table 22.21.

Postural examination

In the thoracic spine, local elevation of the paraspinal musculature is seen at the affected level on the side opposite that of spinous rotation. Subluxation involving the thoracic vertebrae, where a significant rotational component can be shown to exist, tends to cause an increase in the depth of the paraspinal gutter on the side of spinous laterality and a high 'muscle bunch' over the opposite transverse process. This muscle 'bunching' will be significantly accentuated in PRI-T and PLI-T listings.

Muscle bunching over several segments is a frequent finding on the side of scoliotic convexity. It should be noted that primary thoracic subluxation is uncommon from birth to school age and then begins to appear with greater frequency with advancing age throughout adolescence and into adulthood. It is thought that this may be due to the child becoming more physically active for longer periods of time after starting school.

Table 22.21 Relationship of point-specific pain findings and thoracic and upper lumbar listings

Listing	Description of location of pain points
PRS PRI-T or M	Pain over the inferior tip and right side of the spinous and the left transverse process for the thoracic vertebrae and the mamillary process for the lumbar vertebrae
PLS PLI-T or M	Pain over the inferior tip and left side of the spinous and the right transverse process for the thoracic vertebrae and the mamillary process for the lumbar vertebrae
PI	Pain over the inferior tip of the spinous process

The costovertebral subluxation

When examining the thoracic spine it is important to examine the ribs as well as the thoracic vertebrae. When a thoracic vertebra is the site of subluxation, there will be hypomobility in flexion at the involved level, hypermobility at the level above, and normal movement at the adjacent rib angle. The rib angle will, however, be painful when pressure is applied to the sclerotome.

When the subluxation is at the costovertebral articulation, there may be a loss of either flexion or extension at the rib angle and a loss of flexion between the adjacent thoracic vertebrae. Since the ribs attach between two vertebrae there will be a loss of flexion at both vertebral levels but no associated hypermobility at the level above. For example, if the sixth rib (which attaches to the spine between T5 and T6) is subluxated, there will be a loss of flexion at T5/T6 and at T6/T7 but flexion at T4/T5 will be normal. In addition, the rib angle will not be painful. Rather, there will be pain along either the rib's superior or its inferior margin, depending on whether the rib is superior or inferior, as the pain in this case is caused by soft tissue compression, not sclerotomal involvement.

Assessment of thoracic and upper lumbar spine motion

Superiority or inferiority of the rib is determined by motion palpation and will correlate with the pain finding. The palpatory location when assessing the ribs is the intercostal space at the level of the rib angle. If this space fails to open when the patient's head is taken into flexion (ribs 1–6) or they are asked to slump (ribs 6–12), this may be due to either the superior rib being subluxated inferiorly, or the inferior rib being subluxated superiorly. Differentiation is made by palpating the next rib space down while taking the spine into extension. If the motion here is normal, then the loss of flexion at the intercostal space above is due to inferior subluxation of the superior rib. If, however, this space fails to close on extension, then the loss of flexion at the level above is due to superior subluxation of the inferior rib.

Neuropathology

Abduction of the arms at the glenohumeral joint will also be affected by costovertebral subluxation, the degree to which the abduction is impaired being associated with the level of the subluxation in the same way as with thoracic vertebral subluxation. The most reliable pre-test for costovertebral subluxation is to apply gentle pressure to the rib in the direction of vector resolution and retest the glenohumeral abduction.

Myopathology and connective tissue pathology

For each costovertebral subluxation there will be a reliably reproducible pattern of bony and soft tissue point-specific pain findings. In superior subluxation the pain finding will be along the superior margin of the rib, as far laterally as the rib angle, while in inferior subluxation the pain finding will be along the inferior margin of the rib.

Exacerbation and adjustive pre-testing

It has been stated previously that the subluxation is a neurological entity and as such behaves predictably. In order to qualify as a subluxation, the appropriate kinesiopathology, neuropathology, and expected compensation pattern must all be demonstrated. Occasionally there are instances when all of these factors are demonstrable, with the exception of the neuropathology. In such cases, the neurological function cannot be said to be normal until the relevant neurological test has been performed with the nervous system placed under stress in such a way as to exacerbate the putative subluxation.

With spinal subluxation complexes, this is most readily achieved by changing spinal posture in such a way that the subluxation vectors, previously identified on kinesiological examination, will be exacerbated. This represents 'exacerbation testing of the subluxation'. Its basis in neuroscience is found in the assessment protocols employed when neurogenic claudication is suspected. In this condition, which involves mechanical pressure on neurological structures not dissimilar to that caused by the subluxation, it is common for there to be no demonstrable neurological deficit until the patient has walked/exercised to the point of pain, at which point focal neurological signs become readily measurable. This form of testing makes the link between neuropathology and the subluxation complex entirely reliable and has been the missing link in neurological assessment of the subluxation since the inception of chiropractic.

'Adjustive pre-testing' is essentially the opposite of exacerbation testing. It should be performed prior to making the adjustment and is carried out to prove that the area of kinesiopathology being examined does, in fact, represent the area of primary subluxation, and that the proposed adjustment will make the desired change within the nervous system. It is achieved by taking a contact over the subluxated level in such a way as to reduce all the vectors of the subluxation and then retesting an appropriate function. This may take the form of a reflex, a myotome, a sclerotome, or the compensation response.

References

Bergmann, T.F., Peterson, D.H., Lawrence, D.J., 1993. Chiropractic Technique, Principles and Procedures. Churchill Livingstone, New York.

Coggins, W., 1975. Basic Technique: A System of Body Mechanics. ELCO Publishing, Florissant.

Gatterman, M.I., 1990. Chiropractic Management of Spine Related Disorders. Williams and Wilkins, Baltimore.

Gatterman, M.I., 1995. Foundations of Chiropractic: Subluxation. Mosby, St Louis.

Herbst, R.W., 1968. Gonstead Chiropractic Science and Art. Sci Chi Publications, Chicago.

Kirk, C.R., Lawrence, D.J., Valvo, N.L., 1985. State's Manual of Spinal, Pelvic and Extra-vertebral Technic, second ed. Waverly Press, Baltimore.

Logan, V.F., Murray, F.M., (Eds), 1950. Textbook of Logan Basic Methods. LBM, St Louis.

Plaugher, G., 1993. Textbook of Clinical Chiropractic, a Specific Biomechanical Approach. Williams and Wilkins, Baltimore.

Reuter, P., 2005. Springer Universalwarterbuch Medizin, Pharmakologie Und Zahnmedizin. Englisch-Deutsch. Springer, Berlin.

Schwartzman, R.J., 2006. Neurologic Examination. Blackwell Publishing, Oxford.

Shimizu, T., Shimada, H., Shirakura, K., 1993. Scapulohumeral reflex (Shimizu): its clinical significance and testing maneuver. Spine 18 (15), 2182–2190.

Watson, J.C., Broaddus, W.C., Smith, M.M., et al., 1997. Hyperactive pectoralis reflex as an indicator of upper cervical spinal cord compression: report of 15 cases. J. Neurosurg. 86 (1), 159–161.

Adjusting the pediatric spine

Neil J. Davies   Sarah E. Whyatt

The principle of adjusting used in the procedures described in this chapter is the application of impulse to the affected segment in a direction that is in direct reverse to the three-dimensional vectors of dysfunction created by the cortical dysafferentation pattern being addressed. The initial contact should be held as lightly as possible and sustained for a period of 10–15 seconds before the thrust is applied. The thrust should be as shallow and as fast as possible.

The upper cervical complex

Occiput

Adjusting the posterior occiput (PS, PS-RS, PS-LS) requires a precise contact using the tip of the middle finger placed on the superior/medial aspect of the mastoid process on the involved side (Fig. 23.1). The patient is placed prone on the table with the head in the midline position and the thrust is applied in a posterior to anterior, lateral to medial, and superior to inferior direction. In the case of the double PS listing, the contact is applied to both sides simultaneously (Fig. 23.2).

To adjust the anterior occiput (AS, AS-RS, AS-LS) the patient is placed supine on the table. For a bilateral straight AS listing the patient's head is in the midline position, with a bilateral, simultaneous contact (Fig. 23.3). For the unilateral listings the patient's head is turned to the extent needed to acquire a stable contact on the anterior margin of the mastoid process (Fig. 23.4). The tip of the middle finger is placed on the anterior margin of the mastoid at the level of the external auditory meatus. The thrust is applied in an anterior to posterior and superior to inferior direction.

Atlas

For all atlas listings the patient is placed side-lying with the involved side up and the knees and hips comfortably flexed.

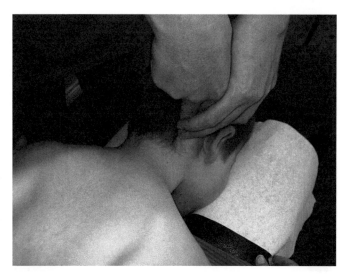

Figure 23.1 • Unilateral posterior occiput adjustment. In this case the listing is PS-RS.

The lower arm is wrapped around the abdomen and the upper arm placed straight down the patient's side. The head should be positioned such that the cervical spine is in its normal continuous contour with the thoracic spine. Contact is taken over the transverse process of the atlas using the tip of the middle finger (Fig. 23.5). Torque is applied through the soft tissues overlying the contact as the adjusting contact is slowly taken to tissue depth. The direction of thrust will vary according to the listing as shown in Table 23.1.

Axis and lower cervical vertebrae

The axis and lower cervical spine behave in a similar manner biomechanically and therefore will be considered together. For all listings the patient is placed prone on the table with the head in the midline position. For PLS, PRS and PI listings contact is taken with the tip of the middle finger

© 2010, Elsevier Ltd, Inc, BV
DOI: 10.1016/B978-0-7020-3129-8.00023-2

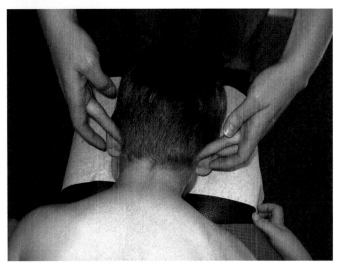

Figure 23.2 • Bilateral straight posterior occiput adjustment. In this case the listing is double PS.

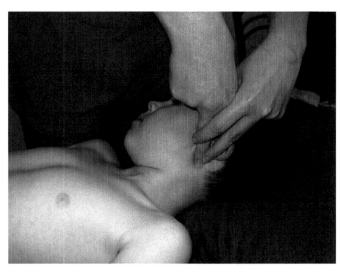

Figure 23.4 • Unilateral anterior occiput adjustment. In this case the listing is double AS.

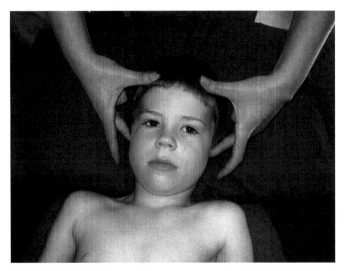

Figure 23.3 • Bilateral anterior occiput adjustment. In this case the listing is AS-LS.

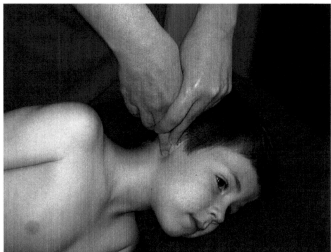

Figure 23.5 • Contact for right atlas adjustment. In this case the listing is either ASRA or AIRA.

Table 23.1 Direction of thrust for atlas listings. With torque, CW = clockwise and CCW = counterclockwise

Rotation	ASLA	AILA	ASLP	AILP	ASRA	AIRA	ASRP	AIRP
z-axis	L-M	L-M	L-M	L-M	L-M	L-M	L-M	L-M
y-axis	A-P	A-P	P-A	P-A	A-P	A-P	P-A	P-A
x-axis	CCW	CW	CCW	CW	CW	CCW	CW	CCW

over the spinous process of the involved vertebra (Figs 23.6, 23.7). For the listings PLI-La and PRI-La, the same contact is taken, this time over the lamina opposite the side of spinous rotation of the involved vertebra (Figs 23.8, 23.9). The direction of thrust will vary with the listing, as shown in Table 23.2.

The thoracic spine

For all adjustments of the thoracic spine the patient is placed prone on the table with the head in the midline position. For PLS, PRS and PI listings contact is taken with the tip of the middle finger over the spinous process of the involved vertebra

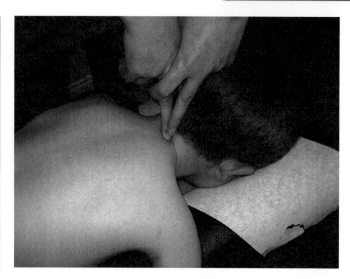

Figure 23.6 • Cervical spinous contact adjustment. In this case the listing is C6 PLS.

Figure 23.8 • Cervical lamina contact adjustment. In this case the listing is C6 PLI-La.

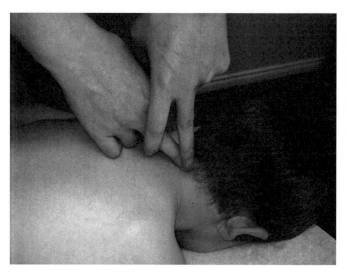

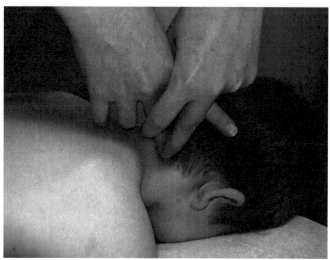

Figure 23.7 • Cervical spinous contact adjustment. In this case the listing is C2 PLS.

Figure 23.9 • Cervical lamina contact adjustment. In this case the listing is C2 PLI-La.

Table 23.2 Direction of thrust for axis and lower cervical listings. With torque, CW = clockwise and CCW = counterclockwise

Rotation	PLS	PRS	PLI-La	PRI-La	PI
y-axis	L-M	L-M	L-M	L-M	Neutral
x-axis	P-A	P-A	P-A	P-A	P-A
z-axis	CCW	CW	CW	CCW	None

as close to the tip of the spinous above as possible (Fig. 23.10). For the listings PLI-T and PRI-T, the contact is taken over the transverse process opposite the side of spinous rotation at the involved level (Fig. 23.11).

The direction of thrust will vary with the listing, as shown in Table 23.3.

The lumbar spine

Adjusting the lumbar spine follows a similar protocol to the low cervical and thoracic spine, with the exception of L5, which presents some special case scenarios arising from its articulation inferiorly with the sacral base which does not behave biomechanically in the same manner as a lumbar vertebra. These special case scenarios, in which the open wedge occurs on the side opposite the scoliotic convexity, are discussed in detail in Chapter 22.

For all listings in the lumbar spine the patient is placed prone on the table with the head in midline position. For PLS, PRS, PLI, PRI and PI listings contact is taken with the tip of the middle finger over the midpoint of the spinous process of the involved vertebra (Fig. 23.12). For the listings PLI-M, PRI-M, L5 PLS-M and L5 PRS-M

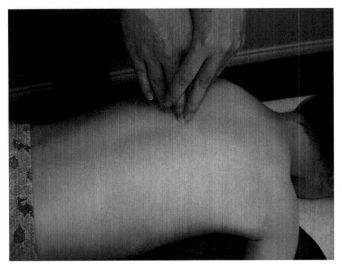

Figure 23.10 • Thoracic spinous contact adjustment. In this case the listing is T6 PLS.

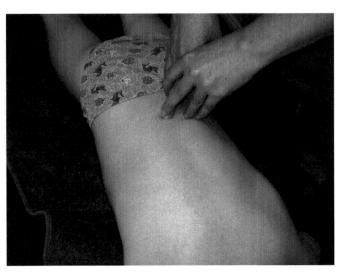

Figure 23.12 • Lumbar spinous contact adjustment. In this case the listing is L4 PLS.

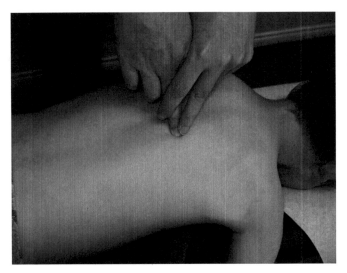

Figure 23.11 • Thoracic transverse process contact adjustment. In this case the listing is T6 PLI-T.

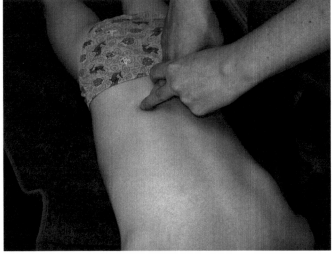

Figure 23.13 • Lumbar mamillary contact adjustment. In this case the listing is L4 PLI-M.

Table 23.4 Direction of thrust for lumbar listings. With torque, CW = clockwise and CCW = counterclockwise

Rotation	PLS	PRS	PLI-M	PRI-M	PI	PLS-M	PRS-M
z-axis	L-M	L-M	Neutral	Neutral	L-M	Neutral	Neutral
y-axis	P-A	P-A	P-A	P-A	P-A	P-A	P-A
x-axis	CCW	CW	CW	CCW	Neutral	CW	CCW

Table 23.3 Direction of thrust for thoracic listings. With torque, CW = clockwise and CCW = counterclockwise

Rotation	PLS	PRS	PLI-T	PRI-T	PI
y-axis	L-M	L-M	L-M	L-M	Neutral
x-axis	P-A	P-A	P-A	P-A	P-A
z-axis	CCW	CW	CW	CCW	None

The sacrum and coccyx

Rotated sacral and coccygeal segments

the contact is taken over the mamillary process opposite the side of spinous rotation of the involved vertebra (Fig. 23.13).

The direction of thrust will vary with the listing, as shown in Table 23.4.

Adjusting the rotated sacral or coccyx segment (P-L, P-R) requires a precise contact using the tip of the middle finger placed

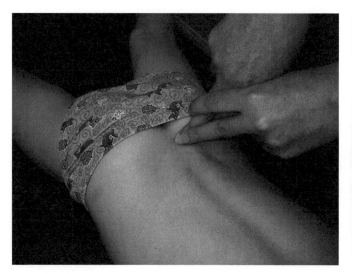

Figure 23.14 • Posteriorly rotated sacral segment adjustment. In this case the listing is S3 P-L.

over the affected sacral or coccyx segment on the posteriorly rotated side (Fig. 23.14). The patient is positioned prone on the table with the head in the midline position for all listings. The thrust is directed in a posterior to anterior direction for all sacral contacts, and a posterior to anterior and slightly superior to inferior direction for the coccyx listings.

In the unusual case where adjacent sacral segments are contralaterally rotated (S2 P-L/S3 P-R), the adjustive contact is applied to both affected segmental levels and the thrust is delivered simultaneously (Fig. 23.15).

Posterior sacral segments and base posterior coccyx

To adjust the posterior sacral segment (S2 P) and base posterior coccyx (BP) the patient is placed prone on the table with

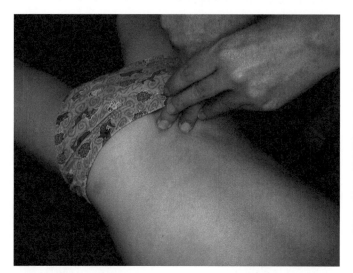

Figure 23.15 • Adjustive contacts for the contralaterally rotated sacral segment adjustment, in this case for the listings S2 P-L and S3 P-R. The adjustive impulse is applied to both the right and the left sides of the sacrum at the same time.

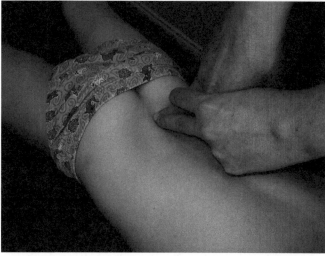

Figure 23.16 • Adjustive contact for the straight posterior sacral segment. In this case the listing is S2 P.

the head in the midline position. The tip of the middle finger is placed over the tubercle of the affected sacral segment (Fig. 23.16) or, in the case of the coccyx, over the midline of the coccygeal base. The thrust is directed in a posterior to anterior direction for all sacral contacts and a posterior to anterior and slightly superior to inferior direction for the base posterior coccyx.

Posteriorly rotated sacrum

The posteriorly rotated sacrum (P-L, P-R) is adjusted with the patient positioned prone on the table with the head in the midline position. A precise contact is taken using the tip of the thumb placed over the musculature inferior and posterior to the greater trochanter on the involved side (Fig. 23.17). A light sustained force is held, with a posterior to anterior vector directed towards the crest of the ilium on

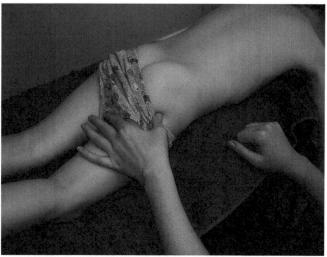

Figure 23.17 • Trochanteric contact adjustment for the posteriorly rotated sacrum. In this case the listing is P-R.

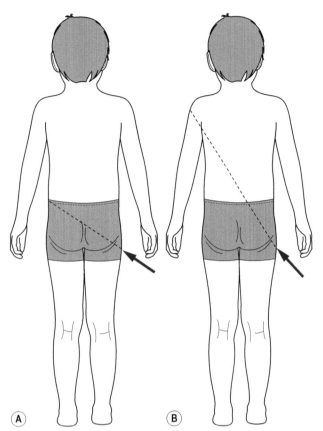

Figure 23.18 • Initial direction of contact (A) and final direction of contact (B) for both the posteriorly and anteriorly rotated sacrum.

the side opposite the contact, until normal pelvic girdle respiratory driven movement is restored (Fig. 23.18A). At that point, which is frequently accompanied by a sigh or change in respiratory depth, the direction of force is altered towards the shoulder on the side opposite the contact (Fig. 23.18B). The occiput is palpated, feeling for the restoration of cranial rhythm. When this is achieved, the contact time is complete and a fast shallow thrust is applied.

Anteriorly rotated sacrum

To adjust the anteriorly rotated sacrum (LAIS, RAIS) the patient is again positioned prone on the table with the head in the midline position. A precise contact is taken using the tip of the thumb placed over the musculature inferior and anterior to the greater trochanter on the involved side (Fig. 23.19). A light sustained force is held, with an anterior to posterior vector directed towards the crest of the ilium on the side opposite the contact (see Fig. 23.18A), until normal pelvic girdle respiratory driven movement is restored. At that point, which is frequently accompanied by a sigh or change in respiratory depth, the direction of force is altered towards the shoulder on the side opposite the contact (see Fig. 23.18B). The occiput is palpated, feeling for the restoration of cranial rhythm. When this is achieved, the contact time is complete and a fast shallow thrust is applied.

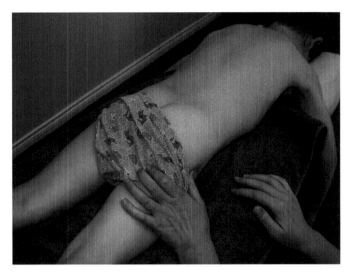

Figure 23.19 • Trochanteric contact adjustment for the anteriorly rotated sacrum. In this case the listing is RAIS.

Base posterior sacrum

Adjusting the base posterior sacrum (BP) may be done with the patient either standing with the trunk very slightly flexed at the lumbosacral junction, or prone on the table with the head in the midline position. The tips of the thumbs are placed over the musculature inferior and posterior to the greater trochanters on both sides simultaneously (Fig. 23.20). A light sustained force is held with both thumbs directed with a posterior to anterior vector towards the crest of each opposite ilium until normal pelvic girdle respiratory driven movement is restored. At that point, which is frequently accompanied by a sigh or change in respiratory depth, the direction of force is altered towards each opposite shoulder. This contact direction is held for a further 60 seconds and then a fast shallow thrust is applied.

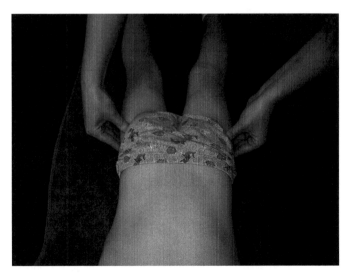

Figure 23.20 • Trochanteric contact adjustment for the base posterior sacrum.

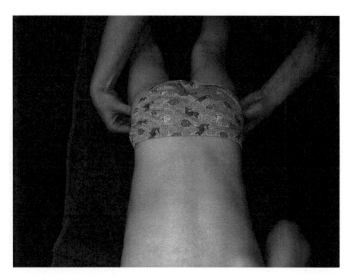

Figure 23.21 • Trochanteric contact adjustment for the base anterior sacrum.

Base anterior sacrum

Adjusting the base anterior sacrum (BA) may also be done with the patient either standing with the trunk very slightly flexed at the lumbosacral junction, or prone on the table with the head in the midline position. The tips of the thumbs are placed over the musculature inferior and anterior to the greater trochanter on both sides simultaneously (Fig. 23.21). A light sustained force is held with both thumbs directed with an anterior to posterior vector towards the crest of each opposite ilium until normal pelvic girdle respiratory driven movement is restored. At that point, which is frequently accompanied by a sigh or change in respiratory depth, the direction of force is altered towards each opposite shoulder. This contact direction is held for a further 60 seconds and then a fast shallow thrust is applied.

Atypical sacral subluxation

The atypical sacral subluxation, also known as a bilateral torsional subluxation, is a situation in which one side of the sacrum is posteriorly rotated and simultaneously the opposite side is anteriorly rotated. The two possible listings are P-R/LAIS and P-L/RAIS.

The adjustment is effected using a simultaneous contact with the tips of the thumbs placed over the musculature inferior and anterior to the greater trochanter on the anteriorly rotated side (RAIS or LAIS) and inferior and posterior to the greater trochanter on the posteriorly rotated side (P-R or P-L). The best position to effect the adjustment is with the patient standing. Very young or small children should be prone across their mother's lap. The standing patient is asked to flex their trunk very slightly at the lumbosacral junction while a light, sustained force is applied through both thumbs directed with an anterior to posterior vector towards the crest of the opposite ilium on the anteriorly rotated side and with a posterior to anterior vector towards the crest of the opposite ilium on the posteriorly rotated side until normal pelvic girdle respiratory driven movement is restored. At that point, which is

frequently accompanied by a sigh or change in respiratory depth, the direction of force is altered towards each opposite shoulder. This contact direction is held for a further 60 seconds and then a fast shallow thrust is applied. It is critical to an efficient adjustment that the appropriate posterior to anterior and anterior to posterior directions are maintained throughout the procedure.

The ilium

The posterior ilium

To adjust the posterior ilium (PIIn, PIEx), contact is taken on the involved side over the posterior surface of the posterior superior iliac spine (PSIS) for the PIEx and over the medial surface of the PSIS for the PIIn. When adjusting the posterior ilium, torque accounts for the rotational (In or Ex) components of the adjustment. The patient is positioned prone with the head in the midline position. For the PIEx ilium, a light sustained force is first held in a posterior to anterior, lateral to medial, and inferior to superior direction. After 10–15 seconds a very fast, light thrust is made in that direction with the addition of counterclockwise torque for the left side and clockwise torque for the right. For the PIIn, a light sustained force is first held in a posterior to anterior, medial to lateral, and inferior to superior direction. After 10–15 seconds a very fast, light thrust is made in that direction with the addition of clockwise torque for the left side and counterclockwise torque for the right.

The anterior ilium

For the anterior ilium (ASIn, ASEx) the torque again accounts for the rotational (In or Ex) components of the adjustment. The patient is positioned prone with the head in the midline position. Contact is taken over the ischial spine on the involved side. For the ASEx ilium, a light sustained force is first held in a posterior to anterior, lateral to medial, and inferior to superior direction. After 10–15 seconds a very fast, light thrust is made in that direction with the addition of counterclockwise torque for the left side and clockwise torque for the right. For the ASIn, a light sustained force is first held in a posterior to anterior, medial to lateral, and superior to inferior direction. After 10–15 seconds a very fast, light thrust is made in that direction with the addition of clockwise torque for the left side and counterclockwise torque for the right.

The internal ilium

To adjust the internal ilium (In) the patient is placed prone with the head in the midline position. Contact is taken over the medial surface of the PSIS at the midpoint of the sacro-iliac joint (Fig. 23.22). A light sustained force is first held in a medial to lateral direction. After 10–15 seconds a very fast, light thrust is made in that direction, without the addition of any torque.

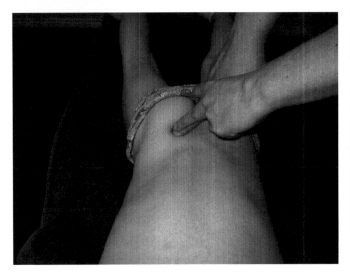

Figure 23.22 • Contact for the In ilium adjustment. In this case the listing is R-In.

The external ilium

In the case of the external ilium (Ex), the patient is again placed prone with the head in the midline position. Contact is taken over the lateral surface of the PSIS at the midpoint of the sacroiliac joint (Fig. 23.23). A light sustained force is first held in a lateral to medial direction. After 10–15 seconds a very fast, light thrust is made in that direction, without the addition of any torque.

The In-Ex pelvis

Adjustment of the In-Ex pelvis (LEx-RIn, REx-LIn) requires a simultaneous contact over the lateral surface of the PSIS at the midpoint of the sacroiliac joint on the Ex side and over the medial surface of the PSIS at the midpoint of the sacroiliac joint on the In side (Fig. 23.24). The patient is positioned

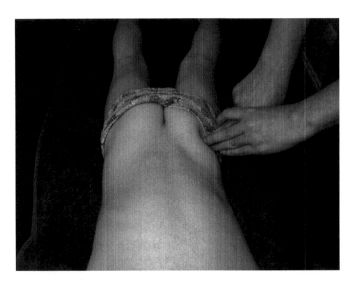

Figure 23.23 • Contact for the Ex ilium adjustment. In this case the listing is L-Ex.

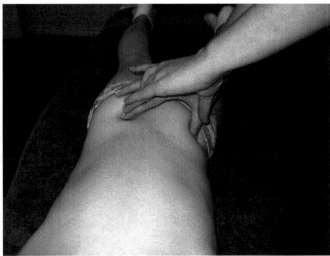

Figure 23.24 • Contact for the Ex-In pelvis adjustment. In this case the listing is L-Ex/R-In.

prone with the head in the midline position. The practitioner stands on the side of the Ex ilium and holds a light sustained force in a lateral to medial direction for the Ex component. After 10–15 seconds a very fast, light thrust is made at both contact points simultaneously in that direction without the addition of any torque.

The pubis

Synchondrosis separation

To adjust the separated pubic synchondrosis the patient is placed supine on the table and contact is taken with the pads of the thumbs placed approximately one finger's width lateral to the pubic synchondrosis on the anterior surface of the pubis on both sides. Gentle lateral to medial pressure is applied through both thumbs to 'close' the synchondrosis on the expiratory phase of respiration. This procedure is performed through five phases of respiration followed by a light, fast thrust at the completion of the fifth cycle.

The superior pubic ramus

For the superior pubic ramus subluxation the patient is placed supine on the table and contact is taken with the pads of the thumbs placed over the superior pubic ramus on the involved side. Gentle superior to inferior pressure is applied to the superior pubic ramus on the expiratory phase of respiration. This procedure is performed through five phases of respiration and a light, fast thrust is made at the completion of the fifth cycle.

The inferior pubic ramus

For the inferior pubic ramus subluxation the patient is placed supine on the table and contact is taken with the pads of the thumbs placed over the inferior pubic ramus on the involved side.

Gentle inferior to superior pressure is applied to the inferior pubic ramus on the inspiratory phase of respiration. This procedure is performed through five phases of respiration and a light, fast thrust is made at the completion of the fifth cycle.

The countertorsional (inferior/superior) pubic rami

Adjustment of the inferior/superior pubic rami, a countertorsional subluxation of the pubic synchondrosis, requires a bilateral contact with the pads of the thumbs with the patient in the supine position. The inferior hand thumb pad is placed over the inferior pubic ramus on the inferior pubic side and the superior hand thumb pad is placed over the superior pubic ramus on the superior pubic side. An alternating gentle pressure is applied with increased inferior to superior pressure to the inferior pubic ramus on the inspiratory phase of respiration followed by an increased superior to inferior pressure to the superior pubic ramus on the expiratory phase of respiration. This procedure is performed through five phases of respiration and at the completion of the fifth cycle a light, fast thrust is delivered simultaneously through both thumbs.

The upper limb subluxation

24

Neil J. Davies   Robert Turner-Jensen

Subluxation in the upper limb is commonly encountered in pediatric practice. It may present as the primary layer of subluxation following trauma, with the child complaining of pain or displaying obvious signs of discomfort, but more often the upper limb subluxation is disguised, regionally asymptomatic, and often overlooked or misdiagnosed as a cervical problem. Subluxation at a distal location in the biomechanical chain will, as a rule, lead to kinesiopathology more proximally. A good example of this linkage phenomenon is the lunate, which, when subluxated, will typically affect the wrist, elbow, shoulder and cervical spine. While this association may seem daunting at first, the principles of adjustive pre-testing in accordance with the vectors of subluxation will demonstrate which of the functionally impaired joints are actually a compensation response. The large representation of the hand on the sensory homunculus in the cerebral cortex may explain the level of dysafferentation seen with upper limb subluxation, and the often dramatic resolution following correction.

Diagnosis of the upper limb subluxation

In order to determine that the upper limb is a possible area of subluxation, a number of key findings should be present on examination of the upper cervical spine and the glenohumeral joint. Subluxation examination of the patient must begin as standard at the upper cervical complex, regardless of symptomatology at any level. It is, however, imperative that a thorough orthopedic examination be performed at the affected joint and subluxation examination should in no way be seen as a replacement for such an examination.

Kinesiopathology

The subluxation examination of the upper limb starts with the standard examination of the upper cervical complex, with the patient seated in an anatomical position neutral to the three axes of rotation. When the primary subluxation is located in the upper extremity, the upper cervical complex will demonstrate diminished lateral flexion on the side of the affected limb, while the remainder of the examination remains within normal limits. This pattern of loss is by far the most common. However, bilateral subluxation of the upper limb can and does occur, and, when it does, the affected joints are usually the same, like a mirror image of each other.

In addition to lateral flexion restriction in the upper cervical complex, shoulder abduction will be universally restricted on the affected side and sometimes on both sides. When the glenohumeral restriction is bilateral, the upper limb subluxation may still be only unilateral, in which case the upper cervical lateral flexion will also be unilateral. It is important to note that no correlation can be drawn between the degree of movement loss in the upper cervical complex and/or the glenohumeral joint and the level or severity of the subluxation in terms of the patient's symptoms.

Neuropathology

Once it has been determined that upper cervical lateral flexion is impaired, either unilaterally or bilaterally, the pattern of neurological deficit will direct the chiropractor to the appropriate anatomical location (Table 24.1). It is noteworthy that the more proximal the subluxation, the more apparent the neuropathology will be. The glenohumeral subluxation requires that the Shimizu reflex be positive, whereas all the other levels in the upper limb, including the acromioclavicular joint, the Shimizu reflex will be normal (See Table 24.1).

The glenohumeral joint

The humeral head subluxation in the glenohumeral cavity is a very common problem in pediatrics, especially in the first year of life. Unilateral glenohumeral subluxation is associated with

© 2010, Elsevier Ltd, Inc, BV
DOI: 10.1016/B978-0-7020-3129-8.00024-4

Table 24.1 Neurological deficits associated with the upper limb subluxation

Structure	Associated neurological deficits
Glenohumeral joint	Shimizu positive Pectoral normal or absent SHR normal
Acromioclavicular joint (clavicle)	Shimizu normal Pectoral normal SHR normal
Acromioclavicular joint (scapula)	Shimizu normal Pectoral normal SHR normal or absent
Elbow, wrist or hand	Shimizu normal Pectoral normal SHR normal

(Scapulohumeral reflex)

sleep dysfunction, breast refusal (when the baby is placed affected side down to feed), fixed head posture syndromes and, by extension, plagiocephaly. Later in the first year of life, glenohumeral subluxation affects the ready adoption of the prone posture, critical to extensor reflex development, rolling over and crawling.

Kinesiopathology

The humeral head is capable of subluxation medially, laterally, anteriorly, posteriorly, and into either internal or external rotation within the glenohumeral cavity. The reference landmark for all movements is the anterior humeral tubercle. When examining the glenohumeral joint it is important to grasp the humerus as close as possible to its proximal end to best appreciate the range of motion (Figs 24.1–24.6).

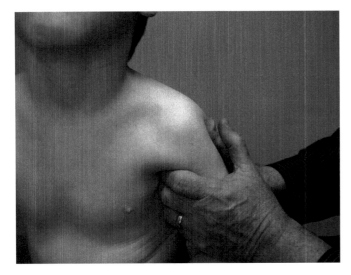

Figure 24.1 • Assessment of the range of motion of the humeral head within the glenohumeral cavity in translation along the x-axis from medial to lateral. Restricted movement suggests a medial humeral head.

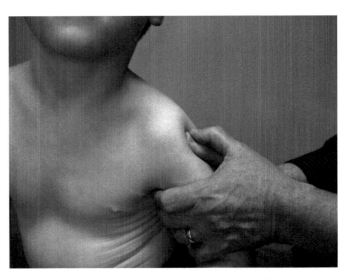

Figure 24.2 • Assessment of the range of motion of the humeral head within the glenohumeral cavity in translation along the x-axis from lateral to medial. Restricted movement suggests a lateral humeral head.

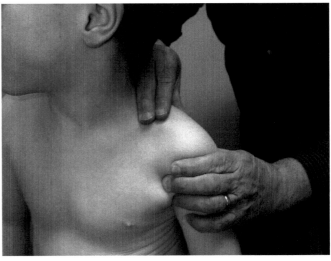

Figure 24.3 • Assessment of the range of motion of the humeral head within the glenohumeral cavity in translation parallel to the z-axis from anterior to posterior. Restricted movement suggests an anterior humeral head.

By far the majority of humeral head subluxations, particularly in the first year of life, have a dominant anterior element; this is usually associated with external rotation subluxation. Any compound combination, however, is possible, making the evaluation of each element critical in establishing the optimal line of adjustive thrust. It should also be noted that the humeral head subluxation, while occurring most commonly as a unilateral phenomenon, can occur simultaneously on both sides, and on occasion exhibits exactly the opposite direction of subluxation. A good example of such a complex bilateral subluxation would be a right anterior/external rotation subluxation concomitant with a left posterior/internal rotation subluxation. Lateral and medial humeral head subluxations are rare at all age levels and, when present, usually suggest an initiating trauma.

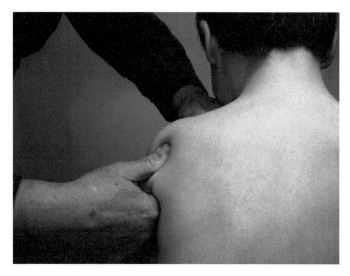

Figure 24.4 • Assessment of the range of motion of the humeral head within the glenohumeral cavity in translation parallel to the z-axis from posterior to anterior. Restricted movement suggests a posterior humeral head.

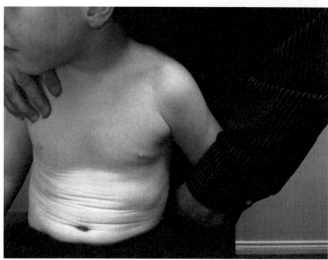

Figure 24.6 • Assessment of the range of motion of the humeral head within the glenohumeral cavity in rotation about an axis parallel to the y-axis. In the above case, internal rotation of the humerus is being assessed. Restricted movement suggests external rotation of the humeral head, usually associated with the posterior humeral head subluxation when present.

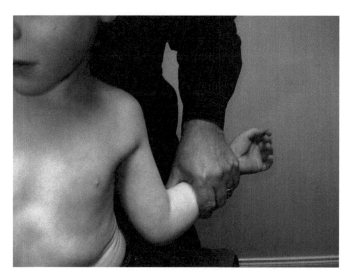

Figure 24.5 • Assessment of the range of motion of the humeral head within the glenohumeral cavity in rotation about an axis parallel to the y-axis. In the above case, external rotation of the humerus is being assessed. Restricted movement suggests internal rotation of the humeral head, usually associated with the anterior humeral head subluxation when present.

Myopathology and connective tissue pathology

The humeral head will exhibit subluxation vector-specific pain findings related to muscle stretch and connective tissue irritation. The exact locations of these pain findings are shown in Table 24.2.

Table 24.2 Location of the point-specific pain findings associated with subluxation of the humeral head

Vector of subluxation	Point-specific pain finding
Lateral	Lateral humeral head
Medial	Medial humeral head high in the lateral axilla wall
Anterior	Anterior humeral tubercle
Posterior	Posterior humeral head
External rotation	Pectoralis major insertion
Internal rotation	Teres minor insertion

Neuropathology

In addition to the reflex changes mentioned earlier in this chapter, the three divisions of the deltoid muscle will be weakened in a pattern specific to the direction of humeral head movement (Table 24.3), and these are tested in age-appropriate

Table 24.3 Weak muscle pattern associated with the humeral head subluxation

Vector of humeral head subluxation	Associated weak muscle
Anterior	Anterior deltoid
Posterior	Posterior deltoid
Medial/lateral	Middle deltoid

patients. The biceps, triceps and coracobrachialis all appear to remain unaffected by glenohumeral subluxation.

As in other regions of the body, adjustive pre-testing using the neuropathology is a valuable clinical tool. However, in young children who have not reached the age where they can be meaningfully and reliably muscle tested, the chiropractor needs to rely on other neurological deficits in the adjustive pre-test. For example, in a baby with an anterior humeral head subluxation, impulse-generating pressure is held over the anterior humeral head in a posterior direction, usually by the caregiver, while the chiropractor re-evaluates cervical lateral flexion, humeral abduction, or the Shimizu reflex.

Corrective procedures

The adjustive procedures are applied to the glenohumeral subluxations according to the vector(s) of movement involved, making precise kinesiopathology identification extremely important. Once identified, adjustive pre-testing is first performed to ensure that correction can be demonstrated with impulse generation at the point of proposed adjustive thrust. Once this has been established, it is appropriate to make the adjustment. The contact point and direction of adjustive thrust for each of the glenohumeral subluxations is shown in Figs 24.7–24.10.

The acromioclavicular joint (clavicle)

The acromioclavicular joint may involve subluxation of the clavicular head or the scapula. The clinical presentation is quite different. In the discussion to follow, the clavicular head subluxation will first be dealt with, then the scapula subluxation.

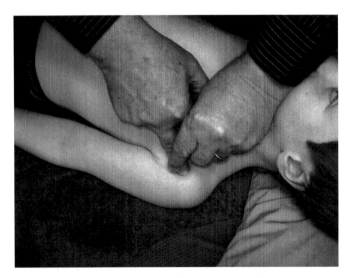

Figure 24.7 • Contact point and direction of thrust for the anterior humeral head subluxation. In the event the anteriority is coupled with external rotation, the forearm is taken across the child's chest to induce internal rotation before the contact is taken.

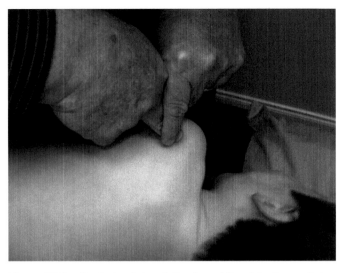

Figure 24.8 • Contact point and direction of thrust for the posterior humeral head subluxation. In the event the posteriority is coupled with internal rotation, the forearm is taken into abduction to induce external rotation before the contact is taken.

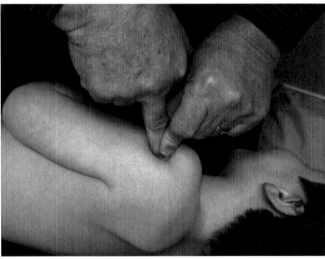

Figure 24.9 • Contact point and direction of thrust for the lateral humeral head subluxation.

Kinesiopathology

It is not unusual for the clavicle to fracture during the events of birth, but while most fractures heal remarkably quickly, subluxation may persist beyond the healing phase.

The clavicular head may subluxate anteriorly, posteriorly, or superiorly. Combinations of superiority with anteriority or posteriority occur with some regularity; however, the straight anterior listing is by far the most common. Within the acromioclavicular joint, the anterior and posterior subluxation vectors are derived by inducing translation of the clavicular head along a line parallel to the z-axis (Figs 24.11 and 24.12). The superior vector is assessed only by pain findings and is frequently not present.

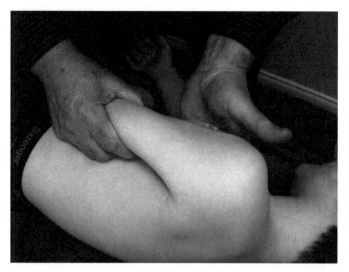

Figure 24.10 • Contact point and direction of thrust for the medial humeral head subluxation.

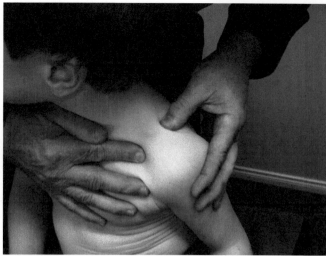

Figure 24.12 • Assessment of translation along a line parallel to the z-axis from posterior to anterior. Restricted movement implies a posterior clavicular head at the acromioclavicular joint.

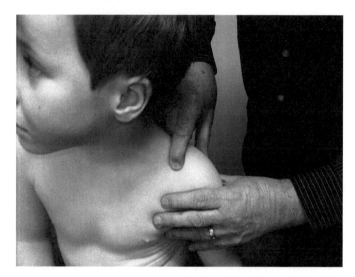

Figure 24.11 • Assessment of translation along a line parallel to the z-axis from anterior to posterior. Restricted movement implies an anterior clavicular head at the acromioclavicular joint.

Myopathology and connective tissue pathology

Point-specific pain findings are seen consistent with the movement of the clavicular head and are probably related to connective tissue stress rather than muscle stretch. The anterior subluxation has a pain finding over the anterior aspect of the clavicular head, the superior subluxation on the superior surface, and the posterior subluxation over the posterior aspect of the clavicular head.

Neuropathology

Irrespective of the direction of movement, the clavicular division of the pectoralis major will usually weaken. It can be strengthened by gently holding pressure on the clavicular head

in a direction to take it out of subluxation. Conversely, if the muscle is not weak when the joint meets all the other criteria of subluxation, holding it gently further into subluxation will indeed cause the muscle to weaken.

Corrective procedures

The adjustive procedures are applied to the acromioclavicular (clavicle) subluxations according to the vector(s) of movement involved, making precise kinesiopathology identification extremely important. Once identified, adjustive pre-testing is first performed to ensure that correction can be demonstrated with impulse generation at the point of proposed adjustive thrust. Once this has been established, it is appropriate to make the adjustment. The contact point and direction of adjustive thrust for each of the acromioclavicular (clavicle) subluxations is shown in Figs 24.13 and 24.14.

The acromioclavicular joint (scapula)

Kinesiopathology

The scapula may subluxate in rotation about either the y-axis or z-axis, or both. The reference point for determining kinesiopathology is the superior scapular angle. The movements into subluxation about the z-axis are therefore superior or inferior and those about the y-axis are internal or external. Combinations of movement about both axes occur with some regularity, but the superior listing is by far the most common. This is thought to be due to the action of the levator scapulae muscle. Once it has been determined that the scapula is the likely site of subluxation, the diagnosis is confirmed by point-specific pain finding, muscle test and neurological pre-test.

Lifting a young child by the arms, or swinging a young child around, causes undue stress to the shoulder girdle, including

307

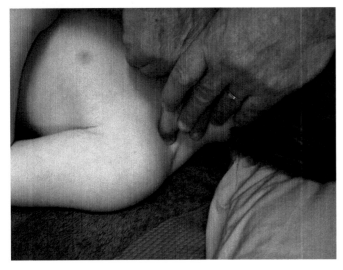

Figure 24.13 • Contact point and direction of thrust for the anterior clavicular head subluxation. When there is a superior element, the line of adjustive thrust is altered from solely A-P to include a S-I vector.

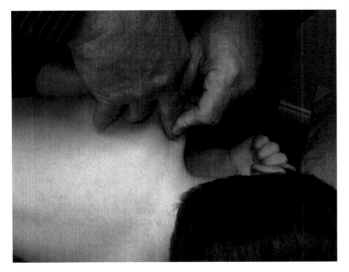

Figure 24.14 • Contact point and direction of thrust for the posterior clavicular head subluxation.

the clavicular and scapular articulations, and if subluxation recurs it is advisable to look for handling errors by caregivers, however unintentional this may have been.

Myopathology and connective tissue pathology

The scapula will exhibit very consistent point-specific pain findings related to the direction of movement (Table 24.4).

Neuropathology

In addition to the reflex changes mentioned earlier, the rhomboids major and minor, subscapularis, teres minor and infraspinatus will be weakened in pattern with the direction of

Table 24.4 Location of the point-specific pain findings associated with subluxation of the scapula

Vector of subluxation	Point-specific pain finding
Superior	Superior scapula angle
Inferior	Lateral aspect of the inferior scapula angle
Internal rotation	Rhomboid major insertion
External rotation	Teres minor insertion

Table 24.5 Weak muscle pattern associated with the scapula subluxation

Vector of scapula subluxation	Associated weak muscle
Superior	Rhomboid major
Inferior	Subscapularis, infraspinatus, supraspinatus and teres minor
Internal rotation	Rhomboid major
External rotation	Subscapularis, infraspinatus, supraspinatus and teres minor

scapular movement (Table 24.5). Obviously these muscles can only be effectively tested with children whose cognitive ability is at an appropriate level.

Corrective procedures

The adjustive procedures are applied to the acromioclavicular (clavicle) subluxations according to the vector(s) of movement involved, making precise kinesiopathology identification extremely important. Once identified, adjustive pre-testing is first performed to ensure that correction can be demonstrated with impulse generation at the point of proposed adjustive thrust. Once this has been established, it is appropriate to make the adjustment. The contact point and direction of adjustive thrust for each of the acromioclavicular (scapular) subluxations is shown in Figs 24.15–24.17.

The elbow joint

The elbow articulations are sensitive to the child being pulled forcefully where the radial head sustains the trauma and can dislocate. Translational and rotational forces also occur during play, gripping, throwing and playing racket sports, to mention just a few. When the primary subluxation is located at the elbow, there will always be a restriction in upper cervical lateral flexion while rotation is maintained as well as a decrease in abduction of the humerus to some extent. The degree of loss does not appear to equate to the severity of the subluxation in terms of the patient's symptoms. Subluxation may occur at the elbow joint involving either x-axis translation, rotation about the y-axis of

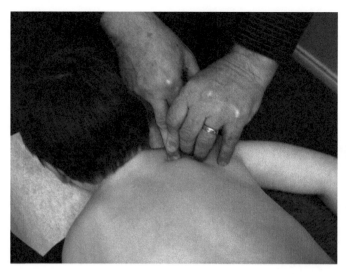

Figure 24.15 • Contact point and direction of thrust for the superior scapular subluxation.

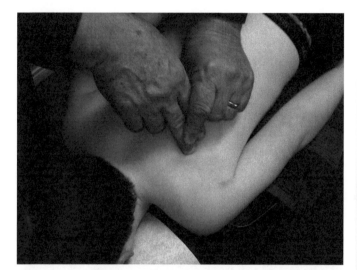

Figure 24.16 • Contact point and direction of thrust for the medial scapular subluxation.

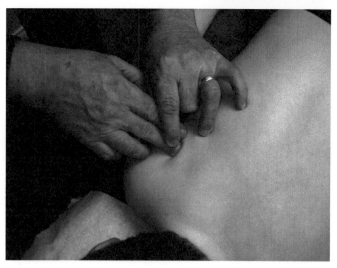

Figure 24.17 • Contact point and direction of thrust for the lateral scapular subluxation. This exact same contact point and direction of thrust applies equally to the inferior scapular subluxation. It is worth noting that inferior and lateral scapular subluxations frequently occur concomitantly.

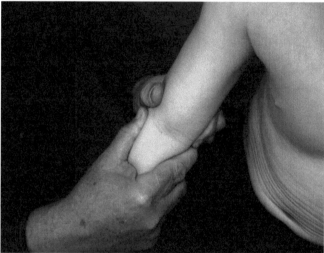

Figure 24.18 • Assessment of lateral to medial translation of the ulna under the humerus along the x-axis.

the ulna under the humerus and of the radial head around the ulna. While most ulnar rotations are unilateral, the elbow joint occasionally exhibits a counter-rotated subluxation.

Kinesiopathology

The ulna needs to be examined in translation and rotation, while the radial head needs to be examined in rotation. The technique of examination for the elbow joints is shown in Figs 24.18–24.23. One must pay particular attention to locate the ulna correctly when examining it from the radial aspect. The majority of radial head subluxations are internally rotated (anterior) and are evidenced by poor supination capability and a very painful point located immediately over the anterior aspect of the radial head. On observation, the patient will also hold the hand at rest in an internally rotated posture, so that the palm of the hand on the affected side will face more to the posterior than medially.

Myopathology and connective tissue pathology

The elbow and radioulnar joints will exhibit very consistent point-specific pain findings related to the direction of movement (Table 24.6).

Neuropathology

The Shimizu reflex is universally absent in elbow subluxation and the pectoral and scapulohumeral reflexes will be normal. Quite specific myotome weakness, however, will be seen which, in older children able to cooperate meaningfully with the examination procedure, will differentiate the elbow joint from the

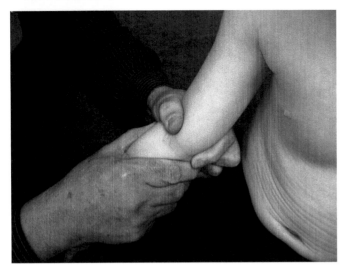

Figure 24.19 • Assessment of medial to lateral translation of the ulna under the humerus along the x-axis.

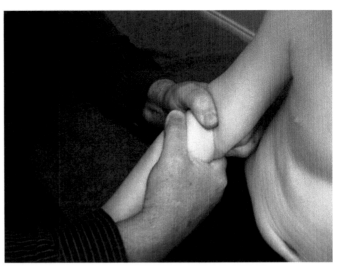

Figure 24.21 • Assessment of internal rotation of the ulna under the humerus about the y-axis.

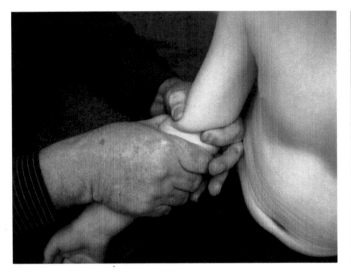

Figure 24.20 • Assessment of external rotation of the ulna under the humerus about the y-axis.

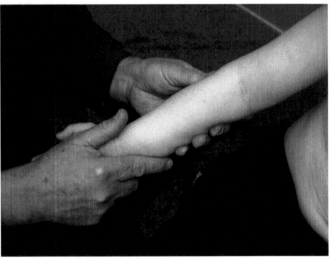

Figure 24.22 • Assessment of external rotation of the radius around the ulna about the y-axis.

radioulnar joint. The test involves assessment of the strength of the triceps muscle, firstly with the hand locked into palmar flexion (Fig. 24.24) and, secondly, with the hand locked into dorsiflexion (Fig. 24.25). Ulnar subluxation at the elbow joint causes the triceps to test weak with the hand locked in palmar flexion, while subluxation at the radioulnar joint causes the triceps to test weak with the hand locked in dorsiflexion.

Corrective procedures

The adjustive procedures are applied to the elbow and radio-ulnar subluxations according to the vector(s) of movement involved, making precise kinesiopathology identification extremely important. Once identified, adjustive pre-testing is first performed to ensure that correction can be demonstrated with impulse generation at the point of proposed adjustive thrust. Once this has been established, it is appropriate to make the adjustment. The contact point and direction of adjustive thrust for each of the elbow joint subluxations is shown in Figs 24.26–24.31 and for the radioulnar subluxation in Figs 24.32 and 24.33.

The wrist and hand

Subluxation at the wrist in children is common, and by nature somewhat complicated. Children examine everything by touch, brace falls on their hands, and put fingers where they should not. The wrists and hands contain a large number of bones and articulations (Fig. 24.34) and the size of these makes investigation difficult. The key to accurate diagnosis is

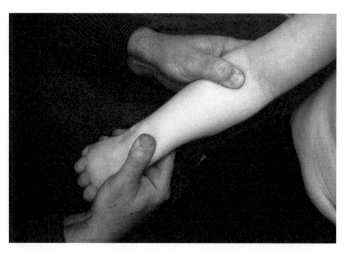

Figure 24.23 • Assessment of internal rotation of the radius around the ulna about the y-axis.

Table 24.6 Location of the point-specific pain findings associated with subluxation of the elbow and radioulnar joints

Vector of subluxation	Point-specific pain finding
Lateral ulna	Lateral aspect of the ulna immediately below the elbow joint line
Medial ulna	Medial aspect of the ulna immediately below the elbow joint line
Internal rotation of the ulna	Anterolateral aspect of the ulna immediately below the elbow joint line
External rotation of the ulna	Anteromedial aspect of the ulna immediately below the elbow joint line
Internal rotation of the radial head (anterior radius)	Anterior aspect of the radial head
External rotation of the radial head (posterior radius)	Posterior aspect of the radial head

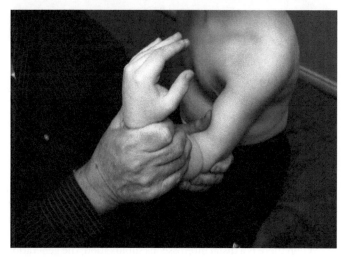

Figure 24.24 • Triceps muscle test with the hand locked into palmar flexion. Weakness in this position implies an ulnar subluxation at the elbow joint.

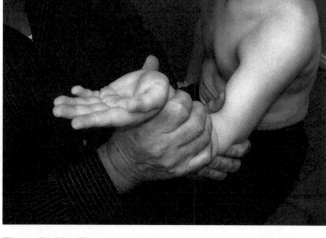

Figure 24.25 • Triceps muscle test with the hand locked into dorsiflexion. Weakness in this position implies a radial head subluxation at the radioulnar joint.

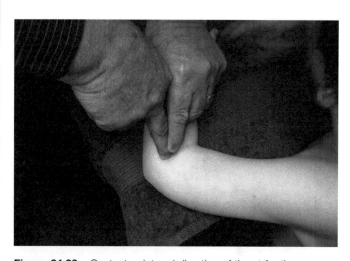

Figure 24.26 • Contact point and direction of thrust for the lateral ulna.

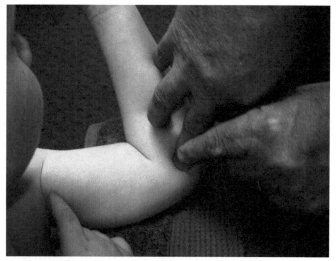

Figure 24.27 • Contact point and direction of thrust for the medial ulna.

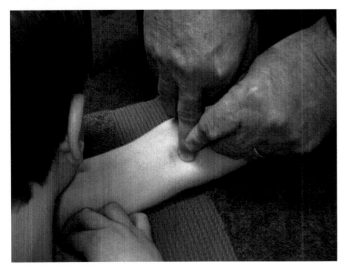

Figure 24.28 • Contact point and direction of thrust for the externally rotated ulna.

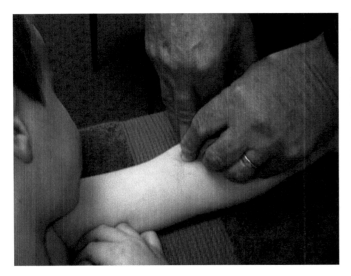

Figure 24.29 • Contact point and direction of thrust for the internally rotated ulna.

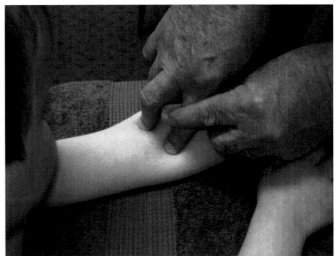

Figure 24.30 • Contact points and direction of thrust for the counter-rotated ulna. In the above case, the ulna is externally rotated and the humerus is internally rotated. This unusual subluxation is seen where there is reciprocal loss of total movement in the elbow joint and pain findings on the ulna and humerus diagonally opposite each other across the joint line, as shown.

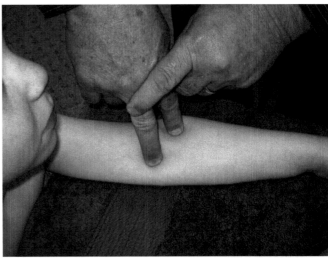

Figure 24.31 • Contact points and direction of thrust for the counter-rotated ulna. In the above case, the ulna is internally rotated and the humerus is externally rotated. This unusual subluxation is seen where there is reciprocal loss of total movement in the elbow joint and pain findings on the ulna and humerus diagonally opposite each other across the joint line, as shown.

careful, thorough, joint-by-joint examination and adjustive pre-testing to make absolutely sure the correct segment has been located. Any of the following structures may constitute the primary subluxation:

- interosseous (distal radius/ulna)
- proximal carpals in their relationship to the radius and ulna
- distal carpals in their relationship to the proximal carpals and metacarpals
- metacarpophalangeal
- interphalangeal.

The interosseous subluxation

Subluxation involving the interosseous articulation at the distal ends of the radius and ulna is uncommon, and can easily create diagnostic confusion when it does occur. The examination is performed by applying pressure in opposite directions at the bony heads of the radius and ulna. Failure of movement to occur when the radial head is being taken posteriorly against the ulna implies an anterior radial head with a concomitant posterior ulna head (Fig. 24.35) and vice versa.

When there is a distal interosseous subluxation, the generation of impulse on only one of the involved bones will usually produce a positive adjustive pre-test and in this case will be the only bone to receive a thrust. When both bones pre-test positively then a

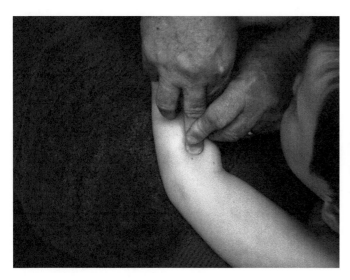

Figure 24.32 • Contact point and direction of thrust for the externally rotated (posterior) radial head.

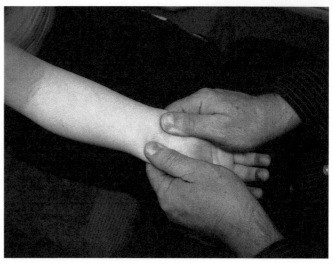

Figure 24.35 • Assessment of translational movement between the radius and ulna along the z-axis at the distal interosseous articulation. The radius and ulna are taken in opposite directions as the examiner feels for translational movement between the heads of the bones.

thrust needs to be made on both. The neuropathology for this subluxation follows the same pattern as that seen in the subluxation complexes involving the proximal row of carpals.

The carpal subluxation

There are four bones in the proximal row of carpals, namely scaphoid, lunate, triquetral and pisiform. The first three articulate with the radius in what is termed the radial condyle, while the pisiform does not articulate directly with the ulna but with the medial side of the triquetral. The distal row of carpals is also made up of four bones, namely the trapezium, trapezoid, capitate and hamate (see Fig. 24.34).

Movement of the scaphoid, lunate and triquetral at the radial condyle involves flexion and extension (x-axis rotation), as well as ulnar deviation (adduction z-axis) and radial deviation (abduction z-axis). There is no axial rotation. The pisiform demonstrates similar movements, but again there is no axial rotation.

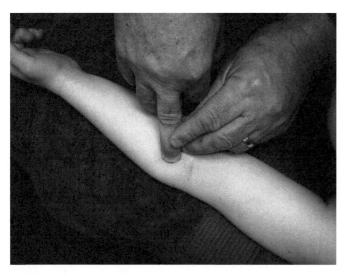

Figure 24.33 • Contact point and direction of thrust for the internally rotated (anterior) radial head.

Kinesiopathology: proximal row of carpals

Anterior subluxation in the scaphoid, lunate and triquetral is evidenced by loss of movement in dorsiflexion between the individual bones in their respective articulations with the radius in the radial condyle. The pisiform subluxates proximally and this movement is evidenced by a loss of separation with the ulna on radial deviation. Posterior subluxation of the scaphoid, lunate and triquetral is evidenced by loss of movement in palmar flexion between the individual bones in their respective articulations with the radius in the radial condyle. The technique of examination for the proximal row of carpals is demonstrated in Figs 24.36 and 24.37. The assessment of the pisiform involves only movement examination on radial deviation (Fig. 24.38).

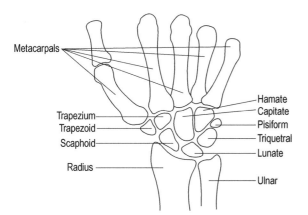

Figure 24.34 • The anatomical arrangement of the bones of the wrist and hand.

313

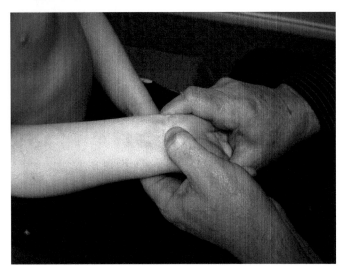

Figure 24.36 ● Assessment of the lunate in palmar flexion. Failure to detect movement during this procedure implies an anterior lunate subluxation. The scaphoid and triquetral are examined in the same manner.

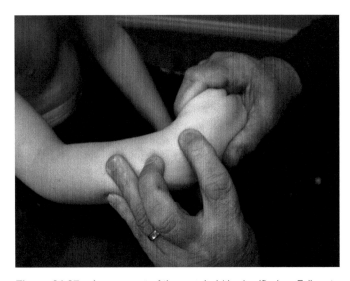

Figure 24.37 ● Assessment of the scaphoid in dorsiflexion. Failure to detect movement during this procedure implies a posterior scaphoid subluxation. The lunate and triquetral are examined in the same manner.

Myopathology and connective tissue pathology

Point-specific pain findings are seen consistent with the movement of the involved bone. In the anterior listings, pain will be seen on the palmar surface of the bones, while in the posterior listings pain will be seen over the dorsal aspects of the bones. The pisiform pain finding is over its proximal surface.

Neuropathology

All proximal carpal subluxations are associated with weakness of the opposition of thumb and finger. It is usually best to use

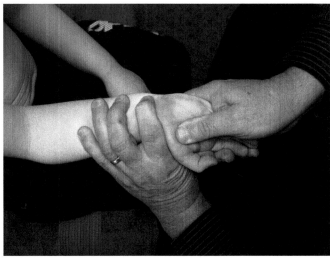

Figure 24.38 ● Assessment of the pisiform involves only palpation in the space between the pisiform bone and the ulna. Failure of this space to open on radial deviation of the wrist implies a proximal pisiform subluxation.

opposition of the thumb and fifth finger, as this position exerts maximum compressive stress on the wrist. The adjustive pre-test impulse will only test positive if the impulse is directed into the correct structure.

Kinesiopathology: distal row of carpals and proximal metacarpal heads

Only posterior subluxation is seen with the trapezium, trapezoid, capitate and hamate. The same is true of the proximal metacarpal heads. The reason for this is thought to be due to the anatomical formation and function of the hand, existing as it does in the neutral or slightly flexed to fully fisted position at all times. This orientation effectively disallows an anterior subluxation. The technique of examination for the distal row of carpals and proximal metacarpal heads involves gliding the bones one at a time posterior to anterior and feeling for movement against each of the adjacent bones (Fig. 24.39). When subluxation exists at a carpal bone, it will demonstrate loss of normal movement against all adjacent bones.

Myopathology and connective tissue pathology

Point-specific pain findings are seen consistent with the movement of the involved bone. Given all listings will be posterior, the point-specific pain finding will be seen over the dorsal aspect of the involved bone.

Neuropathology

All distal carpal and proximal metacarpal head subluxations are associated with weakness of the opposition of thumb and finger. It is usually best to use opposition of the thumb and

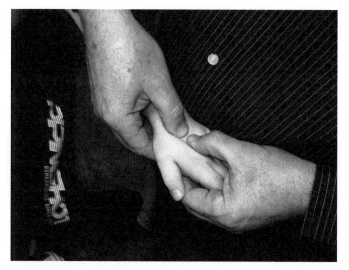

Figure 24.39 • Assessment of the capitate against the adjacent carpal bones. Assessment of the movement against each bone, in this case the hamate, lunate, scaphoid, trapezoid, third and fourth metacarpal. The same assessment procedure applies to all the bones of the distal row of carpals, including the proximal metacarpal heads.

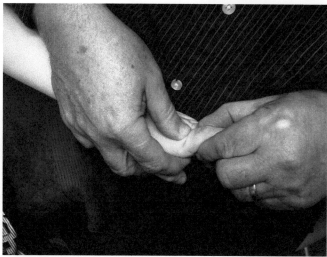

Figure 24.40 • Metacarpophalangeal assessment with the phalange taken into extension. Restricted movement indicates a posterior metacarpal head or anterior phalangeal subluxation. The interphalangeal joints are examined in the same manner.

fifth finger as this position exerts maximum compressive stress on the wrist. The adjustive pre-test impulse will test positive only if the impulse is directed into the correct structure.

Kinesiopathology: distal metacarpal heads and phalanges

The distal end of the metacarpals can subluxate both anteriorly and posteriorly, while the phalanges can subluxate in all manner of directions, that is: flexion, extension, axial rotation, abduction and adduction. This is also true of all the interphalangeal articulations. An important point to note is the orientation of the longitudinal axis of rotation as it relates to the distal metacarpal heads and the phalanges. The axis is defined as lying in the center of the palm and extending to the space between fingers 3 and 4. The practical significance of this is that what represents external rotation in fingers 4 and 5 is actually internal rotation in fingers 2 and 3 and the thumb. The point of reference is, of course, the axis and not the patient's body.

The assessment techniques for the metacarpophalangeal, and indeed the interphalangeal joints, are demonstrated in Figs 24.40–24.45.

Myopathology and connective tissue pathology

Point-specific pain findings are seen consistent with the movement of the involved bone. In these joints the pain will always be found on the side of bony protrusion or rotation.

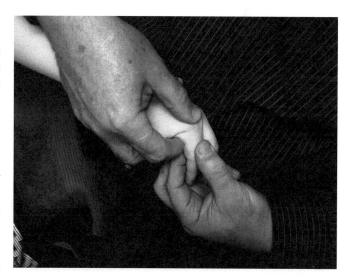

Figure 24.41 • Metacarpophalangeal assessment with the phalange taken into flexion. Restricted movement indicates an anterior metacarpal head or posterior phalangeal subluxation. The interphalangeal joints are examined in the same manner.

Neuropathology

All phalangeal subluxations are associated with weakness of the flexor digitorum muscles at the involved joint (Figs 24.46 and 24.47).

Corrective procedures

The adjustive procedures are applied to the wrist and hand subluxations according to the vector(s) of movement involved, making precise kinesiopathology identification extremely important. Once identified, adjustive pre-testing is first performed

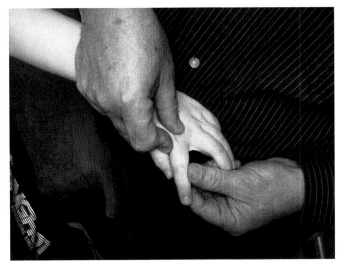

Figure 24.42 • Metacarpophalangeal assessment with the second phalange taken into abduction. Restricted movement indicates a medial metacarpal head or lateral phalangeal subluxation. The interphalangeal joints are examined in the same manner.

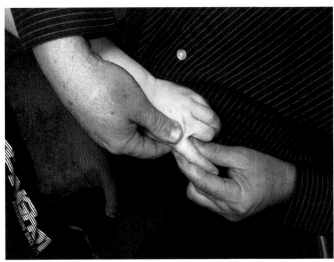

Figure 24.44 • Metacarpophalangeal assessment with the second phalange taken into internal rotation. Restricted movement indicates an externally rotated phalangeal subluxation. The interphalangeal joints are examined in the same manner.

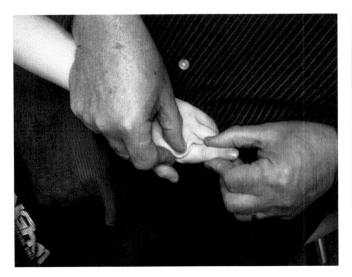

Figure 24.43 • Metacarpophalangeal assessment with the second phalange taken into adduction. Restricted movement indicates a lateral metacarpal head or medial phalangeal subluxation. The interphalangeal joints are examined in the same manner.

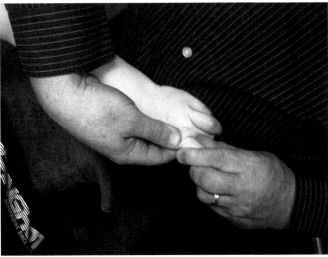

Figure 24.45 • Metacarpophalangeal assessment with the second phalange taken into external rotation. Restricted movement indicates an internally rotated phalangeal subluxation. The interphalangeal joints are examined in the same manner.

to ensure that correction can be demonstrated with impulse generation at the point of proposed adjustive thrust. Once this has been established, it is appropriate to make the adjustment. The contact point and direction of adjustive thrust for each of the wrist and hand subluxations is shown in Figs 24.48–24.57.

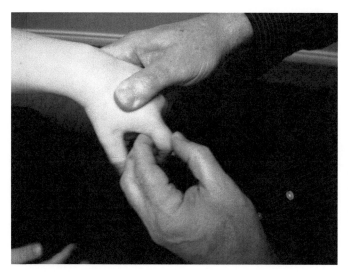

Figure 24.46 • Assessment of the flexor digitorum muscle for weakness at the metacarpophalangeal joint.

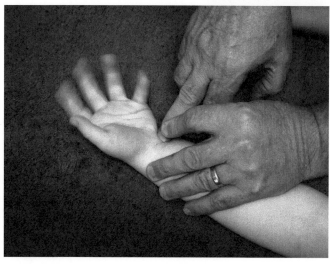

Figure 24.49 • Contact point and direction of thrust for the proximal pisiform subluxation.

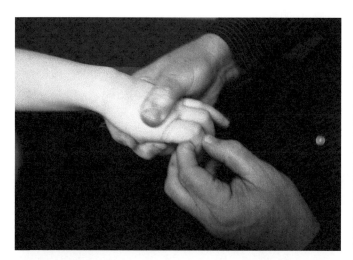

Figure 24.47 • Assessment of the flexor digitorum muscle for weakness at the interphalangeal joint.

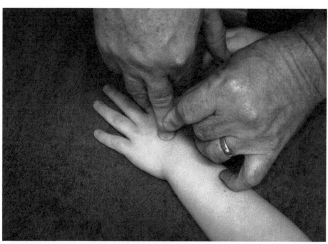

Figure 24.50 • Contact point and direction of thrust for the posterior capitate subluxation. All posterior carpal and proximal metacarpal head subluxations are adjusted in a similar manner.

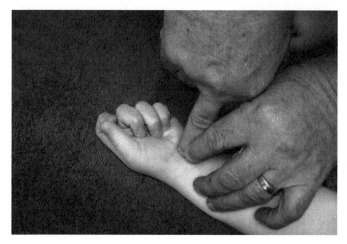

Figure 24.48 • Contact point and direction of thrust for the anterior lunate subluxation. The anterior scaphoid and triquetral are adjusted in a similar manner.

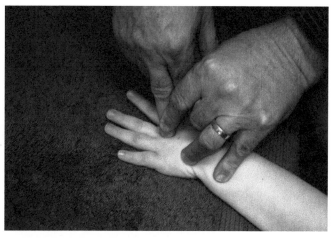

Figure 24.51 • Contact point and direction of thrust for the posterior distal metacarpal head subluxation.

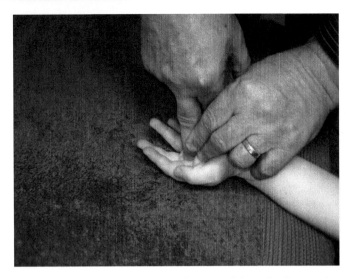

Figure 24.52 • Contact point and direction of thrust for the anterior distal metacarpal head subluxation.

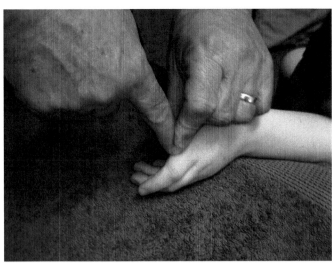

Figure 24.54 • Contact point and direction of thrust for the lateral phalangeal subluxation at the metacarpophalangeal joint. All lateral phalangeal subluxations at the interphalangeal joints are adjusted in a similar manner.

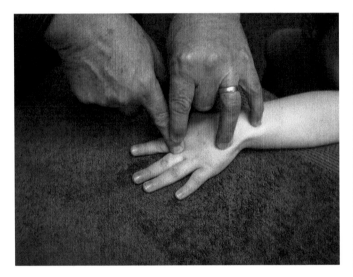

Figure 24.53 • Contact point and direction of thrust for the posterior phalangeal subluxation at the metacarpophalangeal joint. All posterior phalangeal subluxations at the interphalangeal joints are adjusted in a similar manner.

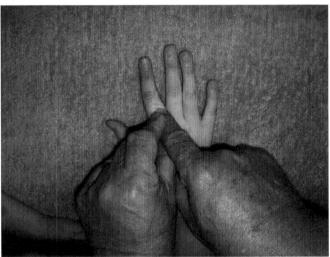

Figure 24.55 • Contact point and direction of thrust for the medial phalangeal subluxation at the metacarpophalangeal joint. All medial phalangeal subluxations at the interphalangeal joints are adjusted in a similar manner.

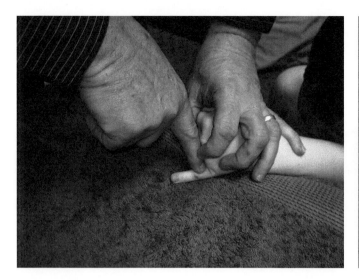

Figure 24.56 • Contact point and direction of thrust for the internally rotated phalangeal subluxation at the metacarpophalangeal joint. All internally rotated phalangeal subluxations at the interphalangeal joints are adjusted in a similar manner.

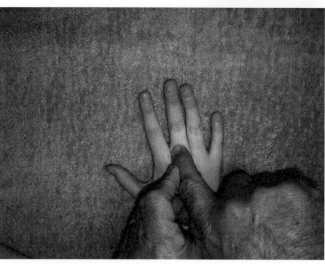

Figure 24.57 • Contact point and direction of thrust for the externally rotated phalangeal subluxation at the metacarpophalangeal joint. All externally rotated phalangeal subluxations at the interphalangeal joints are adjusted in a similar manner.

The lower limb subluxation

Neil J. Davies   Ailsa van Poecke

The lower limb subluxation in the child should be considered a relatively rare phenomenon and the younger the child, the more rare it is. While the lower limb, particularly at the hip and knee, provides for a number of common orthopedic conditions, this is not synonymous with the frequency of subluxation. While the lower limb subluxation is rarely primary, it may provide the key to resolving some recurring subluxation patterns and/or chronic conditions. It is in these cases that satisfactory subluxation management can occur only following resolution of the lower limb subluxation.

An understanding of the effect of the lower limb subluxation can only be achieved by understanding the intimate relationship between subluxation and neurological function. The mechanical findings provide a reflection of brain dysafferentation and it is through this appreciation that it is possible to understand that subluxation of a distal phalanx can have a substantial effect on the functional capacity of the cervical spine.

In general terms, each large joint in the biomechanical chain leading to the subluxated articulation will demonstrate kinesiopathology. Therefore, if subluxation is found at the tibiotalar articulation, both the hip and knee will demonstrate kinesiopathology. It is rare that large joints are free of kinesiopathology when a more distal joint is subluxated. The articulations of the foot are less affected by the kinematic chain and it is thus possible that in the presence of a phalangeal subluxation the bones of the mid-foot are free of kinesiopathology.

Diagnosis of the lower limb subluxation

In order to determine that the lower limb is a possible area of subluxation, a number of key findings will be present on examination of the upper cervical and lumbopelvic regions. Subluxation examination of the patient must begin as standard at the upper cervical complex, regardless of symptomatology at any level. It is, however, imperative that a thorough orthopedic examination be performed at the affected joint and subluxation examination should in no way be seen as a replacement for such an examination.

Kinesiopathology

Examination of the upper cervical complex will reveal both diminished lateral flexion and gross rotation bilaterally. Condylar movement and axis/C3 motion in flexion will be normal. At the upper limb, while the finding is somewhat variable, the majority of cases will demonstrate varying degrees of reduction in shoulder abduction, usually bilaterally.

At the lumbopelvic region there will be paradoxical kinesiopathology typical of that seen in a primary, below the diaphragm, front of body subluxation complex. These subluxation complexes are described in detail in Chapter 26. However, on further examination of the front of body, either no subluxation is identified or there are further paradoxical findings. This confluence of paradoxical findings is suggestive of a lower limb subluxation.

Neuropathology

It is the role of the neurological assessment to determine unilaterality or bilaterality. The patterns of neurological deficit which define the unilaterality or bilaterality of the lower limb subluxation follow the same basic rules as those applicable to the lumbopelvic subluxation. The lower limb subluxation will be bilateral when the Shimizu reflex is positive bilaterally in conjunction with a normal pectoral reflex response. When the Shimizu reflex is unable to be elicited and the pectoral reflex is normal, the lower limb subluxation will be unilateral.

The hip

The hip is a large ball joint that has minimal coverage by the acetabular roof at birth and maximal coverage by age 4 years. While various pathologies can affect the hip during childhood and adult life, the subluxation as a primary entity is very rare at any age. Thorough orthopedic examination is essential in assessing the child in whom hip pathology is suspected.

Loss of movement at the hip in vectors consistent with that seen in genuine subluxation is almost universally related to subluxation elsewhere in the body. Kinesiopathology in the hip features significantly in the pelvic reflection of the cranial subluxation and also as a compensatory response in the link system associated with subluxation of the sacrum, innominate, pubis, knee, ankle and foot.

Kinesiopathology

There have been several models proposed over the years for use in determining loss of motion related to subluxation at the hip. To be certain, the movements of the hip are very broad, of a large magnitude, and occur in multiples of direction at the same time. The hip, however, is such a large joint, and so spherical in construction, that translational movements in the z-axis will produce concomitant rotational movements that are predictable in direction about the y-axis. Examination of the movements of the hip is very simple. A lift and push technique is used.

With the patient supine, the examiner grasps the femur as close to the femoral head as possible with both hands (Fig. 25.1) and draws the hip in a P-A direction and then in an A-P direction to feel the extent of movement. The movement is of large magnitude and obvious, with the P-A movement concomitant with external rotation and the A-P movement concomitant with internal rotation. This is the case because of the sphericity of the femoral head and its articulation within the acetabulum. Failure of the hip to move in an A-P direction implies anterior subluxation of the hip, and vice versa.

In addition to the A-P and P-A movements, the examiner should draw the hip from medial to lateral and compress the joint from lateral to medial. This motion is a true linear or translational motion along the x-axis of the body occasioned by the pliability of the connective tissue in the joint capsule. A failure of the hip to move from medial to lateral implies medial subluxation of the hip, and vice versa.

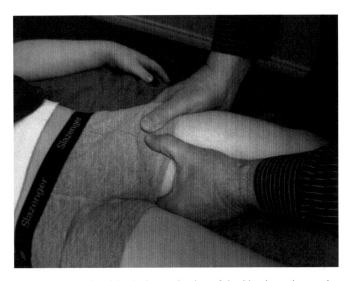

Figure 25.1 ● Kinesiological examination of the hip along the z-axis.

Unlike many other joints in the body, the hip subluxation is consistently associated with positive orthopedic tests. The most likely tests to be positive when the hip is genuinely subluxated are the Patrick Fabere and Thomas tests. One has to be careful not to place too much clinical emphasis on these tests being positive in the subluxation as the loss of movement occurring as a compensatory response, particularly in the pelvic and cranial subluxation patterns, will produce exactly the same positive result. The point here is simple, namely that positive orthopedic tests can be associated with loss of movement due to subluxation rather than necessarily being due to pathology. In diagnosing a hip subluxation it is essential the examiner bear in mind that, as with all subluxation listings, every element of the subluxation must be present and it must pre-test positively before being considered a genuine subluxation. Use of these principles prevents the examiner from reaching incorrect conclusions based on a number of incongruous positive orthopedic tests or signs.

In noting the presence of positive orthopedic tests in the child, the examiner must at all times be aware of the possibility of development dysplasia syndrome (DDS), either unilaterally or bilaterally. A particular awareness of the bilateral condition is required which may present as the older child toe-walking or presenting with an obvious increase in their lumbar lordosis. These children require specific imaging. See Chapter 14 for more information.

Myopathology and connective tissue pathology

Point-specific pain findings will be seen with the hip subluxation in relation to the direction of movement of the femoral head. Both anterior and posterior subluxation produce pain findings over the anterior and posterior aspects of the femoral head respectively. The lateral hip subluxation produces pain over the greater trochanter, and the medial hip subluxation produces pain over the lesser trochanter. The pain finding for the lateral hip subluxation is in exactly the same location as the area of tenderness associated with trochanteric bursitis and, while rare in the young child, it should be excluded in the very athletic teenager.

Neuropathology

In the hip subluxation, neuropathology is related to weak muscles attaching to and acting upon the hip. The specific muscles relating to the hip subluxation patterns are shown in Table 25.1. Of particular note is that weakness of the adductors is not specific to the medial hip subluxation, but is also seen in subluxation of the pelvic floor.

Corrective procedures for the hip subluxation

The NeuroImpulse Protocol (NIP) adjusting procedures are applied to the hip subluxation according to vector listing, as in other parts of the body. Figs 25.2–25.5 illustrate the specific contact points and directions of thrust for the range of hip subluxations.

Table 25.1 Muscle weaknesses associated with the hip subluxation

Subluxation listing of the hip	Associated muscle weakness
Anterior	Piriformis
Posterior	Quadriceps femoris
Lateral	Tensor fascia lata, gluteus minimus
Medial	Hip adductors, gluteus medius, piriformis

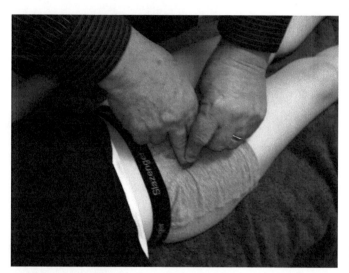

Figure 25.2 • With the anterior hip subluxation, contact is taken over the anterior aspect of the femoral head and the direction of thrust is directly anterior to posterior.

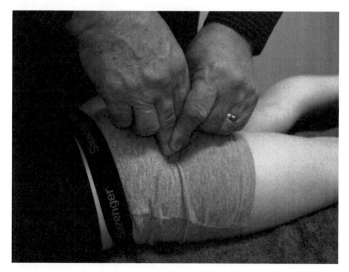

Figure 25.3 • With the posterior hip subluxation, contact is taken over the posterior aspect of the femoral head and the direction of thrust is directly posterior to anterior.

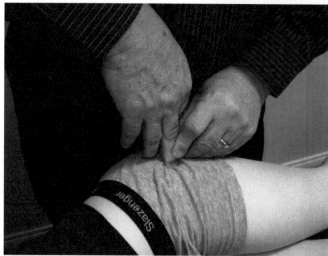

Figure 25.4 • With the lateral hip subluxation, contact is taken over the lateral aspect of the greater trochanter and the direction of thrust is directly lateral to medial.

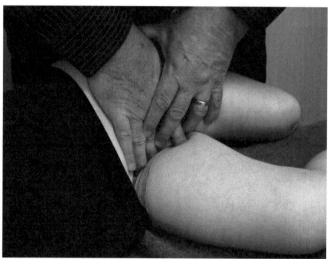

Figure 25.5 • With the medial hip subluxation, contact is taken over the medial aspect of the lesser trochanter and the direction of thrust is directly medial to lateral.

The knee

Subluxation at the knee is a more common phenomenon than that involving the hip. During puberty, the frequently diagnosed Osgood–Schlatter disease can often be more correctly diagnosed as an anterior tibial subluxation. The knee is a joint commonly affected by sporting injury, making a thorough orthopedic examination essential on every child presenting with knee pain prior to subluxation diagnosis. There is, however, some inevitable overlap between the subluxation examination of the knee and the orthopedic evaluation. It is additionally an area which provides for many questions from parents regarding posture and development. These are more fully discussed in Chapter 14.

Subluxation may occur at the tibiofemoral joint involving translation along either the x-axis or z-axis, or rotation of the tibia under the femur about the y-axis. Subluxation can also occur at the tibiofibular joint, with the fibular head moving into rotation about the y-axis around the tibia or in translation inferiorly, parallel to the y-axis, a movement colloquially referred to as the 'dropped fibula'. In rare instances the fibula may also translate superiorly. This extensive motion at the knee joint requires considered examination in order to correctly diagnose the exact vectors of subluxation.

When the primary subluxation is located at the knee, there will always be a restriction in hip movement, usually in the A-P or P-A glide motion, and often both. The degree of loss at the hip does not appear to equate to the severity of the subluxation in terms of the patient's symptoms.

It is of great clinical importance to note that the dropped fibula subluxation is very common and is usually associated with a history of trauma involving forced inversion of the ankle. However, it is critical to understand that it is universally associated with concomitant rotational movement of the fibular head and does not stand alone as a single subluxation vector.

Kinesiopathology: the tibiofemoral joint

The tibia needs to be examined in translation along the z-axis, a movement that equates to the A-P and P-A draw signs respectively in the orthopedic examination. In addition, the tibiofemoral joint must be examined in translation along the x-axis, a motion that equates to the apprehension test in the orthopedic examination. Finally, the tibia also needs to be assessed in rotation. The technique of examination for the tibiofemoral joint is shown in Figs 25.6–25.9.

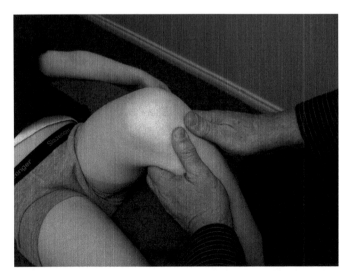

Figure 25.6 • Assessment of translation of the tibia along the z-axis under the femur. Failure of the tibia to move from anterior to posterior (A-P draw sign) implies an anterior tibial subluxation, while failure of the tibia to move from posterior to anterior (P-A draw sign) implies a posterior tibial subluxation.

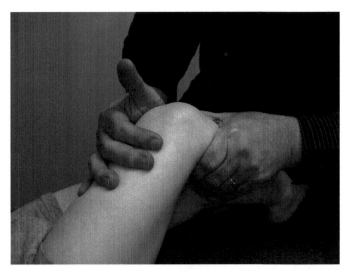

Figure 25.7 • Lateral to medial translation of the tibia along the x-axis under the femur (apprehension test). Failure of the tibia to move from lateral to medial implies a lateral tibial subluxation.

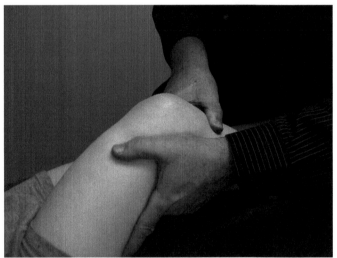

Figure 25.8 • Medial to lateral translation of the tibia along the x-axis under the femur (apprehension test). Failure of the tibia to move from medial to lateral implies a medial tibial subluxation.

Myopathology and connective tissue pathology

The tibia will exhibit point-specific pain findings related to effects exerted on muscle and connective tissue. The relationship between the precise anatomical locations of these points and the vectors of subluxation at the knee are described in Table 25.2.

Neuropathology: the tibiofemoral joint

Weakness will be seen in several muscles in a pattern consistent with the subluxation complex at the tibiofemoral joint. The exact relationship between weak muscles and the vectors of subluxation at the knee are described in Table 25.3.

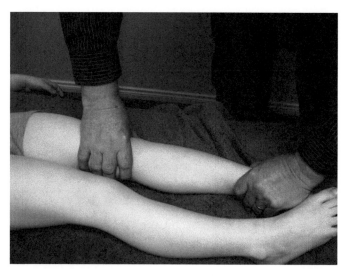

Figure 25.9 • Assessment of y-axis rotation of the tibia under the femur. Failure of the tibia to rotate internally implies an external tibial subluxation, while failure of the tibia to rotate into external rotation implies an internal tibial subluxation.

Table 25.2 Point-specific pain findings associated with the tibiofemoral and tibiofibular subluxation

Subluxation listing at the knee	Associated pain finding
Anterior tibia	Tibial tubercle
Posterior tibia	Popliteal space over the proximal tibia
Lateral translation of the tibia	Lateral aspect of the proximal tibia
Medial translation of the tibia	Medial aspect of the proximal tibia
Internal rotation of the tibia	Anterior aspect of the lateral tibial plateau
External rotation of the tibia	Anterior aspect of the medial tibial plateau
Internal rotation of the fibular head	Anterior surface of the proximal fibular head
External rotation of the fibular head	Posterior surface of the proximal fibular head
Counter-rotational subluxation at the knee joint	Combinations of the above pain findings according to direction of rotation

Table 25.3 Muscle weaknesses associated with tibial subluxation

Subluxation listing of the tibia	Associated muscle weakness
Anterior/posterior, lateral/medial	Quadriceps femoris
Anterior/posterior, lateral/medial, rotational subluxations, internal or external	Tibialis anterior
Rotational subluxations, internal or external	Popliteus

Kinesiopathology: the tibiofibular joint

Subluxation in the tibiofibular joint is less common in the child. Rotations of the proximal fibula head often exist as stand-alone subluxation vectors, but when the fibula has dropped inferiorly it is universally associated with a rotated proximal fibula head, the direction of rotation being unpredictable. The technique of examination is shown in Figs 25.10–25.12.

Myopathology and connective tissue pathology

Point-specific pain findings are seen consistent with the movement of the proximal head of the fibula. The pain finding will

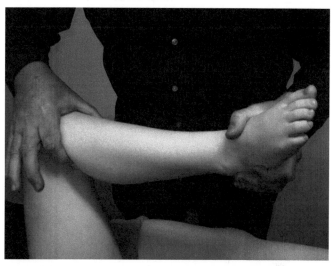

Figure 25.10 • Assessment of external rotation of the fibular head about the tibia. Failure of the fibular head to move into external rotation implies an internal rotation subluxation of the fibular head.

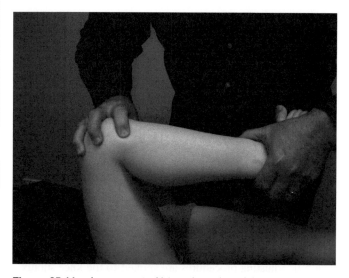

Figure 25.11 • Assessment of internal rotation of the fibular head about the tibia. Failure of the fibular head to move into internal rotation implies an external rotation subluxation of the fibular head.

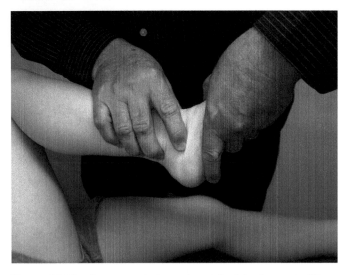

Figure 25.12 • Assessment of eversion at the lateral aspect of the ankle. Failure of the space between the lateral malleolus and the talus to close implies inferiority of the fibula.

Table 25.4 Point-specific pain findings associated with the proximal tibiofemoral interosseous subluxation

Subluxation listing of the proximal tibiofibular interosseus joint	Associated pain finding
Anterior tibia	Anterior/lateral surface of upper ⅓ proximal tibia
Posterior tibia	Posterior/lateral surface of upper ⅓ proximal tibia
Anterior fibula	Anterior/medial surface of upper ⅓ proximal fibula
Posterior fibula	Posterior/medial surface of upper ⅓ proximal fibula

be over the anterior head when it is anterior and the posterior head when it is posterior (Table 25.4). In the case of the dropped fibula, a further pain finding will be found at the pole of the inferior end of the fibula directly under the lateral malleolus, and is often an excruciatingly painful point.

Neuropathology: the tibiofibular joint

The peroneus longus and brevis muscles are weak when the fibula is subluxated in any direction.

Corrective procedures for the knee subluxation

The NIP adjusting procedures are applied to the knee subluxation according to joint and listing, making precise kinesiopathological identification extremely important. Once identified, pre-testing is first performed to ensure that correction can be

demonstrated with impulse generation at the point of proposed intrusion. In the child, accurate pre-testing should occur with the help of an assistant as testing against muscle strength is often difficult in the child under 5 years. In this case the pre-test should involve testing against an improvement in cervical motion or other factor. Once this has been established, it is appropriate to make the adjustment. The contact point and adjustive direction for each of the possible subluxation complexes is shown in Figs 25.13–25.23.

The ankle and foot

Subluxation of the ankle and foot in the baby is a rare occurrence. As the child grows and begins to bear weight, the frequency of subluxation increases but nevertheless remains uncommon. In the school-age child, foot and ankle subluxations may be seen in combination with poor gait patterns, sporting

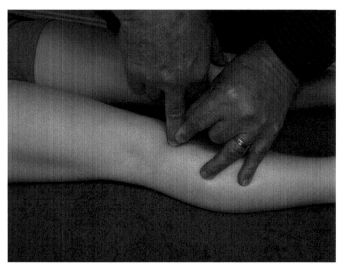

Figure 25.13 • Contact and direction of thrust for the anterior tibial subluxation.

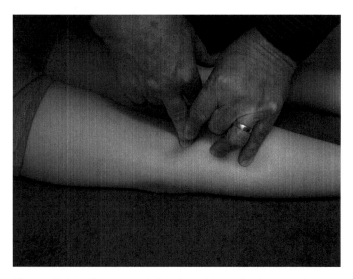

Figure 25.14 • Contact and direction of thrust for the posterior tibial subluxation.

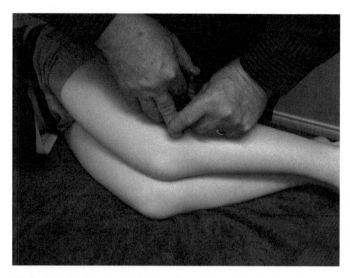

Figure 25.15 • Contact and direction of thrust for the lateral tibial subluxation.

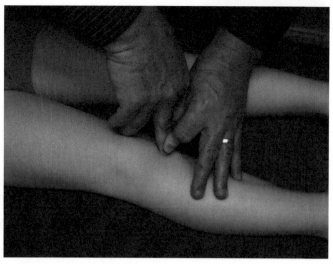

Figure 25.18 • Contact and direction of thrust for the externally rotated tibial subluxation.

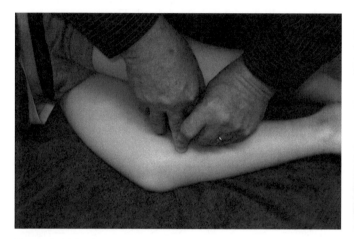

Figure 25.16 • Contact and direction of thrust for the medial tibial subluxation.

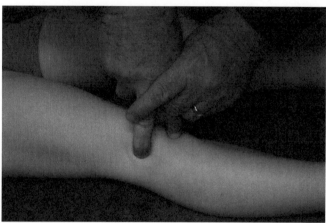

Figure 25.19 • Contact and direction of thrust for the counter-rotated subluxation with the tibia in external rotation and the femur in internal rotation. The contact positions are reversed for the opposite counter-rotational subluxation.

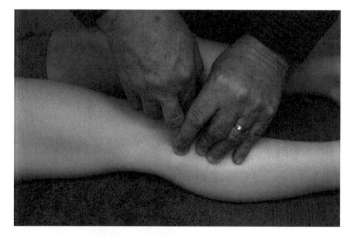

Figure 25.17 • Contact and direction of thrust for the internally rotated tibial subluxation.

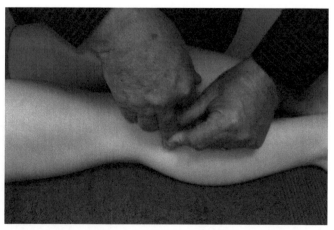

Figure 25.20 • Contact and direction of thrust for the anterior proximal fibular head subluxation.

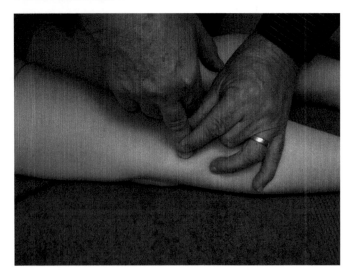

Figure 25.21 • Contact and direction of thrust for the posterior proximal fibular head subluxation.

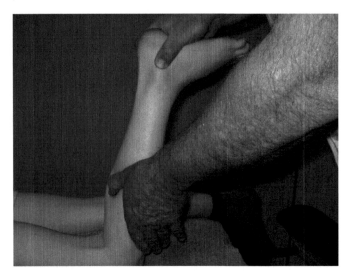

Figure 25.22 • Contact and direction of thrust for the dropped fibular subluxation with the proximal fibular head anterior.

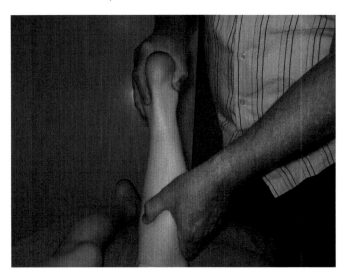

Figure 25.23 • Contact and direction of thrust for the dropped fibular subluxation with the proximal fibular head posterior.

incidents, and as a result of the considerable growth and development in this area up to and beyond puberty. The foot and its posture is an area of considerable concern to many parents, prompting questions regarding the arches of the foot, the shape of the ankles, and the position of the toes. A thorough knowledge of the development, normal variations, and orthopedic conditions of the foot and ankle is essential.

For the purposes of this discussion, the usual anatomical and biomechanical protocol of subdividing the foot and ankle into hindfoot, mid-foot and forefoot for separate consideration will be followed. The reason why this has been done is not for any particular functional reason, but to attempt to make what could be a very complex discussion more readily understandable. The rationale for choosing this categorization of the bones of the ankle and foot is based on the fact that some lie in a vertical plane continuous with the lower leg, while the remaining bones lie in an essentially horizontal plane at right angles to the lower leg (Fig. 25.24). For the purposes of this text, the bones of the foot and ankle have been subdivided as identified in Table 25.5.

Clinically measurable movement is complex at the joints of the hindfoot (talus, calcaneus, distal tibia and fibula) and involves multiple vectors at each level. These movements and their individual assessment are described below.

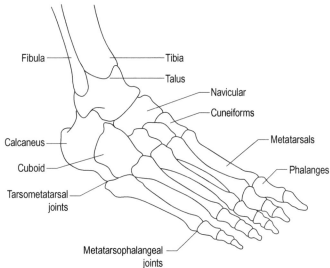

Figure 25.24 • The structural arrangement of the bones of the ankle and foot. Notice the vertical arrangement of the tibia, fibula, talus and calcaneus, and the more horizontal arrangement of the navicular, cuboid, cuneiforms, metatarsals and phalanges.

Table 25.5 Anatomical orientation of the bones of the ankle and foot

Area of the foot and ankle	Associated bones
Hindfoot	Fibula, tibia, talus, calcaneus
Mid-foot	Navicular, cuboid, cuneiforms – medial, intermediate and lateral
Forefoot	Metatarsals and phalanges

Figure 25.25 • Technique of examination for the talus in dorsiflexion. Movement, in the form of the joint space closing, is palpated at the articulation of the talus in the tibiofibular mortise as the ankle is taken into full dorsiflexion. When this motion is restricted, the talus is deemed to be posterior.

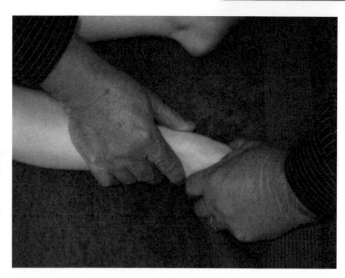

Figure 25.27 • Technique of examination for the talus in eversion. Movement, in the form of the joint space closing, is palpated between the lateral aspect of the talus and the inferior pole of distal fibular head. When this motion is restricted, the talus is deemed to be medial.

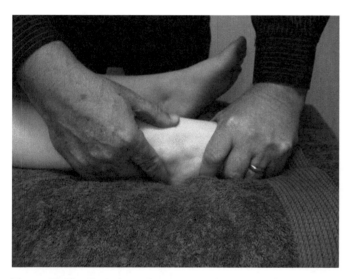

Figure 25.26 • Technique of examination for the talus in plantarflexion. Movement, in the form of the joint space opening, is palpated at the articulation of the talus in the tibiofibular mortise as the ankle is taken into full plantarflexion. When this motion is restricted, the talus is deemed to be anterior.

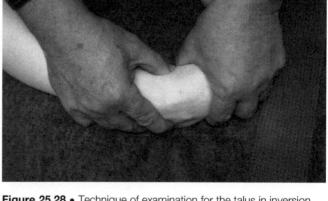

Figure 25.28 • Technique of examination for the talus in inversion. Movement, in the form of the joint space opening, is palpated between the medial aspect of the talus and the inferior pole of distal tibia. When this motion is restricted, the talus is deemed to be lateral.

Kinesiopathology

Talus

The movements which occur between the talus and the tibia (talotibial joint) are dorsiflexion, plantarflexion, eversion and inversion. The tightly packed joint prevents any meaningful translation along the x-axis, and translation along the z-axis is coupled with dorsiflexion and plantarflexion. The techniques used for assessment are shown in Figs 25.25–25.28.

Calcaneus

The movements which occur between the calcaneus and the talus are in translation along both the z-axis and x-axis, meaning that, in relation to the talus, the calcaneus can be found to be anterior, posterior, lateral or medial. The technique of examination is shown in Figs 25.29–25.32.

Distal fibular head

The distal fibular head is capable of a small degree of movement in translation along the z-axis, giving rise to anterior or posterior movement against the tibia. This movement is best appreciated by simply grasping the fibular head and moving

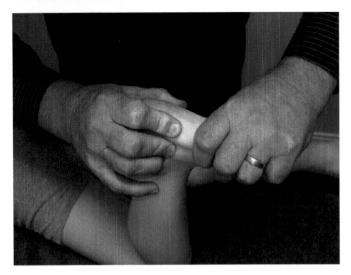

Figure 25.29 ● Failure of the calcaneus to move in translation along the z-axis from anterior to posterior implies an anterior calcaneus. This movement is best appreciated by grasping the calcaneus as shown above and moving the entire segment from anterior to posterior under the talus. As pressure is applied to the calcaneus from anterior to posterior, the calcaneus will be felt to move posteriorly under the talus.

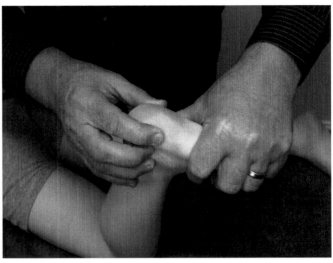

Figure 25.31 ● Failure of the calcaneus to move in translation along the x-axis from lateral to medial implies a lateral calcaneus. This movement is best appreciated by grasping the calcaneus as shown above and applying pressure to its lateral aspect, literally pushing the calcaneus medially across the talus. As pressure is applied to the calcaneus from lateral to medial, the calcaneus will be felt to move medially under the talus.

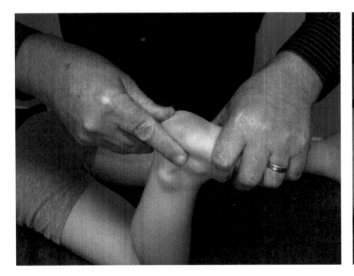

Figure 25.30 ● Failure of the calcaneus to move in translation along the z-axis from posterior to anterior implies a posterior calcaneus. This movement is best appreciated by applying pressure to the posterior aspect of the calcaneus, as shown above, while applying pressure in an anterior direction, literally pushing the calcaneus forward under the talus. As pressure is applied to the calcaneus from posterior to anterior, the calcaneus will be felt to move anteriorly under the talus.

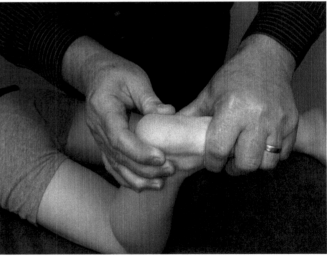

Figure 25.32 ● Failure of the calcaneus to move in translation along the x-axis from medial to lateral implies a medial calcaneus. This movement is best appreciated by grasping the calcaneus as shown above and applying pressure to its medial aspect, literally pushing the calcaneus laterally across the talus. As pressure is applied to the calcaneus from medial to lateral, the calcaneus will be felt to move laterally under the talus.

it in translation from anterior to posterior and then from posterior to anterior. It is deemed to be anterior when it will not move to the posterior and posterior, when it will not move toward the anterior.

Distal tibiofibular interosseus joint

The distal tibiofibular interosseus joint is capable of a small degree of movement in translation along the z-axis in the form of a shearing motion between the tibia and fibula as they are tractioned in opposite directions. If the motion is restricted when the fibular head is moved posteriorly as the tibia is moved anteriorly, then the fibula is denoted to be anterior and the tibia posterior. Alternatively, if the motion is restricted when the fibular head is moved anteriorly as the tibia is moved posteriorly, then the fibula is denoted to be posterior and the tibia anterior.

Myopathology and connective tissue pathology

Point-specific pain findings are seen in listings at the ankle as elsewhere in the body, and for the same basic anatomical reasons. The subluxation vector-specific pain locations for subluxation involving the bones of the hindfoot and the distal interosseous joint are described in Table 25.6.

Neuropathology

In the ankle subluxation, neuropathology is related to weak muscles, specifically those crossing the affected joint. The relationship of bone/joint to muscle is distributed according to the location of the muscle being medial or lateral as it

Table 25.7 Muscle weaknesses associated with ankle and foot subluxation

Muscle weakness	Associated subluxation
Tibialis anterior	Lateral talus Anterior distal tibia at the distal tibiofibular interosseous joint
Tibialis posterior	Medial talus Posterior distal tibia at the distal tibiofibular interosseous joint
Flexor digitorum brevis	Calcaneus subluxation, not listing specific Metartarsophalangeal and interphalangeal at digits II–V
Flexor digitorum longus	Anterior and posterior talus
Flexor and extensor hallucis longus	Metartarsophalangeal and interphalangeal at digit I
Peroneus longus and brevis	Lateral talus Anterior and posterior distal fibular head Anterior and posterior distal fibula at the distal tibiofibular interosseous joint
Flexor digitorum longus and brevis	Mid-foot bones subluxated superiorly
Extensor digitorum longus and brevis	Mid-foot bones subluxated inferiorly

Table 25.6 Point-specific pain findings associated with the hindfoot subluxations

Subluxation listing of the hindfoot	Associated pain finding
Anterior talus	Anterosuperior aspect of the talus high in the tibiofibular mortise
Posterior talus	Posterior aspect of the talus in the line of the Achilles tendon
Lateral talus	Lateral aspect of the talus immediately below the lateral malleolus
Medial talus	Medial aspect of the talus immediately below the medial malleolus
Anterior calcaneus	Anterior pole of the calcaneus in the midline
Posterior calcaneus	Posterior aspect of the calcaneus at the attachment of the Achilles tendon
Lateral calcaneus	Lateral aspect of the calcaneus in a line immediately below the lateral malleolus
Medial calcaneus	Medial aspect of the calcaneus in a line immediately below the medial malleolus
Distal interosseous	Pain will be over the anterior aspect of the malleolus of the bone which has moved anteriorly and the posterior aspect of the malleolus of the bone which has moved posteriorly

crosses the ankle. The relationships in Table 25.7 have been established as being clinically predictable.

Corrective procedures for the ankle subluxation

The NIP adjusting procedures are applied to ankle subluxations according to joint and listing as in other parts of the body. Once identified, adjustive pre-testing is first performed to ensure that correction can be demonstrated with impulse generation at the point of proposed intrusion. In the child, accurate pre-testing should occur with the help of an assistant or the attending caregiver as testing against muscle strength is often difficult or not possible in the child under 5 years. In this case, the pre-test should involve testing against an improvement in cervical motion or other compensatory factor such as arm abduction. In the case of the older child, it is a simple matter to apply pre-adjustive impulse generating impulse to a segment and retest the weak muscle. Once this has been established, it is appropriate to make the adjustive thrust. Specific contact points and precise directions of thrust are shown in Figs 25.33–25.42. In the interosseous subluxation, correction is achieved by grasping both malleoli and making a gentle thrust which produces a shearing movement in the joint in a direction appropriate to the vectors of kinesiopathology established previously by examination.

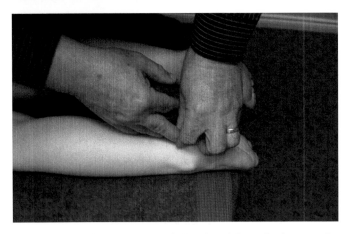

Figure 25.33 • Contact point and direction of thrust for the posterior talus subluxation.

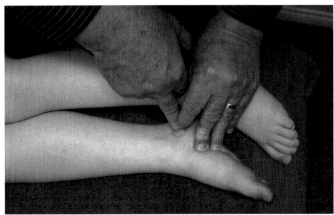

Figure 25.36 • Contact point and direction of thrust for the medial talus subluxation.

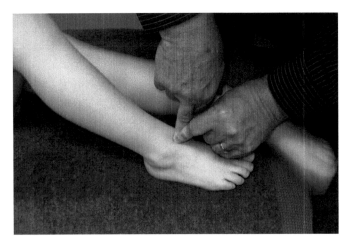

Figure 25.34 • Contact point and direction of thrust for the anterior talus subluxation.

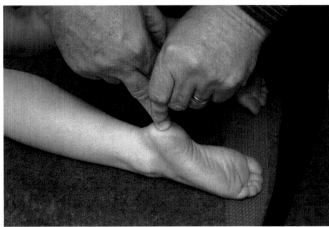

Figure 25.37 • Contact point and direction of thrust for the posterior calcaneus subluxation.

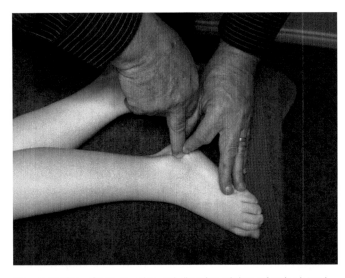

Figure 25.35 • Contact point and direction of thrust for the lateral talus subluxation.

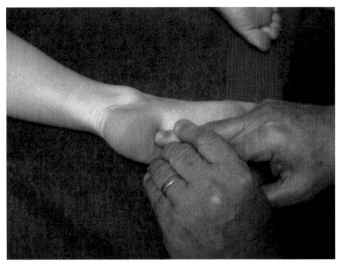

Figure 25.38 • Contact point and direction of thrust for the anterior calcaneus subluxation.

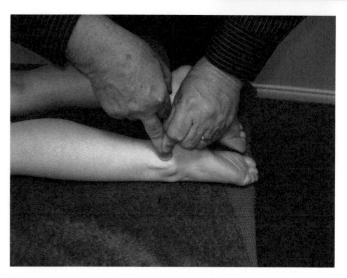

Figure 25.39 • Contact point and direction of thrust for the lateral calcaneus subluxation.

Figure 25.41 • Contact point and direction of thrust for the posterior distal fibular head subluxation.

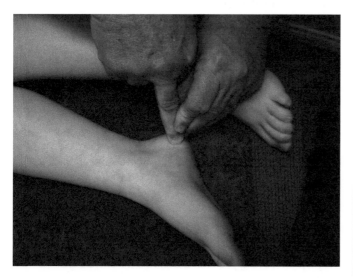

Figure 25.40 • Contact point and direction of thrust for the medial calcaneus subluxation.

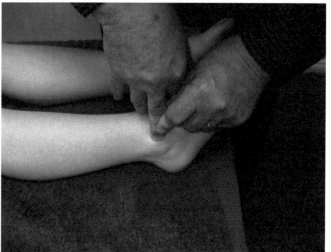

Figure 25.42 • Contact point and direction of thrust for the anterior distal fibular head subluxation.

The mid-foot, made up of the navicular, cuboid and cunei-forms, is an uncommon area for subluxation in the child. It becomes slightly more frequent in the weight-bearing and pre-adolescent child and can be associated with pes planus. It is often necessary to co-manage children with postural deformity of the ankle and mid-foot with a podiatrist. Subluxation stabilization is essential prior to the specialist fitting of any footwear or insoles.

Kinesiopathology

The tarsal bones

Clinically measurable movement involves translation parallel to the y-axis of the body in both a superior and inferior direction. The method of assessment of these movements at the individual joints is discussed below.

Navicular

The navicular is the key to understanding all the possible subluxation complexes affecting the mid-foot as it articulates with the talus, cuboid, and all three cuneiforms. It is therefore essential that superior and inferior translational movement parallel to the y-axis be assessed at each of these articulations to ensure that any adjustive thrust made is at exactly the right location. Given the diversity of the articulations of the navicular, when it is the affected segment, all the articulations in which it is involved will demonstrate a consistent pattern of motion restriction. However, when one of the bones with which it articulates is the affected segment, only that particular joint will demonstrate restricted motion. The navicular will subluxate inferiorly or superiorly and the technique of examination is shown in Fig. 25.43.

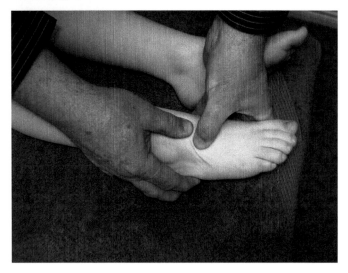

Figure 25.43 ● Assessment of motion between the navicular and the third cuneiform. Care must be taken to examine the motion of the navicular against all three cuneiforms, the talus, and the cuboid before it is determined that the navicular is the affected segment. In the event the navicular is subluxated, each of the bones surrounding the navicular will demonstrate normal movement in their articulations with their adjacent segments, other than the navicular. When one of the bones adjacent to the navicular is subluxated, it will demonstrate restricted movement against the navicular and the other bones which surround it.

Cuboid

The cuboid is a commonly subluxated mid-foot segment. Its movement must be assessed against the calcaneus, fourth and fifth metatarsal bases, the navicular, and lateral or third cuneiform. Again, given the diversity of the articulations of the cuboid, when it is the affected segment, all the articulations in which it is involved will demonstrate a consistent pattern of motion restriction. When examining the bones surrounding the cuboid they will demonstrate normal superior and inferior translational movement parallel to the y-axis in their articulations with the adjacent segments, other than the cuboid. However, when one of the bones with which the cuboid articulates is the affected segment, only that particular joint will demonstrate restricted motion. The cuboid may subluxate either inferiorly or superiorly.

The first cuneiform

The first (or medial) cuneiform is also a commonly subluxated mid-foot segment. Its movement must be assessed against the first and second metatarsal bases, the navicular, and the second (or intermediate/middle) cuneiform. Again, given the diversity of the articulations of this first cuneiform, when it is the affected segment, all the articulations in which it is involved will demonstrate a consistent pattern of motion restriction. When examining the bones surrounding the first cuneiform, they will all demonstrate normal superior and inferior translational movement parallel to the y-axis in their articulations with their adjacent segments, other than the first cuneiform. However, when one of the bones with which it articulates is the affected segment, only that particular joint will

demonstrate restricted motion. The first cuneiform may subluxate inferiorly or superiorly.

The second cuneiform

The second (or intermediate/middle) cuneiform is not a commonly subluxated mid-foot segment. Its movement must be assessed against the first cuneiform, second metatarsal base, third cuneiform (or lateral), and the navicular. Again, given the diversity of the articulations of this second cuneiform, when it is the affected segment, all the articulations in which it is involved will demonstrate a consistent pattern of motion restriction. When examining the bones surrounding the second cuneiform they will all demonstrate normal superior and inferior translational movement parallel to the y-axis in their articulations with their adjacent segments, other than the second cuneiform. However, when one of the bones with which it articulates is the affected segment, only that particular joint will demonstrate restricted motion. The second cuneiform may subluxate inferiorly or superiorly.

The third cuneiform

The third (or lateral) cuneiform is not a commonly subluxated mid-foot segment. Its movement must be assessed against the second cuneiform, third metatarsal base, cuboid, and navicular. Again, given the diversity of the articulations of this third cuneiform, when it is the affected segment, all the articulations in which it is involved will demonstrate a consistent pattern of motion restriction. When examining the bones surrounding the third cuneiform, they will all demonstrate normal superior and inferior translational movement parallel to the y-axis in their articulations with their adjacent segments, other than the third cuneiform. However, when one of the bones with which it articulates is the affected segment, only that particular joint will demonstrate restricted motion. The third cuneiform may subluxate inferiorly or superiorly.

Myopathology and connective tissue pathology

Point-specific pain findings are seen consistent with the movement of the involved bone. In each case the pain finding will be located on the superior surface of the bone on the dorsum of the foot with superior subluxation and, conversely, over the inferior surface of the affected bone on the plantar aspect of the foot with inferior subluxation.

Neuropathology

In superior mid-foot subluxation, the extensor digitorum longus and brevis muscles are weak. In inferior mid-foot subluxation, the flexor digitorum longus and brevis muscles will be weak.

Corrective procedures for the mid-foot

The NIP adjusting procedures are applied to mid-foot subluxations according to joint and listing, making precise kinesiopathological identification extremely important. Once identified, pre-testing is first performed to ensure that correction can be demonstrated with impulse generation at the point of proposed intrusion. In the child, accurate pre-testing should occur with the help of an assistant as testing against muscle strength is often difficult in the child under 5 years. In this case, the pre-test should involve testing against an improvement in cervical motion or other factor. In the case of the older child, it is a simple matter to apply pre-adjustive impulse-generating force to a segment and retest the weak muscle. Once this has been established, it is appropriate to make the adjustment. The contact points and adjustive direction for each of the possible mid-foot subluxations are shown in Figs 25.44 and 25.45.

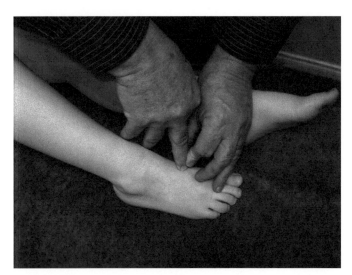

Figure 25.44 • Contact and direction of thrust for the superior first cuneiform subluxation. The contact is held for the usual 10–15 seconds and is followed by a very fast, shallow thrust. The same procedure is applied to all superior mid-foot subluxations.

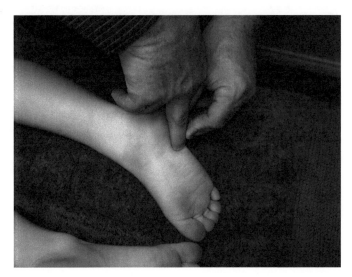

Figure 25.45 • Contact and direction of thrust for the inferior cuboid subluxation. The contact is held for the usual 10–15 seconds and is followed by a very fast, shallow thrust. The same procedure is applied to all inferior mid-foot subluxations.

The forefoot, consisting of the metatarsals and phalanges, is an uncommon area for subluxation in children. It does, however, require specific attention as it occasionally will be the reason for recurring dural tension subluxation patterns.

Kinesiopathology

Clinically measurable movement at the metatarsophalangeal and interphalangeal joints involve flexion, extension, abduction, adduction, and a small degree of rotation.

At the metatarsal bases

These were discussed in the section on the mid-foot as part of the description of the movements of the tarsal bones in their respective relationships to the cuneiforms and cuboid.

At the metatarsal heads and phalanges

The metatarsal heads can subluxate anteriorly or posteriorly, while the phalange articulating with it can subluxate in flexion, extension, rotation, abduction or adduction. The same is true of all the interphalangeal articulations. When assessing the rotation and abduction/adduction motion of the phalanges, it is essential to recognize that the conventional axis of motion for the foot occurs between digits II and III. Therefore adduction of the toes is movement towards the axis between digits II and III, and abduction is movement away from the axis between these same digits. Internal rotation describes motion inwardly towards the axis of motion and external rotation describes motion outwardly away from the axis. Each direction of the motion examination is carried out by grasping the bones on each side of the joint to be examined with the thumb and forefinger kept as close to the joint line as possible. Examination of the interphalangeal articulations follows exactly the same pattern.

Myopathology and connective tissue pathology

Point-specific pain findings are seen consistent with the movement of the involved bone. In these joints, the pain finding will always be on the side of bony protrusion/rotation.

Neuropathology

All phalangeal and metatarsal head subluxations at digits II–V are associated with weakness of the flexor digitorum brevis muscles at the involved joint in the case of inferior subluxation and extensor digitorum longus in the case of superior and rotary phalangeal subluxation. In the unlikely event there is abduction or adduction subluxation, the flexor digitorum longus and brevis and/or the extensor digitorum longus can both be used and will also test positive on adjustive pre-test.

The flexor hallucis longus and extensor hallucis longus will be weak with inferior, superior and rotary subluxation of digit I respectively.

Corrective procedures for the forefoot

The adjusting procedures are applied to forefoot subluxations according to joint and listing, making precise kinesiopathology identification extremely important. Once identified, pre-testing is first performed to ensure that correction can be demonstrated with impulse generation at the point of proposed intrusion. Once this has been established, it is appropriate to make the adjustment. Examples of contact points and adjustive directions of thrust at the metatarsophalangeal joints are shown in Figs 25.46–25.50.

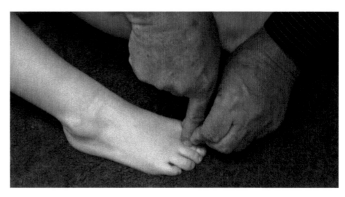

Figure 25.48 ● Contact and direction of thrust for the superior phalangeal head subluxation at the metatarsophalangeal joint of digit I.

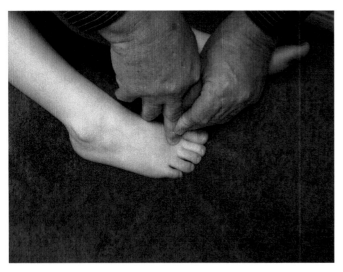

Figure 25.46 ● Contact and direction of thrust for the superior metatarsal head subluxation at the metatarsophalangeal joint of digit II.

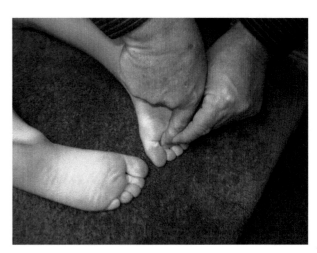

Figure 25.49 ● Contact and direction of thrust for the inferior phalangeal head subluxation at the metatarsophalangeal joint of digit II.

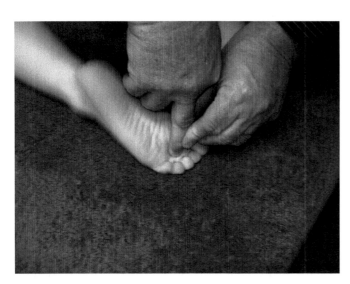

Figure 25.47 ● Contact and direction of thrust for the inferior metatarsal head subluxation at the metatarsophalangeal joint of digit III.

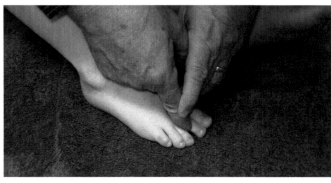

Figure 25.50 ● Contact and direction of thrust for the rotated first phalangeal segment at the metatarsophalangeal joint of digit II. In this case, the phalangeal segment is in external rotation as it has rotated away from the central axis which is sited between digits III and IV.

Front of body subluxation syndromes

Neil J. Davies   Kimberley Tuohey

Subluxation can occur absolutely anywhere in the body, including the structures of the front of the body that demonstrate functional capability. In terms of subluxation, these structures should be considered as those lying above the diaphragm and those below. The reason for this division is not arbitrary, but is indeed based upon the observation of which structures in the axial skeleton they are associated with. Those structures lying above the diaphragm are related in subluxation pattern and effect to the upper cervical complex, and, in particular, to the loss of gross rotation when it exists alongside relatively normal lateral flexion. The diaphragm itself and those structures below it, however, are related in subluxation pattern and effect to the pelvis, and will therefore be associated with a loss of both gross rotation and lateral flexion at the upper cervical complex. Of interest is the fact that the one common denominator is the loss or restriction of abduction at the glenohumeral joint.

Structures located above the diaphragm

The hyoid

Subluxation of the hyoid is uncommon in children, but by no means rare. To be sure it is largely ignored, or may be unrecognized, despite its highly specific and characteristic effects on both kinesiopathology and neuropathology. Given that it is almost invariably posterior, its genesis in babies is presumed to be due to pressure from the anterior, possibly due to the cord being around the neck. In the event the hyoid is anterior, it is presumed to be due to the action of the digastric muscle which, due to its lie in the anterior neck, has the capacity to pull one or both sides anteriorly.

The characteristic clinical findings associated with the hyoid subluxation are an ipsilateral loss of gross rotation at the upper cervical complex with normal lateral flexion, a positive Shimizu reflex, and a hyperactive pectoral reflex. The hyoid subluxation may be mistaken for a cranial problem, but careful and thorough examination will differentiate them on the basis of incomplete neuropathology for the latter, especially the ocular signs described in Chapter 27.

The diagnosis can be confirmed by neurological pre-testing. The hyoid is distracted from posterior to anterior and held gently in order to generate pre-adjustive impulse while the Shimizu reflex is retested. If the direction of impulse application is correct, the Shimizu reflex will diminish or disappear and the gross rotation restriction will normalize.

The adjustive procedure for the hyoid subluxation is to initiate pre-adjustive impulse in the direction of correction, neurologically pre-test, sustain the hold for 10–15 seconds, and then make a fast, very low-amplitude thrust. The possible listings are unilateral posterior (P-L/P-R), bilateral posterior (BP), unilateral anterior (A-L/A-R), bilateral anterior (BA), and in rare instances, usually precipitated by rotational trauma, reverse rotation (P-L/A-R, P-R/A-L). The adjustive set-ups for the typical hyoid listings are shown in Figs 26.1–26.4.

Hyoid subluxations, even in the very young, seldom stand alone. They are commonly associated with second-layer cranial subluxation and, in particular, the dropped sphenoid. It is not uncommon for the second-layer subluxation to manifest immediately after the correction of the hyoid, making post-adjustive assessment a critical part of the patient consultation.

The first rib

In terms of rib subluxation, the first rib is unique in that it only subluxates in a superior direction, into the anterior cervical triangle, presumably under the influence of the anterior neck flexors which attach directly on to the superior margin of the bone. For all the other ribs, the direction of subluxation can and does vary with an apparent lack of predictability.

Subluxation of the first rib is less common than that of the sternoclavicular joint (SCJ), despite the fact that they are in

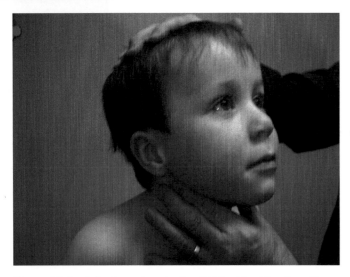

Figure 26.1 • Adjustive set up for the P-R hyoid subluxation. The contact is taken over the greater horn of the hyoid and the direction of impulse generation is straight P-A on the right side only.

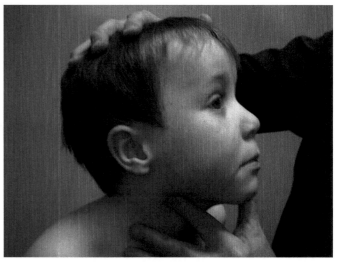

Figure 26.3 • Adjustive set up for the A-R hyoid subluxation. The contact is taken over the body of the hyoid bone immediately anterior to the greater horn and the direction of impulse generation is straight A-P on the right side only.

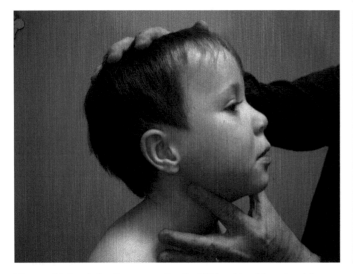

Figure 26.2 • Adjustive set up for the BP hyoid subluxation. The contact is taken over the greater horn of the hyoid bilaterally and the direction of impulse generation is straight P-A, simultaneously and equally applied to both sides.

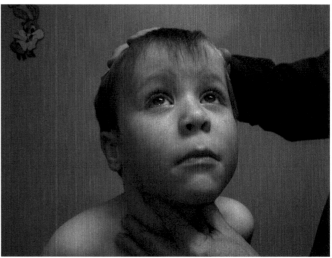

Figure 26.4 • Adjustive set up for the BA hyoid subluxation. The contact is taken over the body of the hyoid bone immediately anterior to the greater horn bilaterally and the direction of impulse generation is straight A-P, simultaneously and equally applied to both sides.

some ways very similar in that both involve restricted gross cervical rotation, while lateral flexion of the upper cervical complex, as well as flexion/extension at C0/C1 and flexion at C2/C3, are largely preserved. One salient difference is the fact that gross cervical rotation is restricted towards the affected side when the first rib is subluxated, but away from the affected side when the sternoclavicular joint is subluxated.

Once this typical pattern of kinesiopathology has been identified, the rib should be examined at its costovertebral joint. Given the tightly curved shape and relative shortness of the bone, any movement of the head of the rib against the sternum will be reflected as restricted movement at the costovertebral joint, the rib head being inferior. This is identified as a loss of widening of the first intercostal space at end-range on the affected side when the cervical spine is taken into full flexion (Fig. 26.5).

Specific pain points will be found in this subluxation complex over the rib in the anterior cervical triangle. There will be a palpatory sense of fullness in this tightly packed area and the anterior cervical muscle attachments will often feel rope-like and taut. The inferior aspect of the head of the rib at the costovertebral joint is also often tender, a finding consistent with the inferior subluxation.

Neurologically, it is characteristic for the first rib subluxation to be associated with weakness of the ipsilateral anterior neck flexors and a positive Shimizu reflex, also ipsilateral. Changes in the pectoral reflex are variable and not considered part of the characteristic subluxation pattern.

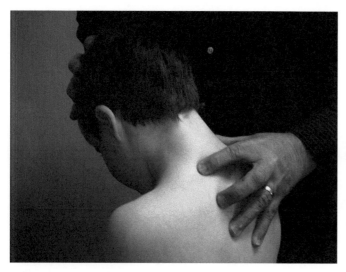

Figure 26.5 • Identification of the inferior rib head at the costovertebral joint. The intercostal space fails to widen at end-range on full cervical flexion.

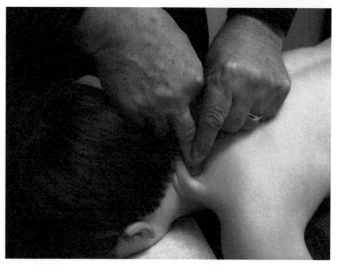

Figure 26.7 • Contact and line of thrust at the first rib head at the costovertebral joint in a patient with a first rib subluxation.

Subluxation correction is achieved by first applying the usual pre-adjustive hold for 10–15 seconds followed by a fast, shallow thrust applied over the most medial possible aspect of the first rib in the anterior cervical triangle, followed by the same procedure applied to the inferior aspect of the first rib head at the costovertebral joint. The direction of impulse generation is S-I over the rib in the anterior cervical triangle (Fig. 26.6), and P-A/I-S over the rib head at the costovertebral joint (Fig. 26.7).

The costochondral subluxation

The costochondral subluxation is highly pain specific and indeed rare to nonexistent in the very young. In the pediatric age group, one would expect to see this subluxation only in the school-age child and adolescent. The diagnosis is characterized by normal

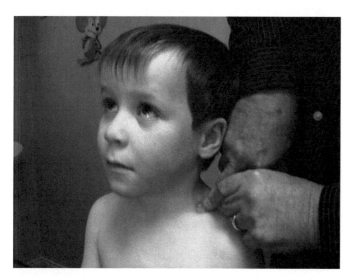

Figure 26.6 • Contact and line of thrust in the anterior cervical triangle in a patient with a first rib subluxation.

upper cervical motion in all directions, a reduction in arm abduction consistent with the level of subluxation, a pattern that follows that of the thoracic spine, and point-specific pain over the affected costochondral junction. Once the affected joint has been identified, the application of pre-adjustive impulse in the direction of correction will restore normal shoulder abduction.

Subluxation correction is obtained by holding pre-adjustive contact over the affected joint for 10–15 seconds followed by the usual fast, shallow thrust.

The sternal subluxation

The sternum is formed by the manubrium, body and xiphisternum. The manubrium is notched on its superior margin forming the jugular notch. The upper lateral angles are notched for articulation with the clavicles. The first ribs articulate immediately below the sternoclavicular joints. The second rib articulates at the manubriosternal joint. Because of the angle at which the manubrium and body meet, a ridge is formed, the sternal angle or angle of Louis. This joint lies in the same plane as the disc between the fourth and fifth thoracic vertebrae.

Subluxation involving the sternum is complex and may involve the entire sternal body, the sternoclavicular joint, individual or multiple chondrosternal joints, the angle of Louis, and the xiphoid process at its junction with the sternal apex. The characteristic feature of all these subluxation complexes is restricted upper cervical rotation, normal lateral flexion, restricted shoulder abduction, positive Shimizu reflex, normal pectoral reflexes, and highly specific pain points. All the sternal subluxation complexes accurately pre-test against both shoulder abduction and upper cervical rotation.

The sternoclavicular joint

Subluxation of the sternoclavicular joint (SCJ) is common in children and by far the most common of the front of body subluxation syndromes. It characteristically reduces rotation to the side opposite the affected joint while having no effect on lateral flexion, condylar movement or axis/C3 flexion. The joint itself is complex and many of the movements that are impaired by the subluxation are compound in nature. While simple, unidirectional subluxation patterns can and do occur, it is more common to encounter compound, multidirectional vectors at the SCJ. The SCJ subluxation is frequently associated with fixed fetal position (hands under chin and adducted humeri), often seen when there is reduced amniotic levels at the end of the third trimester of pregnancy, parents using the axillae as a point of contact to lift the child, and where there has been a history of non-accidental injury.

The first motion to be examined is designed to identify the superior and inferior subluxation vectors of the clavicular head. The technique of examination involves first abducting the arm to 90° and then flexing the elbow, also to 90°. Using the forearm as a lever, the humerus is taken into external rotation followed by internal rotation as the examiner palpates the SCJ. Failure of the SCJ to move when the humerus is externally rotated (Fig. 26.8) implies a superior subluxation of the sternal head, while failure to move when the humerus is taken into internal rotation (Fig. 26.9) implies a superior subluxation of the sternal head.

The second motion to be examined is designed to identify the lateral and medial subluxation vectors of the clavicular head. The technique of examination involves first abducting the arm to 90°, then taking the whole arm in an arc posteriorly and in the transverse (xz) plane. Failure of the SCJ to separate at end-range of motion (Fig. 26.10) implies a medial subluxation of the humeral head. The arm is then taken across the front of the body in the transverse plane while continuing to palpate the SCJ. Failure of the SCJ to compress or close at end-range of arm motion (Fig. 26.11) implies a lateral subluxation of the humeral head.

Anterior and posterior movement of the clavicular head against the sternum and the SCJ is not able to be readily appreciated by motion palpation techniques. Specific pain

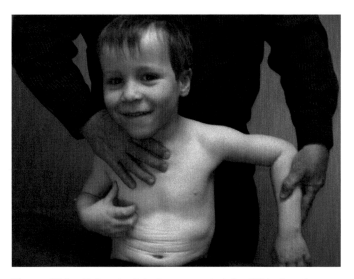

Figure 26.9 • Failure to detect movement at the SCJ when the humerus is internally rotated as shown implies a superior subluxation of the humeral head.

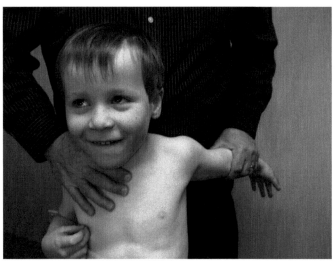

Figure 26.10 • Failure of the SCJ to separate at end range of arm extension as shown implies a medial subluxation of the humeral head.

findings and positive pre-testing appear to be the only reliable way to determine these vectors of subluxation in children.

Specific pain findings associated with the various vectors of subluxation at the SCJ follow simple rules of compression of soft tissues by bony prominences associated with the joint structures. The relationship of pain location and subluxation vectors are described in Table 26.1.

Neurologically, in children old enough to cooperate cognitively with muscle testing techniques, weakness will be seen ipsilaterally in the pectoralis major clavicular division, sternocleidomastoid, and somewhat more variably the anterior neck flexors.

Subluxation correction is achieved by first applying the usual pre-adjustive hold for 10–15 seconds followed by a fast, shallow thrust over the clavicular head in a direction consistent with the subluxation vector(s). In both simple and compound listings, the exact direction of impulse generation should be established by adjustive pre-test using the loss of shoulder abduction as an

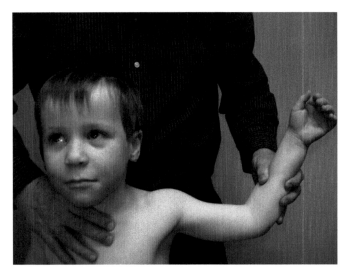

Figure 26.8 • Failure to detect movement at the SCJ when the humerus is externally rotated as shown implies an inferior subluxation of the humeral head.

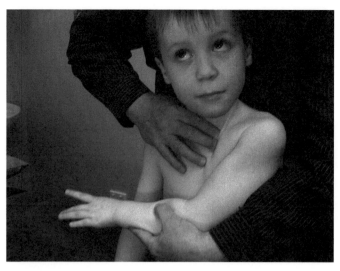

Figure 26.11 • Failure of the SCJ to compress or close at end-range of arm motion as shown implies a lateral subluxation of the humeral head.

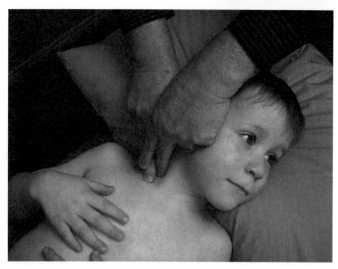

Figure 26.12 • Contact and line of thrust used for correction when the clavicular head is subluxated superiorly.

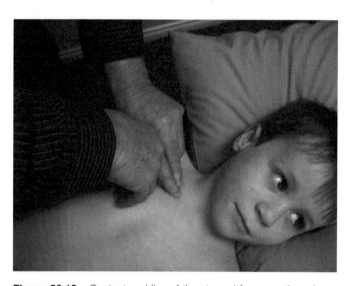

Figure 26.13 • Contact and line of thrust used for correction when the clavicular head is subluxated inferiorly.

Table 26.1 Specific pain findings and their relationship to sternoclavicular joint vectors of subluxation

Vector of subluxation of the clavicular head	Location of pain finding
Superior	Along the superior margin of the clavicle at its medial end
Inferior	Along the inferior margin of the clavicle at its medial end
Medial	At the medial end of the clavicle at its articulation with the sternum
Lateral	In the joint space between the clavicular head and the sternum
Anterior	Over the medial head of the clavicle on its anterior surface
Posterior	Over the sternum immediately adjacent to the sternoclavicular joint

indicator. The directions of impulse generation for all the simple listings are shown in Figs 26.12–26.17. A description of the vectors of correction for some of the more commonly occurring compound listings are described in Table 26.2.

The angle of Louis

Subluxation at the angle of Louis is more commonly seen in adolescents and adults, but while uncommon in children, especially the very young, it is not rare. The movements in subluxation are complex and varied. The body may rotate about the x-axis in such a way that it is either anterior or posterior to the manubrium in the midline, or it may rotate about the y-axis in such a way that it will be anterior or posterior in relation to the manubrium on one side. To complicate matters a little

more, it sometimes rotates about the y-axis in such a way that it is posterior on one side and anterior on the opposite side in its relationship to the manubrium as a composite subluxation complex, in much the same way as the sacrum counter-rotates.

Typically the angle of Louis subluxation, regardless of the vectors involved, causes loss of full rotational capacity of the upper cervical complex accompanied by a positive Shimizu reflex and, variably, a hyperactive pectoral reflex. Failure to identify the angle of Louis subluxation, which is usually primary when it exists, results in a frustrating clinical experience for the patient and the chiropractor and much unnecessary impulse generation at the upper cervical complex. The angle of Louis subluxation produces characteristic point-specific pain findings (Table 26.3), and on that basis alone will not be mistaken for the hyoid, sternoclavicular, or first rib subluxation. It also positively pre-tests consistently and predictably against the affected reflexes and the rotational capacity of the upper cervical complex.

341

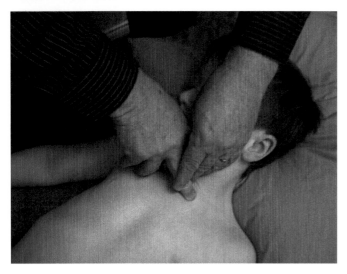

Figure 26.14 • Contact and line of thrust used for correction when the clavicular head is subluxated medially.

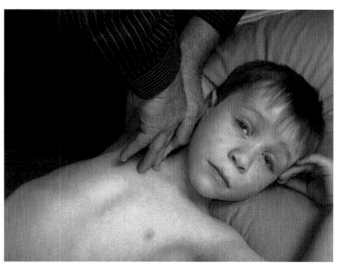

Figure 26.16 • Contact and line of thrust used for correction when the clavicular head is subluxated anteriorly.

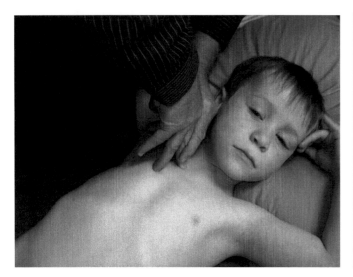

Figure 26.15 • Contact and line of thrust used for correction when the clavicular head is subluxated laterally.

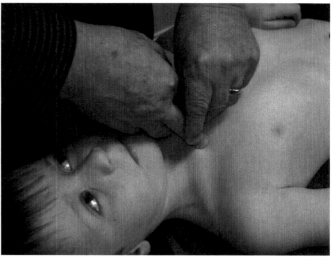

Figure 26.17 • Contact and line of thrust used for correction when the clavicular head is subluxated posteriorly. Note that, in this case, the contact is actually taken on the sternum as close to the clavicular head as possible.

Like all subluxations exerting an effect at the upper cervical complex, the angle of Louis subluxation produces a positive Shimizu reflex ipsilateral to the involved side, or bilateral when it is affected on both sides, and, variably, a hyperactive pectoralis reflex following the same pattern.

The neurological pre-testing procedure involves the initiation of impulse in the direction of subluxation vector correction while either the affected reflexes or kinesiopathology are retested. All the elements of both kinesiopathology and neuropathology which are characteristic of this subluxation complex can be predictably normalized by neurological pre-testing.

Subluxation correction is achieved by first applying the usual pre-adjustive hold for 10–15 seconds followed by a fast, shallow thrust over the appropriate anatomical location at the angle of Louis consistent with the involved subluxation vector(s). The exact direction of impulse generation should be established by adjustive pre-test using any of the characteristic subluxation elements. The contact points for all the angle of Louis listings are shown in Fig. 26.18 and the directions of thrust are described in Table 26.4.

The sternal body and chondrosternal subluxation

The sternal body at all ages in life is very mobile owing to its attachments to the costal cartilages. It is, of course, most mobile during the early years of life, and therefore less susceptible to subluxation. However, trauma to the chest is capable of causing sternal body subluxation even in an infant, and in fact a small number of newborns will exhibit this problem arising from their birth experience.

Table 26.2 Directions of thrust for the simple sternoclavicular joint listings and some of the more commonly occurring compound listings

Listing	Direction of adjustive thrust
Superior	S-I
Inferior	I-S
Medial	M-L
Lateral	L-M
Superior/lateral	S-I/L-M
Inferior/medial	I-S/M-L
Medial/anterior	M-L/A-P
Superior/anterior	S-I/A-P

Table 26.3 Characteristic point-specific pain findings for the angle of Louis subluxation vectors

Listing	Location of pain finding
Sternal body posterior (unilateral)	On the manubrium at the angle of Louis immediately adjacent to the joint line on the affected side
Sternal body posterior (midline)	Midline of the manubrium immediately adjacent to the joint line
Sternal body anterior (unilateral)	On the sternal body at the angle of Louis immediately adjacent to the joint line on the affected side
Sternal body anterior (midline)	Midline of the sternal body immediately adjacent to the joint line
Counter-rotation of the sternum about the y-axis	Combinations of the above according to the vectors involved

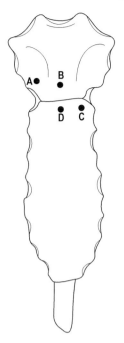

Figure 26.18 • Contact points for adjusting the various angle of Louis subluxations: (A) right posterior sternal body, (B) midline posterior sternal body, (C) left anterior sternal body, and (D) midline anterior sternal body.

Table 26.4 Directions of thrust for the angle of Louis subluxation vectors

Listing	Direction of adjustive thrust
Sternal body posterior (unilateral)	A-P with manubrium contact
Sternal body posterior (midline)	A-P with manubrium contact
Sternal body anterior (unilateral)	A-P with sternal contact
Sternal body anterior (midline)	A-P with sternal contact
Counter-rotation	A-P with contact on the manubrium (posteriorly rotated side) and on the sternum (anteriorly rotated side)

The sternal body can subluxate anteriorly in translation along the z-axis, posteriorly, also in translation along the z-axis and in rotation about the y-axis, either unilaterally or in reverse rotation. When rotation is being considered, a clinical decision identifying the direction of rotation must be made. Fortuitously, this area of the body is very pain sensitive, making the point-specific pain findings a very useful and reliable diagnostic tool.

Typically the sternal body and chondrosternal subluxation, regardless of the vectors involved, causes loss of full rotational capacity of the upper cervical complex and reduction of shoulder abduction to approximately 135° accompanied by a positive Shimizu reflex and, variably, a hyperactive pectoral reflex. The pain findings will then be absolutely characteristic of the exact vectors of sternal subluxation. Pain to light palpation will be found in the midline of the sternal body along its entire length in the anterior subluxation and at the chondrosternal junctions over the terminal end of the cartilages on both sides, again along

the entire length of the sternal body in the posterior subluxation. In rotation, the pain findings will be at the chondrosternal junctions over the terminal end of the cartilages on the side corresponding to posterior rotation of the sternal body, and in the case of the anterior sternal body the pain findings will be along the lateral edge of the sternum. In the event the sternum is held in a counter-rotation, the pain findings will be on both sides of the sternal body and will be located according to anterior/posterior position of that side of the sternum.

The differentiating feature of the single chondrosternal subluxation lies in the specificity of the point-specific pain finding. Pain will be located at the subluxated level only over

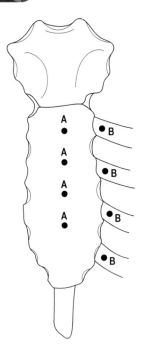

Figure 26.19 ● Contact points for adjusting the translated sternal body subluxations: (A) anterior sternal body and (B) posterior sternal body.

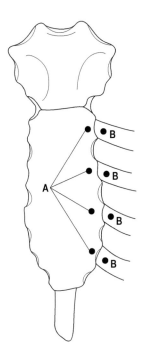

Figure 26.20 ● Contact points for adjusting the rotated sternal body subluxations: (A) anterior sternal body and (B) posterior sternal body.

the terminal end of the cartilage at the chondrosternal junction. Importantly, pre-adjustive impulse testing will only be successful when applied at that one point in this particular subluxation, whereas it needs to be applied more diffusely along the length of the sternal edge if it is to be clinically significant in the sternal body subluxation.

The neurological pre-testing procedure involves the initiation of impulse in the direction of subluxation vector correction while either the affected reflexes or kinesiopathology are retested. All the elements of both kinesiopathology and neuropathology which are characteristic of this subluxation complex can be predictably normalized by neurological pre-testing.

Subluxation correction is achieved by first applying the usual pre-adjustive hold for 10–15 seconds followed by a fast, shallow thrust over the appropriate anatomical location according to subluxation vectors identified by point-specific pain findings and adjustive pre-testing. The precise contact points are shown in Figs 26.19 and 26.20, and the directions of adjustive thrust for all the sternal body and chondrosternal listings are described in Table 26.5.

Structures located at or below the diaphragm

The diaphragm and xiphoid process subluxation

The diaphragm and xiphoid process are intimately linked in the subluxation complex. The xiphoid, in particular, will always need to be differentiated from the diaphragm subluxation irrespective of whether it occurs as a midline or torsional

Table 26.5 Directions of thrust for the sternal body subluxation vectors

Listing	Direction of adjustive thrust
Anterior sternal body	A-P with contact along the sternal body midline
Posterior sternal body	P-A with contact over the chondrosternal junction just lateral to the sternal edge
Anterior sternal body rotation	A-P with contact along the sternal edge on the affected side
Posterior sternal body rotation	P-A with contact over the chondrosternal junctions just lateral to the sternal edge on the affected side
Counter-rotation	A-P with contact along the sternal edge on the anterior side and at the same time over the chondrosternal junctions just lateral to the sternal edge on the posterior side
Anterior cartilage at the chondrosternal junction	A-P over the terminal end of the cartilage
Posterior cartilage at the chondrosternal junction	A-P on the sternal edge immediately opposite the affected cartilage

phenomenon. The xiphoid subluxation will always exist in close connection to diaphragmatic dysfunction, evidenced by restriction in the z-axis movement at the lower end of the thoracic cage, in addition to reduced chest expansion measured at the lower end of the thoracic cage. The expected measurement in an adolescent ranges between 7 and 11 cm, while in school-age children it usually ranges between 5 and 7 cm, depending upon body type and height (endomorphic and tall at the higher end of the scale with ectomorphic and short at the lower end). This measurement can be as low as 2–3 cm when the diaphragm is involved in the subluxation process.

It should also be noted that whenever the sacrum is subluxated the diaphragm will show negative functional changes and there will be a reduction in the chest expansion capability of the patient. The diaphragm and/or xiphoid should only be considered to be a potential subluxation in the event that there is paradoxical kinesiopathology in the posterior elements of the pelvis, as described in Chapter 22.

In the event that the xiphoid or diaphragm is involved as a primary subluxation complex, the kinesiopathology that will be seen will be a restriction of upper cervical lateral flexion and rotation, reduced abduction capability at the glenohumeral joint, paradoxical kinesiopathology between L5/S1 and the sacroiliac joints, and a demonstrable loss of z-axis movement at the lower end of the thoracic cage on the involved side. It should be noted that the diaphragm and xiphoid subluxation is sometimes associated with a unilateral reduction in humeral abduction when the diaphragm subluxation is unilateral. This is one of the defining features of a diaphragm subluxation, as opposed to the sacrum or xiphoid, both of which are associated with a bilateral reduction in humeral abduction.

Precise definition of the subluxation vectors involved in the xiphoid subluxation can only be determined by the pattern of point-specific pain findings, similar to those seen at the angle of Louis. The exact locations of these precise pain points are described later in this chapter.

The midline subluxation, as is the case with the sacral midline subluxation, is associated with a positive Shimizu reflex but a normal pectoral reflex. There is absolutely no variability in this pattern. Again, as is the case with the sacrum, the unilateral subluxation is associated with no Shimizu reflex response.

In addition to the reflexes at the shoulder (Shimizu and pectoral), the psoas muscle will universally test weak on the side of subluxation due to either the xiphoid or diaphragm. It is always possible, as is the case with subluxation in other parts of the body, that neuropathology will not be evident until the subluxation vectors are exacerbated. In the case of the diaphragm the most effective way to demonstrate a latent neuropathology is to perform a Valsalva maneuver. After performing the Valsalva maneuver, the psoas muscle is retested and a latent weakness will become very obvious on the affected side. In the very young child, crying creates a window of opportunity to test for latency as it raises intra-abdominal pressure.

Diaphragmatic myopathology is rather simple and straightforward. The diaphragmatic attachments to the anterior costal arch will be tender to palpate, as will the origin of the rectus abdominis muscle. In the event that the diaphragm is the primary subluxation and there is no involvement of the xiphoid, the only pain finding will be that described for the diaphragm. When the xiphoid is the primary subluxation, however, quite a specific pattern of pain findings will be present at the articulation of the xiphoid process with the body of the sternum at its apex. This pattern of pain findings is described in Table 26.6.

As a midline subluxation, the base of the xiphoid process is capable of rotating positively or negatively about the x-axis,

Table 26.6 Characteristic point-specific pain findings for the xiphoid subluxation vectors

Listing	Location of pain finding
Xiphoid body rotated posteriorly about the y-axis on one side (P-R, P-L)	On the lateral edge of the apex of the sternum on the involved side immediately adjacent to the joint line
Xiphoid body rotated posteriorly about the x-axis (BP)	Midline of the apex of the sternum immediately adjacent to the joint line
Xiphoid body rotated anteriorly about the y-axis (A-R, A-L)	On the lateral edge of the xiphoid base on the affected side immediately adjacent to the joint line
Xiphoid body rotated anteriorly about the x-axis (midline)	Midline of the xiphoid base immediately adjacent to the joint line
Counter-rotation about the y-axis	Combinations of the above according to the vectors involved

creating the possibility of a base anterior or a base posterior subluxation complex. It is also capable of rotating anteriorly or posteriorly on one side, and, finally, can counter-rotate in such a way that one side is anterior and the other side is posterior in relation to the apex of the body of the sternum. The range of possible listings for the xiphoid subluxation is shown in Table 26.7.

The neurological pre-testing procedure involves the initiation of impulse in the direction of subluxation vector correction while either the affected reflexes or kinesiopathology are retested. All the elements of both kinesiopathology and neuropathology which are characteristic of either the diaphragm or xiphoid subluxation complex can be predictably normalized by neurological pre-testing.

Subluxation correction is achieved by first applying the usual pre-adjustive hold for 10–15 seconds followed by a fast, shallow thrust over the appropriate anatomical location

Table 26.7 Directions of thrust for the xiphoid listings

Listing	Direction of adjustive thrust
Xiphoid body rotated posteriorly about the y-axis on one side (P-R, P-L)	A-P with sternal apex contact
Xiphoid body rotated posteriorly about the x-axis (BP)	A-P with sternal apex contact
Xiphoid body rotated anteriorly about the y-axis (A-R, A-L)	A-P with xiphoid base contact
Xiphoid body rotated anteriorly about the x-axis (midline)	A-P with xiphoid base contact
Counter-rotation about the y-axis	A-P with contact on the sternal apex (posteriorly rotated side) and on the xiphoid base (anteriorly rotated side)
Diaphragm	A-P and I-S

according to subluxation vectors identified by point-specific pain findings and adjustive pre-testing. It is only ever necessary to make one adjustive impulse generation in this subluxation complex, irrespective of whether it is a xiphoid or diaphragm subluxation. When the xiphoid is subluxated, adjusting will only take place at the xiphoid, and never at the xiphoid and diaphragm. When the xiphoid is subluxated, the diaphragm must be considered to be a compensatory response.

When the diaphragm is subluxated and the xiphoid has been shown not to be involved, the adjustive thrust is applied to the anterior attachments of the diaphragm at the costal arch at the point of maximal pain intensity, which is usually found to be approximately one-third of the way between the mid-sternal line and the mid-clavicular line. At times, however, this point can be located quite laterally. The directions of impulse generation for all the diaphragm and xiphoid listings are shown in Figs 26.21 and 26.22.

Pubic symphysis subluxation

The pubic symphysis subluxation is relatively common, even in young children. It is readily recognized as the location of the subluxation by the paradoxical kinesiopathology at the posterior elements of the pelvis and the neuropathology characteristic of the front of body subluxation syndromes below the diaphragm. Definition of the precise listing is afforded the examiner by the very specific pain point pattern and the reliable adjustive pre-testing procedures.

The most common pubic subluxations involve separation of the synchondrosis (Fig. 26.23), torsion of the synchondrosis with one ramus superior and one inferior (Fig. 26.24), or a non-torsional, unilateral subluxation in which the ramus has

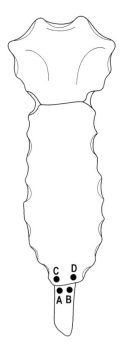

Figure 26.22 • Contact points for adjusting the rotated xiphoid subluxations: (A) right anterior rotation (A-R), (B) left anterior rotation (A-L), (C) right posterior rotation (P-R), and (D) left posterior rotation (P-L).

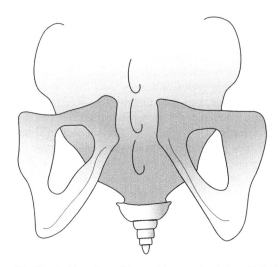

Figure 26.23 • Subluxation of the pubic symphysis in which the synchondrosis has uniformly separated.

gone either inferior (Fig. 26.25) or superior (Fig. 26.26). When the pubic synchondrosis is uniformly separated, the pain finding will be along the entire length of the joint. When the ramus is superior, the point-specific pain finding will be over the superior pubic tubercle, where the rectus abdominis inserts, and when it is inferior, the point-specific pain finding will be over the pubic arch, just lateral to the most inferior aspect of the synchondrosis. Combinations of these pain findings will accompany the various listings.

Less commonly, it is possible to see a number of more complex subluxation patterns at the pubic symphysis. The first of

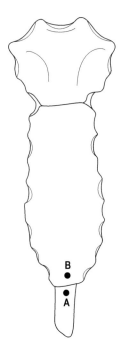

Figure 26.21 • Contact points for adjusting the midline xiphoid subluxations: (A) base anterior and (B) base posterior.

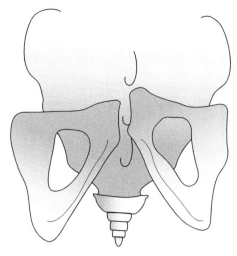

Figure 26.24 • Subluxation of the pubic symphysis in which the synchondrosis is in torsion. In the above case the right pubic ramus is inferior and the left is superior. In this case, the upper cervical and glenohumeral kinesiopathology, when taken together with the presence of the Shimizu reflex bilaterally, suggests a midline problem.

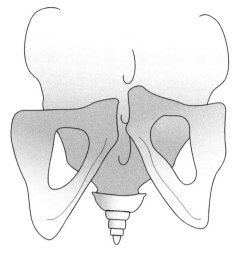

Figure 26.26 • Subluxation of the pubic symphysis in which the synchondrosis is in torsion. In the above case, the left pubic ramus is superior. In this case, the upper cervical and glenohumeral kinesiopathology, when taken together with the absence of the Shimizu reflex, suggests a unilateral problem.

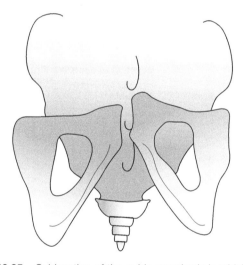

Figure 26.25 • Subluxation of the pubic symphysis in which the synchondrosis is in torsion. In the above case the right pubic ramus is inferior. In this case, the upper cervical and glenohumeral kinesiopathology, when taken together with the absence of the Shimizu reflex, suggests a unilateral problem.

The second of these patterns involves asymmetrical separation of the pubic synchondrosis at either end. The first of these patterns involves separation of the superior aspect of the synchondrosis, while the inferior aspect remains in normal relationship (Fig. 26.27). In this case, the point-specific pain finding will be over the synchondrosis at its superior end with a normal sensory load at the inferior end. Conversely, the inferior aspect of the synchondrosis can separate while the superior aspect remains normal (Fig. 26.28). In this situation, the point-specific pain finding will be evident over the synchondrosis at its inferior end, while the superior end of the synchondrosis maintains a normal sensory load.

these is the superior pubic ramus on both sides at once. This subluxation complex meets the criteria for a true midline subluxation and is invariably associated with a bilateral PI innominate. The point-specific pain finding will be consistent with the superior ramus subluxation at the pubic tubercle. It is also possible to see a situation where the rectus abdominis muscles have become flaccid and a bilaterally inferior pubic ramus occurs, which also meets the criteria for a true midline subluxation and is universally associated with a bilateral AS innominate. The point-specific pain finding will be consistent with the inferior ramus subluxation just lateral to the inferior aspect of the synchondrosis.

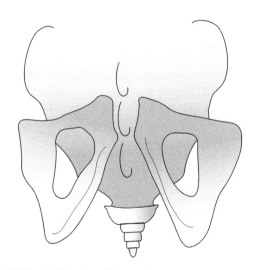

Figure 26.27 • Subluxation of the pubic symphysis in which the synchondrosis has separated at its superior end while remaining in normal relationship at its inferior end. In this case, the upper cervical and glenohumeral kinesiopathology, when taken together with the presence of the Shimizu reflex bilaterally, suggests a midline problem.

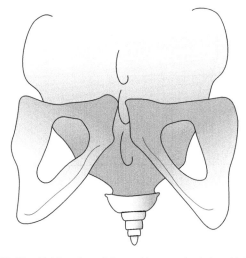

Figure 26.28 • Subluxation of the pubic symphysis in which the synchondrosis has separated at its inferior end while remaining in normal relationship at its superior end. In this case, the upper cervical and glenohumeral kinesiopathology, when taken together with the presence of the Shimizu reflex bilaterally, suggests a midline problem.

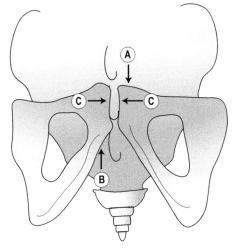

Figure 26.29 • Contact points for adjusting pubic symphysis subluxations: (A) superior ramus, (B) inferior ramus, (C) synchondrosis separation. When the separation is uniform, the contact is taken at the midpoint of the joint; when it is separated at its superior end, the contacts are taken at the superior end of the joint, and vice versa for the inferior separation.

Adjustive pre-testing for the pubis is performed in much the same way as for any other subluxation complex. Impulse generation is initiated in the direction of vector correction, and in children old enough to cooperate the psoas is retested. The previously weak muscle will strengthen. In younger children, impulse generation is initiated by the mother or other caregiver and the upper cervical motion or Shimizu reflex is reassessed.

Subluxation correction is achieved by first applying the usual pre-adjustive hold for 10–15 seconds followed by a fast, shallow thrust over the appropriate anatomical location, according to subluxation vectors identified by point-specific pain findings and adjustive pre-testing. The various listing specific contact points are shown in Fig. 26.29 and the specific directions of thrust for each of the possible pubic symphysis subluxations are described in Table 26.8.

As a final word on the pubic symphysis subluxation, while it is very uncommon, combinations of any of the possible subluxation vectors may occur. For example, one may see a superior ramus existing alongside a superior separation. Unless both subluxations are corrected, the full range of kinesiopathology

Table 26.8 Directions of thrust for the pubic symphysis listings

Listing	Direction of adjustive thrust
Pubic synchondrosis separation	A-P, L-M
Superior pubic ramus	S-I
Inferior pubic ramus	I-S
Bilateral pubic torsion	S-I on the superior ramus and I-S on the inferior ramus

and neuropathology that led to the pubic subluxation in the first place will not be adequately eliminated. To guard against this eventuality, when the pubic symphysis is indicated as the primary subluxation, a careful search of all the point-specific pain findings, followed by adjustive pre-testing, is warranted and appropriate.

The cranial subluxation in children

Neil J. Davies   Kimberley Tuohey

Like all other adjustive procedures in chiropractic, the goal of cranial adjusting is to restore functional neurological balance. Neurological deficits demonstrated on the standard, orthodox neurological examination, coupled with precise, detailed patterns of kinesiopathology, now dictate the need to apply the adjustment to the bones of the cranium. A cranial adjustment is a potent neurological stimulus and should be performed only when the confluence of examination findings indicates the need for such a procedure. The cranium is a very delicate structure. It should be handled with the greatest possible care, based on a thorough understanding of its mechanics; thus a technique that is gentle and without force is used in normalizing the position of the cranial structure (Wales 1990).

The primary respiratory mechanism (PRM)

Dr WG Sutherland observed five basic elements at work in the human body and he called these the 'five phenomena of the primary respiratory mechanism'. The word 'primary' was used as it indicated something that was basic or first. The word 'respiratory' referred to metabolism or physiological respiration. He considered the human body to be a complex 'mechanism' (a grouping of parts working together towards a definite action), hence the use of this word. Though primary respiration has two phases, inhalation and exhalation, this is a separate concept from and not to be confused with *secondary respiration*. Secondary respiration refers to the process produced by movement of the primary and secondary muscles of respiration that results in the exchange of oxygen for carbon dioxide at the pulmonary alveoli. Primary respiration is a deeper, more basic process to life. The primary respiratory mechanism has two alternating phases, the inspiratory and the expiratory phases, also respectively known as the flexion and extension phases (Magoun 1951). For the sake of study and the ease of clinical application, the cranial bones are grouped into those that principally flex and extend (occiput and sphenoid) and those that externally and internally rotate as they flex and extend (temporal, parietal and frontal).

During the inspiratory phase of primary respiration, as the midline bones flex, the peripheral bones externally rotate, resulting in an increase in the transverse cranial diameter and a decrease in the anteroposterior diameter (DiGiovanna & Schiowitz 1997). In addition, the basicranium and foramen magnum move superiorly, which in turn draws the sacral base posterosuperiorly as a result of the changing tensions in the dural sac. During the expiratory phase of primary respiration, the midline bones extend and the peripheral bones internally rotate, resulting in a decrease in the transverse cranial diameter and an increase in the anteroposterior diameter, while the basicranium and foramen magnum move inferiorly, thus drawing the sacral base anteroinferiorly.

The five phenomena of the PRM described by Sutherland (1988) are as follows:

- fluctuation of the cerebrospinal fluid (CSF)
- mobility of the intracranial and intraspinal membranes and the function of the reciprocal tension membrane (RTM)
- the inherent motility of the central nervous system (CNS)
- articular mobility of the cranial bones
- the involuntary mobility of the sacrum between the ilia.

The rhythmic fluctuation of the cerebrospinal fluid

CSF fluctuation is considered the first principle of the PRM. Movement of the CSF involves both circulation and fluctuation. Circulation occurs as a result of hydrostatic forces at the choroid plexus and arachnoid granulations (DiGiovanna & Schiowitz 1997). However, forces generated by hydrostatic gradients are not sufficient in and of themselves to account for the exchange of CSF with the circulation of the body. Indeed, fluctuation within the CSF provides this force. The CSF fluctuates, or moves back and forth, within a relatively closed container, the central nervous system. As the brain and spinal cord change shape with the cycles of inhalation and exhalation, the CSF fluctuates back and forth in the spaces in the brain and spinal cord. As the brain is constantly producing CSF, a small excess travels out along the channels around the peripheral nerve trunks during the exhalation phase of primary respiration.

The CSF plays an important role in circulation and nourishment of body tissues. Fluctuation of the CSF has now been documented in MRI studies. This fluctuation provides a continuous mixing which, combined with the small circulatory forces, allows for adequate exchange of the CSF with the circulation of the body. The fluctuation of the CSF and cranial articular motion coincide under normal resting conditions. In addition, CSF fluctuation, changes in the contours of the central nervous system, and motion of the craniosacral mechanism are synchronous at such times.

The motion of the dural membranes

The second principle of the PRM involves the reciprocal tension membranes (RTM), otherwise known as the meninges, which are made up of the dura mater, arachnoid mater and pia mater. Together they are the agencies for articular mobility of the cranial and craniosacral mechanisms, creating balance in all dimensions – aiding, controlling and limiting motion. Basically, the intracranial and intraspinal membranes allow a range of motion in the bones that are suspended within them in much the same way as ligaments allow a range of motion of the joints of the spine and extremities.

All membranes change shape during the phases of the PRM. During the inspiratory phase, the anterior end of the falx cerebri moves slightly posteriorly and inferiorly, the tentorium shifts slightly anteriorly, and the craniosacral mechanism functions so that the spinal dura lifts the sacrum around its axis, so that the base is superior and the apex anterior. The exact opposite occurs during the expiratory phase, to complete the cycle.

Membranous structures in the body are all composed of connective tissue and are derived from the embryological mesenchymal layer. They are all continuous with one another, with the intracranial membranes closely related to the rest of the body via fascial connections from the cranial base throughout the entire spine, the diaphragm, the extremities and the viscera.

In the neonate, and beyond into infancy, there are no interlocking sutures in the skull. The only functional joints in the neonatal skull are those of the occiput with the atlas vertebra (occipitoatlantal). The cranial bones of the newborn are suspended in space by the dural membrane and the pressure applied by the CSF. Developmentally, prior to completed bone formation, it is the membranes that house, protect, guide and limit motion.

Inherent motility of the central nervous system (CNS)

The third principle of the PRM concerns the brain and spinal cord. The CNS has a 'jellyfish' type of mobility which has long been recognized by the scientific community (Magoun 1951).

This mobility has a mechanical function in the operation of the PRM. The mobility of the bones of the skull is accommodative to that motility and therefore to the subsequent fluctuation of the cerebrospinal fluid.

This jellyfish mobility is evident as a very slight coiling (roughly mimicking its embryological state) during the inhalation phase of primary respiration, with a shortening from top to bottom (decreased cephalad to caudad length) of the spinal cord. The transverse diameter of the cranium becomes slightly wider (increased) and shorter from front to back (decreased A-P diameter). The exhalation phase of primary respiration produces the exact opposite (DiGiovanna & Schiowitz 1997, Magoun 1951). This expansion and contraction of the cranium is not large, but it is physiologically significant. Estimates place the change at hundredths of an inch, but it varies according to where it is measured. There are cavities and spaces in and around the CNS, and as the brain and spinal cord change shape with the inherent rhythmic motion, the volume of these spaces and hence the amount of fluid that they hold will change. This type of motion is not limited to humans, but is a basic and vital property of any living organism with a nervous system.

Articular mobility of the cranial bones

The fourth principle of the PRM involves the articular mobility of the cranial bones. The cranium is made up of 26 bones in total and they are all in slight rhythmic motion along with the CNS, CSF, membranes and sacrum. These bones all fit together like the gears of a watch and influence one another. Within the joints in the head (sutures) are contained connective tissue, nerves and blood vessels. This is like any other joint in the body and as such is designed for motion.

The cranium of the newborn is predominantly cartilage and membrane without sutures between the bones as in the adult. By 13 years of age there is a moderate degree of suture formation and this is complete by approximately 18 years of age. As the skull ossifies, sutures are formed in response to forces exerted by adjacent bones on each other, the shape of the suture being consistent with the direction of inherent mobility. Hence, the motion of a bone may be deduced by the shape of its suture with adjacent bones. When an axis of motion crosses a suture line, that suture will form in the shape of a bevel (e.g. the squamosal suture), since motions on the opposite sides of an axis are different. These points are called pivots.

Cranial bone motion will also exert a developmental effect on the shape of the facial bones (Magoun 1951), but for the purposes of this chapter, only the occiput, sphenoid, temporal, parietal and frontal bones will be discussed in detail.

The sphenoid

The sphenoid bone consists of the body, the greater and lesser wings laterally, and the pterygoid plates inferiorly. The sphenoid articulates with 12 other cranial bones, being the occiput, temporal bones (2), parietal bones (2), frontal bone, ethmoid, palatine bones (2), vomer, and zygomae (2). The palatine bones, the vomer and the zygomae are intermediary between the sphenoid and the maxillae, making the sphenoid influential in the motion of the frontal and facial bones.

Although all the cranial bones move together during respiration, the sphenoid and occiput principally work together to induce flexion and extension about the midline.

The occiput

The occiput is in four parts at birth, namely the squamous, basilar, and two lateral condylar parts. The base of the occiput articulates anteriorly with the base of the sphenoid. The occiput articulates with six other bones, namely the sphenoid, the parietal bones (2), the temporal bones (2), and the atlas vertebra. The occiput, like the sphenoid, moves primarily into flexion during inspiration and extension during expiration.

The temporal

At birth, the temporal bone consists of the petromastoid portion and the squamous portion. The petromastoid part is developed in cartilage that projects obliquely between the occiput and the greater wing of the sphenoid to articulate at its apex with the body of the sphenoid. This portion contains the auditory and vestibular apparatus. The squamous part is developed in membrane and forms the greater part of the lower lateral wall of the skull (Fryman 1976). The squamous and tympanic parts unite just prior to birth. The temporal bone forms articulation with the sphenoid, occiput, parietal, zygoma, maxilla, and nasal bones on each side of the cranium. The temporal bones primarily externally rotate during inspiration, and internally rotate during expiration.

The parietal

The parietal bone only ever has one part. The parietal bones articulate at the sagittal suture with each other along with the frontal, sphenoid, temporal and occiput. Like the temporal it moves into external rotation during inspiration and internal rotation during expiration.

The frontal

The frontal bone consists of the squama, orbital and nasal parts. The external or frontal surface of the squama is divided by the metopic suture, running from the nasion through the glabella to the bregma. The frontal bone articulates with the sphenoid, parietal bones, ethmoid, lacrimal bones, maxillae, nasal bones and zygomae. Like all peripheral plates, the frontal bone primarily externally rotates during inspiration and internally rotates during expiration. It should be noted that as the peripheral bones externally and internally rotate it is within the context of flexion and extension. Therefore, they primarily externally rotate while flexing (inspiration) and internally rotate while extending (expiration).

The articular mobility of the sacrum between the ilia

The fifth and final principle of the PRM involves the articular mobility between the sacrum and the ilia. The dural membrane is firmly attached to the base of the skull, the sacrum and coccyx, resulting in the motion of the cranial mechanism to be transmitted to the sacrum. The end result of this is that the cranium and the sacrum work together as a functional unit.

The involuntary motion of the sacrum is about a transverse axis anterior to the sacral canal, through the body of S2 at the junction of the short and long arms of the L-shaped sacroiliac joints (DiGiovanna & Schiowitz 1997). The anterosuperior movement of the foramen magnum during the inspiratory phase of the PRM lifts the spinal dural membrane, a function referred to as the 'core link' between the cranial and pelvic bowls (Magoun 1951). The effect of the lift is to rotate the sacrum about the transverse axis at S2 whereby the base of the sacrum moves posterosuperiorly and the apex moves towards the pubic symphysis. The opposite occurs in the expiratory phase to complete the cycle.

Principles of diagnosis

The principal diagnostic decision that needs to be made is whether or not a given patient has need of a cranial adjustment as the primary approach to their pattern of dysafferentation. In its original concept, the decision to make a cranial adjustment depended upon the ability of the individual clinician to feel the various rhythms of movement inherent within the PRM. Recent research has seriously called into question the validity of a palpatory cranial diagnostic method based on the ability of the clinician to appreciate the rhythm of movement inherent within the PRM (Hanten et al 1998, Moran & Gibbons 2001, Sommerfeld et al 2004, Wirth-Pattullo & Hayes 1994).

The diagnostic methodology utilized in adjusting the child in today's world of neurological chiropractic is based on a far more sophisticated protocol which involves the identification of specific patterns of kinesiopathology which are then cross-referenced to a series of orthodox neurological tests.

Key patterns of kinesiopathology

The method of biomechanical assessment that leads to the identification of patterns of kinesiopathology has been exhaustively covered in Chapter 22. From that examination, the four patterns of kinesiopathology detailed in Fig. 27.1 emerge as being highly suggestive of a cranial problem. Bear in mind that, once identified, specific patterns of neurological deficit also need to be demonstrated before a definitive diagnosis is arrived at.

Neuropathology

When a cranial subluxation is the cause of one of the four patterns of kinesiopathology described in Fig. 27.1, various combinations of the following neurological deficits will be seen.

Shimizu reflex

The Shimizu reflex will be universally present (normally not able to be elicited) in the presence of the cranial subluxation. This reflex response (otherwise known as the 'scapulohumeral reflex of Shimizu') is elicited by striking the lateral third of the spine of the scapula in an anteroinferior direction and the acromion process in a caudal direction. The Shimizu reflex is classified as hyperactive when elevation of the scapula,

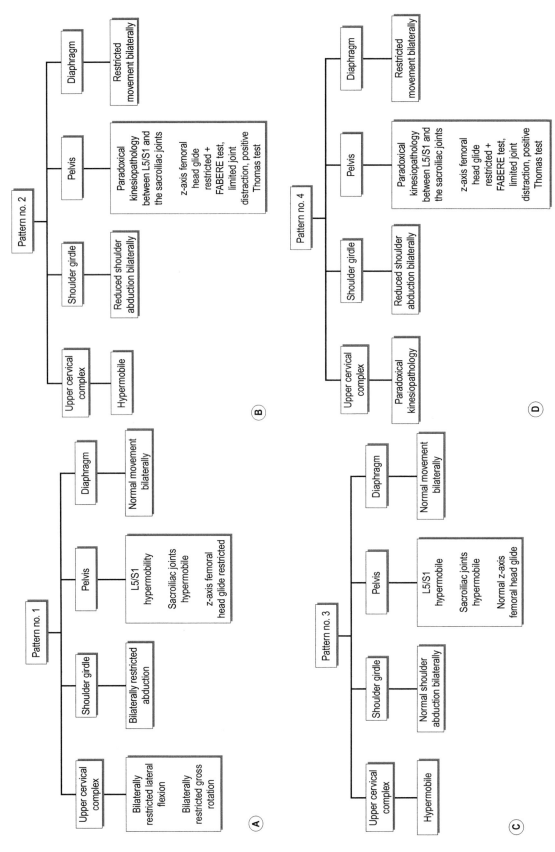

Figure 27.1 ● The four patterns of kinesiopathology associated with the cranial subluxation.

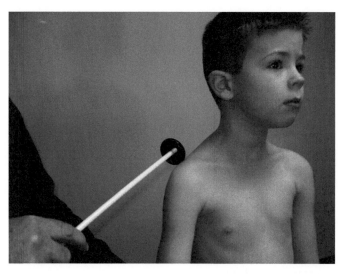

Figure 27.2 • Technique for the performance of the Shimizu reflex. When the lateral one-third of the spine of the scapula or the acromion process is struck, humeral abduction and elevation of the shoulder are deemed to be positive responses.

abduction of the humerus, or both, appear following the strike of the reflex hammer (Shimizu et al 1993). The methodology of performing the Shimizu reflex test is shown in Fig. 27.2.

Pectoral reflex

This reflex is elicited by striking the tendon of the pectoralis major tendon at the anterior margin of the axilla, as shown in Fig. 27.3. A hyperactive pectoral reflex, like the Shimizu reflex, is suggestive of upper cervical cord compression (Watson et al 1997). The pectoral reflex will be universally hyperactive in the presence of the cranial subluxation, with the noticeable and important exception of the dropped sphenoid, either unilaterally or bilaterally.

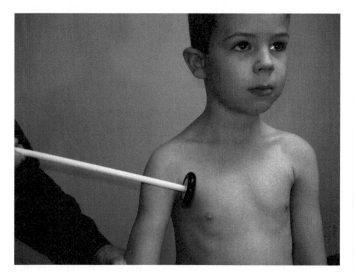

Figure 27.3 • Technique for the performance of the pectoral reflex. When the inferior margin of the pectoral tendon is struck, slight forward and medial movement of the shoulder is the expected appropriate response.

Cranial nerve XI deficit

In children who are of school age and older, the XIth cranial nerve may be tested and will be found to be universally weak in the presence of the cranial subluxation. The preferred method for testing the XIth cranial nerve is by direct evaluation of the upper trapezius muscle as shown in Fig. 27.4.

Intraocular pressure changes

It is common to see asymmetrical intraocular pressure when there is a cranial subluxation. The technique for assessing intraocular pressure is shown in Fig. 27.5.

Circular ocular tracking

Ask the child to follow your finger as you trace out a circle, as shown in Fig. 27.6. Poor performance on this test and the observation of circular nystagmus is common in children with cranial subluxations.

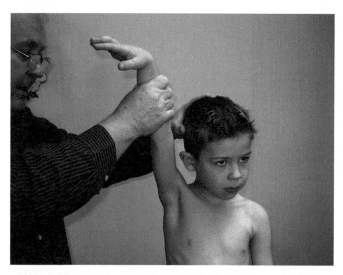

Figure 27.4 • Testing procedure for cranial nerve XI. The patient's arm is pulled away from the midline in the xy plane against resistance.

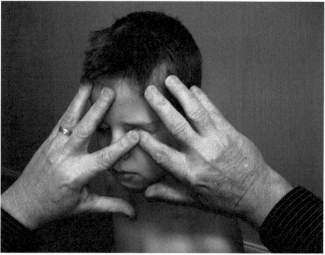

Figure 27.5 • Technique for assessing intraocular pressure. Very gentle pressure is applied to the closed eye and the resistance to that pressure is assessed.

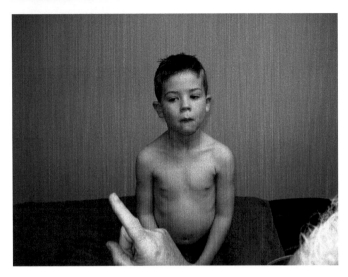

Figure 27.6 • Ocular tracking using a circular pattern. Nystagmus is considered a positive finding.

Asymmetry in the accommodation response

Hold your finger 50 cm in front of the child's face and ask them to focus on it (Fig. 27.7). Carefully observe the width between the medial edge of the iris and the medial epicanthus. Asymmetry is common and strongly associated with the cranial subluxation. In addition to initial asymmetry, as the clinician moves their finger toward the child's face, the eyes may converge at different rates.

Making the cranial diagnosis

Within the context and framework of the adjusting the child, protocols detailed in Chapter 22, certain distinct patterns of functional loss, kinesiological and neurological, need to be demonstrated. The absolute bedrock of diagnosis is the demonstration of all elements of one of the four patterns of

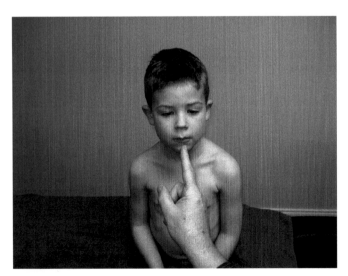

Figure 27.7 • Assessment of the accommodation response for symmetry. Asymmetrical movement of the eyes is considered a positive finding.

kinesiopathology coupled with the presence of the Shimizu and hyperactive pectoralis reflex, both bilaterally, and any combination of the other neurological findings described previously in this chapter.

Clinical correlations

While it is always precarious to relate specific patterns of patient symptoms to particular subluxation complexes, it is reasonable to identify the following as being often associated with persistent cranial subluxation, presumably as reflex triggers:

- trauma
- congestive disorders
- infection
- emotional stress
- environmental stress.

The cranial subluxation is often seen to exist as secondary to spinal and extremity subluxation and, in adolescents, to diaphragm and pelvic floor muscle compartment syndromes. In practice, what this means is that the characteristic cranial findings are not in evidence until the primary subluxation is corrected. The cranial subluxation is very commonly associated with the sacrum, sacral segment, coccyx, diaphragm, and pelvic floor problems.

The cranial adjusting protocols

Basic respiratory assisted techniques

Magoun (1951) made the point that no cranial bone moves independently of the other bones. The underlying principle of respiratory assisted adjusting is to apply very gentle pressure in the direction that each bone will normally move on each phase of respiration. The intent is to work with the inherent movements of the body, not against them. These adjusting protocols have been designed to offer the chiropractor a method of affecting cranial/membranous function without being able to appreciate by palpation the underlying cranial rhythm. This is particularly important in the light of recent studies that have cast grave doubts on the interexaminer and intraexaminer reliability of this palpatory method (Hanten et al 1998, Moran & Gibbons 2001, Sommerfeld et al 2004, Wirth-Pattullo & Hayes 1994). Any chiropractor can effectively use these adjusting protocols as they depend for their successful application on an understanding of bone movement patterns as they relate to the phases of respiration.

For the purpose of this chapter, the bones of the cranium are divided into those which move principally in flexion/extension (occiput and sphenoid) and those which move into rotation as they flex and extend (temporal, parietal and frontal). This anatomical division of cranial areas is not completely random. The great majority of cranial problems in children are those affecting the sphenobasilar mechanism, so named because of the flexion/extension movements of the sphenoid at its articulation with the basilar portion of the occiput. Maximal reduction of the kinesiopathological pattern and restoration of the neurological deficits is often accomplished by simple normalization of the sphenobasilar mechanism.

All the cranial procedures are performed with the patient fully clothed and placed in the supine position with a pillow placed comfortably under the head. In the case of infants, particularly if they are unsettled and crying, the procedures are best performed while nursing. The rhythmical sucking action may be used as one uses inspiration (sucking in) and expiration (relaxing) in the older, more compliant child.

The adjusting protocol requires that the chiropractor apply the protocol at each of the bones, the direction of adjustive pressure being consistent with bone movement in the two phases of respiration. While it is a random figure, application throughout five respiratory cycles is appropriate in children. The success or otherwise of the total procedure will be determined by the reduction of the kinesiopathological factors and restoration of the neurological deficits. These must be retested after the completion of the total procedure at all five bones to be sure a correction has been attained.

Adjusting the occiput

In the inspiratory phase, the chiropractor applies very gentle pressure in an anteroposterior direction equally over the anterior aspect of both mastoid processes, as shown in Fig. 27.8.

In the expiratory phase, the chiropractor applies very gentle pressure in a posterosuperior direction equally over each side of the lateral aspect of the base of the occiput, as shown in Fig. 27.9.

Adjusting the sphenoid

In the inspiratory phase, the chiropractor applies very gentle pressure with the tips of the fingers to gently lift the greater wing of the sphenoid equally on each side while simultaneously applying torque in a forward direction to assist flexion

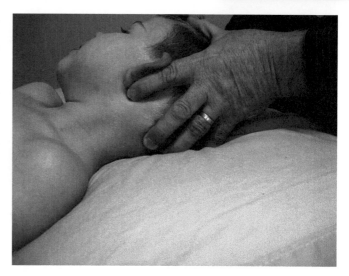

Figure 27.9 • Adjustive contacts for the expiratory phase of the occipital adjustment.

of the sphenobasilar mechanism (Fig. 27.10). Care must be taken to maintain a steady cephalad pressure throughout the procedure.

In the expiratory phase, the lift of the sphenoid equally on each side is maintained while simultaneously applying torque in a backward direction to assist extension of the sphenobasilar mechanism (Fig. 27.11). Again, care must be taken to maintain a steady cephalad pressure throughout the procedure.

Adjusting the temporal

In the inspiratory phase, the chiropractor uses the tips of the index and middle fingers to gently lift the temporal bone in a cephalad direction while compressing the lower regions of the temporal bone in order to assist external rotation. At the same time, a slight torque motion towards the occiput is applied to assist flexion of the sphenobasilar mechanism (Fig. 27.12).

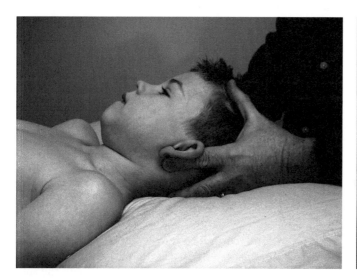

Figure 27.8 • Adjustive contacts for the inspiratory phase of the occipital adjustment.

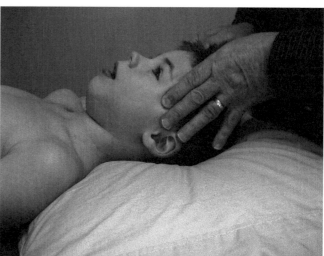

Figure 27.10 • Adjustive contacts for the inspiratory phase of the sphenoid adjustment.

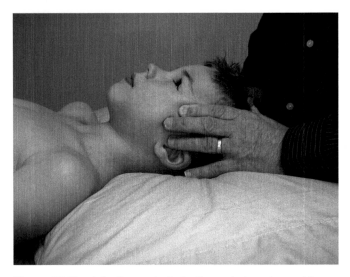

Figure 27.11 ● Adjustive contacts for the expiratory phase of the sphenoid adjustment.

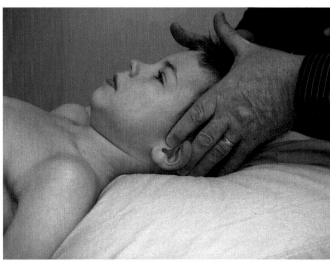

Figure 27.13 ● Adjustive contacts for the expiratory phase of the temporal adjustment.

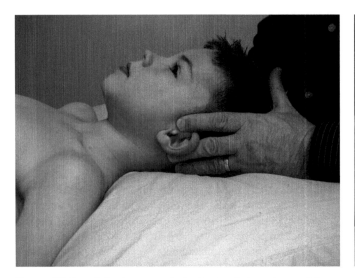

Figure 27.12 ● Adjustive contacts for the inspiratory phase of the temporal adjustment.

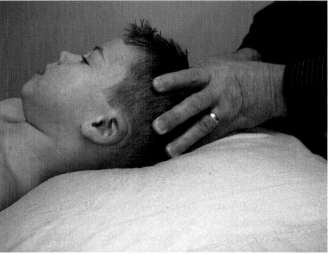

Figure 27.14 ● Adjustive contacts for the inspiratory phase of the parietal adjustment.

Both temporal bones are adjusted simultaneously and care must be taken to maintain a steady cephalad pressure throughout the procedure.

In the expiratory phase, the lift of the temporal bone in a cephalad direction is maintained while compressing the upper regions of the temporal bone in order to assist internal rotation. At the same time, a slight torque motion towards the sphenoid is applied to assist extension of the sphenobasilar mechanism (Fig. 27.13). Both temporal bones are adjusted simultaneously and care must be taken to maintain a steady cephalad pressure throughout the procedure.

Adjusting the parietal

In the inspiratory phase, the chiropractor uses the tips of the second, third and fourth fingers to gently lift the parietal bones simultaneously on both sides. The thumbs are crossed in the

midline across the sagittal suture (Fig. 27.14), but apply no pressure at all in this phase.

In the expiratory phase, the chiropractor uses the pads of the thumbs to gently depress and separate the sagittal suture (Fig. 27.15). The second, third and fourth fingers remain in contact with the lower regions of the parietal bones on both sides, but apply no pressure whatsoever during this phase of the procedure.

Adjusting the frontal

In the inspiratory phase, the chiropractor uses the tips of the second, third and fourth fingers to gently lift the frontal bones simultaneously on both sides. The thumbs are crossed in the midline over the sagittal suture near to its entry into the anterior fontanel (Fig. 27.16), but apply no pressure at all in either phase.

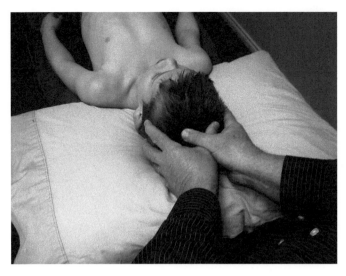

Figure 27.15 • Adjustive contacts for the expiratory phase of the parietal adjustment.

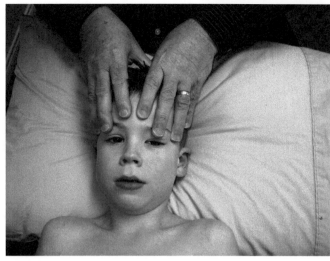

Figure 27.17 • Adjustive contacts for the expiratory phase of the frontal adjustment.

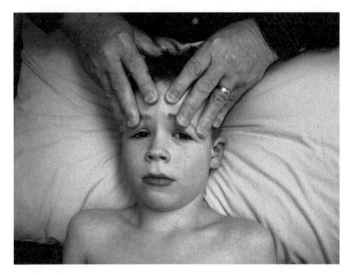

Figure 27.16 • Adjustive contacts for the inspiratory phase of the frontal adjustment.

In the expiratory phase, the chiropractor uses the tips of the second, third and fourth fingers to gently depress the frontal bones simultaneously on both sides. The thumbs are crossed in the midline over the sagittal suture near to its entry into the anterior fontanel (Fig. 27.17), but apply no pressure at all in either phase.

The intraoral techniques

Intraoral techniques have the capability of making profound neurological change. In pediatric cranial adjusting, as in all other areas of the body, the principle of always choosing to do the least invasive procedure is sacrosanct. These intraoral procedures should therefore be reserved for the most intractable cases where sustainable change has been unachievable using the basic adjusting procedures.

As is the case with the basic respiratory assisted procedures, the intent is to work with the inherent movements of the body, not against them. With the exception of the temporomandibular joint (TMJ) adjustment, one does not have to be able to appreciate cranial rhythm to successfully perform these advanced level adjusting procedures which are applied synchronously with the respiratory cycle. The objective is to influence the flexion/extension functional capability of the cranium, in particular the sphenobasilar mechanism. Taking the decision to perform an intraoral adjustment is based on the failure of sustainable response when using the less invasive basic respiratory assisted procedures. Once the clinical decision has been taken to apply an intraoral adjustment, the order of procedure is the molar contact, followed by the sphenobasilar release and the TMJ release. The total adjustment is made up of all three procedures.

The molar contact

Contact is taken on the medial surface of the molar teeth or, in the very young, over the gum area where the molars will eventually appear. Gentle lateral pressure is applied during inspiration only in order to decompress the palatine suture and allow for normal function. No pressure is ever applied during the expiration phase.

The sphenobasilar release in flexion

A bimanual contact is taken with the middle finger of the right hand placed over the hard palate while the left hand cradles the occiput as shown in Fig. 27.18. On inspiration, gentle pressure is applied in a cephalad direction toward the sella turcica with the right hand contact while the left hand applies pressure caudally.

The sphenobasilar release in extension

A bimanual contact is taken with the pad of the middle finger of the right hand placed over the posterior surface of the medial incisors while the left hand cradles the occiput in the

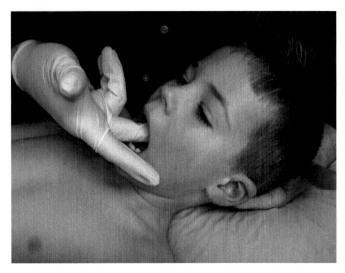

Figure 27.18 • Adjustive contacts for intraoral correction of the sphenobasilar mechanism during the inspiration/flexion phase.

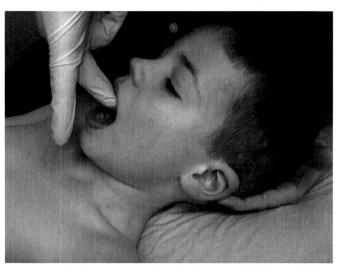

Figure 27.19 • Adjustive contacts for intraoral correction of the sphenobasilar mechanism during the expiration/extension phase.

same manner as that used for the inspiration phase. On expiration, gentle pressure is applied to draw the medial incisors directly forward while the occiput is lifted in a cephalad direction (Fig. 27.19).

The temporomandibular joint release

Before the TMJ correction is made, it is appropriate to feel the symmetry of opening and closing movement. This is achieved by placing the index fingers in the patient's external ear canal and, with the pads of the fingers oriented anteriorly, feel for the symmetry of movement as the jaw is slowly opened and closed. It is important to determine which side moves last when the jaw is opened.

Contact is taken over the superior end of the mandibular ramus as shown in Fig. 27.20. On inspiration, gentle pressure is applied in a cephalad direction on both sides when the opening of the jaw has been shown to be symmetrical. When it is asymmetrical, pressure is still applied to both sides, but maximally to the side which was slow to open. On expiration, the pressure is relaxed to zero.

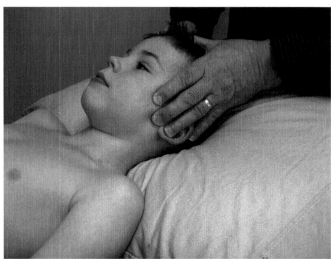

Figure 27.20 • Adjustive contacts for the temporomandibular joint correction.

References

DiGiovanna, E.L., Schiowitz, S., 1997. An Osteopathic Approach to Diagnosis and Treatment, second ed. Lippincott-Raven, New York.

Fryman, V.M., 1976. The trauma of birth. Osteopathic Annals (May), 197–205.

Hanten, W.P., Dawson, D.D., Iwata, M., et al., 1998. Craniosacral rhythm; reliability and relationships with cardiac and respiratory rates. J. Orthop. Sports Phys. Ther. 27 (3), 213–218.

Magoun, H.I., 1951. Osteopathy in the Cranial Field, original ed. (As approved by William Garner Sutherland.). Journal Printing Company, Kirksville, Missouri.

Moran, R.W., Gibbons, P., 2001. Intraexaminer and interexaminer reliability for palpation of the cranial rhythm impulse at the head and sacrum. J. Manipulative Physiol. Ther. 24 (3), 183–190.

Shimizu, T., Shimada, H., Shirakura, K., 1993. Scapulohumeral reflex (Shimizu): its clinical significance and testing maneuver. Spine 18 (15), 2182–2190.

Sommerfeld, P., Kaider, A., Klein, P., 2004. Inter- and intraexaminer reliability in palpation of the 'primary respiratory mechanism' within the 'cranial concept.' Man. Ther. 9 (1), 22–29.

Sutherland, S., 1988. Notes – a manual for the Osteopathic College of Osteopathic Medicine of the Pacific. Osteopathy in the Cranial Field. Department of Osteopathic Principles and Practice, College of Osteopathic Medicine of the Pacific, California.

Wales, A.L., 1990. WG Sutherland Teachings in the Science of Osteopathy. Sutherland Cranial Teaching Foundation, Texas.

Watson, J.C., Broaddus, W.C., Smith, M.M., et al., 1997. Hyperactive pectoralis reflex as an indicator of upper cervical spinal cord compression: report of 15 cases. J. Neurosurg. 86 (1), 159–161.

Wirth-Pattullo, V., Hayes, K.W., 1994. Interrater reliability of craniosacral rate measurements and their relationship with subjects' and examiners' heart and respiratory rate measurements. Phys. Ther. 74 (10), 908–916.

Care of the pregnant patient

Kimberley Tuohey   Kyla Sheridan   Neil J. Davies

28

The preconception period

The preconception period is that period of time immediately prior to the advent of pregnancy. It is a period of time which offers the patient a unique opportunity to implement intentional, well planned, healthy life choices which carry the potential to positively impact the health and developmental status of the newborn. The family care oriented chiropractor is well placed in the community of health care professionals to guide the prospective parents through this vital period in their lives.

The scope of preconception care

Preconception health care focuses on the clinical conditions and risk factors that could affect a woman if she becomes pregnant. The key to promoting preconception health is to develop a plan that seeks to combine the best available health care with healthy behaviours, strong family support, and a safe environment at both home and work.

Effective preconception health care focuses on managing current clinical conditions and implementing an action plan to take control over any health issues prior to pregnancy. Such a strategy offers the would-be mother the best chance of preventing problems for both herself and her baby. Preconception health care is an individually customized strategy based around the needs, choices and cultural issues affecting intending mothers to be. It means helping women and their partners to minimize risks and access appropriate ongoing care. Men and other family members are also very important in supporting the goals of preconception health.

Planning and implementing preconception care

As a guide to the chiropractor providing family oriented care, the following seven elements are important in planning and implementing preconception care:

- Provision of regular chiropractic check-ups. Carefully implemented chiropractic care will help to facilitate optimal body performance through balanced and stable neurological function. Having a nervous system that has normal tone limits musculoskeletal pain, including back pain, headaches, leg and pelvic pain, that often ensues following the advent of a normal pregnancy.
- Prescribing of 500 µg of folic acid daily to be taken for at least 3 months prior to becoming pregnant. This helps to reduce the risk of birth defects, as folic acid supplementation in the preconception period has been shown to significantly reduce the incidence of low birth weight and small for gestational age (SGA) babies (Timmermans et al 2009). Periconceptional use of folic acid has also been shown to reduce the incidence of neural tube defects which lead to brain and spine abnormalities such as spina bifida (Blom 2009, Massi Lindsey et al 2009).
- Encouraging stopping smoking. Smoking is known to increase the risk of having a baby of low birth weight (Vlajinac et al 1997). Low birth weight babies have increased risks of a range of other clinical problems, and generally require a longer hospital stay and a greater level of medical intervention.
- Encouraging stopping any alcohol consumption. The US Centers for Disease Control and Prevention currently recommends complete abstention from alcohol while pregnant. Current research suggests that even small amounts of alcohol may lead to fetal alcohol syndrome. At this stage, no safe level for alcohol consumption has been established (CDCP 2009).
- In the event there are current clinical problems best managed by a physician, be sure these conditions are kept under control. Such conditions would include, but are not limited to, asthma, diabetes, oral health, obesity and epilepsy. Encourage the patient to consult their family physician or obstetrician to discuss their plans to start a family so medical assistance can be accessed in a timely

DOI: 10.1016/B978-0-7020-3129-8.00028-1

manner to provide an adequate level of control in relation to any current clinical problems.

- Investigate with the patient any over-the-counter or prescription medicines they may be taking, including vitamins, dietary supplements and herbal remedies. Around 4% of pregnant women are taking prescription or over-the-counter medication which could increase the risk of birth defects, without knowing it (CDCP 2009).
- Advise on the avoidance of exposure to toxic environmental substances or potentially infectious materials at work or at home. Examples of such substances would include organic and inorganic chemicals, spray-can propellants, air and water pollutants, animal and rodent feces.

It is important to ensure that the future mother has an adequate and well balanced diet, is getting 30 minutes of vigorous exercise daily, is kept well hydrated with clean water, maintains adequate sleep, and controls stress.

The pregnancy period

The pregnancy period is obviously the time from conception to delivery. It is broken into three trimesters of 13 weeks each. As is the case for any patient, a detailed health history, physical examination and clinical investigations constitute an appropriate approach to the patient. In the pregnant patient, of course, there are a number of special clinical considerations to take into account.

The patient history

As is always best, this should be carried out in a quiet, unhurried private environment. The history of a pregnant patient needs to include personal details, family history, social history, previous medical history, surgical history, previous chiropractic history, and the obstetrical history.

Personal details

As with all patients, the patient's full name, date of birth, address and occupation should be noted.

Family history

It is important to record any condition affecting the three generational family (siblings, parents, grandparents) which may be inherited by the patient and have capacity to affect the growth and development of the fetus. Important clinical conditions affecting the mother would include diabetes, hypertension, psychiatric disorders, twinning, deafness, blindness, chromosomal or metabolic disorders.

The general medical history

Particular attention should be directed towards the presence of any known allergies, cardiac disease, hypertension, renal disease, central nervous system disorders (especially epilepsy), psychoses, gastrointestinal disorders, metabolic conditions (especially thyroid disorders and diabetes), previous blood transfusions and any medications.

The pregnancy-specific history

Details that should be covered in the pregnancy-specific history include sexually transmitted diseases, nausea and vomiting, alcohol and drug history, dizziness and lightheadedness, sleep patterns, pain, fetal movements, heartburn (reflux), varicosities, bleeding/spotting, and diet.

Sexually transmitted diseases (STDs)

These occur across all social strata, making their presence, or possibility, an important element to explore during history-taking. STDs affect not only the mother but can also affect the baby. The harmful effects of STDs in babies may include stillbirth, low birth weight (<5 lb/2.25 kg), conjunctivitis, pneumonia, neonatal sepsis (infection in the baby's bloodstream), neurological damage, blindness, deafness, acute hepatitis, meningitis, chronic liver disease including cirrhosis, and death in the first year of life (Bobat et al 1999, Jain et al 2009). Most of these problems can be prevented if the mother receives routine prenatal care, which includes screening tests for STDs starting early in pregnancy and repeated close to delivery, if necessary. Other problems can be treated if the infection is found at birth.

Nausea and vomiting

The presence of nausea and vomiting should be assessed and recorded. Nausea and vomiting of pregnancy is the most common condition affecting pregnant women, with a prevalence of 50–90%. Persistent vomiting that leads to a weight loss of >5% is uncommon and affects only about 1% of pregnant women. When this occurs it is referred to as hyperemesis. This is a significant clinical issue as it is often associated with electrolyte imbalance and dehydration. Nausea and vomiting usually begin by the ninth week of gestation, peaking at 10–11 weeks and usually resolving by 12–14 weeks. Nausea and vomiting can have a profound effect on the pregnant woman as well as her family, so early identification and management is important (Gadsby et al 1993).

There are many reasons why a woman might experience nausea and vomiting during first trimester of pregnancy. Some of the important clinical conditions that may lead to hyperemesis include gastrointestinal causes (e.g. peptic ulcer, pancreatitis), genitourinary, metabolic (e.g. adrenocortical insufficiency, thyroid disease) and central nervous system disorders. It is therefore important in cases of hyperemesis to ensure that the relevant prenatal health care providers are aware of the presence and severity of the symptoms to ensure that appropriate care and management is afforded the pregnant patient. Other, less common, causes of pregnancy-related hyperemesis that need to be considered are gestational trophoblastic disease and multiple pregnancy (Goh & Flynn 1996, Lane 2007, Pearlman & Tintinalli 2004).

Alcohol and drug history

Authorities both at the US Centers for Disease Control and Prevention and in Australia are now recommending a zero level of alcohol intake during pregnancy. They have found that fetal alcohol syndrome can occur at relatively low levels of alcohol intake, and have now recommended that the pregnant woman abstain from drinking alcohol completely. The pregnancy-specific history needs to include how much alcohol the woman is drinking and at what frequency. The time spent with the pregnant patient taking the history offers the clinician an ideal opportunity to educate the mother-to-be on what the current guidelines are in relation to alcohol and pregnancy.

Drugs are very prevalent in our society, making it entirely appropriate to enquire directly about drug abuse in the pregnant woman. It is estimated that around 4% of expectant women are taking medications that are teratogenic. These include prescribed, over-the-counter, non-restricted medication, and illicit drugs.

Dizziness and lightheadedness

It very common for pregnant women to feel dizzy or lightheaded. This appears to be related to changes in hormone levels occurring with the developing pregnancy and blood pressure. Low blood pressure is more likely to cause dizziness or lightheadedness than is high blood pressure, but the clinician needs to remain alert to the possibility that high blood pressure may also cause these symptoms and this could be due to something more dangerous such as pre-eclampsia (depending on the stage of pregnancy). There are some management options that can be implemented with the patient who has dizziness due to low blood pressure, for example increased fluid intake, increased salt intake, and regular chiropractic care.

Sleep patterns

An increase in progesterone is suspected to disturb sleep patterns. Insomnia is a common complaint of pregnancy and needs to be enquired about. Fatigue resulting from sleep deprivation is also a factor known to exacerbate the symptoms of morning sickness.

Pain

It is important to determine if the patient has any pain. Pain needs to be very precisely identified as to location, severity, timing, exacerbation, remission, any known onset factors, and whether it correlates with any other known clinical condition.

Fetal movements

A minimum of 10 fetal movements should be felt every 24 hours once the patient is past 26 weeks of gestation. It is one of the most important clinical factors to enquire about at history. A reduction in fetal movements can mean infection (chorioamnionitis) which could lead to a growth disorder or fetal death. Placental insufficiency or pre-eclampsia can also cause a reduction in fetal movements. Each of these conditions can endanger the life of the baby, and potentially also the mother.

Heartburn (reflux)

Hormonal changes during pregnancy cause relaxation of the ligaments which normally keep the lower esophageal sphincter closed. If it relaxes, the stomach contents may pass back up the esophagus, causing 'heartburn' or reflux. The key to managing heartburn is to avoid the triggers which cause it. These will be discussed later, in management.

Varicosities

During pregnancy, varicosities may appear in the form of hemorrhoids, vulvar varicosities, and lower limb varicosities. Varicosities usually appear later in pregnancy and arise from the growing pressure of the uterus. Varicosities can occur anywhere, but are most commonly in the lower limbs, the anus (hemorrhoids), and the perineum/vulva (vulvar varicosities). Varicosities can cause pain during intercourse or during a bowel motion and may cause some bleeding. If they are in the lower limb, they are clearly seen, and can also cause pain and 'tired' legs.

Bleeding/spotting

Bleeding or spotting is never considered normal during pregnancy. There are many reasons why bleeding or spotting may occur, but the appearance of blood always requires prompt medical referral. There is never a reason for a chiropractor to delay medical referral when a pregnant patient reports blood loss of any kind.

Diet

It is an old wives' fable to say that a pregnant woman needs to 'eat for two'. It is important, however, to give the pregnant patient information about what constitutes a healthy diet for her and her baby, as unhealthy dietary habits lead to inappropriate weight gain during pregnancy (Uusitalo et al 2009), which is a well-known risk factor for gestational diabetes. It is good clinical practice also to discuss what represents appropriate weight gain during pregnancy. Many women have concerns about putting on too much weight and this can lead to an inadequate food intake. Excessive weight gain, however, can lead to the development of gestational diabetes. The key is to give accurate and balanced information.

Surgical history

All surgical procedures performed on the patient should be recorded.

Previous chiropractic history

If the patient has had chiropractic care before, it is important to ascertain what the reasons were for the care, how successful it was and if there have been any ongoing issues. It is also often helpful to be aware of patient response to particular techniques.

Obstetrical history

Details of previous pregnancies should be obtained with particular focus on the patient's general health while pregnant, pain syndromes experienced, and perinatal details.

Social history

While this should include information on family adjustment and living conditions, particular attention should be paid to any unusual level of stress in addition to the use of alcohol and drugs of addiction including tobacco, prescribed medications, and illegal substances.

Current prenatal care

In most western countries, pregnant patients usually have a number of options to choose from in terms of the management of their pregnancy, the place and mode of delivery of their baby, and the health professionals involved in the process. Despite all this, some pregnant patients remain very much uninformed in relation to these choices and the time spent with the patient at history affords the clinician an excellent opportunity to educate her (and her partner) and offer guidance. The choices an expectant mother has for management of her delivery are usually either medically managed hospital birth, midwife-managed hospital birth, or midwife-managed home birth.

Medically managed hospital birth
This is one of the most popular choices. The patient will consult with an obstetrician (private care) or a registrar in obstetrics and gynecology (public care). That doctor will then manage the prenatal care and birth.

Midwife-managed hospital birth
In a lot of the major hospitals, patients, now have the option of seeing a midwife or a team of midwives through the course of their pregnancy and labor. This is a great option for the uncomplicated, low-risk birth.

Midwife-managed home birth
In order to qualify for a home birth, the patient must have an uncomplicated, low-risk pregnancy. A qualified midwife will attend at the patient's home for regular antenatal appointments and will be on call to attend the birth of the baby.

Physical examination of the pregnant woman

The physical examination of the pregnant woman presenting to the chiropractic clinic should be as complete as possible. The elements that should be considered routine are discussed under various headings below.

Vital signs

It is appropriate on the initial visit to measure height, weight, pulse rate and respiratory rate. From the height and weight, the body mass index (BMI) should be calculated as this offers a guide to weight gain in particular individuals. Patients with a higher starting BMI should aim to gain 6–9 kg during their pregnancy; patients starting with an average BMI should aim to gain 9–14 kg; and those starting with a low BMI should aim to gain up to 19 kg.

Heart and lungs

Included in this examination would be blood pressure, pulse assessment, cardiac and respiratory sounds.

Hypertension is one of the three cardinal signs of pre-eclampsia, the other two being proteinuria and edema at the ankles. Pre-eclampsia may go on to fully developed eclampsia and the HELLP syndrome. HELLP syndrome is a triad of red blood cell hemolysis (H), elevated liver enzymes (EL) and low platelet count (LP). Hypotension is often associated with electrolyte imbalance due to vomiting.

It is also appropriate to check for the physical signs of anemia.

Neurology

A routine neurological examination should be conducted which would include cranial nerves, motor and sensory evaluation, and reflexes. Hyperreflexia is often seen with the progression of pre-eclampsia or the sudden onset of the HELLP syndrome. This examination is essential in the evaluation of the state of afferentation of the patient and therefore their need for chiropractic care.

Genitourinary system

In the chiropractic office, it is always appropriate to perform a chemical assessment of a fresh urine sample. Protein may indicate the development of pre-eclampsia, glucose may indicate the presence of gestational diabetes, and blood may indicate the presence of infection. Nitrites and white blood cells may also indicate infection.

Fundal height and baby's position

While it has always been the domain of the attending medical professional to determine the baby's presenting part (Fig. 28.1) and the fundal height (Fig. 28.2), it is entirely appropriate, and indeed desirable, for the chiropractor to do the same. The purpose is to establish a baseline throughout pregnancy of the fundal height of the uterus which is a reliable indicator of the period of gestation (Fig. 28.3) in addition to being the baseline from which sudden decreases and increases of uterine size may be estimated. The development of a sudden decrease could indicate fluid resorption due to fetal death, and a sudden increase (polyhydramnios) may indicate fetal abnormality or a large fetus.

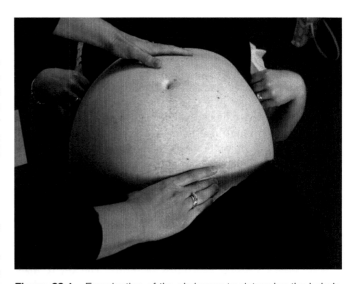

Figure 28.1 • Examination of the abdomen to determine the baby's presenting part.

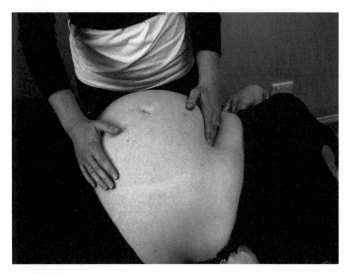

Figure 28.2 • Examination of the abdomen to determine the fundal height.

Percentile charts for uterine fundal heights may also be used to record and assess values on patients and these are widely available through both print and electronic media. However, as a clinical rule of thumb, when performing fundal height measurement, locate the top of the symphysis pubis and the top of the fundus, measure between these two points with a tape measure (cm side down to avoid bias). The measurement in centimeters should correlate to the number of weeks' gestation (i.e. at 32 weeks of pregnancy, measurement from the pubic symphysis to the top of the fundus should measure 32 cm). It is acceptable for this measurement to vary with the gestational period by ± 2 cm. Any deviation >2 cm requires a referral for further investigation (Fraser & Cooper 2003, Wheeler 2002).

The subluxation examination

The subluxation examination should be carried out as part of the normal routine physical examination and in preparation

for the implementation of chiropractic care. The authors recommend the system of examination and assessment described in Chapters 21 and 22 be applied to the pregnant woman.

The chiropractic review visit with the pregnant patient

The pregnant patient is like no other in terms of what constitutes due clinical diligence in their day-to-day care. It is appropriate, as a minimum, to do the following on each chiropractic review visit:

- weight
- blood pressure
- chemical urine analysis
- fundal height assessment
- subluxation assessment and correction.

Diagnosis and management of pregnancy-specific conditions

Morning sickness

No one knows for sure the causes of morning sickness. It is known that the neurological 'control' for nausea and vomiting is located in the brainstem. A myriad of physical reasons why this area may be overstimulated during pregnancy have been suggested, including the high level of the pregnancy hormone HCG (human chorionic gonadotropin) in the blood in the first trimester, rapid stretching of the uterine muscles, relaxation of the muscle in the digestive tract (which makes digestion less efficient), and excess acid in the stomach caused by not eating or by eating the wrong foods. It is also reasonable to suggest that neurological dysafferentation, particularly when the upper cervical complex and pelvis are involved, may affect both the integrity of the dural lie and tension and CSF pressure, which in turn may influence the brainstem.

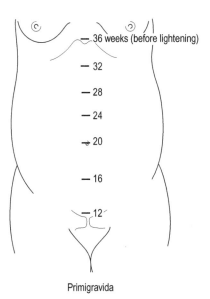

Primigravida

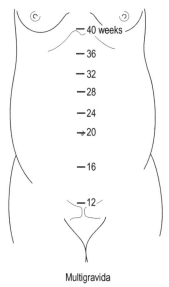

Multigravida

Figure 28.3 • Height of the uterine fundus is a guide to the period of gestation, as shown. Nulliparas experience lightening at 36–38 weeks when the fundal height reverts to the 34–36 week level (Beisher et al 1987).

Emotional factors may also influence morning sickness, which has been reported to be virtually unknown in some more primitive societies where lifestyles are simpler, more relaxed, and less emotionally demanding.

The following guidelines may assist with advising patients on how to minimize morning sickness:

- Maintain regular chiropractic check-ups.
- Eat four to six small meals per day, instead of three heavy meals. An empty stomach and low blood sugar resulting from long stretches without food can trigger nausea, as can eating too much at one meal.
- Eat crackers or dry toast 20–30 minutes before getting up in the morning, while slightly propped up in bed. Bland foods such as crackers or pretzels may help at any time of the day when the patient feels nauseated.
- Minimize the intake of fluids with meals. Instead, drink small amounts of fluids frequently between meals.
- Eat a diet high in protein and complex carbohydrates, both of which tend to prevent nausea.
- Drink plenty of fluids, especially if you are losing them through vomiting. If they are easier to get down than solids when your stomach is upset, use them to get your nutrients.
- Herbal teas, fruit juices and popsicles are helpful in combating the nauseated feeling.
- Take a prenatal vitamin supplement to compensate for nutrients missed through not eating. Studies have shown that vitamin B_6, in particular, may assist with reducing morning sickness (Power et al 2007).
- Avoid the sight, smell and taste of foods that lead to nausea.
- Eat before nausea appears. Food will be easier to get down and may prevent an episode.
- Eat in bed to avoid an empty stomach and to keep the blood sugar as stable as possible. Dry crackers or toast are a good choice.
- Before retiring at night, have a snack that is high in protein and complex carbohydrates.
- Get extra sleep and relaxation. Both emotional and physical fatigue can exacerbate morning sickness.
- Greet the morning in slow motion – rushing tends to aggravate nausea.
- Brush teeth with a toothpaste that does not increase the feeling of nausea and rinse the mouth after each bout of vomiting, as well as after each meal. Not only will this keep the mouth fresh and reduce nausea, it will also decrease the risk of damage to teeth and gums that can occur when bacteria start working on the regurgitated material in the mouth.
- Minimize stress. Morning sickness is more common among women who are under a great deal of stress, at either work or home.
- Sugar solution, available over the counter from your pharmacy, may be useful.
- Some women have found that the acupressure wristbands, available for seasickness, can also help with morning sickness.

If none of the above suggestions is helping to make the patient's morning sickness more manageable, she may need to consult her medical professional. She will particularly need to do so if the vomiting is intractable, if she is having difficulty keeping fluid down, or losing weight. In this situation, a prescription medication may be helpful while still being safe for the baby (Arsenault & Lane 2002, Koren & Maltepe 2004, Lane 2007, Pearlman & Tintinalli 2004).

Heartburn

The key to managing heartburn is to avoid the foods which trigger it and to eat smaller quantities of food but at greater frequency. The foods which most commonly act as an irritant to produce heartburn include tomato-based foods, vinegar, mustard, chocolate, citrus fruits and juices, highly spiced foods, and fatty fried foods. If avoiding food triggers fails to reduce the heartburn, there are some medications which can be used safely during pregnancy. A pharmacist should always be consulted before a patient is advised to take any medication during pregnancy.

Liver cholestasis

Pregnancy hormones affect gallbladder function, resulting in biliary stasis, which causes a build-up of bile in the liver which can enter the bloodstream. Patients with liver cholestasis present with itching, particularly on the hands and feet, which is often is the only symptom, darkly colored urine, light coloring of bowel movements, fatigue or exhaustion, loss of appetite or depression.

The incidence of liver cholestasis is 1–2 per 1000 pregnancies. Risk factors include:

- women carrying multiples
- women who have previous liver damage
- women whose mother or sisters had cholestasis.

Hypertension, HELLP syndrome, pre-eclampsia/eclampsia

Pregnancy-induced hypertension (PIH) is classified as new arterial hypertension when diagnosed after 20 weeks of pregnancy. The signs and symptoms may include:

- rapid weight gain, 4–5 lb (1.8–2.2 kg) in a single week
- a rise in the blood pressure
- proteinuria
- severe headaches
- blurry vision
- seeing spots in front of the eyes
- severe pain
- epigastric pain
- decrease in the amount of urine.

It is very important to take the blood pressure of your pregnant patients at every visit. Hypertension can come on quickly between visits with the prenatal care provider. It can cause prematurity or even the death of the baby. PIH can progress to pre-eclampsia, or eclampsia which is life-threatening.

It is essential that the hypertension be found and treated as early as possible. This allows the best possible outcome for the patient.

Gestational diabetes

Gestational diabetes occurs in about 4% of all pregnancies. It is characterized clinically by the presence of glucose in the urine. Bear in mind that trace glucose can be normal.

The absolute cause of gestational diabetes is still unknown. Hormonal changes associated with pregnancy can cause problems with the mother's ability to block insulin, a condition referred to as insulin resistance syndrome. Therefore, the body does not have its normal ability to utilize insulin appropriately. This means the patient needs up to three times the amount of insulin as would normally be the case. So when the body is unable to make and use the insulin in pregnancy it is called gestational diabetes. When there is an inability to use insulin, glucose metabolism is affected and the blood sugar level rises. This makes routine, regular chemical urine analysis during pregnancy absolutely non-negotiable.

Gestational diabetes is more prevalent in women carrying multiples, in African-American women and in younger women (Rauh-Hain et al 2009), while obesity remains a major risk factor (Schrauwers & Dekker 2009, Uusitalo et al 2009).

Pelvic instability

Pelvic instability (PI) is a condition that causes pain around the joints of the pelvis (pelvic girdle) during and after pregnancy. In normal pregnancy, a hormone called relaxin softens the ligaments around the joints of the pelvis. This is a natural process which prepares the maternal pelvis for childbirth and does not usually cause lasting discomfort. For some women this natural process seems to go wrong, causing the joints of the pelvis to become too lax. This can result in the pelvis becoming unstable. The degree of instability will vary for individual patients.

Pregnancy can also put strain on the muscles of the back, stomach, pelvic floor, hips and pelvic girdle which may also lead to the pelvic joints becoming less stable. Pelvic instability can also occur due to a previous fall or injury to the pelvis and, in rare cases, by complications in labor or the postnatal period.

The pain experienced by a pregnant woman can include any of the joints of the low back and pelvis, including the pubis, the sacroiliac joints, or the L5/S1 junction. The symptoms of PI include the following:

- pain in the front or back of the pelvis, groin, buttocks, thighs, hips or lower back
- difficulty walking, or a waddling gait
- pain felt when turning, twisting or bending – this will be felt or noted in many day-to-day activities
- women may feel and/or hear a clicking, clunking or grinding sensation in their pelvis
- some women find it difficult to part their legs without severe pain
- pain and difficulty with sexual intercourse – this will correlate with several other problems that have been discussed earlier in this chapter which may cause pain during intercourse

- women with PI can suffer from incontinence and/or bowel problems
- pain and difficulty squatting – note that this symptom is particularly prevalent with women with pubic dysfunction, and is readily treatable. Often if you have a patient with any of the other symptoms, and you ask them to squat, they will not be able to or will have difficulty doing it. These women will often have pubic subluxation.

Previously, these women have all required a support belt and/or a walking aid, or even a wheelchair (depending upon the severity). The authors have found, however, that if the pelvis and low back, as well as any relevant muscle compartment syndromes, are carefully examined and treated with appropriate chiropractic techniques, most patients will experience satisfactory relief. Most women treated this way report a significant improvement in their symptoms and mobility. This allows them to get on with their everyday activities without the need for aids or support belts. However, if at the very end of pregnancy there is difficulty in stabilizing the pelvis, and the pain is significant, a pelvic support belt is a good option. It will decrease the pain while still allowing a satisfactory level of function. It is better, however, if the patient has an increased frequency of chiropractic care during this time.

Common subluxation patterns in the pregnant patient

In Chapters 21 and 22 a highly sophisticated system of subluxation examination and clinical interpretation based on the best available current evidence was presented. It was presented as it relates to the child patient, but it equally applies to the adult and especially the pregnant patient. The information which follows is built around the subluxation protocol detailed in those chapters.

In the first and even early second trimester of pregnancy, the chiropractic subluxation patterns encountered do not vary greatly from those seen in the general population. However, as pregnancy progresses, several intrinsic and extrinsic factors come to bear on the pregnant woman which leads to the evolution of predictable subluxation patterns which are not usually seen in any other population group, making the management of the pregnant woman a rather special clinical situation. Changing hormone levels, especially relaxin, leads to increased motion in the joints and as the uterus expands and projects forwards, gait, posture and centre of gravity all shift, often leading to varying degrees of back pain and discomfort.

In advancing pregnancy

Typical pelvic subluxation patterns in late pregnancy are characterized by an increase in the sacral angle and posterior/inferior rotation of the ilia about the x-axis. This phenomenon leads to any combination of the following subluxation patterns:

- base anterior sacrum
- posterior innominate, usually accompanied by internal rotation
- double posterior and internally rotated innominates

- coccyx base posterior
- pubic separation, often in combination with external rotation
- all upper cervical complex patterns.

Typical cranial patterns include:

- dropped sphenoid, often bilaterally
- sphenobasilar flexion subluxation, commonly concomitant with the coccyx.

Typical muscle compartment syndromes, which are often seen bilaterally, include:

- quadratus lumborum
- psoas
- piriformis
- gluteus medius and maximus
- gluteus minimus and tensor fascia lata
- quadriceps
- hamstrings
- hiatal hernia subluxation syndrome
- diaphragm
- pelvic floor
- apex anterior xiphoid, more common in very late pregnancy and cases where the fundus is late in lightening (i.e. remains high late into pregnancy).

In the postpartum period

While any of the subluxation patterns which had been troublesome during later pregnancy can persist initially, the most common problems encountered in the immediate postpartum period are as follows:

- rectus abdominis separation syndrome
- pubic separation, often associated with bilateral superiority of the pubic rami.

The perinatal period

Preparation for delivery

During the third trimester of pregnancy, there is a window of opportunity for the chiropractor to assist the expectant mother to prepare her body for the impending birth. The abdomen grows very rapidly, resulting in an increase in the lumbar lordosis and other postural changes detailed previously in this chapter. In addition to the postural changes, the ligaments will become more elastic under the influence of the hormone relaxin, making the joints more mobile than normal. Relaxin reaches its highest levels inside the first 12 weeks of pregnancy and then begins to increase again at around 36 weeks in preparation for the birth. The pubic symphysis will widen, allowing for easier separation during labor to make room for the passage of the baby.

The role of the chiropractor in preparing the expectant mother's body for birth is to provide regular chiropractic care to help her maintain a healthy structural balance. Not only will this help her pelvis function better, but also allow her to be more mobile and to feel more comfortable.

In the birthing room

Having their chiropractor attend the birth of their child can provide the mother and her partner with great encouragement and support. Women in labor will vary greatly in what their needs are, so it is very important to let the mother dictate what she feels she needs for support. The birth of a child is such a momentous and private occasion, it remains imperative for the chiropractor attending a birth to make sure the birthing couple have space and are made to feel like they are in total control of what support they receive. They need to feel they have support, but that this experience is theirs to share together.

It is appropriate to examine the woman in labor every couple of hours to optimize the efficiency and progression of the labor. Rotated sacral subluxation is by far the most common pattern seen during labor and correction should be made between contractions. It may not follow a typical pattern normally seen during pregnancy. Mostly the sacrum will rotate anteriorly, then in a couple of hours' time becomes a rotated or posterior sacrum. This phenomenon is largely due to the internal forces of the uterus, and the positioning of the baby. Ipsilateral muscle compartment syndromes are also common in labor, as the baby is generally positioned across on to one side.

Facilitating natural pain control is a very positive and supportive function the chiropractor can perform in the birthing room. The applications of heat, warm water and massage are very useful pain control techniques. In addition, cranial holds during contraction and sacral holds between contractions may provide great relief from the pain associated with the contraction and the referred pain to the low back respectively. Most partners can be trained to effect these holds themselves, thus increasing their active involvement level in the birthing process.

The cranial hold is applied as soon as a contraction begins. A pisiform contact is applied to the glabella with one hand, while the pisiform of the other hand is placed over the external occipital protuberance. Cranial pressure is slowly increased by approximating the two contacts until critical pressure is reached and the perceived pain level associated with the contraction suddenly drops. Visual analog scale assessments performed during labor have shown 10/10 pre-hold pain assessment values to consistently drop to 4–5/10 when critical pressure is reached. In some patients this procedure ceases to be effective after a couple of hours. When this happens, it is appropriate to switch to a normal parietal respiratory assisted procedure (see Chapter 27) for one contraction and then return to the original contact at the next contraction.

The sacral hold is effected by positioning the patient side-lying and placing the pisiform of the inferior hand over the sacral base. Using the flexed knees as a lever, extension of the L5/S1 junction is initiated with pressure to pain relief level.

The postnatal period

Following the birth of the baby, the mother needs chiropractic care as soon as possible to address the issues which may arise in her pelvis and contiguous structures in addition to the possibility of suboccipital and intracranial strain produced by the labor. There are, however, a number of clinical issues which may arise in the postnatal period that a chiropractor needs to be aware of.

Dural puncture headache

Headache following dural puncture generally comes on within 48 hours following epidural anesthesia and presents with vomiting, nausea and severe headache. It can also be associated with dizziness, and a general feeling of being unwell. Dural puncture headaches are commonly associated with cranial, sacral and coccygeal subluxation patterns.

Pelvic instability

The withdrawal of pregnancy-related hormones in the immediate postnatal period can be associated with instability in the pelvis. Also, the obvious extreme changes in weight and center of gravity following the delivery of the baby will also contribute to instability. On examination, the patient's pelvic joints will be hypermobile and pelvic belt support for a short time may be necessary to achieve a satisfactory result.

Bleeding

Bleeding following birth is normal. However, the chiropractic clinician caring for a postnatal mother needs to be watchful for bleeding with the passage of clots (small or large), ongoing heavy bleeding, bleeding that is foul smelling, and pain or fever. Any of these symptoms and signs could indicate infection or retained products of pregnancy, making an urgent medical referral a necessity.

Postnatal depression

It is very common for a new mother to experience the 'blues' for the first few days following the birth experience. This is completely normal and is not postnatal depression (PND).

While some women may be depressed antenatally, and continue to be depressed postnatally, their symptom profile is not the same as the woman who was not depressed antenatally but is now suffering from PND (Kammerer et al 2009).

The sudden withdrawal of pregnancy-related hormones in the first few days after birth, when combined with various feelings and factors intrinsic to the individual mother, can, however, lead to the onset of PND, which is characterized by fatigue, insomnia, withdrawal from relationship with the baby or significant others, loss of personal confidence, and psychomotor slowing, evidenced by the inability to organize herself or her home environment. Fatigue, of course, may be due to sleep deprivation or reaction to the effort of labor and not related to PND at all. When this is the case, the patient's symptoms will abate as the fatigue is relieved and this has been shown to be an accurate diagnostic indicator for determining when fatigue is a symptom of PND (Runquist 2007).

While the symptoms of PND may abate under chiropractic care, it remains a potentially dangerous situation for both the mother and her baby. PND may last for many months and women with persistent or recurrent depressive symptoms need forms of preventive intervention that cover at least the first postpartum year (Monti et al 2008), making concomitant referral by the chiropractor to an appropriate mental health professional a wise course of action.

Feeding difficulties

It is not uncommon for new breastfeeding mothers to experience feeding difficulties. These can arise from inappropriate nursing technique, poor nipple health, inadequate milk supply, maternal anxiety, and physical problems related to the baby. Often the baby will nurse well on one side and be fussy and irritable on the other. Subluxation in either the mother or the baby is a common cause of feeding difficulty and may lead to a failed breastfeeding experience. While the early implementation of chiropractic care is critical in these cases, it remains best practice to refer the mother to an appropriately qualified lactation consultant or the breastfeeding clinic at the local hospital.

References

Arsenault, M., Lane, C.A., 2002. The management of nausea and vomiting of pregnancy. Clinical Practice Guideline no. 120. Society of Obstetricians and Gynaecologists of Canada (SOGC). J. Obstet. Gynaecol. Can. 24 (10), 817–823.

Beisher, N.A., Mackay, E.V., Purcal, N.K., 1987. Care of the Pregnant Woman and her Baby, second ed. WB Saunders/Baillière Tindall, Sydney.

Blom, H.J., 2009. Folic acid, methylation and neural tube closure in humans. Birth Defects Res. A Clin. Mol. Teratol. 85 (4), 295–302.

Bobat, R., Coovaadia, H., Moodley, D., et al., 1999. Mortality in a cohort of children born to HIV-1 infected women in Durban, South Africa. S. Afr. Med. J. 89 (6), 646–648.

Centers for Disease Control and Prevention (CDCP), Department of Health and Human Services, USA, 2009. Fetal Alcohol Spectrum Disorders. Available at: http://www.cdc.gov/ncbddd/fas/ (accessed April 2009).

Fraser, D.M., Cooper, M.A., 2003. Myles Textbook for Midwives, fourteenth ed. Churchill Livingstone, Edinburgh.

Gadsby, R., Barnie-Adshead, A.M., Jagger, C., 1993. A prospective study of nausea and vomiting during pregnancy. Br. J. Gen. Pract. 43, 245–248.

Goh, J., Flynn, M., 1996. Examination Obstetrics and Gynaecology. Maclennan and Petty, Sydney.

Jain, M., Chakravarti, A., Verma, V., et al., 2009. Seroprevalence of hepatitis viruses in patients

infected with the human immunodeficiency virus. Indian J. Pathol. Microbiol. 52 (1), 17–19.

Kammerer, M., Marks, M.N., Pinard, C., et al., 2009. Symptoms associated with the DSM-IV diagnosis of depression in pregnancy and post partum. Arch. Womens Ment. Health 12 (3), 135–141.

Koren, G., Maltepe, C., 2004. Pre-emptive therapy for severe nausea and vomiting of pregnancy and hyperemesis gravidarum. J. Obstet. Gynaecol. 24 (5), 530–533.

Lane, C.A., 2007. Nausea and vomiting of pregnancy: a tailored approach to treatment. Clin. Obstet. Gynecol. 50 (1), 100–111.

Massi Lindsey, L.L., Silk, K.J., Von Friedrichs-Fitzwater, M.M., et al., 2009. Developing effective campaign messages to prevent neural tube defects: a qualitative assessment of women's reactions to advertising concepts. J. Health Commun. 14 (2), 131–159.

Monti, F., Agostini, F., Marano, G., et al., 2008. The course of maternal depressive symptomatology during the first 18 months postpartum in an Italian sample. Arch. Womens Ment. Health 10 (6), 267–275.

Pearlman, M.D., Tintinalli, J.E., 2004. Nausea and vomiting of pregnancy. ACOG Practice Bulletin. No. 52 (April), 103.

Power, M.L., Milligan, L.A., Schulkin, J., 2007. Managing nausea and vomiting of pregnancy: a survey of obstetrician-gynecologists. J. Reprod. Med. 52 (10), 922–928.

Rauh-Hain, J.A., Rana, S., Tamez, H., et al., 2009. Risk for developing gestational diabetes in women with twin pregnancies. J. Matern. Fetal Neonatal Med. 25, 1–7.

Runquist, J.J., 2007. A depressive symptoms responsiveness model for differentiating fatigue from depression in the postpartum period. Arch. Womens Ment. Health 11 (3), 231–238.

Schrauwers, C., Dekker, G., 2009. Maternal and perinatal outcome in obese pregnant patients. J. Matern. Fetal Neonatal Med. 22 (3), 218–226.

Timmermans, S., Jaddoe, V.W., Hofman, A., et al., 2009. Periconception folic acid supplementation, fetal growth and the risks of low birth weight and preterm birth: the generation R study. Br. J. Nutr. 102 (5), 777–785.

Uusitalo, U., Arkkola, T., Ovaskainen, M.L., et al., 2009. Unhealthy dietary patterns are associated with weight gain during pregnancy among Finnish women. Public Health Nutr. 27, 1–8.

Vlajinac, H., Petrovic, R., Marinkovic, J., et al., 1997. The effect of cigarette smoking during pregnancy on fetal growth. Srp. Arh. Celok. Lek. 125 (9–10), 267–271.

Wheeler, L.A., 2002. Nurse-Midwifery Handbook: A Practical Guide to Prenatal and Postpartum Care, second ed. Lippincott Williams & Wilkins, Philadelphia.

Appendix 1: Anthropometric percentile charts used in pediatric assessment

© 2010, Elsevier Ltd, Inc, BV
DOI: 10.1016/B978-0-7020-3129-8.00039-6

BOYS	In utero 24–42 wks
	Postnatal 0–3 years

Surname _____

Given names _____

Identification number _____

Date of birth _____

Interauterine growth curves (Composite male/female)

Measuring techniques: (as for ages 0–36 months – see over page)

Additional Note: Gestational ages are recorded in completed weeks from the first ay of the mother's last menstual period. Fetal growth is influenced by many factors including age, body weight, height, parity, ethnic origin of the mother and sex of the fetus. Corrections for some of these factors are found in the quoted reference

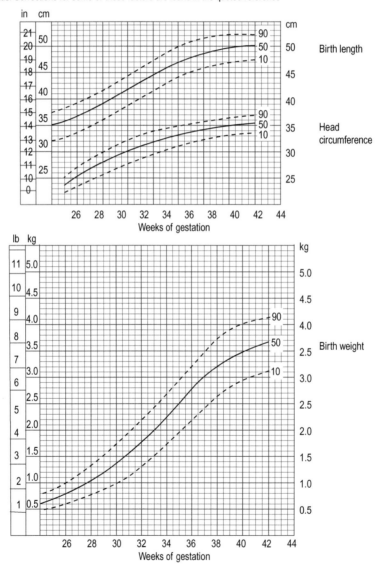

Boys 0–3 years
Length percentile chart

Mother's height ————————————— Father's height ————————————— cm in

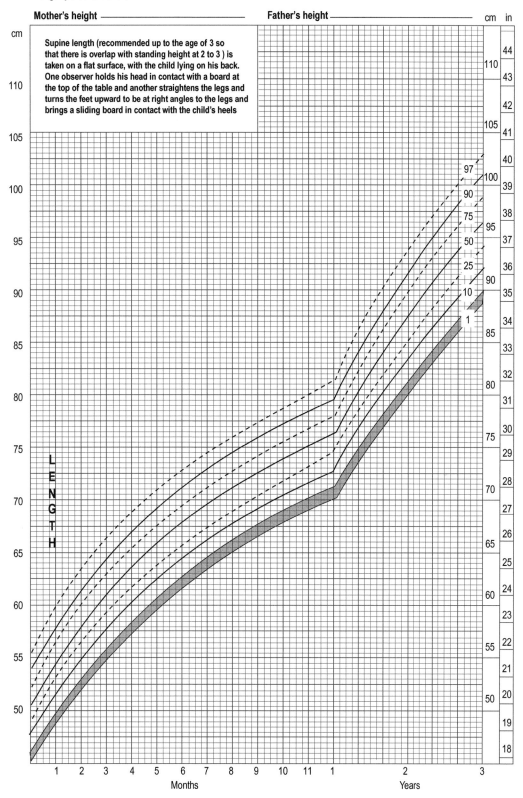

Supine length (recommended up to the age of 3 so that there is overlap with standing height at 2 to 3) is taken on a flat surface, with the child lying on his back. One observer holds his head in contact with a board at the top of the table and another straightens the legs and turns the feet upward to be at right angles to the legs and brings a sliding board in contact with the child's heels

Months

Years

Boys 0–3 years Weight percentile chart

Weight should be taken in the nude, or as near thereto as possible.
If a surgical gown or minimal underclothing (vest and pants) is worn,
then the estimated weight (about 0.1 kg) must be subtracted before
weight is recorded. Weights are conveniently recorded to the completed
0.1 kg above the age of 6 months. The bladder should be empty.

Date	Age	Length	Weight	Head circum.

DATE OF BIRTH _____ / _____ / _____

Simplified calculation of body surface area (BSA)

$$\text{BSA (m}^2) = \sqrt{\frac{\text{Ht (cm) x Wt (kg)}}{3600}}$$

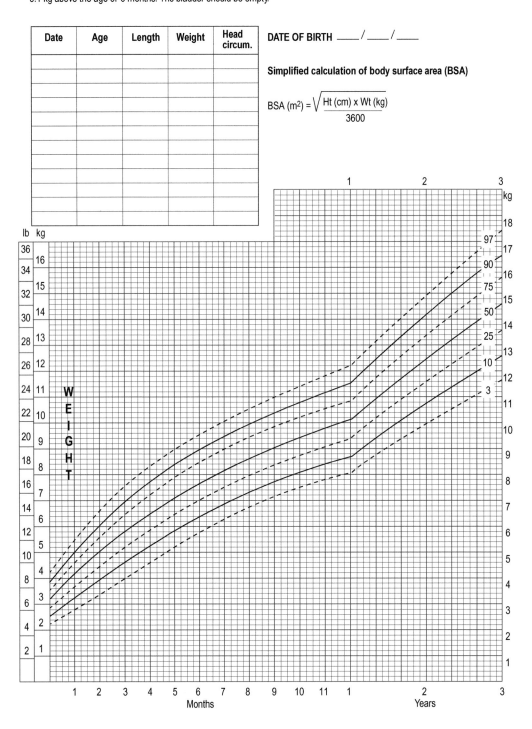

Head circumference
Boys
In utero 28–40 weeks, 0–12 months

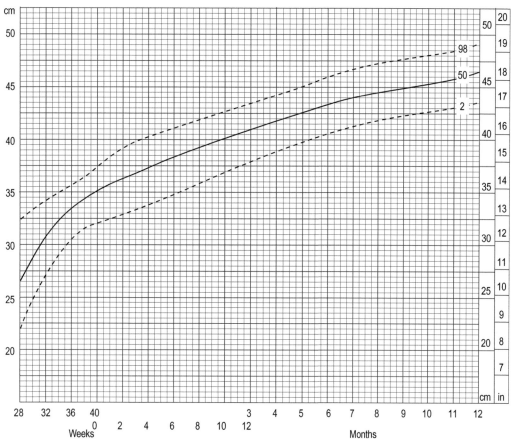

1–3 years

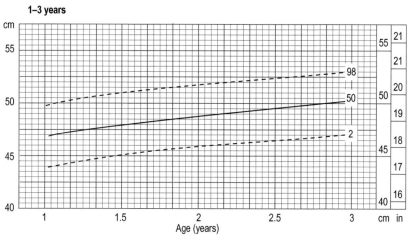

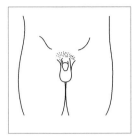

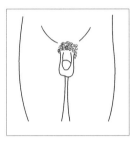

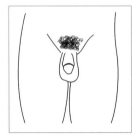

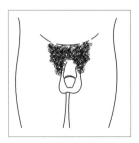

Boys 2–18

Surname _____

Given names _____

Identification number _____

Date of birth _____

Stages of puberty

Ages of attainment of successive stages of pubertal sexual development are given in the height centiles chart overpage. The stage Pubic Hair 2+ represents the state of a child who shows the pubic hair appearance stage 2 but not stage 3 (see below). The centiles for age at which this state is normally seen are given, the 97th centile being considered as the early limit, the 3rd centile as the late limit. The child's puberty stages may be plotted at successive ages (Tanner, *Growth at Adolescence*, 2nd Ed., 1962). Testis sizes are judged by comparison with the Prader orchidometer (Zachmann, Prader, Kind, Haflinger and Budliger, *Helv. Paediatr. Acta* 29, 61–72, 1974)

Genital (penis) development:

Stage 1. Pre-adolescent. Testes, scrotum and penis are of about the same size and proportion as in early childhood.

Stage 2. Enlargement of scrotum and testes. Skin of scrotum reddens and changes in texture. Little or no enlargement of penis at this stage.

Stage 3. Enlargement of the penis which occurs at first mainly in length. Further growth of the testes and scrotum.

Stage 4. Increased size of penis with growth in breadth and developement of glans; testes and scrotum larger; scrotal skin darkened

Stage 5. Genitalia adult in size and shape.

Pubic hair:

Stage 1. Pre-adolescent. The vellus over the pubes is not further developed than that over the abdominal wall, i.e. no pubic hair.

Stage 2. Sparse growth of long, slightly pigmneted, downy hair, straight or slightly curled at the base of the penis.

Stage 3. Considerably darker, coarser and more curled. The hair spreads sparsely over the junction of the pubes.

Stage 4. Hair now adult in type, but area covered is still considerably smaller than in the adult. No spread to the medial surface of thighs.

Stage 5. Adult in quantity and type with distribution of the horizontal (or classically 'feminine') pattern. Spread to medial surface of thighs but not up linea alba or elsewhere above the base of the inverse triangle (spread up linea alba occurs late and is rated stage 6).

Stretched penile length

Measured from the pubo-penile skin junction to the tip of the glans.

(Schonfeld and Beebe, *J. Urol.* 48, 759-777, 1942)

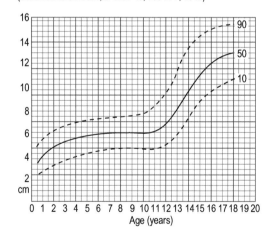

Boys: 2–18 years
Height percentile

Mother's height _____

Father's height _____

Simplified calculation of body surface area (BSA)

$$BSA\ (m^2) = \sqrt{\dfrac{Ht\ (cm)\ \times\ Wt\ (kg)}{3600}}$$

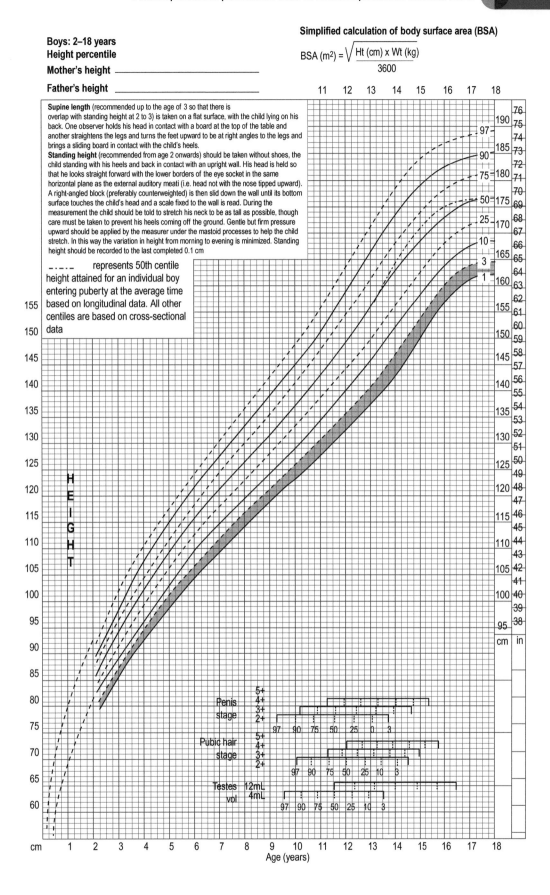

Supine length (recommended up to the age of 3 so that there is overlap with standing height at 2 to 3) is taken on a flat surface, with the child lying on his back. One observer holds his head in contact with a board at the top of the table and another straightens the legs and turns the feet upward to be at right angles to the legs and brings a sliding board in contact with the child's heels.

Standing height (recommended from age 2 onwards) should be taken without shoes, the child standing with his heels and back in contact with an upright wall. His head is held so that he looks straight forward with the lower borders of the eye socket in the same horizontal plane as the external auditory meati (i.e. head not with the nose tipped upward). A right-angled block (preferably counterweighted) is then slid down the wall until its bottom surface touches the child's head and a scale fixed to the wall is read. During the measurement the child should be told to stretch his neck to be as tall as possible, though care must be taken to prevent his heels coming off the ground. Gentle but firm pressure upward should be applied by the measurer under the mastoid processes to help the child stretch. In this way the variation in height from morning to evening is minimized. Standing height should be recorded to the last completed 0.1 cm.

_ _ _ _ represents 50th centile height attained for an individual boy entering puberty at the average time based on longitudinal data. All other centiles are based on cross-sectional data

Boys: 2–18 years Weight percentile

Weight should be taken in the nude, or as near thereto as possible. If a surgical gown or minimal underclothing (vest and pants) is worn, then its estimated weight (about 0.1 kg) must be subtracted before weight is recorded. Weights are conventionally recorded to the last completed 0.1 kg above the age of 6 months. The bladder should be empty.

Body mass index

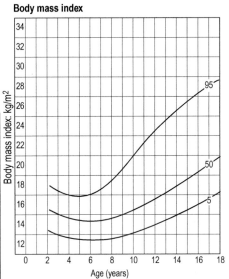

DATE OF BIRTH ____ / ____ / ____

Date	Age	Length	Weight	Head circum.	Genital	Pubic hair	Testes R	L

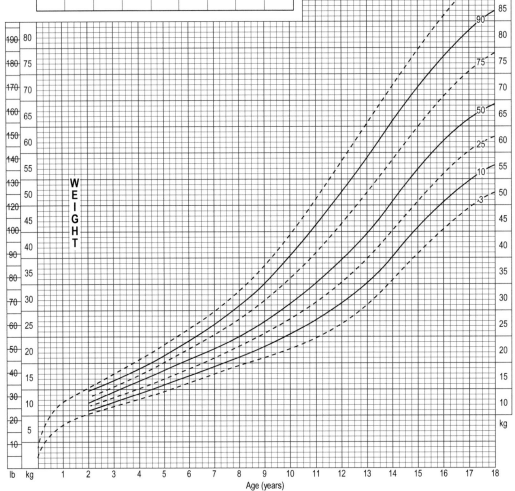

Head circumference, boys
Head circumference: The tape should be placed over the eyebrows, above
the ears and over the most prominent part of the occiput taking a direct route.
A paper tape is preferable to plastic, which stretches unacceptably under tension.
The maximum measurement should be recorded to the nearest 0.1 cm.

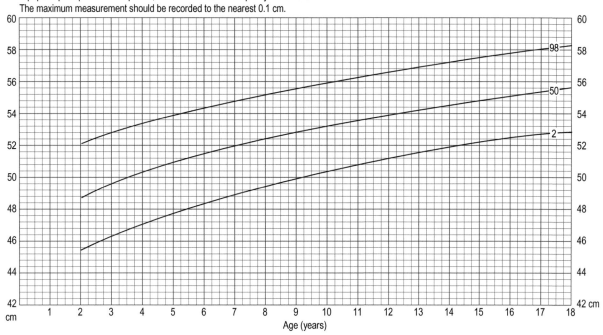

Height velocity, boys

The standards are appropriate for velocity calculated over a whole year, not less, since a small period requires wider limits (the 3rd and 95th centiles for months). The yearly velocity should be plotted at the mid point of the year. The centiles given in black are appropriate to children of average maturational tempo, who have their peak velocity at the average of this event. The line marked A `is the 50th centile line for the child who is 2 years early in maturity and age at peak height velocity, and the line marked B refers to a child who is 50th centile in velocity for early and late maturers.

Centile of whole-year velocity for maturers at average time

97th and 3rd centiles at peak height velocity
Early (+2SD) maturers
Late (−2SD) maturers

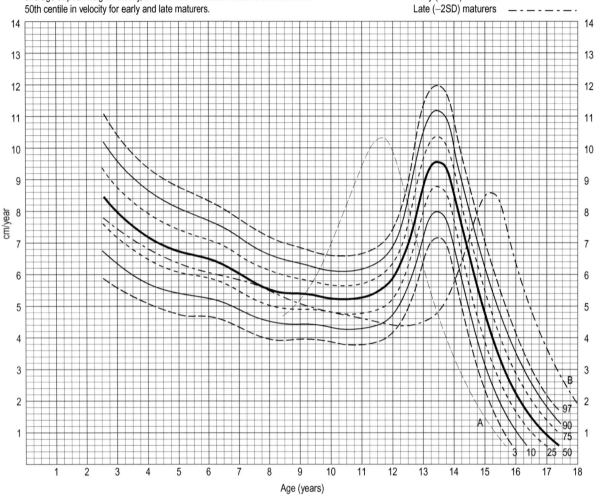

Intrauterine growth curves (composite male/female)
Measuring techniques: (as for ages 0–36 months – see over page)

Additional Notes: Gestational ages recorded in completed weeks from the first day of the mother's last menstrual period. Fetal growth is influenced by many factors including age, body weight, height, parity, ethnic origin of the mother and sex of the fetus. Corrections for some of these factors are found in the quoted reference.

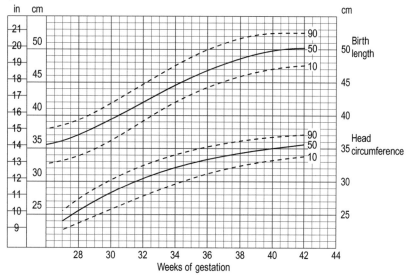

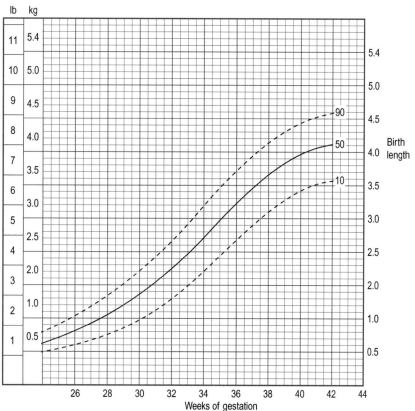

Girls 0–3 years
Length percentile chart

Mother's height ————————————   Father's height —————————————————   cm   in

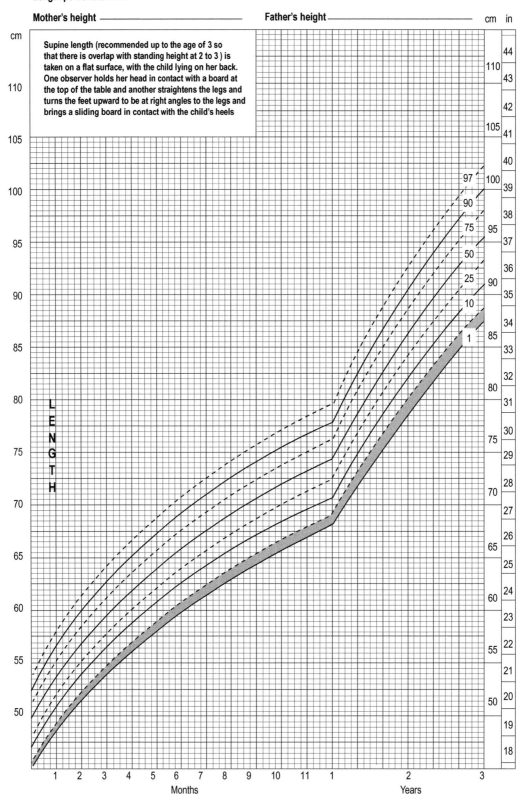

Supine length (recommended up to the age of 3 so that there is overlap with standing height at 2 to 3) is taken on a flat surface, with the child lying on her back. One observer holds her head in contact with a board at the top of the table and another straightens the legs and turns the feet upward to be at right angles to the legs and brings a sliding board in contact with the child's heels

Girls 0–3 years Weight percentile chart

Weight should be taken in the nude, or as near there to as possible.
If a surgical gown or minimal underclothing (vest and pants) is worn,
then its estimated weight (about 0.1 kg) must be subtracted before
weight is recorded. Weights are conveniently recorded to the completed
0.1 kg above the age of 6 months. The bladder should be empty.

Date	Age	Length	Weight	Head circum.

DATE OF BIRTH ____ / ____ / ____

Simplified calculation of body surface area (BSA)

$$BSA\ (m^2) = \sqrt{\frac{Ht\ (cm) \times Wt\ (kg)}{3600}}$$

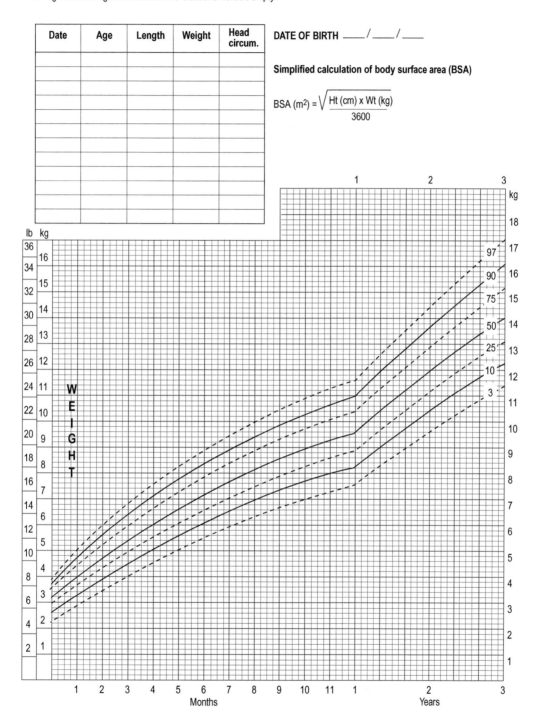

Head circumference
Girls
In utero 28–40 weeks, 0–12 months

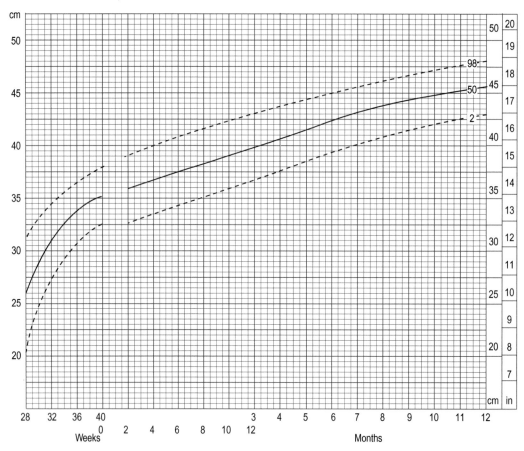

1–3 years

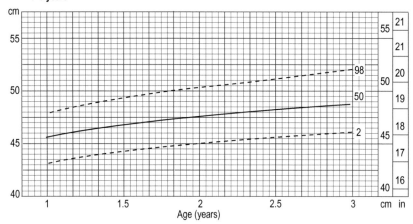

Breast development

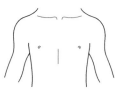

Stage 1 – prepubertal

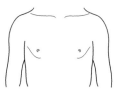

Stage 2 – elevation of breasts and papilla

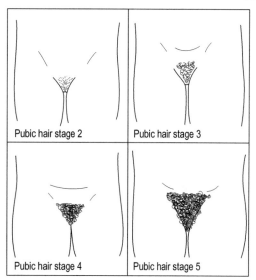

| Pubic hair stage 2 | Pubic hair stage 3 |
| Pubic hair stage 4 | Pubic hair stage 5 |

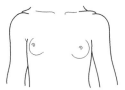

Stage 3 – further elevation and areola but no separation of contours

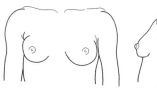

Stage 4 – areola and papilla form a secondary mound above level of the breast

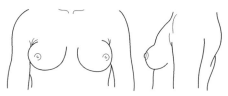

Stage 5 – areola recesses to the general contour of the breast

Stages of puberty

Ages of attainment of successive stages of pubertal sexual development are given in the height centile chart overpage. The stage Pubic Hair 2+ represents the state of a child who shows the pubic hair appearance stage 2 but not stage 3 (see below). The centiles for age at which this state is normally seen are given, the 97th centile being considered as the early limit, the 3rd centile as the late limit. The child's puberty stages may be plotted at successive ages (Tanner, *Growth at Adolescence*, 2nd Ed., 1962).

Pubic hair:

Stage 1. Pre-adolescent. The vellus over the pubes is not further developed than that over the abdominal wall, i.e. no pubic hair.

Stage 2. Sparse growth of long, slightly pigmented, downy hair, straight or slightly curled, chiefly along labia.

Stage 3. Considerably darker, coarser and more curled. The hair spreads sparsely over the junction of the pubes.

Stage 4. Hair now adult in type, but area covered is still considerably smaller than in the adult. No spread to the medial surface of thighs.

Stage 5. Adult in quantity and type with distribution of the horizontal (or classically 'feminine') pattern. Spread to medial surface of thighs but not up the linea alba or elsewhere above the base of the inverse triangle (spread up linea alba occurs late and is rated stage 6).

Girls: 2–18 years
Height percentile
Mother's height —————————————

Father's height —————————————

Simplified calculation of body surface area (BSA)

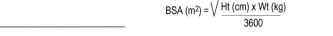

$$BSA \ (m^2) = \sqrt{\frac{Ht \ (cm) \times Wt \ (kg)}{3600}}$$

Supine length (recommended up to the age of 3 so that there is overlap with standing height at 2 to 3) is taken on a flat surface, with the child lying on her back. One observer holds her head in contact with a board at the top of the table and another straightens the legs and turns the feet upward to be at right angles to the legs and brings a sliding board in contact with the child's heels.

Standing height (recommended from age 2 onwards) should be taken without shoes, the child standing with her heels and back in contact with an upright wall. Her head is held so that she looks straight forward with the lower borders of the eye socket in the same horizontal plane as the external auditory meati (i.e. head not with the nose tipped upward). A right-angled block (preferably counterweighted) is then slid down the wall until its bottom surface touches the child's head and a scale fixed to the wall is read. During the measurement the child should be told to stretch her neck to be as tall as possible, though care must be taken to prevent her heels coming off the ground. Gentle but firm pressure upward should be applied by the measurer under the mastoid processes to help the child stretch. In this way the variation in height from morning to evening is minimized. Standing height should be recorded to the last completed 0.1 cm

–·–·– represents 50th centile height attained for an individual girl entering puberty at the average time based on longitudinal data. All other centiles are based on cross-sectional data

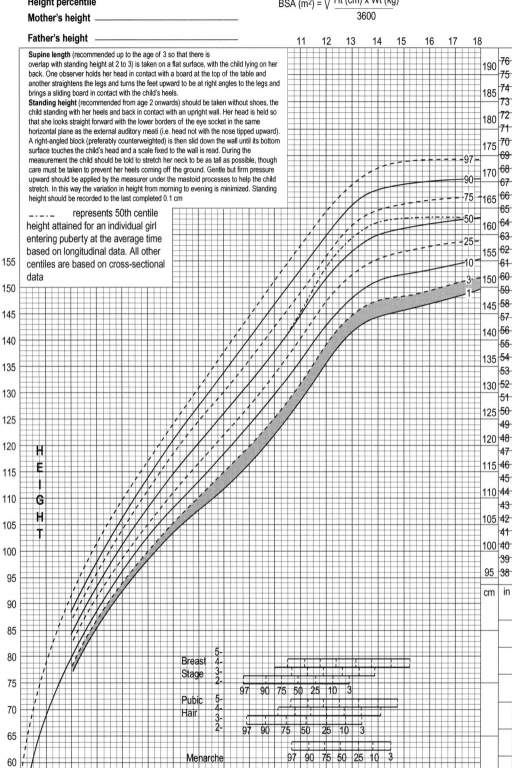

Girls: 2–18 years Weight percentile

Weight should be taken in the nude, or as near thereto as possible. If a surgical gown or minimal underclothing (vest and pants) is worn, then its estimated weight (about 0.1 kg) must be subtracted before weight is recorded. Weights are conventionally recorded to the last completed 0.1 kg above the age of 6 months. The bladder should be empty.

DATE OF BIRTH ___ / ___ / ___

Date	Age	Length	Weight	Head circum.	Breast	Pubic hair	Men- arche

Body-mass index

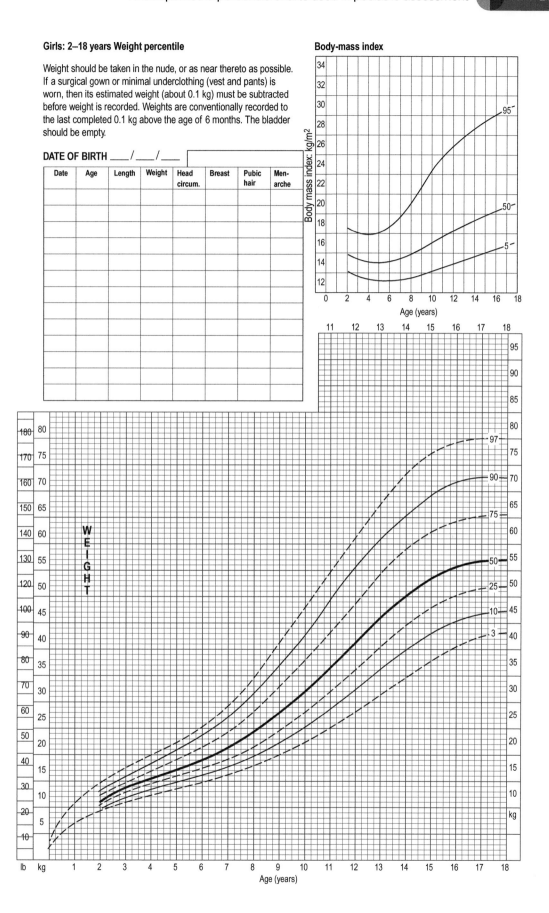

Head circumference, girls

Head circumference: The tape should be placed over the eyebrows, above
the ears and over the most prominent part of the occiput taking a direct route.
A paper tape is preferable to plastic, which stretches unacceptably under tension.
The maximum measurement should be recorded to the nearest 0.1 cm.

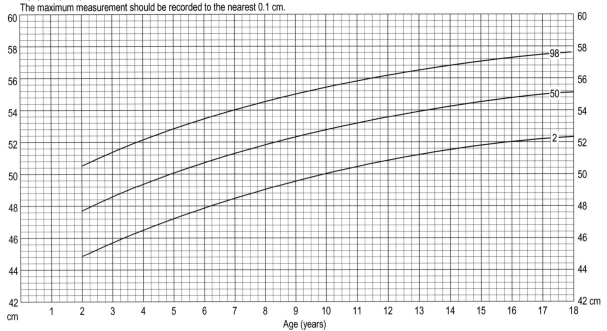

Height velocity, girls

The standards are appropriate for velocity calculated over a whole year, not less, since a small period requires wider limits (the 3rd and 95th centiles for months). The yearly velocity should be plotted at the mid point of the year. The centiles given in black are appropriate to children of average maturational tempo, who have their peak velocity at the average of this event. The line marked A is the 50th centile line for the child who is 2 years early in maturity and age at peak height velocity, and the line marked B refers to a child who is 50th centile in velocity for early and late maturers.

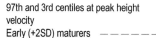

Centile of whole-year velocity for maturers at average time

97th and 3rd centiles at peak height velocity

Early (+2SD) maturers — — — — —
Late (−2SD) maturers — · — · — · —

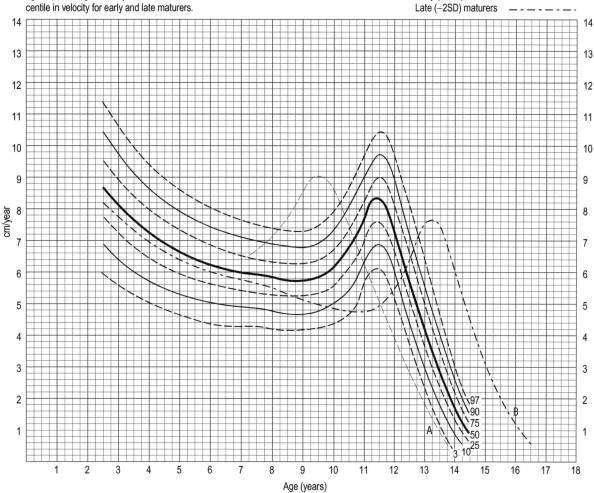

Age (years)

Appendix 2: Adult head circumference percentiles

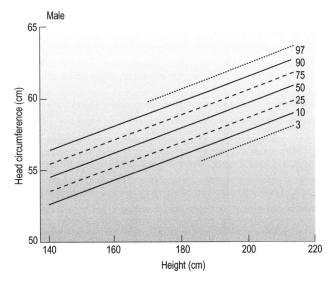

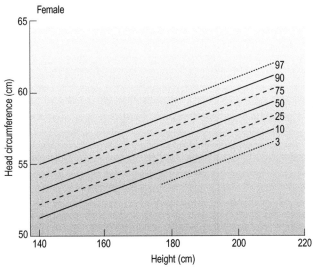

Appendix 3: Blood pressure levels for girls by age and height percentile

© 2010, Elsevier Ltd, Inc, BV
DOI: 10.1016/B978-0-7020-3129-8.00041-4

Blood pressure levels for girls by age and height percentile

Age year	BP percentile	SBP, mmHg Percentile of height							DBP, mmHg Percentile of height						
		5th	10th	25th	50th	75th	90th	95th	5th	10th	25th	50th	75th	90th	95th
1	50th	83	84	85	89	85	89	90	38	39	39	40	41	41	42
	90th	97	97	98	100	101	102	103	52	53	53	51	55	55	56
	95th	100	101	102	104	105	106	107	56	57	57	58	59	59	60
	99th	108	108	109	111	112	113	114	64	64	65	65	66	67	67
2	50th	85	85	87	88	89	91	91	43	44	44	45	46	46	47
	90th	98	99	100	101	103	104	105	57	58	58	59	60	61	61
	95th	102	103	104	105	107	108	109	61	62	62	63	64	65	65
	99th	109	110	111	112	114	115	116	69	69	70	70	71	72	72
3	50th	86	87	88	89	91	92	93	47	48	48	49	50	50	51
	90th	100	100	102	103	104	106	106	61	62	62	63	64	64	65
	95th	101	104	105	107	108	109	110	65	66	66	67	68	68	69
	99th	111	111	113	114	115	116	117	73	73	74	74	75	76	76
4	50th	88	88	90	91	92	94	94	50	50	51	52	52	53	54
	90th	101	102	103	104	106	107	108	64	64	65	66	67	67	68
	95th	105	106	107	108	110	111	112	68	68	69	70	71	71	72
	99th	112	113	114	115	117	118	119	76	76	76	77	78	79	79
5	50th	89	90	91	93	94	95	96	52	53	53	54	55	55	56
	90th	103	103	105	106	107	109	109	66	67	67	68	69	69	70
	95th	107	107	108	110	111	112	113	70	71	71	72	73	73	74
	99th	114	114	116	117	118	120	120	78	78	79	79	80	81	81
6	50th	91	92	93	94	96	97	98	54	54	55	56	56	57	58
	90th	104	105	106	108	109	110	111	68	68	69	70	70	71	72
	95th	108	109	110	111	113	114	115	72	72	73	74	74	75	76
	99th	115	116	117	119	120	121	122	80	80	80	81	82	83	83
7	50th	93	93	95	96	97	99	99	55	56	56	57	58	58	59
	90th	106	107	108	109	111	112	113	69	70	70	71	72	72	73
	95th	110	111	112	113	115	116	116	73	74	74	75	76	76	77
	99th	117	118	119	120	122	123	124	81	81	82	82	83	84	84
8	50th	95	95	96	98	99	100	101	57	57	57	58	59	60	60
	90th	108	109	110	111	113	114	114	71	71	71	72	73	74	74
	95th	112	112	114	115	116	118	118	75	75	75	76	77	78	78
	99th	119	120	121	122	123	125	125	82	82	83	83	84	85	86
9	50th	96	97	98	100	101	102	103	58	58	58	59	60	61	61
	90th	110	110	112	113	114	116	116	72	72	72	73	74	75	75
	95th	114	114	115	117	118	119	120	76	76	76	77	78	79	79
	99th	121	121	123	124	125	127	127	83	83	84	84	58	86	87
10	50th	98	99	100	102	105	104	105	59	59	59	60	61	62	62
	90th	112	112	114	115	116	118	118	73	73	73	74	75	76	76
	95th	116	116	117	119	120	121	122	77	77	77	78	79	80	80
	99th	123	123	125	126	127	129	129	84	84	85	86	86	87	88
11	50th	100	101	102	103	105	106	107	60	60	60	61	62	63	63
	90th	114	114	116	117	118	119	120	74	74	74	75	76	77	77
	95th	118	118	119	121	122	123	124	78	78	78	79	80	81	81
	99th	125	125	126	128	129	130	131	85	85	86	87	87	88	89
12	50th	102	103	104	105	107	108	109	61	61	61	62	63	64	64
	90th	116	116	117	119	120	121	122	75	75	75	76	77	78	78
	95th	119	120	121	123	124	125	126	79	79	79	80	81	82	82
	99th	127	127	128	130	131	132	133	86	86	87	88	88	89	90
13	50th	104	105	106	107	109	110	110	62	62	62	63	64	65	65
	90th	117	118	119	121	122	123	124	76	76	76	77	73	79	79
	95th	121	122	123	124	126	127	128	80	80	80	81	82	83	83
	99th	128	129	130	132	133	134	135	87	87	88	89	89	90	91
14	50th	106	106	107	109	110	111	112	63	63	63	64	65	66	66
	90th	119	120	121	122	124	125	125	77	77	77	78	79	80	80
	95th	123	123	125	126	127	129	129	81	81	81	82	83	84	84
	99th	130	131	132	133	135	136	136	88	88	89	90	90	91	92
15	50th	107	108	109	110	111	113	113	64	64	64	65	66	67	67
	90th	120	121	122	123	125	126	127	78	78	78	79	80	81	81
	95th	124	125	126	127	129	130	131	82	82	82	83	84	85	85
	99th	131	132	133	134	136	137	138	89	89	90	91	91	92	93
16	50th	108	108	110	111	112	114	114	64	64	65	66	66	67	68
	90th	121	122	123	124	126	127	128	78	78	79	80	81	81	82
	95th	125	126	127	128	130	131	132	82	82	83	84	85	85	86
	99th	132	133	134	135	137	138	139	90	90	90	91	92	93	93
17	50th	108	109	110	111	113	114	115	64	65	65	66	67	67	68
	90th	122	122	123	125	126	127	125	78	79	79	80	81	81	82
	95th	125	126	127	129	130	131	132	82	83	83	84	85	85	86
	99th	133	133	134	136	137	138	139	90	90	91	91	92	93	93

Appendix 4: Varni/Thompson Pediatric Pain Questionnaires

© 2010, Elsevier Ltd, Inc, BV
DOI: 10.1016/B978-0-7020-3129-8.00042-6

Form C (Child) _____

Name: _____

Age: _____

Date: _____

What words would you use to describe pain or hurt?

_____

_____

_____

From the words listed below, circle the ones that best describe the way it feels when you are hurt or are in pain.

cutting	pounding	tingling	tiring	deep
beating	squeezing	throbbing	horrible	stabbing
burning	pulling	sickening	biting	screaming
scraping	aching	uncomfortable	cold	tugging
pricking	cruel	warm	miserable	stretching
pinching	unbearable	sad	itching	terrible
stinging	cool	sore	flashing	pressing
fearful	pins & needles	sharp	jumping	tight
hot	spreading	punishing	scared	lonely
				bad

From the words you circled, which three words best describe the pain you are feeling right now?

_____

_____

Put a mark on the line that best shows *how you feel now.* If you have no pain or hurt, you would put a mark at the end of the line by the happy face. If you have some pain or hurt, you would put a mark near the middle of the line. If you have a whole lot of pain or hurt, you would put a mark by the sad face.

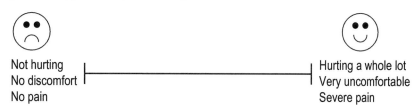

Not hurting
No discomfort
No pain

Hurting a whole lot
Very uncomfortable
Severe pain

Put a mark on the line that best shows what was the *worst pain you had this week.* If you had no pain or hurt this week, you would put a mark at the end of the line by the happy face. If the pain or hurt you had was some hurting, you would put a mark by the middle of the line. If the worse pain you had was a whole lot of pain or hurt, you would put a mark by the sad face.

No pain
No hurt

Mild pain
A little hurt

Moderate pain
More hurt

Severe pain
A lot of hurt

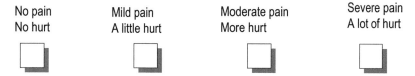

Pick the colors that mean *No hurt, A little hurt, More hurt* and *A lot of hurt to you* and color in the boxes. Now, using those colors, color in the body to show how you feel. Where you have no hurt, use the *no hurt* color to color in your body. If you have hurt or pain, use the color that tells how much hurt you have.

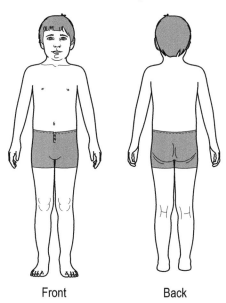

Front   Back

Form P (Parent)

The purpose of this questionnaire is to help us to obtain a comprehensive history of your child's pain problems. All information obtained from this questionnaire and in interviews will remain strictly confidential. If you do not wish to answer a particular question, for any reason, please write 'Do not wish to answer' in the space provided. Please print or write clearly.

Today's date: _____

Your name: _____

Address: _____

_____

Phone number: _____

Relationship to child of person completing this form: _____

Child Information

Name: _____

Age: _____ Date of birth: _____

Sex: _____

Grade in school: _____

Home Information

Please list the name, age and sex of all individuals living in the home.

Name	Age	Sex

Please list any health problems that your child has.

_____

_____

_____

If any one else in the family has health problems please list the person and the health problem. Example: son with asthma, husband with arthritis.

_____

_____

_____

Please list all severe or chronic family illnesses that your child has been aware of.

Family member	Dates	Type of illness	Outcome

Please list all severe and/or chronic pain problems experienced by other family members that your child has observed.

Family member	Dates	Type of pain	Outcome

Are there currently any major life stresses in the family situation (e.g. divorce, separation, difficult financial burden, illness)? If yes, please list.

_____

_____

_____

When did your child's present pain problem begin? Please also explain the symptoms, exact locations of pain and whether the pain has been on or off over the months and years?

_____

_____

_____

_____

_____

What was your reaction to the pain at that time? Please explain.

_____

_____

Were any major changes in your or your child's life occurring then?
Please explain.

_____

_____

Is your child's current pain constant or does it appear to come and go?

_____

_____

Is your child's pain accompanied by nausea, vomiting, dizziness, feeling faint, anxiety, rapid breathing or other symptoms? If so, please list the symptoms.

_____

_____

When your child has pain how do you react? Please explain.

_____

_____

_____

If your child's pain were to suddenly disappear, how would it change his/her life?

_____

_____

_____

How would it change your life?

_____

_____

_____

How would it change family relationships?

_____

_____

_____

Assuming that the pain continues, what kinds of things do you think your child should do *now,* which will help him/her later on?

_____

_____

_____

Is there anything else you would like to tell us about your child's pain and the effect it has on your child, yourself or the family?

_____

_____

_____

_____

What words would you use to describe your child's pain?

_____

_____

_____

Please circle any of the words listed below that you feel describe your child's pain.

cutting	pounding	tingling	tiring	deep
beating	squeezing	throbbing	horrible	stabbing
burning	pulling	sickening	biting	screaming
scraping	aching	uncomfortable	cold	tugging
pricking	cruel	warm	miserable	stretching
pinching	unbearable	sad	itching	terrible
stinging	cool	sore	flashing	pressing
fearful	pins & needles	sharp	jumping	tight
hot	spreading	punishing	scared	lonely
				bad

What day of the week does your child have the most pain? _____

What week of the month does your child have the most pain? _____

What season or month does your child have the worst pain? _____

Have you ever noticed something that tells you your child is about to experience a pain episode (e.g. stiffness, particular thoughts or statements, physical sensations or irritability)?

_____

_____

_____

How many hours a day does your child have pain now? _____

How long does a single pain episode last (minutes, hours)? _____

What do you label your child's pains as (e.g. 'headache', 'joint pain', 'stomach ache', 'backache', etc.)? Please list them in order of severity, #1 being the most severe pain.

Pain problem #1: _____

Pain problem #2: _____

Pain problem #3: _____

On a scale of 0–10	6 a.m.	_____	6 p.m.	_____
(0 = no pain, 10 = severe pain),	9 a.m.	_____	9 p.m.	_____
how severe is your child's	12 noon	_____	12 midnight	_____
pain at the following	3 p.m.	_____	3 a.m.	_____
times of the day?				

What is the worst time of the day? _____

What is the best time of the day? _____

Is your child currently taking medication for the pain?

Yes _____   No _____

If yes, please complete the following information.

Medication	Dose	#Times/day	When	How effective (0 = not effective, 10 = very effective)

What medications or other treatments have been tried in the past? On a scale of 0–10 (0 = not effective, 10 = very effective), how effective has each one been?

_____

_____

_____

_____

_____

What do you currently do, besides giving medication, to relieve your child's pain?

_____

_____

_____

Does your child seem worse when he/she is?

	Yes	No		Yes	No
tired	_____	_____	angry	_____	_____
anxious	_____	_____	busy	_____	_____
bored	_____	_____	lonely	_____	_____
happy	_____	_____	arguing	_____	_____
unhappy	_____	_____	upset	_____	_____

Other situations is which your child's pain is worse? Please describe

_____

_____

_____

Does your child's pain interfere with any of the following? Please circle the most correct number.

	Never	Rarely	Sometimes	Often	Always
Enjoying the family	1	2	3	4	5
Eating/appetite	1	2	3	4	5
Seeing friends	1	2	3	4	5
Sports	1	2	3	4	5
Sleeping	1	2	3	4	5
Watching TV	1	2	3	4	5
Reading	1	2	3	4	5
Schoolwork	1	2	3	4	5
Attending school	1	2	3	4	5
Going to the movies	1	2	3	4	5
Favorite activities	1	2	3	4	5
Unliked activities	1	2	3	4	5

Comments?

_____

_____

_____

_____

During the past 3 months, did your child's pain limit him/her from doing things which he/she wanted to do?

1.＿＿＿＿＿＿ Yes

2.＿＿＿＿＿＿ No

If yes, please explain

＿＿＿＿＿＿＿＿＿＿＿＿＿＿＿＿＿＿＿＿＿＿＿＿＿＿＿＿＿＿＿

＿＿＿＿＿＿＿＿＿＿＿＿＿＿＿＿＿＿＿＿＿＿＿＿＿＿＿＿＿＿＿

＿＿＿＿＿＿＿＿＿＿＿＿＿＿＿＿＿＿＿＿＿＿＿＿＿＿＿＿＿＿＿

＿＿＿＿＿＿＿＿＿＿＿＿＿＿＿＿＿＿＿＿＿＿＿＿＿＿＿＿＿＿＿

During the past 3 months of the school year, how often did your child's pain keep him/her from going to school?

0. ＿＿＿＿＿＿＿＿＿ Not at all
1. ＿＿＿＿＿＿＿＿＿ 1 day only
2. ＿＿＿＿＿＿＿＿＿ 2–3 days
3. ＿＿＿＿＿＿＿＿＿ 4–7 days
4. ＿＿＿＿＿＿＿＿＿ more than 1 week
5. ＿＿＿＿＿＿＿＿＿ more than 2 weeks
6. ＿＿＿＿＿＿＿＿＿ more than 3 weeks
7. ＿＿＿＿＿＿＿＿＿ more than 1 month

During the past 3 months, how often did your child's pain limit him/her from *vigorous* activities such as running, bicycling, lifting heavy objects, or participating in strenuous sports?

0. ＿＿＿＿＿＿＿＿＿ Not at all
1. ＿＿＿＿＿＿＿＿＿ 1 day only
2. ＿＿＿＿＿＿＿＿＿ 2–3 days
3. ＿＿＿＿＿＿＿＿＿ 4–7 days
4. ＿＿＿＿＿＿＿＿＿ more than 1 week
5. ＿＿＿＿＿＿＿＿＿ more than 2 weeks
6. ＿＿＿＿＿＿＿＿＿ more than 3 weeks
7. ＿＿＿＿＿＿＿＿＿ more than 1 month

During the past 3 months, how often did your child's pain limit him/her from *moderate* activities such as climbing several flights of stairs, bending, walking several blocks, lifting or stooping?

0. _____ Not at all
1. _____ 1 day only
2. _____ 2–3 days
3. _____ 4–7 days
4. _____ more than 1 week
5. _____ more than 2 weeks
6. _____ more than 3 weeks
7. _____ more than 1 month

During the past 3 months, how often did your child's pain limit him/her from *mild* activities such as walking one block, climbing one flight of stairs, sitting, or standing?

0. _____ Not at all
1. _____ 1 day only
2. _____ 2–3 days
3. _____ 4–7 days
4. _____ more than 1 week
5. _____ more than 2 weeks
6. _____ more than 3 weeks
7. _____ more than 1 month

Please rate how much pain you think your child is *having at the present time* by placing a mark somewhere on the line.

Not hurting		Hurting a whole lot
No discomfort	————————————————	Very uncomfortable
No pain		Severe pain

Please rate how much pain you think your child has *on an average* each day by placing a mark somewhere on the line.

Not hurting		Hurting a whole lot
No discomfort	————————————————	Very uncomfortable
No pain		Severe pain

Please rate how severe was the *worst pain* your child had *in the past week* (7 days) by placing a mark somewhere on the line.

Not hurting		Hurting a whole lot
No discomfort	————————————————	Very uncomfortable
No pain		Severe pain

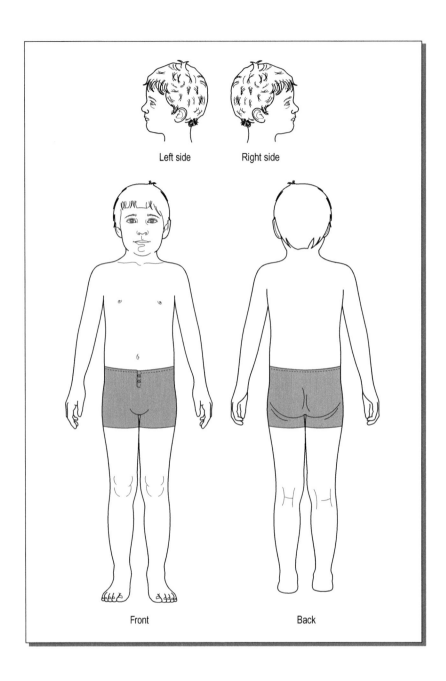

Left side   Right side

Front   Back

Index

NB: Page numbers in *italics* refer to boxes, figures and tables.

Edwards Brothers Malloy
Ann Arbor MI. USA
August 8, 2017